**Critical Decisions in Emergency and
Acute Care Electrocardiography**

Dr Brady's dedication – To my wife, King, for her constant support, patience, and guidance; and for my children, Lauren, Anne, Chip, and Katherine, for their love.

Dr Truwit's dedication – To my wife Jeanne and my children, Jason, Matthew and Lauren without whom I could not be personally or professionally fulfilled nor accomplish as much.

Critical Decisions in Emergency and Acute Care Electrocardiography

EDITED BY

William J. Brady | MD

Professor of Emergency Medicine and Medicine Ice Chair, Department of Emergency Medicine
Medical Director, Life Support Learning Center
University of Virginia Health System
Charlottesville, VA, USA

Jonathon D. Truwit | MD

Senior Associate Dean for Clinical Affairs
E. Cato Drash Professor of Medicine
Pulmonary and Critical Care Medicine
University of Virginia Health System
Charlottesville, VA, USA

WILEY-BLACKWELL

A John Wiley & Sons, Ltd., Publication

Library of Congress Cataloging-in-Publication Data
Critical decisions in emergency and acute care electrocardiography / edited by William Brady, Jonathon Truwit.
    p. ; cm.
    Includes bibliographical references.
    ISBN 978-1-4051-5906-7
    1. Electrocardiography. 2. Critical care medicine. I. Brady, William, 1960– II. Truwit, Jonathon Dean.
    [DNLM: 1. Electrocardiography. 2. Critical Care. 3. Decision Making. 4. Emergency Medical Services. WG 140 C934 2009]
    RC683.5.E5C75 2009
    616.1'207547—dc22

                                                                                      2008030326

ISBN: 9781405159067

A catalogue record for this book is available from the British Library.

Set in 9/12pt Meridien by Graphicraft Limited, Hong Kong

1 2009

Contents

Section Editors

Ellen C. Keeley, MD
Associate Professor of Internal Medicine, Department of
Internal Medicine, Division of Cardiology, University of Virginia,
Charlottesville, VA, USA

Andrew Perron, MD
Program Director, Department of Emergency Medicine, Maine Medical
Center, Portland, ME, USA

Stephen W. Smith, MD
Faculty Emergency Physician, Hennepin County Medical Center,
Associate Professor of Emergency Medicine, University of Minnesota
School of Medicine, Minneapolis, MN, USA

Amal Mattu, MD, FAAEM, FACEP
Director, Emergency Medicine Residency Associate Professor,
Department of Emergency Medicine, University of Maryland School of
Medicine, Baltimore, MD, USA

Ajeet Vinayak, MD
Assistant Professor of Medicine, Pulmonary and Clinical Care Division,
Department of Medicine, University of Virginia, Charlottesville, VA, USA

Christopher P. Holstege, MD
Associate Professor, Department of Emergency Medicine; Director,
Division of Medical Toxicology, University of Virginia School of
Medicine, Charlottesville, VA, USA

Theodore C. Chan, MD
Professor and Medical Director, Department of Emergency Medicine,
University of California, San Diego, CA, USA

Richard A. Harrigan, MD
Professor, Department of Emergency Medicine, Temple University,
Philadephia, PA, USA

Contributors

Michael Abraham, MD
Attending Physician, Department of Emergency Medicine, Upper Chesapeake Medical Center, Bel Air, MD, USA

Khaled Bachour, MD
Fellow, Division of Cardiology, Department of Internal Medicine, Harper Hospital, Wayne State University School of Medicine, Detroit, MI, USA

Billie Barker, MD, USA
Pulmonary & Critical Care Fellow, Department of Internal Medicine, Division of Pulmonary & Critical Care, University of Virginia, Charlottesville, VA, USA

Stefan C. Bertog, MD
Interventional Cardiology Veterans Administration Medical Center, University of Minnesota, Minneapolis, MN, USA

Michael A. Bohrn, MD, FAAEM, FACEP
Associate Residency Program Director, Clinical Assistant Professor, Department of Emergency Medicine, York Hospital, York, PA, USA

Michael C. Bond, MD, FAAEM
Assistant Residency Program Director, Assistant Professor, Department of Emergency Medicine, University of Maryland School of Medicine, Baltimore, MD, USA

Christopher T. Bowe, MD, FACEP
Associate Residency Program Director, Assistant Professor, Emergency Medicine, Department of Emergency Medicine, Maine Medical Center, Portland, ME, USA

David Burt, MD
Assistant Professor, Medical Director, Chest Pain Center, Department of Emergency Medicine, University of Virginia, Charlottesville, VA, USA

Claire C. Caldwell, MD
Department of Emergency Medicine, UMDNJ-Robert Wood Johnson Medical School, Camden, NJ, USA

Clay A. Cauthen, MD, MA
Chief Medical Resident, Department of Internal Medicine, University of Virginia, Charlottesville, VA, USA

Theodore C. Chan, MD
Professor and Medical Director, Department of Emergency Medicine, University of California, San Diego, CA, USA

Nathan P. Charlton, MD
Medical Toxicology Fellow, Division of Medical Toxicology, Department of Emergency Medicine, University of Virginia School of Medicine, Charlottesville, VA, USA

Mark D. Connelly, MD
Emergency Medicine Department, Regions Hospital, St Paul. MN, USA

Andrew Darby, MD
Cardiology Fellow, Department of Medicine, Division of Cardiovascular Medicine, University of Virginia, Charlottesville, VA, USA

John Ferguson, MB ChB, MD
Assistant Professor of Internal Medicine, Department of Medicine, Division of Cardiovascular Medicine, University of Virginia, Charlottesville, VA, USA

Lisa M. Filippone, MD
Assistant Professor of Emergency Medicine, Department of Emergency Medicine, UMDNJ-Robert Wood Johnson Medical School, Camden, NJ, USA

Carl A. Germann, MD
Attending Phsyician, Department of Emergency Medicine, Maine Medical Center, Portland, ME, USA

Chris Ghaemmaghami
Associate Professor, Vice Chair of Academics, and Program Director, Department of Emergency Medicine, University of Virginia, Charlottesville, VA, USA

Daniel Grinnan, MD
Assistant Professor of Medicine, Department of Internal Medicine, Division of Pulmonary & Critical Care, Virginia Commonwealth University, Richmond, VA, USA

Richard A. Harrigan, MD
Professor, Department of Emergency Medicine, Temple University, Philadelphia, PA, USA

Adam Helms, MD
Chief Medical Resident, Department of Internal Medicine, University of Virginia, Charlottesville, VA, USA

Steve Herndon MD
Pulmonary & Critical Care Fellow, Department of Internal Medicine, Division of Pulmonary & Critical Care, University of Virginia, Charlottesville, VA, USA

D. Kyle Hogarth, MD
Assistant Professor of Medicine, Department of Internal Medicine, Division of Pulmonary & Critical Care, University of Chicago, Chicargo, IL, USA

Joel S. Holger, MD
Assistant Professor of Emergency Medicine, University of Minnesota Medical School, Senior Staff Physician, Regions Hospital, St Paul, MN, USA

Benjamin Holland MD
Medical Resident, Department of Internal Medicine, University of Virginia, Charlottesville, VA, USA

Christopher P. Holstege, MD
Associate Professor, Departments of Emergency Medicine & Pediatrics; Director, Division of Medical Toxicology, University of Virginia School of Medicine, Charlottesville, VA, USA

Colin G. Kaide, MD, FACEP, FAAEM, UHM
Associate Professor of Emergency Medicine, Specialist in Hyperbaric Medicine and Wound Care, Department of Emergency Medicine, The Ohio State University, Columbus, OH, USA

Ellen C. Keeley, MD
Associate Professor of Internal Medicine, Department of Medicine, Division of Cardiovascular Medicine, University of Virginia, Charlottesville, VA, USA

Vipin Khetarpal, MD
Fellow in Cardiology, Division of Cardiology, Department of Internal Medicine, Harper Hospital Wayne State University School of Medicine, Detroit, MI, USA

Michael Christopher Kurz, MD, MS-HES
Assistant Professor, Department of Emergency Medicine, Virginal Commonwealth University Medical Center, Richmond, VA, USA

David M. Larson, MD
Clinical Associate Professor, University of Minnesota Medical School, St Paul, MN, USA

David T. Lawrence, DO
Assistant Professor, Department of Emergency Medicine, Division of Medical Toxicology, University of Virginia School of Medicine, Charlottesville, VA, USA

Stephen D. Lee, MD
Emergency Medicine Resident, Department of Emergency Medicine, University of Virginia School of Medicine, Charlottesville, VA, USA

Joseph E. Levitt, MD
Assistant Professor of Medicine, Department of Internal Medicine, Division of Pulmonary & Critical Care, Stanford University Medical Center, Stanford, CA, USA

D. Scott Lim, MD
Assistant Professor of Pediatrics, Department of Pediatrics, University of Virginia, Charlottesville, VA, USA

Michael J. Lipinski, MD
Resident in Medicine, Department of Medicine, University of Virginia, Charlottesville, VA, USA

Amal Mattu, MD, FAAEM, FACEP
Director, Emergency Medicine Residency, Associate Professor, Department of Emergency Medicine, University of Maryland School of Medicine, Baltimore, MD, USA

Michael A. McCulloch, MD
Pediatric Resident, Department of Pediatrics, University of Virginia, Charlottesville, VA, USA

Franklin R. McGuire, MD
Assistant Professor of Medicine, Department of Internal Medicine, Division of Pulmonary & Critical Care, University of South Carolina, Colombia, SC, USA

Robert O'Connor, MD, MPH
Professor and Chair, Department of Emergency Medicine, University of Virginia, Charlottesville, VA, USA

Daniel T. O'Laughlin, MD, FACEP
Emergency Medicine Faculty, Abbott Northwestern Hospital, Assistant Professor of Emergency Medicine, University of Minnesota School of Medicine, Minneapolis, MN, USA

Michael Osmundson, MD, MBA, FACEP
Associate Clinical Professor, Mercer University School of Medicine, Savannah, GA, USA

Rajan A.G. Patel, MD
Cardiology Fellow, Department of Medicine, Division of Cardiovascular Medicine, University of Virginia, Charlottesville, VA, USA

Tamas R. Peredy, MD
Medical Director, Northern New England Poison Center, Maine Medical Center, Portland, ME, USA

Andrew Perron, MD
Program Director, Department of Emergency Medicine, Maine Medical Center, Portland, ME, USA

Peter M. Pollak, MD
Internal Medicine Resident, Department of Medicine, University of Virginia, Charlottesville, VA, USA

Michael Ragosta, MD
Associate Professor of Internal Medicine, Department of Medicine, Division of Cardiovascular Medicine, University of Virginia, Charlottesville, VA, USA

Kevin C. Reed, MD, FACEP, FAAEM
Assistant Clinical Professor, Department of Emergency Medicine, Georgetown University, Attending Physician, Department of Emergency Medicine, Washington Hospital Center, Washington, DC, USA

Christopher M. Rembold, MD
Professor of Internal Medicine, Department of Medicine, Division of Cardiovascular Medicine, University of Virginia, Charlottesville, VA, USA

John R. Saucier, MD, FACEP
Attending Physician, Maine Medical Center, Portland, ME; Assistant Professor of Emergency Medicine, Department of Emergency Medicine; Clinical Assistant Professor in Surgery, University of Vermont, College of Medicine, Burlington, VT, USA

Jason T. Schaffer, MD, FAAEM
Assistant Clinical Professor of Emergency Medicine, Department of Emergency Medicine, Indiana University School of Medicine, Indianapolis, IN, USA

Joseph Shiber, MD, FAAEM, FACEP
Associate Professor of Emergency Medicine, University of Central Florida School of Medicine, Research Director, Florida Hospital Emergency Medicine Residency, Orlando, FL, USA

Allan G. Simpson, MD
Associate Professor of Internal Medicine, Department of Medicine, Division of Cardiovascular Medicine, University of Virginia, Charlottesville, VA, USA

Stephen W. Smith
Faculty Emergency Physician, Hennepin County Medical Center, Associate Professor of Emergency Medicine, University of Minnesota School of Medicine, Minneapolis, MN, USA

Samuel J. Stellpflug, MD
Emergency Medicine Department, Regions Hospital, St Paul, MN, USA

Nima Taha, MD
Resident in Internal Medicine, Department of Internal Medicine, Los Angeles County / University of California Medical Center, Los Angeles, CA, USA

Traci Thoureen, MD, MHS-CL, FACEP, FAAEM
Assistant Professor, Department of Emergency Medicine, Director, Emergency Medicine Simulation Program, University of Maryland School of Medicine, Baltimore, MD, USA

Ajeet Vinayak, MD
Assistant Professor of Medicine, Director of Medical Intensive Care Unit, Department of Medicine, Division of Pulmonary & Critical Care, University of Virginia, Charlottesville, VA, USA

Raed Wahab, MD
Pulmonary & Critical Care Fellow, Department of Medicine, Division of Pulmonary & Critical Care, University of Virginia, Charlottesville, VA, USA

J. Jason West, MD
Cardiology Fellow, Department of Medicine, Division of Cardiovascular Medicine, University of Virginia, Charlottesville, VA, USA

Wayne Whitwam, MD
Physician, Cardiac Electrophysiology, Department of Internal Medicine, Cardiovascular Division, University of California, San Diego, CA, USA

Preface

Electrocardiography is performed widely throughout medicine, ranging from the clinician's office in a scheduled, routine application to the critical care unit with an unanticipated decompensation during active resuscitation. And, of course, a multitude of other areas rely heavily on the ECG as valuable tool in the patient evaluation – the prehospital setting in an EMS unit, the emergency department, the surgical suite and post-anesthesia care area, among many others. In fact, it is appropriate to state that some form of electrocardiographic monitoring is one of the most widely applied diagnostic tests in clinical medicine today. Electrocardiography, whether single-lead monitoring for rhythm disorders or 12-lead analysis for ACS or other morphologic abnormality, remains one of the most cost-effective and useful tests in medicine – rapid, non-invasive, inexpensive, portable, easily interpreted – often providing clinical information that will make the difference between life and death.

In acute care medicine, whether it be the acute care ward, emergency department, or critical care unit, the ECG can assist in establishing a diagnosis, ruling-out various ailments, guiding the diagnostic and management strategies in the evaluation, providing indication for certain therapies, determining inpatient disposition location, offering risk assessment, and assessing end-organ impact of a syndrome. In more routine, though no less crucial, settings, the ECG assists in disease surveillance and screening in office-based evaluations as well as risk stratification in pre-operative assessments.

The ECG, similar to other clinical investigations, must be interpreted within the context of the clinical presentation.

An understanding of this concept and its application at the bedside is crucial for the appropriate use of the ECG in clinical practice – and is the focus of this textbook, *Critical Decisions in Emergency and Acute Care Electrocardiography*. This textbook focuses on the breadth of acute care medicine – the ward, ED, OR, and critical care unit. Each section is organized around traditional topics such as acute coronary syndrome or dysrhythmia. Within each section, however, are a range of chapters, focusing on a specific use or clinical situation, involving the ECG; each chapter is presented in the form of an inquiry, followed by a series of cases, illustrating the issues, controversies, or questions. For instance, what are the electrocardiographic indications for urgent reperfusion therapy in ACS, can the ECG guide the clinician in the management of the patient with wide complex tachycardia, or what is the value of the 12-lead ECG in the poisoned patient? The chapter itself is the answer to the question with appropriate electrocardiographic examples and adequate supporting evidence.

This work stresses the value of the ECG in the range of clinical situations encountered daily by healthcare providers – it illustrates the appropriate applications of the electrocardiogram in acute care medicine today. We have enjoyed its creation – we hope that you the clinician will find it of value in your care of the patient.

William J Brady & Jonathon D Truwit
Charlottesville, VA, USA
September 2008

Foreword 1

In clinical medicine, there are a finite number of clinical skills that are considered essential areas of expertise in the management of critically ill patients. Such a short list might include advanced physical assessment, airway management, critical care problem solving, initiation of resuscitation efforts, identification of the need for early surgical intervention, and the immediate diagnostic interpretation of tests. One of the earliest and most common diagnostic studies performed in the critically ill patient is the electrocardiogram. The tremendous value of the electrocardiogram in the acutely and critically ill patient is unequivocally established – in fact, it is considered essential in management. Certainly, the basic electrocardiographic skill set is considered fundamental; the intricacies and nuances of advanced interpretation offers an abundance of clinical data that can alter patient course and outcome – and should also be considered fundamental in acute, emergency, and critical care settings. Drs. Brady and Truwit have assembled such a text which very nicely explores and reviews the impact of the electrocardiogram, from the prehospital arena and emergency department to the inpatient ward and critical care unit.

Patient safety and outcome goals have moved electrocardiographic analysis from the sole responsibility of the cardiologist to the point of care contact for our patients. Expertise in electrocardiographic interpretation is considered the standard of training in emergency medicine and critical care. Appropriately, there has been mounting pressure on acute care and critical care clinicians to rapidly and accurately assess electrocardiograms in a time dependent fashion. Critical time points have been established for electrocardiographic interpretation in acute ST segment elevation myocardial infarctions that directly impact patient treatment strategies, hospital resources and outcomes. Correct interpretation of the electrocardiogram alter treatment decisions for the management of non-ST elevation myocardial infarctions, dysrhythmias, undifferentiated cardiovascular diseases, and poisoning and ingestions. Additionally, electrocardiograms offer insights into other medical conditions that place acutely and critically ill patients in life threatening situations.

Developing expertise in electrocardiographic analysis requires dedicated study, practice and review. The management of critically ill patients at risk for cardiovascular compromise requires not just a basic familiarity in electrogardiography, but an advanced interpretation skill level. Failure to develop expertise in the area of electrocardiography places patients at risk. Acute care electrocardiographic expertise is developed through meaningful self-education, clinical practice, and thoughtful review. Standardizing this process is essential because clinical experience alone is inadequate in addressing the breadth and extent of the required knowledge base.

This textbook on Critical Decisions in Electrocardiography represents an excellent example of standardizing the educational process of electrocardiography. By reviewing case scenarios, learners can explore and actively participate in critical decision making that is required for developing these essential diagnostic skills. The breadth of clinical presentations offers the learner an opportunity to review and reflect on high risk cardiovascular disease states that may not frequently present in their own clinical practice. The text allows for independent study and reflection that can lead to expertise in the field of electrocardiography, providing an integral component in the pursuit of a competency that our patients rely on and deserve.

Peter Delieux, MD
Professor of Clinical Medicine
Director of Emergency Medicine Services
Emergency Medicine Director of Resident and Faculty
Development
Louisiana State University Health Sciences Center
New Orleans, LA, USA

Foreword 2

William Brady and Jon Truwit have done a masterful job at taking a topic that, while central to the Operating Room, ICU, Emergency Department environments, it is not usually the focus for the personnel regularly working in these areas. As a practicing pulmonary-intensivist, I know that when it comes to ECG abnormalities in the ICU we are exposed to anything and everything, often with very short notice and little time for diagnosis or to think about the most appropriate therapeutic interventions. The common problems such as atrial tachy arrhythmias, ischemic changes, ventricular tachycardia and signs of myocardial infarction occur with such frequency that it is relatively easy to maintain skills necessary to recognize and treat them. However, the uncommon problems are often seen so infrequently that recognition and treatment can be much more of a challenge. Thus Brady and Truwit in *Critical Decisions in Emergency and Acute Care Electrocardiography* have created a text that makes common and obscure ECG findings relevant and accessible.

Intensivists and others who do not regularly work in cardiac units must still maintain skills sufficient to recognize and provide at least the initial management of serious and/or life-threatening diseases manifesting in or resulting from abnormal ECGs. Though complex and challenging, these clinical problems are systematically dealt with by Brady and Truwit in a practical, easily readable format. The format of case presentations followed by a complete and systematic well-organized discussion is designed to give the reader information in a natural flow that facilitates assimilation into practice. The concise but very meaningful discussions of the controversies that loom large in some areas are well-articulated and serve to place much of the information into proper context. The fact that a whole chapter is devoted to the limitations of the ECG in clinical practice is a refreshing testament the pragmatism this volume brings to the field.

The ECG has been around a long time, has many limitations and must be interpreted in the light of the overall clinical presentation including prior probabilities. While the shape of the squiggles on the paper strips have not changed since Einthoven's work in 1895, the true underlying diseases or processes (diagnoses) these represent have been greatly clarified. In addition the prognostic value of the ECG has greatly improved and we are still learning. Brady and Truwit efficiently takes us right up to the edge of the current state of knowledge.

Peter Delieux, MD
Professor of Clinical Medicine
Director of Emergency Medicine Services
Emergency Medicine Director of Resident and Faculty Development
Louisiana State University Health Sciences Center
New Orleans, LA, USA

Part 1 | **The ECG in Clinical Practice**

Chapter 1 | What are the clinical applications of the ECG in emergency and critical care?

Rajan A.G. Patel, Christopher M. Rembold
University of Virginia, Charlottesville, VA, USA

Case presentations

Case 1: A 56-year-old man with a history of hypertension and chronic kidney disease is brought to the emergency department (ED) by his wife, with a chief complaint of progressive lethargy and fatigue over several days. On physical exam the patient appears ill. His blood pressure is 90/50 mmHg. The electrocardiogram (ECG) (Figure 1.1a) demonstrates a regular wide complex QRS rhythm with a right bundle branch-like morphology. The QRS complex is not preceded by P waves and occurs at a rate of approximately 48 beats per minute (bpm). The emergency physician initiates appropriate treatment based upon the electrocardiographic findings; laboratory findings confirmed the diagnosis. Four hours later, the ECG (Figure 1.1b) demonstrates sinus tachycardia at a rate of 103 bpm. Note that the P waves have returned and the QRS complex is now narrow.

Case 2: A 24-year-old graduate student is brought to the ED after calling 911 stating that she overdosed on her antidepressant medication. She is alert, crying, and complains of a dry mouth. Her initial heart rate is 96 bpm with a blood pressure of 120/80 mmHg. Her examination is remarkable for dilated pupils, flushed skin, and occasional twitching of muscles in her arms and legs. The baseline ECG demonstrates sinus rhythm with a markedly prolonged QT interval. The patient suddenly becomes lethargic and a 12-lead ECG (Figure 1.2) prompts the emergency physician to consider urgent therapy.

Case 3: A 59-year-old woman with a history of diabetes, hypertension and hyperlipidemia is brought to the ED having experienced increased difficulty breathing and neck discomfort. On physical examination, the patient is tachypneic with a respiratory rate of 30 breaths per minute. Her heart rate is 106 bpm with a blood pressure of 100/60 mmHg.

Critical Decisions in Emergency and Acute Care Electrocardiography,
1st edition. Edited by W.J. Brady and J.D. Truwit. © 2009 Blackwell Publishing, ISBN: 9781405159067

An ECG (Figure 1.3) is obtained. The patient is emergently taken to the cardiac catheterization lab for primary percutaneous coronary intervention (PCI). Repeat ECG after the procedure demonstrates resolution of all electrocardiographic abnormalities.

Case 4: A 74-year-old woman with a history of tobacco use, hypertension, and hyperlipidemia presents with nausea and an episode of syncope. The initial ECG (Figure 1.4) in the ED shows sinus tachycardia and an inferior ST elevation myocardial infarction (STEMI). She presented 4 hours after the onset of symptoms. The cardiac catheterization laboratory is activated to perform primary PCI. Prior to transfer, the patient suddenly becomes diaphoretic and lethargic. Her heart rate decreases to 30 bpm and her blood pressure is 70/50 mmHg. The patient is treated promptly with intravenous atropine, and the sinus tachycardia returns.

Clinical applications of the ECG

Electrocardiography is performed widely throughout emergency and critical care medicine. In fact, some form of electrocardiographic monitoring is one of the most widely applied diagnostic tests in clinical medicine today – including both single- and multiple-lead analysis as well as the 12-lead ECG. The ECG can assist in establishing a diagnosis, ruling-out various ailments, guiding the diagnostic and management strategies in the evaluation, providing indication for certain therapies, determining inpatient disposition location, and assessing end-organ impact of a syndrome. In the ED environment, the ECG less often provides a specific diagnosis.

Metabolic abnormalities: The surface 12-lead ECG is a reflection of the changes in the transmembrane potential of cardiac myocytes that occur with atrial and ventricular depolarization and repolarization. The transmembrane potential is the electrical gradient from the interior to the exterior of cardiac myocytes. This gradient results from differences in the extracellular and intracellular concentrations of specific anions and cations as determined by the Nernst equation. The cations that contribute significantly to the creation or

(a)

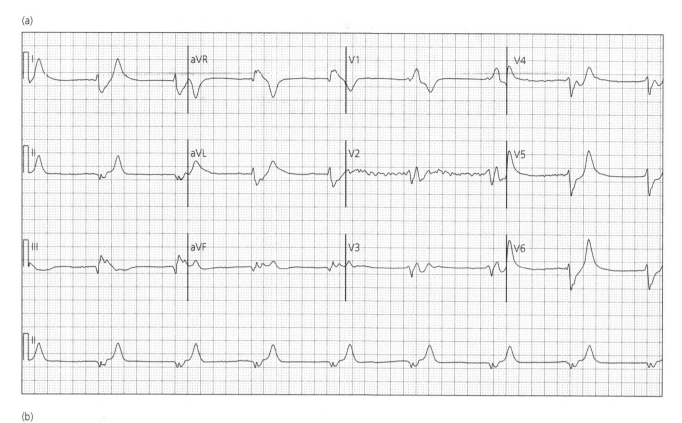

(b)

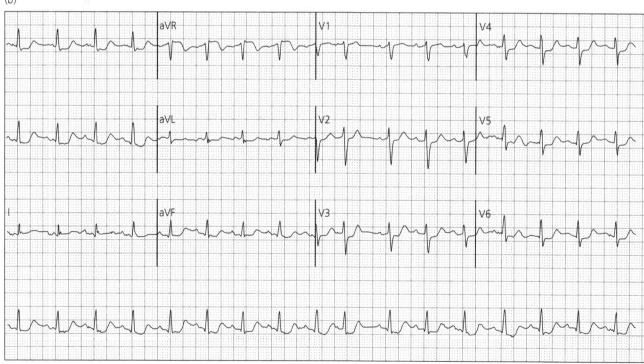

Figure 1.1 (a) Wide QRS complex bradycardia without P wave activity. (b) Improvement in the ECG from (a) with narrowing of the QRS complex, development of P waves, and increase in the rate. These ECGs are consistent with profound hyperkalemia that has markedly improved with therapy.

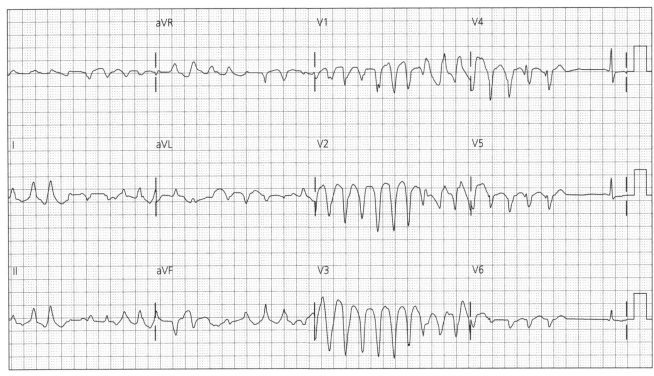

Figure 1.2 Polymorphic ventricular tachycardia (PVT). With review of the ECG in sinus rhythm, a prolonged QT interval was noted. With this additional finding, the PVT can be termed torsade de pointes. Note the varying QRS complex morphology (axis, amplitude, and contour) in a pattern suggesting "twisting about a fixed point."

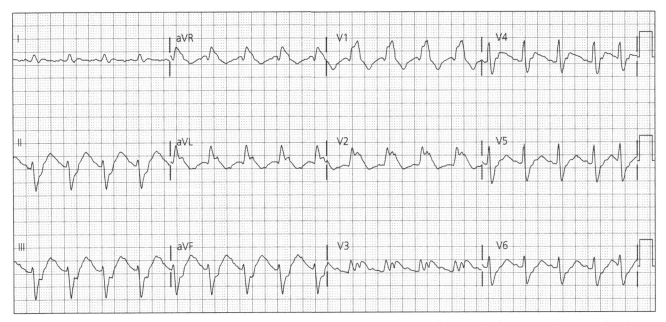

Figure 1.3 Sinus tachycardia with anterolateral wall STEMI, first-degree AV block, and right bundle branch block. Note the ST segment elevation in leads aVl, V2 and V3, consistent with anterolateral wall STEMI. The ST segment elevation in these leads is concordant with the major, terminal portion of the QRS complex – indicative of STEMI in RBBB.

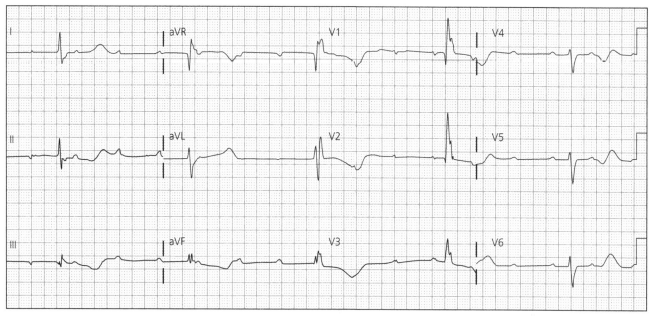

Figure 1.4 Complete heart block with no association of the atria with the ventricles. The P waves are occurring independently of the QRS complexes. Also note that atrial rate is greater than the ventricular rate.

maintenance of this gradient include potassium, sodium, calcium, and magnesium. As such, shifts in the extracellular or plasma concentrations of these cations may result in changes in the surface ECG. These changes are readily appreciated when the baseline ECG is completely normal. However, abnormalities from infarction/ischemia can make changes from electrolyte shifts more difficult to appreciate. In critically ill patients, two or more electrolyte abnormalities may co-exist, resulting in several changes in the ECG, some of which may mask each other.

Hyperkalemia: The electrocardiographic hallmarks of moderate hyperkalemia are symmetric, tall, peaked T waves and low amplitude P waves. Severe hyperkalemia produces a widened QRS complex without P waves. The electrocardiographic changes associated with hyperkalemia are a reflection of changes in the depolarization/repolarization waveform of the cardiac myocytes. One of the first changes observed on the surface ECG when the extracellular potassium ion concentration increases above 6.0 mM is narrow, peaked, tall T waves. This phenomenon occurs because repolarization of the ventricles occurs more synchronously [1]. As the extracellular potassium ion concentration increases further (6.5–8.0 mM), the resting membrane potential of the cardiac myocytes depolarizes, resulting in a slower conduction velocity. Slow depolarization across the atria is appreciated on the surface ECG as prolonged P wave duration with low amplitude. The HV interval also increases further, contributing to the lengthening of the PR interval. Slow depolarization across the ventricles results in prolongation of the QRS complex. If the extracellular potassium ion concentration increases beyond 8.0 mM, then the P wave may be visible for longer on the surface ECG. In canine models of hyperkalemia, once SA node block occurs, action potential propagation from the atrial pacemaker site to the ventricles may occur via atrianodal pathways [2]. At high extracellular potassium ion concentrations, the QRS complex may resemble a left bundle branch-like or right bundle branch-like waveform. With further increases in extracellular potassium ion concentration, activation of multiple pacemaker foci may result in an irregular rhythm. The QRS complex may become so wide that it takes on the appearance of a sine wave. An explanation of this phenomenon is that cardiac myocytes in one area of the ventricle may repolarize before the action potential wavefront has traversed and depolarized the more distant cardiac myocytes. Once the plasma potassium ion concentration rises to 12–14 mM, ventricular fibrillation and asystole may occur [3]. This phenomenon is exploited during on-pump cardiac surgery by bathing or perfusing the heart with a cardioplegia solution.

Hypokalemia: The electrocardiographic hallmarks of hypokalemia are a prominent U wave and prolongation of the QT(U) interval. With profound hypokalemia or with hypokalemia in the presence of cardiac toxic medications, torsade de pointes may be precipitated. As with hyperkalemia, the electrocardiographic changes associated with hypokalemia can be correlated with changes in the cardiac myocyte action potential waveform. Because the changes observed with hypokalemia affect the QT(U) portion of the ECG, it is changes in the ventricular action potential waveform that provide insight into the surface electrocardiographic changes. Hypokalemia results in prolongation of phase 3 repolarization. As the extracellular potassium ion concentration drops, the U wave amplitude increases and the T wave amplitude decreases. With a further decrease in potassium ion concentration, the U wave may begin to fuse with the preceding T wave. Hypokalemia can also result in increased arrhythmia. Davidson and Surawicz reported that the incidence of ectopic complexes was three times higher among patients who had a potassium ion concentration of ≤ 3.2 mEQ/L than control subjects [4]. Paroxsymal atrial tachycardia with block can also be observed in patients with hypokalemia. Severe hypokalemia can also precipitate ventricular tachycardia (VT), ventricular fibrillation (VF), or torsade de pointes [5]. Important non-cardiac manifestations of severe hypokalemia include rhabdomyocytis, metabolic alkalosis, and ascending paralysis.

Hypercalcemia: During phase 2 depolarization of the cardiac myocyte action potential, calcium slowly enters the cell. The duration of phase 2 correlates directly with the duration of the ST segment [6]. When the extracellular calcium ion concentration is elevated, phase 2 occurs relatively rapidly, producing a short ST segment [7]. Nierenberg and Ransil [8] reported a series in which the Q to apex of T wave interval corrected for rate was 0.27 seconds or less in over 90% of hypercalcemia cases.

The presence of hypercalcemia and hypokalemia produces an interesting ECG. This can be seen with multiple myeloma. The hypercalcemia results in a short ST segment and the hypokalemia results in a prominent U wave. Tachyarrhythmias due to hypercalcemia are uncommon in the literature. However, bradyarrhythmias with hypercalcemia are well described [9]. The classic case of hypercalcemia is that of patients presenting with metastatic non-parathyroid cancer that secretes recombinant parathyroid hormone (rPTH).

Hypocalcemia: The surface electrocardiographic changes associated with hypocalcemia are the opposite of those associated with hypercalcemia. Phase 2 depolarization of the cardiac myocyte action potential is lengthened, so the ST segment is prolonged. Suriwicz and Knilans [10] state that hypothermia and hypocalcemia are the only two conditions that increase the length of the ST segment without changing the T wave duration. Suriwicz and Lepeschkin [11] report that isolated hypocalcemia rarely causes the QTc interval to lengthen beyond 140% of normal. If the calculated QTc interval is over 140% of normal, then the measured QT interval may actually be the QU interval due to concomitant hypokalemia. Early after-repolarizations may be observed with hypocalcemia. Importantly, life-threatening arrhythmias can be precipitated with hypocalcemia in the presence of digoxin.

Vigilance for hypocalcemia is critical after thyroidectomy in the case of unintentional parathyroidectomy and, of course, after parathyroidectomy. Clinical scenarios other than primary parathyroidism in which hypocalcemia may occur include acute pancreatitis, rhabdomyositis, and other specific endocrine disorders involving calcium ion metabolism. Carlstedt and Lind [12] report that as many as 50% of critical care patients may have hypocalcemia. The classic clinical features of hypocalcemia include neuromuscular irritability, tetany, and tonic clonic seizure activity. Bedside tests consistent with hypocalcemia include Chvostek's and Trousseau's signs. Therapy for life-threatening arrhythmias and severe symptoms secondary to hypocalcemia includes intravenous calcium solution infusion along with treatment for any other co-existing electrolyte and metabolic conditions.

Other syndromes: Magnesium is largely an intracellular cation. Approximately 1% of total body magnesium is in the extracellular space [13]. No specific arrhythmias are associated with hyper- or hypomagnesemia. However, hypomagnesemia may occur in the context of hypokalemia. Intravenous magnesium sulfate is part of the recommended therapy for torsade de pointes after defibrillation. Additionally, intravenous magnesium sulfate is often given routinely prior to administration of ibutilide for chemical cardioversion of atrial fibrillation.

The presence of isolated hyper- or hyponatremia within the limits compatible with human life is not associated with any specific ECG changes that are well described in the literature. It is noteworthy that hypernatremia in the context of severe hyperkalemia, that would otherwise cause an intraventricular conduction delay, results in a relatively shorter QRS duration than predicted by the degree of hyperkalemia alone. Conversely, the QRS duration is further lengthened in severe hyperkalemia with an intraventricular conduction delay if hyponatremia is present.

Torsade de pointes: Torsade de pointes is a syndrome of ventricular tachycardia in which the electrical axis "twists" around. The QRS complex exhibits a crescendo-decrescendo variation in amplitude. The R-R interval is frequently in the range of 200–250 bpm. One of the characteristic features of torsade is a long period of ventricular repolarization so that the QT interval is typically at least 500 ms long. This prolonged QT interval is most readily observed in the QT interval immediately prior to the onset of torsade. Most cases of torsade are preceded by long-short R-R cycles [14]. For example, after a premature ventricular complex a compensatory pause will occur, and then a sinus beat with a long QT interval will occur. If another PVC occurs, torsade may be initiated. If a premature stimulus occurs near the zenith of the T wave, it may be more likely to induce a ventricular arrhythmia [15]. However, a short couple variant with a particularly high mortality has been described [16, 17]. It is important to distinguish polymorphic VT with a normal QT interval from torsade as the treatment and prognosis may be different.

The QT interval is measured from the onset of the Q wave to the end of the T wave [18]. The QT interval can vary with heart rate. Bradycardia is often associated with a prolonged QT interval while tachycardia is associated with a shortened QT interval. The QT interval can be corrected (QTc) for heart rate using Bazett's formula (the QTc equals the longest QT interval divided by the square root of the preceding R-R interval [19]). If atrial fibrillation is present, the QTc should be measured for 10 consecutive beats and averaged. Correct assessment of the QTc is critical during initiation of sotalol in patients with atrial fibrillation.

Torsade may devolve into ventricular fibrillation, return to the baseline rhythm, or end with asystole. Therefore, the first line of therapy is usually defibrillation followed by intravenous magnesium sulfate. Once the patient has hemodynamics that allow perfusion of vital organs, the goal is identifying the underlying cause. Common causes include extreme bradycardia, congenital causes of long QT syndrome, anti-arrhythmic drugs, and one or more combinations of drugs that prolong the QT interval. Both drug overdose and reduced drug clearance can prolong the QTc sufficiently to cause torsade. In a retrospective study of 249 cases of torsade not attributed to cardiac drugs, Zeltser and colleagues [20] noted that 71% of the cases involved female patients. Other risk factors in this series included hypokalemia, the use of multiple drugs that prolong the QT interval, increased drug dosage, a history of prior torsades, and a family history of long QT syndrome. Among cardiac medications, the class IA and class III anti-arrhythmics are associated with the development of torsade. The class IA drugs are most well known for blocking sodium channels. However, at low serum drug concentrations, potassium ion current blockage occurs. The association of quinidine is well described in the literature. Disopyramide has also been implicated. N-acteylprocainamide, a metabolite or procainamide, can cause torsade via QT prolongation by blocking the I_{kr} channel. Class III anti-arrthymics are potent I_{kr} channel-blockers. High serum concentrations of these drugs, either due to overdose or decreased clearance, can result in torsade. As these drugs exhibit reverse use dependence, I_{kr} is more effectively blocked at slow heart rates. Thus, bradycardia increases the risk of torsade with class III agents [21–23]. Interestingly, the class III agent amiodarone is rarely associated with torsade [24]. Drouin and colleagues [25] demonstrated that amiodarone decreases heterogeneous repolarization, thus reducing the susceptibility of re-entry. Torsade is also associated with overdose of tricyclic anti-depressants [26] and with use of the neuroleptins, including phenothiazines and haloperidol [27,28]. Among antimicrobials, the macrolides erythromycin and clarithromycin have been reported to prolong the QT interval and cause torsade [29,30]. Both of these medications inhibit the CYP3A4 system. Therefore, QT prolongation may occur in a patient taking either of these antibiotics with another drug that is metabolized by the CYP3A4 system. Such drugs will cause QT prolongation with increasing serum concentrations. The incidence of torsade among patients taking azithromycin is substantially less than

that of patients taking erythromycin [31]. An interesting historical footnote is cisapride, a promotility drug withdrawn from the U.S. market because it has a high incidence of QT prolongation and arrhythmia. Cisapride blocks the I_{kr} channel. Finally, in the case of bradycardia with long QT, temporary pacing may be necessary to prevent recurrence until the etiology of the slow heart rate can be diagnosed and treated.

Acute anterior myocardial infarction and right bundle branch block: The formal criteria for right bundle branch block (RBBB) are as follows: (1) the QRS duration must be ≥ 120 ms; (2) an rSR' pattern must be present in lead v1 or v2; (3) the S wave in V6 and I must be longer than 40 ms or at least longer than the R wave duration; and (4) the time to the peak of the R wave must be ≥ 50 ms in v1, but within normal limits in v5–6 [32]. With RBBB, the secondary (R') deflection is typically of greater amplitude than the first (R) deflection. Furthermore, there may be associated T wave inversion. Sometimes downsloping ST segments are observed. The presence of RBBB does not prevent the diagnosis of anterior MI. ST segment elevation and Q waves may be observed in V_1–V_3 precordial leads despite the presence of high amplitude R waves. The Q waves of an anterior infarct can obscure the initial R of a RBBB pattern, so that there is a qR in V_1 rather than an RSR'.

The incidence of RBBB in the population has been reported to be approximately 1.8/1000 people [33]. In patients with isolated RBBB and a structurally normal heart, the conduction delay does not portend a worse prognosis. However, there are many pathologic conditions that may cause RBBB including Ebstein's anomaly, cor pulmonale, myocarditis, hypertensive heart disease, Lenegre's disease, and Lev's disease. RBBB may also occur in patients with repaired tetralogy of Fallot who are left with significant pulmonary valve insufficiency resulting in right ventricular volume overload [34]. The development of RBBB in the context of acute MI occurs more frequently than left bundle branch block (LBBB). This may be due to the fact that the right bundle is a smaller, more discrete structure relative to the left bundle.

Prior to the thrombolytic era, the development of RBBB in the context of acute MI was associated with increased mortality [35]. Among patients who received thrombolysis, Go and colleagues [36] reported that the presence of RBBB was associated with a 69% increase in the risk of in-hospital death compared with acute MI patients who did not have RBBB and ST segment elevation. Moreno and colleagues [37] reported data from 681 patients with acute MI (74 had RBBB). Those with new irreversible RBBB had a 1-year mortality of 73%. The mortality of acute MI patients has decreased with advances in medical and mechanical therapy. More recently, Wong and colleagues [38] reported a 30-day mortality of 27.2% in patients with RBBB and a QRS duration < 160 ms. If the QRS duration was ≥ 160 ms, then the

30-day mortality was 37.2%. If new RBBB developed within 60 minutes of treatment, then the mortality was 24.5% if the QRS duration was less than 160 ms and 46.2% if the QRS duration was ≥ 160 ms. The development of a new bundle branch block in the context of an acute MI is generally a consequence of a large area of necrosis. If a new bundle branch block is a surrogate for a large MI, this explains, in part, the worse prognosis with the development of a new RBBB in the context of an acute MI. By the same logic, a longer QRS duration implies more myocardium is involved in the infarction. Nonetheless, the mortality of acute MI patients continues to decrease with early ECG recognition and treatment of STEMI.

Complete heart block: Complete heart block, also called third-degree heart block, describes a condition in which atrial depolarization is not conducted to the ventricles. Without action potential propagation from the atria through the atrioventricular (AV) node via the conduction system to the ventricles, the ventricular rate falls to that of automatic pacemakers located in the ventricular tissue. The ventricular rate will be in the range of 20 to 40 bpm or sometimes slower. The ventricular escape rate depends on the location of the ectopic escape pacemaker site. The atrial rate will generally be that of the sinus node (i.e., faster than the ventricular rate). As such, the atria and the ventricles are asynchronous. This phenomenon is referred to as AV dissociation. In patients with complete heart block, AV dissociation can be observed on the surface ECG as independent P waves that are not associated to QRS complexes in the usual 1 : 1 relationship. Furthermore, the atrial rate is faster than the ventricular rate. Therefore, the P waves are described as "marching though" the ECG with no fixed relationship to the QRS complexes [39]. Not all patients with AV dissociation have complete heart block. For example, sometimes in ventricular tachycardia P waves can be observed that are slower than the ventricular rate.

The etiology of complete heart block can be considered as primary or secondary. Primary complete heart block is due to pathology intrinsic to the conduction system. Secondary heart block is due to primary pathology outside the conduction system that affects the conduction system. Examples of secondary cases include permanent electronic pacemaker malfunction, neurologic causes, metabolic etiology, and medication toxicity due to overdose or reduced clearance. Iatrogenic complete heart block is a rare complication of aortic valve replacement surgery or atrioventricular nodal re-entry tachycardia catheter ablation. For this reason, temporary epicardial pacing leads are placed in patients undergoing cardiac surgery and transvenous pacing leads are paced in patients undergoing certain catheter ablation procedures in the electrophysiology lab.

Myocardial infarction is an important etiology of complete heart block. The infarct-related artery responsible for inferior infarction is often the right coronary artery (RCA). The AV nodal branch artery is often derived from the RCA, therefore inferior infarctions may cause heart block at the level of the AV node. As such, the escape rhythm will often originate directly below the AV node, from the His bundle. This mechanism generally provides a narrow QRS complex rhythm with a rate of at least 40 bpm. Another etiology of complete heart block with inferior MI is vasovagal reaction. Both are effectively treated with atropine [40]. Heart block secondary to inferior MI is usually transient and generally does not require permanent pacemaker placement unless the heart block persists. In contrast, if complete heart block occurs in the context of an anterior MI, the infarct zone is usually very large. The mechanism of complete heart block with an anterior MI is infarction of the infra-nodal conduction system, therefore the escape rhythm is wide, complex, and slow, typically less than 40 bpm. In the past, when a patient presented sufficiently early in the course of an evolving MI, progressive degrees of AV block were observed prior to complete heart block. As such, the American Heart Association/American College of Cardiology have given temporary pacemaker placement a class I indication for anterior MI patients with progressive AV block. Today, with early reperfusion via primary PCI or fibrinolytic agents, this complication is rarely seen. However, given the risk to the patient, it is critical to recognize progressive heart block in the context of an anterior MI early in the course of treatment so that a temporary pacemaker can be placed before a patient's life depends on emergency pacing [41].

Case conclusions

Case 1 represents a common presentation of severe hyperkalemia. The history suggests a patient with chronic kidney disease. Patients with chronic kidney disease are unable to efficiently excrete excess potassium ion in the urine. It is critical to make the diagnosis of hyperkalemia from an ECG, particularly in the setting of a sinusoidal QRS complex, in that treatment needs to be initiated immediately.

Case 2 presents a common scenario of tricyclic anti-depressant overdose. The patient presented with anti-cholinergic symptoms. Intravenous sodium bicarbonate is the antidote for this type of ingestion with a widened QRS complex – this patient received multiple doses of sodium bicarbonate coupled with endotracheal intubation and other critical management supportive care. Occasionally, the medication or medications upon which the patient overdosed are known. When the drugs are not known, the health care provider must rely on the history and examination for clues. The patient must be stabilized and monitored closely while the laboratory is performing a toxicology or overdose panel. The baseline ECG may provide clues regarding the drugs on which the patient overdosed, and for what acute or sub-acute adverse effects the patient may be at risk.

Case 3 is a classic presentation of an acute MI. This patient was experiencing a large anterior STEMI with RBBB; the patient underwent PCI with stenting of the left anterior descending artery with good outcome. It is critical to recognize the presence of an anterior MI in the presence of RBBB. The presence of RBBB should not distract the health care provider from the diagnosis of MI – as is the case in patients with LBBB presentations. Such infarctions are typically larger and patients have the potential to receive significant benefit from early recognition and treatment.

Case 4 represents a common situation in which complete heart block may occur. Regardless of the clinical context it is important to recognize complete heart block and immediately initiate treatment to stabilize the patient. In this case, the underlying etiology was the inferior MI. If the underlying etiology is not known, once the patient has been stabilized, the patient should be admitted and considered for a permanent pacemaker.

References

1 Surawicz B. Relationship between electrocardiogram and electrolytes. *Am Heart J* 1967;**73**(6):814–34.

2 Hariman RJ, Chen CM. Effects of hyperkalaemia on sinus nodal function in dogs: sino-ventricular conduction. *Cardiovasc Res* 1983;**17**(9):509–17.

3 Mattu A, Brady WJ, Robinson DA. Electrocardiographic manifestations of hyperkalemia. *Am J Emerg Med* 2000;**18**(6):721–9.

4 Davidson S, Surawicz B. Ectopic beats and atrioventricular conduction disturbances in patients with hypopotassemia. *Arch Intern Med* 1967;**120**(3):280–5.

5 Kunin A, Surawicz B, Sims E. Decrease in serum potassium concentrations and appearance of cardiac arrhythmias during infusion of potassium with glucose in potassium-depleted patients. *N Engl J Med* 1962;**266**:228–33.

6 Hoffman B, Suckling E. Effect of several cations on transmembrane potentials of cardiac muscle. *Am J Physiol* 1956;**186**(2):317–24.

7 Saikawa T, Tsumabuki S, Nakagawa M, *et al.* QT intervals as an index of high serum calcium in hypercalcemia. *Clin Cardiol* 1988;**11**(2):75–8.

8 Nierenberg DW, Ransil BJ. Q-aTc interval as a clinical indicator of hypercalcemia. *Am J Cardiol* 1979;**44**(2):243–8.

9 Ziegler R. Hypercalcemic crisis. *J Am Soc Nephrol* 2001;**12** Suppl 17:S3–S9.

10 Surawicz B, Knilans T. Electrolytes, Temperature, Central Nervous System Diseases. In: Surawicz B, Knilans T, editors. *Chou's Electrocardiography in Clinical Practice*. Philadelphia: W.B. Saunders Company, 2001:516–39.

11 Surawicz B, Lepeschkin E. The electrocardiographic pattern of hypopotassemia with and without hypocalcemia. *Circulation* 1953;**8**(6):801–28.

12 Carlstedt F, Lind L. Hypocalcemic syndromes. *Crit Care Clin* 2001;**17**(1):139–viii.

13 Agus MS, Agus ZS. Cardiovascular actions of magnesium. *Crit Care Clin* 2001;**17**(1):175–86.

14 Schwartz PJ, Stramba-Badiale M, Napolitano C. The Long QT Syndrome. In: Zipes Dp, Jalife I, editors. *Cardiac Electrophysiology: From Bench to Bedside*. Philadelphia: WB Saunders, 2000:788–811.

15 Swerdlow CD, Martin DJ, Kass RM, *et al.* The zone of vulnerability to T wave shocks in humans. *J Cardiovasc Electrophysiol* 1997;**8**(2):145–54.

16 Leenhardt A, Glaser E, Burguera M, Nurnberg M, Maison-Blanche P, Coumel P. Short-coupled variant of torsade de pointes. A new electrocardiographic entity in the spectrum of idiopathic ventricular tachyarrhythmias. *Circulation* 1994;**89**(1):206–15.

17 Viskin S, Belhassen B. Polymorphic ventricular tachyarrhythmias in the absence of organic heart disease: classification, differential diagnosis, and implications for therapy. *Prog Cardiovasc Dis* 1998;**41**(1):17–34.

18 Sadanaga T, Sadanaga F, Yao H, Fujishima M. An evaluation of ECG leads used to assess QT prolongation. *Cardiology* 2006;**105**(3):149–54.

19 Bazett H. An analysis of the time-relations of the electrocardiogram. *Heart* 1920;**7**:353–62.

20 Zeltser D, Justo D, Halkin A, Prokhorov V, Heller K, Viskin S. Torsade de pointes due to noncardiac drugs: most patients have easily identifiable risk factors. *Medicine (Baltimore)* 2003;**82**(4):282–90.

21 Ellenbogen KA, Stambler BS, Wood MA, *et al.* Efficacy of intravenous ibutilide for rapid termination of atrial fibrillation and atrial flutter: a dose-response study. *J Am Coll Cardiol* 1996;**28**(1):130–6.

22 Lazzara R. Antiarrhythmic drugs and torsade de pointes. *Eur Heart J* 1993;14 Suppl H:88–92.

23 Torp-Pedersen C, Moller M, Bloch-Thomsen PE, *et al.* Dofetilide in patients with congestive heart failure and left ventricular dysfunction. Danish Investigations of Arrhythmia and Mortality on Dofetilide Study Group. *N Engl J Med* 1999;**341**(12):857–65.

24 Hohnloser SH, Klingenheben T, Singh BN. Amiodarone-associated proarrhythmic effects. A review with special reference to torsade de pointes tachycardia. *Ann Intern Med* 1994;**121**(7):529–35.

25 Drouin E, Lande G, Charpentier F. Amiodarone reduces transmural heterogeneity of repolarization in the human heart. *J Am Coll Cardiol* 1998;**32**(4):1063–7.

26 Vieweg WV, Wood MA. Tricyclic antidepressants, QT interval prolongation, and torsade de pointes. *Psychosomatics* 2004;**45**(5):371–7.

27 Glassman AH, Bigger JT, Jr. Antipsychotic drugs: prolonged QTc interval, torsade de pointes, and sudden death. *Am J Psychiatry* 2001;**158**(11):1774–82.

28 Haddad PM, Anderson IM. Antipsychotic-related QTc prolongation, torsade de pointes and sudden death. *Drugs* 2002;**62**(11):1649–71.

29 Ray WA, Murray KT, Meredith S, Narasimhulu SS, Hall K, Stein CM. Oral erythromycin and the risk of sudden death from cardiac causes. *N Engl J Med* 2004;**351**(11):1089–96.

30 Shaffer D, Singer S, Korvick J, Honig P. Concomitant risk factors in reports of torsades de pointes associated with macrolide use: review of the United States Food and Drug Administration Adverse Event Reporting System. *Clin Infect Dis* 2002;**35**(2):197–200.

31 Kim MH, Berkowitz C, Trohman RG. Polymorphic ventricular tachycardia with a normal QT interval following azithromycin. *Pacing Clin Electrophysiol* 2005;**28**(11):1221–2.

32 The Criteria Committee of the New York Heart Association. *Nomenclature and criteria for the diagnosis of diseases of the heart and great vessels.* 7th ed. Boston: Little, Brown, 1973.

33 Hiss R, Lamb L. Electrocardiographic findings in 122,043 individuals. *Circulation* 1962;**25**:947–61.

34 Gatzoulis MA, Till JA, Somerville J, Redington AN. Mechanoelectrical interaction in tetralogy of Fallot. QRS prolongation relates to right ventricular size and predicts malignant ventricular arrhythmias and sudden death. *Circulation* 1995;**92**(2):231–7.

35 Scheidt S, Killip T. Bundle-branch block complicating acute myocardial infarction. *JAMA* 1972;**222**(8):919–24.

36 Go AS, Barron HV, Rundle AC, Ornato JP, Avins AL. Bundle-branch block and in-hospital mortality in acute myocardial infarction. National Registry of Myocardial Infarction 2 Investigators. *Ann Intern Med* 1998;**129**(9):690–7.

37 Moreno AM, Alberola AG, Tomas JG, *et al.* Incidence and prognostic significance of right bundle branch block in patients with acute myocardial infarction receiving thrombolytic therapy. *Int J Cardiol* 1997;**61**(2):135–41.

38 Wong CK, Gao W, Stewart RA, *et al.* Risk stratification of patients with acute anterior myocardial infarction and right bundle-branch block: importance of QRS duration and early ST-segment resolution after fibrinolytic therapy. *Circulation* 2006;**114**(8): 783–9.

39 Brady WJ, Swart G, DeBehnke DJ, Ma OJ, Aufderheide TP. The efficacy of atropine in the treatment of hemodynamically unstable bradycardia and atrioventricular block: prehospital and emergency department considerations. *Resuscitation* 1999;**41**(1): 47–55.

40 Feigl D, Ashkenazy J, Kishon Y. Early and late atrioventricular block in acute inferior myocardial infarction. *J Am Coll Cardiol* 1984;**4**(1):35–8.

41 Birnbaum Y, Sclarovsky S, Herz I, *et al.* Admission clinical and electrocardiographic characteristics predicting in-hospital development of high-degree atrioventricular block in inferior wall acute myocardial infarction. *Am J Cardiol* 1997;**80**(9): 1134–8.

Chapter 2 | What are the indications for the ECG in the pediatric emergency department?

Michael A. McCulloch, D. Scott Lim
University of Virginia, Charlottesville, VA, USA

Case presentations

Case 1: A 14-year-old female presents to the emergency department (ED) with a chief complaint of chest pain for 1 hour. The pain is characterized as crushing in nature without radiation. There are no other associated symptoms. This is the third such episode since joining the soccer team. She does not take any medications. There is no family history of sudden, unexplained death or congenital heart disease. On examination, her heart rate is 90 beats per minute (bpm), blood pressure is 110/68 mmHg, and oxygen saturation is 95% on room air. Her physical examination is unremarkable and you are unable to reproduce her pain. Her electrocardiogram (ECG) is shown in Figure 2.1.

Case 2: A 10-year-old male presents to the ED after a syncopal episode while running at school. The patient has no memory of the event. Witnesses deny any seizure-type activity. He has no significant past medical history and no habitual medication use. His family history is significant for a distant relative who died suddenly of unknown causes. On examination his heart rate is 85 bpm, blood pressure is 95/53 mmHg, and oxygen saturation is 100% on room air. His physical exam is unremarkable. An ECG is performed, shown in Figure 2.2.

Case 3: A 4-year-old male presents to the ED with a complaint of episodic chest pain that started while watching television. According to the patient's mother, the pain starts and stops abruptly and lasts between 1 and 5 min. The child has not had syncope. His mother reports six of these episodes this morning and denies any such episodes prior to today. He has no significant past medical history, takes no habitual medications, and has a non-contributory family history. On examination, his heart rate suddenly increases to > 250 bpm, his ECG is shown in Figure 2.3. You have the child perform a valsalva maneuver and his heart rate decreases to 120 bpm and the repeat ECG is demonstrated in Figure 2.4.

Clinical indication for the ECG in pediatric emergency and critical care medicine

Clinical indications for the electrocardiogram (ECG) are well documented for adult patients [1,2]; however, studies evaluating its efficacy in the pediatric population are lacking. A systematic approach to ECG interpretation in the pediatric population is required to minimize the occurrence of misdiagnosis. Familiarity with the indication for and interpretation of the pediatric ECG is critical to the clinician managing children with acute illness and injury, as misdiagnosis may lead to mismanagement [3–5]. Based on the literature, ECGs should be considered in the pediatric emergency department in the following scenarios: chest pain with a supportive history, palpitations with a supportive history, most instances of syncope, most cases of apparent life-threatening event (ALTE) or near-miss sudden infant death syndrome (SIDS), ingestions, suspected metabolic derangements, and patients with an episode of commotio cordis; of course, other presentations are appropriate and ECGs may also be performed in these other settings.

Chest pain: Unlike the adult population, fewer than 5% of cases of chest pain in children and adolescents are of cardiac etiology [7–11]. Chest pain in this population, however, has been shown to account for nearly 20% of all new pediatric cardiology consults in the ED [11]. It commonly accounts for more than 50% of all ECGs obtained in pediatric EDs [5], yet accounts for less than 1% of all visits to the pediatric ED [7, 9, 10], and often does not demonstrate any changes even when cardiac pathology is present [10,12,13]. Costochondritis, asthma, gastroesophageal reflux, trauma, and anxiety constitute the majority of presentations for chest pain in this population [7–11,14].

When evaluating chest pain in a pediatric ED, the clinician should consider myocardial ischemia or infarction; refer to

Critical Decisions in Emergency and Acute Care Electrocardiography,
1st edition. Edited by W.J. Brady and J.D. Truwit. © 2009 Blackwell Publishing, ISBN: 9781405159067

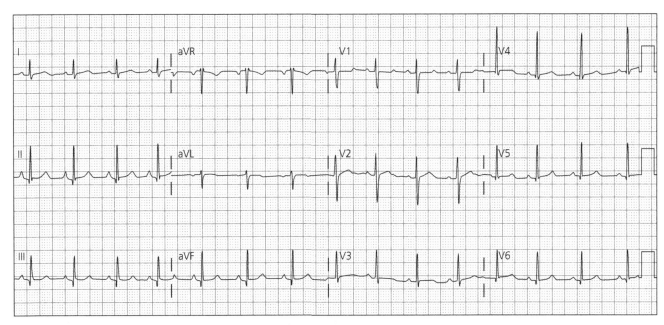

Figure 2.1 This ECG demonstrates upright P waves in leads I, aVF, and V3 to V6, consistent with a sinus rhythm. Her rate of 85 bpm is appropriate for her age. The predominant QRS voltages are upright in leads I and aVF, consistent with a leftward QRS axis that is normal for her age. There is no evidence for ventricular hypertrophy by voltage criteria, no ST segment or T wave abnormalities and no evidence of pre-excitation or "delta waves." The QT interval is less than one-half of the R to R interval, best seen in leads II and aVF, which is typically consistent with a normal corrected QT interval. This is a normal ECG for this girl who was found to have exercise-induced asthma.

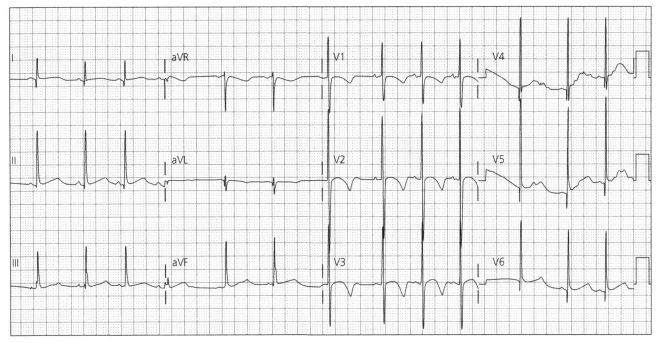

Figure 2.2 As in Figure 2.1, there is normal sinus rhythm and an appropriate heart rate and leftward QRS axis. There are inverted T waves in the early precordial leads (V1 to V3), which is normal into late adolescence. There is no ST segment elevation or depression or pre-excitation. The QT interval is at least one-half the R to R interval, which is typically consistent with long QT syndrome, this patient's diagnosis. The QTc is calculated by dividing the QT interval in leads II or V5 by the square root of the preceding R to R interval; normal values are less than 460 ms.

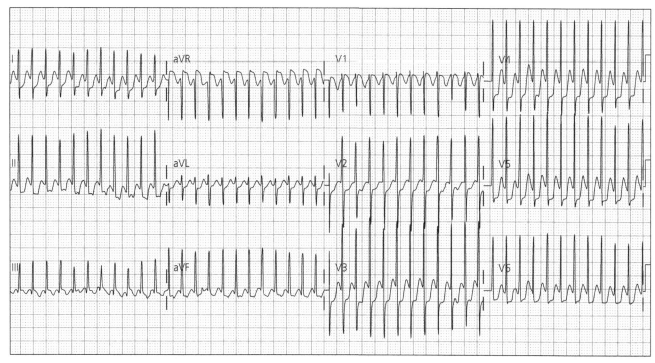

Figure 2.3 The most striking aspect of this ECG is the heart rate of nearly 300 bpm, which is never physiologic. This is a narrow complex tachycardia without clear evidence of P waves.

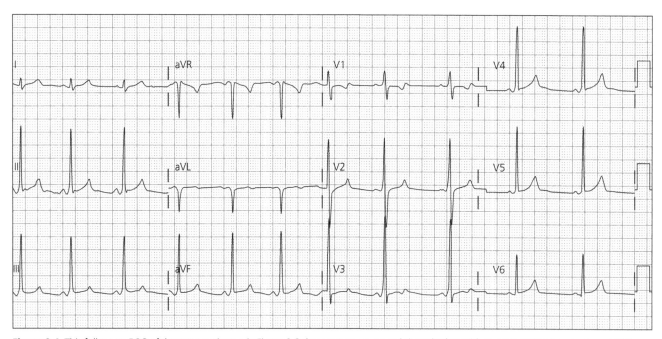

Figure 2.4 This follow-up ECG of the same patient as in Figure 2.3 demonstrates a normal sinus rhythm with an appropriate heart rate and QRS axis. The most notable aspect of this ECG is the pre-excitation or delta waves seen in leads II, III, aVF, and V2 through V4. This patient was diagnosed as having Wolff-Parkinson-White syndrome.

Table 2.1 for a listing of possible causes of myocardial ischemia. The differential diagnosis for myocardial ischemia is more diverse in the pediatric patient, as obstruction of a coronary artery lumen by an atherosclerotic plaque is extremely rare. Severe left ventricular hypertrophy (i.e.,

aortic stenosis, coarctation of the aorta, or hypertrophic cardiomyopathy) can exhibit large QRS voltages and T wave inversions in the lateral precordial leads with or without ST segment changes. "Kinking" of transplanted coronary arteries can produce ST segment changes consistent with ischemia

Table 2.1a Possible causes of myocardial ischemia in the pediatric patient

Congenital heart diseases
    Anomalous left coronary artery arising from the pulmonary artery (ALCAPA)
    Coarctation of the aorta
    Aortic stenosis
    Hypertrophic cardiomyopathy

Congenital heart disease – postoperative
    Transposition of the great arteries status postarterial switch operation
    Single ventricle physiology (i.e., hypoplastic left heart syndrome)
    Aortic stenosis status post-balloon valvuloplasty

Acquired heart disease
    History of Kawasaki's disease with or without echocardiographic evidence of coronary artery involvement

Other
    Cocaine abuse
    Pulmonary hypertension

Table 2.1b Possible causes of myocardial ischemia in the pediatric patient by age

0–6 months
    Anomalous left coronary artery arising from the pulmonary artery (ALCAPA)
    Coarctation of the aorta prior to intervention
    Aortic stenosis
    Cyanotic congenital heart disease – preoperative
    Cyanotic congenital heart disease – postoperative
    Transposition of the great arteries status postarterial switch operation
    Aortic stenosis status post-balloon valvuloplasty

Greater than 5 years old
    History of Kawasaki's disease with or without echocardiographic evidence of coronary artery involvement
    Cocaine abuse

of the affected coronary artery. This pattern can also occur years after the diagnosis of Kawasaki's disease from the thrombosis of coronary arteries. Lastly, ST segment changes may be seen in the setting of cocaine overdose.

As noted, most chest pain in children is not cardiac in origin and several authors have found chest pain associated with psychogenic manifestations in children > 12 years and respiratory diseases in those < 12 years [7,8,10]. Wiens and colleagues were able to reproduce chest pain with an exercise stress test and alleviate symptoms with albuterol in 64 of 88 children with a presenting complaint of chest pain [14]. A history of chest pain with palpitations, syncope, progressive exercise intolerance, prior Kawasaki's disease, or a positive family history of sudden death or defibrillator implantation should raise suspicion for cardiac pathology. However, information regarding chest pain duration, location, and frequency has limited diagnostic utility in the pediatric population [7,8,10]. A focused physical examination should confirm their original suspicions. Evidence of wheezing, decreased breath sounds, stridor, or chest wall tenderness during the examination suggest non-cardiac chest pain. [8,9]. In 168 consecutive patients evaluated in an ED for chest pain, Massin and colleagues reported a friction rub, murmur, pallor, abnormal heart rhythm, or signs of decreased cardiac output in all seven patients ultimately diagnosed with a cardiac etiology [10]. Although 83 ECGs were ordered during this retrospective study, the ECG was abnormal in only seven patients.

Chest pain is a common problem in the pediatric population, which is only rarely associated with myocardial ischemia. Considering the variability in ECG interpretation, its use should be limited to those patients with both a positive history and physical exam. Any patient producing a high index of suspicion, as well as ECG evidence for myocardial ischemia, should undergo prompt evaluation by a pediatric cardiologist.

Syncope and presyncope: Syncope is a transient, self-limited loss of consciousness caused by global cerebral hypoperfusion; presyncope is the feeling that syncope is imminent. As with chest pain, syncope is common in the pediatric population, occurring in up to 15% of adolescents [12,15,16], and is also rarely cardiac in origin. However, with subsequent annual mortality rates of 24% in those with cardiac syncope [15], a thorough evaluation of this presenting symptom is justified.

Any syncopal episode in the setting of known cardiac disease should be considered an aborted sudden death until proven otherwise. Ventricular tachycardia, ventricular fibrillation, or torsade de pointes are the three dysrhythmias most commonly cited as the cause of cardiac syncope, but are only rarely documented in patients who survive to receive emergency medical care. Severe pulmonary hypertension, long QT syndrome, hypertrophic cardiomyopathy, and Wolff-Parkinson-White syndrome are the most likely substrates leading to these ventricular dysrhythmias. In order to properly recognize these rare disease states, the clinician must familiarize him/herself with the most common findings on history, physical exam, and ECG.

A history of dehydration, dizziness, fatigue, vertigo, medication use, or intentional termination of activities prior to the loss of consciousness all suggest a vasovagal etiology. Conversely, syncope during exercise or exertion, or when immediately preceded by palpitations or chest pain is consistent with dysrhythmia. It is generally agreed that all patients with an episode of exercise-induced syncope should be evaluated by a pediatric cardiologist [13,17]. To assess the risk for long QT syndrome and hypertrophic cardiomyopathy (HCM), the clinician should explore any family history of syncope, sudden unexplained deaths particularly with exercise, and defibrillator and, pacemaker placements [18].

A cardiac examination will often be normal in patients with cardiogenic syncope. Two notable exceptions can occur in HCM with left ventricular outflow tract obstruction and severe pulmonary hypertension. In general, however, patients with long QT syndrome, pulmonary hypertension, Wolff-Parkinson-White syndrome, or HCM without left ventricular outflow tract obstruction will have unremarkable physical examination. This fact underscores the importance of a thorough medical and family history, as well as appropriate ordering and interpretation of the ECG. Most pediatric patients referred for a syncopal episode should undergo an ECG. A normal ECG, however, does not rule out a cardiac cause as studies have demonstrated significant variability in ECG interpretation and the common finding of normal QTc intervals on resting ECGs of individuals with long QT syndrome [13].

ECG interpretation in this setting must focus on identifying findings suggestive of HCM, long QT syndrome, Wolff-Parkinson-White syndrome, or pulmonary hypertension with right ventricular hypertrophy. Patients with HCM may demonstrate large R wave voltages in leads I, II, III, aVF, and V3 through V6, consistent with left ventricular hypertrophy; ischemia or left ventricular "strain" may also be seen as ST segment changes or T wave inversion in the lateral precordial leads. Though often normal at rest, long QT syndrome is diagnosed as having a corrected QT interval of greater than 460 ms.

Syncope in patients found to have Wolff–Parkinson-White syndrome is thought to occur due to rapid conduction of atrial fibrillation across the accessory pathway with resultant ventricular fibrillation. The incidence of spontaneous atrial fibrillation is thought to be higher in these patients as compared with the general population, but the incidence of sudden cardiac death is estimated to occur in only 1 of 10,000 patients [19,20]. A short PR interval, along with evidence of pre-excitation, is required to make the diagnosis of this conduction anomaly [21] and should prompt consultation with a pediatric cardiologist.

Severe pulmonary hypertension can result in syncope through two possible mechanisms. In one scenario, right ventricular strain against an acutely elevated pulmonary artery pressure could result in myocardial ischemia and ventricular dysrhythmias. Alternatively, acute right ventricular failure in the setting of elevated pulmonary artery pressures would impede left ventricular preload and systemic cardiac output, ultimately producing cerebral hypoperfusion. Regardless of the mechanism, severe right ventricular hypertrophy can produce large R waves in the early precordial leads (V1 to V3) in addition to a rightward deviation of the QRS axis. T wave inversion in these leads may also be seen, but this finding is normal into adolescence. While these findings could be considered strong evidence in support of the respective diagnoses, their absence does not exclude them. For example, the pre-excitation or "delta wave" seen in Wolff-Parkinson-White syndrome can be intermittently expressed [20]. The corrected QT interval is commonly normal in patients with documented abnormalities in the identified electrolyte channels, the pathologic hallmark of long QT syndrome. Thus, as a screening test for cardiac causes of syncope, the surface ECG is a relatively specific test with poor sensitivity. The clinician should recognize this limitation, and therefore focus attention on the history and physical examination to screen for those patients at most risk for having a cardiac etiology for their syncope.

Palpitations and supraventricular dysrhythmia: Palpitations are the perception of an abnormal heart rate or rhythm. Assessment by both 24-h Holter monitors and event monitors frequently demonstrates this sensation to be associated with premature atrial and ventricular contractions, as well as sinus tachycardia. Sustained periods of abnormal cardiac conduction are relatively uncommon. Primary ventricular dysrhythmias (i.e., ventricular tachycardia) are rare in pediatric patients without congenital or acquired heart disease, and are typically associated with syncope or chest pain. Simple palpitations with a true cardiac etiology are most commonly associated with ventricular electrical conduction via the His-Purkinje fibers and effective ventricular contractions. This scenario occurs in the setting of either normal sinus tachycardia or supraventricular tachycardia. Supraventricular tachycardia is the most common cause of palpitations from a primary cardiac dysrhythmia in pediatric patients [21]; fortunately, less than 1 in 10,000 [20] of such patients are estimated to be at risk for degenerating into a lethal ventricular dysrhythmia.

There are 11 different types of supraventricular tachycardia. These conduction disturbances manifest at a rate faster than that of the sinoatrial node, and are intrinsically unresponsive to the needs of the body. Patients subjected to the persistent state of any one of these dysrhythmias can develop a dilated cardiomyopathy over time; nearly 50% of infants will exhibit signs of congestive heart failure in as little as 48 h of a continuous non-sinus rhythm [22]. While important to make a timely diagnosis, the incidence of sudden cardiac death associated with true supraventricular tachycardia is exceedingly rare and has only been associated with one type: Wolff-Parkinson-White syndrome (WPW).

The electrocardiographic findings necessary to make the diagnosis of Wolff-Parkinson-White syndrome include a PR interval that is shortened due to aberrant prograde conduction over an accessory pathway [21]. This finding is not present during the typical tachycardia cycle, as conduction is prograde down the atrioventricular (AV) node, into the His-Purkinje fibers, and retrograde up the accessory pathway back into the atria – perpetuating the cycle until some part of the circuit is made refractory to further conduction. Most commonly, the AV node is the focus of interventions through either vagal maneuvers or adenosine, which both slow conduction through this structure and terminate the circuit. Unlike in the other 10 types of supraventricular tachycardia, the accessory pathway in Wolff-Parkinson-White syndrome has the potential to allow rapid prograde conduction into the ventricles. In the setting of atrial fibrillation with rates up to 300 bpm, this will quickly degenerate into an unstable ventricular rhythm.

Paul and colleagues [19] published a landmark study about patients with Wolff-Parkinson-White syndrome, linking a predisposition to atrial fibrillation with syncope. Of 74 adolescents with this diagnosis who underwent formal electrophysiology testing, 14 presented with a history of syncope. This subset demonstrated a significantly increased ability to be induced into atrial fibrillation as compared with the other 60 patients who did not present with a history of syncope. Prograde conduction down the accessory pathway in patients with Wolff-Parkinson-White syndrome places them at increased risk for sudden cardiac death.

Psychiatric history should be thoroughly addressed, as studies have demonstrated non-cardiac palpitations to be present in nearly half of all patients suffering from anxiety disorders [23]. As physical examination is unlikely to guide the diagnosis, the clinician must rely on ECG interpretation to detect underlying processes. After determining whether the absolute heart rate is appropriate for the particular patient, the clinician must focus attention on the cardiac rhythm. Sinus rhythm is a heart rate that is being controlled by the rightward, superior, and posteriorly located sinoatrial node. This anatomic position can be verified by the P wave axis. When originating from the sinoatrial node, there should exist upright P waves in leads I, II, III, aVF, and the precordial leads V3 through V6. Any variation from this pattern implies that another region of the atria is controlling the heart rate. Once the rhythm is determined, attention should be given to the presence of pre-excitation. This will produce a gradual upstroke that terminates into the rapid upstroke of the QRS complex, signifying the less efficient conduction through the accessory pathway as compared with the His-Purkinje fibers. In patients with Wolff-Parkinson-White syndrome this pattern should be seen in more than one lead, but typically will not be seen in all leads.

Apparent life-threatening event (ALTE) and near-miss sudden infant death syndrome (SIDS): Formerly known as "crib death," SIDS is a devastating loss of life that classically occurs in the first 5–12 weeks [24] in an estimated 7 out of 10,000 live births [25]. Several authors have suggested a correlation between SIDS and the long QT syndrome by citing that 14% of all patients with long QT syndrome will die with their sentinel event, of which 30% occur in the first year of life [25].

Schwartz and colleagues [25] prospectively followed more than 33,000 infants who underwent a resting ECG on day three or four of life. A QT interval was measured in lead II and corrected for heart rate (QTc). The mean QTc was 400 ms and the 97.5th percentile was 440 ms. At 1-year follow-up, the overall risk of non-traumatic death was 1.53% in those infants with a QTc greater than 440 ms, compared with 0.037% in those with a QTc < 440 ms. None of the infants with the longer QTc had a positive family history for long QT syndrome. An ECG should be considered as a portion of the initial evaluation of any patient with a suspected ALTE or near-miss SIDS [26].

Brugada syndrome is another electrocardiographic diagnosis that has been suggested to have a link to sudden cardiac death in children. The findings of a right bundle branch block (RBBB) pattern and ST segment elevation in precordial leads V1 to V3 are necessary for this diagnosis, which occurs most commonly in Asian and South American males, with an overall estimated prevalence of 1 in 5000 [27]. Priori and colleagues [27] reported a family in which four children died between 2 and 36 months of age. Though less likely in the United States, this diagnosis should also be considered in the setting of ALTE.

Commotio cordis: Commotio cordis is the onset of cardiovascular collapse immediately following a blunt, non-penetrating blow to the chest, in the absence of underlying cardiovascular abnormalities. In patients who have survived long enough to receive prompt medical attention, the three most commonly documented rhythms are ventricular tachycardia, ventricular fibrillation and asystole. Animal studies have suggested the mechanism is similar to the R-on-T phenomenon that destabilizes patients with long QT syndrome into unstable ventricular dysrhythmias [28]. In the largest retrospective study on the subject, 84% of the 128 patients identified over a 16-year period died as a consequence of their event; more than 75% of these victims received appropriate resuscitative measures in under 3 min [29]. Despite these results, death is not universal if the problem is identified quickly [30]. Therefore, any pediatric patient presenting to the ED following an episode of significant chest trauma should have an ECG to confirm a normal sinus rhythm.

Case conclusions

Case 1, a normal ECG in a child with non-cardiac chest pain, was discharged from the ED without consequence. Case 2 illustrates a potential long QT syndrome presentation; this child was admitted for further monitoring. The child in Case 3 presented with symptomatic paroxysmal supraventricular tachycardia. With resolution of the tachycardia, a 12-lead ECG in sinus rhythm demonstrated Wolff-Parkinson-White syndrome. Due to this finding, he was admitted for further therapy and monitoring. No recurrence was found and he was ultimately discharged without therapy.

References

1 Antman EM, Anbe DT, Armstrong PW, *et al.* ACC/AHA guidelines for the management of patients with ST-elevation myocardial

infarction – executive summary. A report of the American College of Cardiology/American Heart Association Task Force on Practice Guidelines (Writing Committee to revise the 1999 guidelines for the management of patients with acute myocardial infarction). *J Am Coll Cardiol* 2004;**44**(3):671–719.

2 Pollack CV, Jr., Diercks DB, Roe MT, *et al.* 2004 American College of Cardiology/American Heart Association guidelines for the management of patients with ST-elevation myocardial infarction: implications for emergency department practice. *Ann Emerg Med* 2005;**45**(4):363–76.

3 Westdrop EJ, Gratton MC, Watson WA. Emergency department interpretation of electrocardiograms. *Ann Emerg Med* 1992;**21**(5): 541–4.

4 Erling BF, Perron AD, Brady WJ. Disagreement in the interpretation of electrocardiographic ST segment elevation: a source of error for emergency physicians? *Am J Emerg Med* 2004;**22**(2): 65–70.

5 Horton LA, Mosee S, Brenner J. Use of the electrocardiogram in a pediatric emergency department. *Arch Pediatr Adolesc Med* 1994;**148**(2):184–8.

6 Giuffre RM, Nutting A, Cohen J, *et al.* Electrocardiogram interpretation and management in a pediatric emergency department. *Pediatr Emerg Care* 2005;**21**(3):143–8.

7 Selbst SM. Chest pain in children. *Pediatrics* 1985;**75**(6):1068–70.

8 Selbst SM, Ruddy RM, Clark BJ, *et al.* Pediatric chest pain: a prospective study. *Pediatrics* 1988;**82**(3):319–23.

9 Zavaras-Angelidou KA, Weinhouse E, and Nelson DB. Review of 180 episodes of chest pain in 134 children. *Pediatr Emerg Care* 1992;**8**(4):189–93.

10 Massin MM, Bourguignont A, Coremans C, *et al.* Chest pain in pediatric patients presenting to an emergency department or to a cardiac clinic. *Clin Pediatr (Phila)* 2004;**43**(3):231–8.

11 Geggel RL. Conditions leading to pediatric cardiology consultation in a tertiary academic hospital. *Pediatrics* 2004;**114**(4):e409–17.

12 Driscoll DJ, Jacobsen SJ, Porter CJ, Wollan PC. Syncope in children and adolescents. *J Am Coll Cardiol* 1997;**29**(5):1039–45.

13 McHarg ML, *et al.* Syncope in childhood. *Pediatr Cardiol* 1997; **18**(5):367–71.

14 Wiens L, Sabath R, Ewing L, *et al.* Chest pain in otherwise healthy children and adolescents is frequently caused by exercise-induced asthma. *Pediatrics* 1992;**90**(3):350–3.

15 Brignole M, Alboni P, Benditt D, *et al.* Guidelines on management (diagnosis and treatment) of syncope. *Eur Heart J* 2001; **22**(15):1256–306.

16 McLeod KA. Syncope in childhood. *Arch Dis Child* 2003;**88**(4); 350–3.

17 Sapin SO. Autonomic syncope in pediatrics: a practice-oriented approach to classification, pathophysiology, diagnosis, and management. *Clin Pediatr (Phila)* 2004;**43**(1):17–23.

18 Johnsrude CL. Current approach to pediatric syncope. *Pediatr Cardiol* 2000;**21**(6): 522–31.

19 Paul T, Guccione P, and Garson A, Jr. Relation of syncope in young patients with Wolff-Parkinson-White syndrome to rapid ventricular response during atrial fibrillation. *Am J Cardiol* 1990;**65**(5):318–21.

20 Munger T, Packer DL, Hammill SC, *et al.* A population study of the natural history of Wolff-Parkinson-White syndrome in Olmsted County, Minnesota, 1953–1989. *Circulation* 1993;**87**(3):866–73.

21 Nehgme R. Recent developments in the etiology, evaluation, and management of the child with palpitations. *Curr Opin Pediatr* 1998;**10**(5):470–5.

22 Doniger SJ, Sharieff GQ. Pediatric dysrhythmias. *Pediatr Clin North Am* 2006;**53**(1):85–105, vi.

23 Pantell RH and Goodman BW, Jr. Adolescent chest pain: a prospective study. *Pediatrics* 1983;**71**(6):881–7.

24 Schwartz PJ, Stramba-Badiale M, Segantini A, *et al.* A molecular link between the sudden infant death syndrome and the long-QT syndrome. *N Engl J Med* 2000;**343**(4):262–7.

25 Schwartz PJ, *et al.* Prolongation of the QT interval and the sudden infant death syndrome. *N Engl J Med* 1998;**338**(24):1709–14.

26 Kahn A. Recommended clinical evaluation of infants with an apparent life-threatening event. Consensus document of the European Society for the Study and Prevention of Infant Death, 2003. *Eur J Pediatr* 2004;**163**(2):108–15.

27 Priori SG, Nopolitano C, Giordano U, *et al.* Brugada syndrome and sudden cardiac death in children. *Lancet* 2000;**355**(9206):808–9.

28 Link MS, Maron BJ, VanderBrink BA, *et al.* Impact directly over the cardiac silhouette is necessary to produce ventricular fibrillation in an experimental model of commotio cordis. *J Am Coll Cardiol* 2001;**37**(2):649–54.

29 Maron BJ, Gohman TE, Kyle SB, *et al.* Clinical profile and spectrum of commotio cordis. *JAMA* 2002;**287**(9):1142–6.

30 Maron BJ, Strasburger JF, Kugler JD, *et al.* Survival following blunt chest impact-induced cardiac arrest during sports activities in young athletes. *Am J Cardiol* 1997;**79**(6):840–1.

Chapter 3 | **What are the limitations of the ECG in clinical practice?**

J. Jason West, Allan G. Simpson
University of Virginia, Charlottesville, VA, USA

Case presentations

Case 1: A 52-year-old man presents to the emergency department (ED) following a motor vehicle accident. The man had been the restrained driver involved in a head-on collision. The man was found by first responders at the scene to be lethargic but responsive. The man's medical history is significant for diabetes, hypertension and hypercholesterolemia. Further evaluation demonstrates a fractured sternum and ecchymoses across his chest. Given the man's medical history and the extent of his injuries, an electrocardiogram (ECG) was obtained (Figure 3.1).

Case 2: A 67-year-old woman with a history of systemic lupus erythematosus and hypertension presents to the ED complaining of shortness of breath and chest pain. She denies any previous history of similar complaints. The pain and shortness of breath began approximately 2 h previously. The pain is sharp and located in the center of her chest without radiation. Despite taking aspirin and antacids, the pain is persistent. Her blood pressure is 88/60 mmHg and her pulse is 86 beats per minute (bpm). She is pale and diaphoretic on examination, and appears uncomfortable. An ECG is obtained (Figure 3.2).

Limitations of the ECG

The ECG is a potentially valuable diagnostic tool that is limited by issues of sensitivity, specificity, and pretest probability. Sensitivity is the measure of true positive results achieved by the testing method. Specificity is the measure of true negative results returned by the test. These measures determine the value and usefulness of a given test. Ideally, any test should have both perfect sensitivity and specificity. In reality, there is often a tradeoff between the two measures (increasing one will decrease the other). Pretest probability is the ultimate determinant of the value of testing. If there is a

Critical Decisions in Emergency and Acute Care Electrocardiography,
1st edition. Edited by W.J. Brady and J.D. Truwit. © 2009 Blackwell Publishing, ISBN: 9781405159067

very high likelihood of an event being a true positive, then even a test with a fairly marginal sensitivity is likely to produce a positive result. Conversely, a test can have exceedingly good sensitivity, but if the pretest probability of a true event is low, then any positive test result is more likely to be a false-positive than a true-positive.

It is with these limitations in mind that the clinician must approach diagnostic problems in clinical medicine. The 12-lead ECG is a widely available test, useful in the differentiation of many cardiac conditions. We will re-examine the two clinical scenarios described above in the context of the fundamental concepts of sensitivity, specificity, and pretest probability.

The patient in Case 1 presents to the ED following a motor vehicle accident with significant traumatic injuries. He may have sustained several different thoracic injuries, some benign and others life-threatening. Blunt cardiac injury may result in myocardial contusion, hemopericardium, coronary artery injury with infarction, and cardiac rupture. An ECG should be obtained as part of the patient's initial assessment. Its usefulness, however, is dependent upon its sensitivity to detect or exclude significant blunt cardiac injury, its specificity, and the pretest probability that significant injury is indeed present.

There is no single ECG abnormality diagnostic of myocardial contusion. Changes observed can be categorized as those due to myocardial injury or inflammation, conduction system abnormalities, and arrhythmias [1]. The most frequent abnormalities are non-specific ST and T wave changes. These include ST segment elevation or depression, and T wave inversions, especially across the anterior precordium. These most often represent contusion of the right ventricle (the most anterior chamber). They may also be due to left ventricular contusion, pericarditis from hemopericardium, and ischemia or infarction from coronary artery injury.

In myocardial contusion, conduction system abnormalities comprise nearly 25% of abnormalities detected on ECG. The most common is transient right bundle branch block (RBBB). Other conduction system findings include left bundle branch block (LBBB), non-specific intraventricular conduction delay, and atrioventricular (AV) nodal block (first-, second-, and third-degree). A variety of arrhythmias have been reported as well, with up to 70% of patients experiencing some type of arrhythmia. Premature ventricular complexes comprise

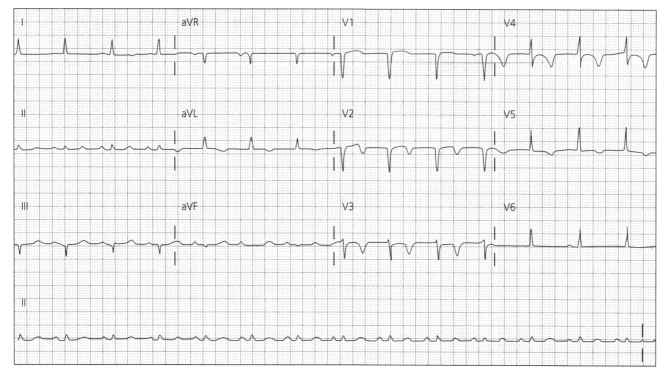

Figure 3.1 ECG in the patient with blunt chest injury. Note the inverted T waves in the anterior leads. These electrocardiographic abnormalities are likely associated with myocardial contusion.

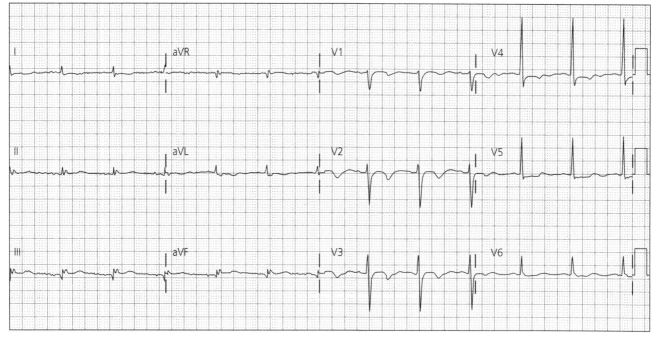

Figure 3.2 Twelve-lead ECG in the chest pain patient. Note the insignificant Q waves in leads III and aVf as well as inverted T waves in leads aVl, and V1 to V4. Prominent R waves are seen in lead V2. Closer inspection reveals approximately 1 mm of ST segment elevation in leads III and aVf, consistent with early inferior wall STEMI.

about half the arrhythmias noted. Other arrhythmias included ventricular tachycardia, ventricular fibrillation, atrial fibrillation, premature atrial complexes, sinus tachycardia and sinus bradycardia.

Thus, the usefulness of the ECG for the evaluation of myocardial contusion is limited by both the low incidence of contusion resulting from chest trauma, and a lack of specific electrocardiographic changes. A meta-analysis of 41 studies of myocardial contusion (analyzing a total of 4681 patients) found that an abnormal ECG and/or elevated cardiac enzyme levels correlated with complications, while a normal ECG and/or normal cardiac enzyme levels correlated with an absence of complications [2]. Several prospective studies have addressed this issue. In one study, 115 patients were admitted with evidence of significant blunt thoracic trauma [3]. Electrocardiographic abnormalities were found in 58 patients. Although sensitive, the ECG positive predictive value (the number of true-positives/the total number of positives) was only 28%. Conversely, the negative predictive value (the number of true-negatives/the total number of negatives) was 95%. In this study, a normal ECG effectively identified a low-risk group of patients for early discharge from the emergency room. In another study, 333 patients were admitted with significant blunt thoracic trauma and serial ECG cardiac enzymes were monitored [4]. Cardiac contusion was diagnosed in 44 patients (13%). The ECG alone had a positive predictive value of only 29%, but a negative predictive value of 98%. Combined with normal cardiac biomarkers, the negative predictive value was 100%.

In Case 2, the patient presents to the ED with the chief complaints of chest pain and shortness of breath. These two common complaints have several potential etiologies, some of which are benign, and some of which are life-threatening. It is important to create a differential diagnosis based upon the pretest probabilities.

This woman has a history of lupus and hypertension, both of which are risk factors for coronary artery disease. Other possible etiologies include pulmonary embolism and pericarditis. Importantly, the ECG is often used in the work-up of all three conditions. Coronary artery disease is quite common, particularly in older individuals and those with cardiovascular risk factors. Individuals with coronary artery disease can present with stable angina, unstable angina, non-ST elevation myocardial infarction (NSTEMI), and ST elevation myocardial infarction (STEMI). The ECG is very helpful in differentiating between these conditions. There are limitations to this test, both in terms of sensitivity (failure to detect true-positives) and specificity (failure to exclude true-negatives).

Use of the ECG in STEMI: ST segment elevation on the ECG of at least 1 mm in two contiguous leads is necessary for the diagnosis of STEMI. Patients with STEMI represent a high-risk population that require immediate assessment and treatment to restore perfusion to their ischemic myocardium.

While the electrocardiogram reliably detects STEMI resulting from occlusion of the left anterior descending and right coronary arteries (sensitivities of 96% and 90%, respectively), it is not reliable for the left circumflex coronary artery (abnormal in only 30–61% of patients) [5]. The left circumflex coronary artery subtends the lateral and posterior walls of the left ventricle. While the lateral wall is reflected in leads V6 and aVL, the posterior wall is very poorly represented by the standard 12-lead ECG. Ischemia of the posterior wall is reflected by ST *depression* in the anterior leads. This finding, however, is present in only 42% of patients [6]. The ECG, therefore, represents a fairly insensitive tool for the detection of posterior infarction. Investigators have sought to overcome this limited sensitivity through the application of posterior chest leads. Posterior chest leads V7–V9 provide ECG coverage of the posterior wall. Studies have demonstrated a modest increase in the sensitivity of circumflex occlusion with this method [5–7]; however, determining the pretest probability is crucial [8].

Use of the ECG in non-STEMI: In their study of 1416 patients presenting with non-ST elevation myocardial infarction, Cannon and colleagues reported that 60% of patients had no ECG changes at the time of presentation [9]. The remaining 40% of the patients had ST depression, T wave inversion, or a LBBB on ECG. While ST depression and LBBB predicted increased 1-year mortality, T wave changes had no influence on mortality. Others demonstrated sensitivity and specificity of prehospital ECGs in detecting acute coronary syndrome as 80% and 60%, respectively. The presence of dynamic ECG changes increased the specificity of the test to 68%, sensitivity decreased to 57% [10].

Use of the ECG in pulmonary embolism: The ECG has been used as a screening tool for pulmonary embolism (PE) because it is cheap and readily available. Investigators first described ECG changes, the "S1Q3T3 pattern," associated with PE in 1935 [11]. Subsequently, others have reported ECG changes in 90 patients with angiographically confirmed PE. Only 13% of the cohort had a normal ECG. The ECG was abnormal in 87%: T wave changes were the most common abnormality (occurring in 42% of patients), while only 7% of patients exhibited the "classic" finding of S1Q3T3 (Figure 3.3) [12]. These findings have been confirmed by others [13].

Kosuge and colleagues compared ECG findings of patients with PE and those with coronary ischemia [14]. These investigators found that while troponin was not predictive between the two groups, the location of T wave inversion was: cardiac ischemia was more commonly associated with T inversion involving the anterolateral leads, while in patients with PE, T wave inversions were found in the inferior and septal leads. When present on the ECG, T wave inversion has a high sensitivity and specificity, 88% and 99%, respectively. However, most patients do not manifest T wave inversions, thus limiting the overall value of this ECG finding.

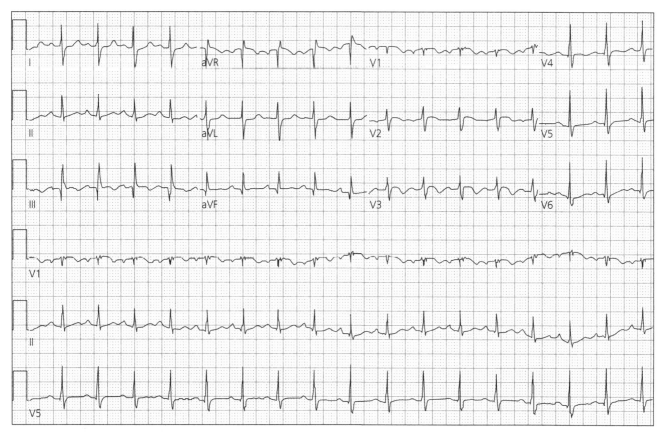

Figure 3.3 Note the sinus tachycardia with deep S wave in lead I, Q wave in lead III, and inverted T wave in lead III – the so-called S1Q3T3, suggestive of pulmonary embolism. Also note the prominent R wave in leads V2 And V3.

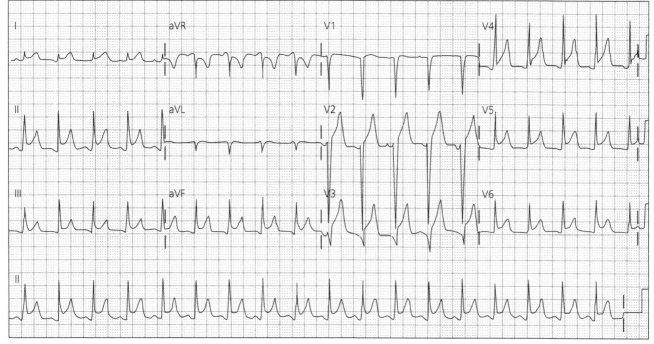

Figure 3.4 Note the widespread ST segment elevation in the anterior, inferior, and lateral leads. Also note the PR segment depression in the inferior leads and, importantly, the "reciprocal" PR segment elevation in lead aVr. This ECG demonstrates findings suggestive of myopericarditis.

Use of the ECG in pericarditis: Pericarditis is a common cause of atypical chest pain and has classically been associated with multiple ECG changes: PR segment depression had a sensitivity of 27.8% and a specificity of 95% for the detection of pericarditis. Low T wave amplitude in Lead I (< 0.2 mV) was associated with a sensitivity of 86% and a specificity of 82% [15]. Widespread ST segment elevation and PR segment depression has been reported in 80% of patients early in the course of pericarditis (Figure 3.4) [16]. These ECG changes resolve in a predictable fashion (first resolution of the ST and PR segments, then resolution of the T wave inversion), eventually leading to a normal ECG. However, such classic resolution of the ECG findings occurs in only 50% of cases [17]. Despite the fact that multiple ECG changes have been linked with various stages of the clinical course of pericarditis, no ECG finding reliably predicts the disease.

Case conclusions

The patient in Case 1 was diagnosed with numerous traumatic injuries. He was admitted to the hospital for additional management. The ECG demonstrates findings consistent with myocardial contusion. The echocardiogram performed on the first day in hospital day demonstrated no significant abnormality. Case 2 demonstrates an early inferior STEMI; the patient was managed with intravenous fibrinolytic agent with resolution of the chest pain and electrocardiographic findings.

The ECG is an important tool in modern medicine. It is cheap, readily available, and reproducible. The ECG is limited by sensitivity and specificity inherent to the detection of certain diseases. Nevertheless, when the ECG is used in the appropriate clinical setting it can confirm or rule out a diagnosis. The pretest probability of the diagnosis is important when interpreting the results of the ECG.

References

1 Potkin R, Werner J, Trobaugh G, Chestnut C, 3d, Carrico C, Hallstrom A, Cobb L. Evaluation of noninvasive tests of cardiac damage in suspected cardiac contusion. *Circulation* 1982;**66**:627–31.

2 Maenza RL, Seaberg D, D'Amico F. A meta-analysis of blunt cardiac trauma: Ending myocardial confusion. *Am J Emerg Med* 1996;**14**:237–41.

3 Salim A, Velmahos GC, Jindal A, *et al.* Clinically significant blunt cardiac trauma: role of serum troponin levels combined with electrocardiographic findings. *J Trauma-Injury Infect Crit Care* 2001;**50**(2):237–43.

4 Velmahos GC, Karaiskakis M, Toutouzas KG, *et al.* Normal electrocardiography and serum troponin i levels preclude the presence of clinically significant blunt cardiac injury. *J Trauma* 2003;**54**(1):45–51.

5 Schmitt C, Lehmann G, Schmieder S, Karch M, Neumann F, Schomig A. Diagnosis of acute myocardial infarction in angiographically documented occluded infarct vessel: limitations of ST-segment elevation in standard and extended ECG leads. *Chest* 2001;**120**(5):1540–6.

6 Khaw K, Moreyra AE, Tannenbaum AK, Hosler MN, Brewer TJ, Agarwal JB. Improved detection of posterior myocardial wall ischemia with the 15-lead electrocardiogram. *Am Heart J* 1999; **138**(5 Pt 1):934–40.

7 Zalenski RJ, Rydman RJ, Sloan MPH, *et al.* Value of posterior and right ventricular leads in comparison to the standard 12-lead electrocardiogram in evaluation of ST-segment elevation in suspected acute myocardial infarction. *Am J Cardiol* 1997;**79**(12):1579–85.

8 Ganim RP, Lewis WR, Diercks DB, Kirk D, Sabapathy R, Baker L, Amsterdam EA. Right precordial and posterior electrocardiographic leads do not increase detection of ischemia in low-risk patients presenting with chest pain. *Cardiology* 2004; **102**(2):100–3.

9 Cannon C, McCabe C, Stone P, *et al.* The electrocardiogram predicts one-year outcome of patients with unstable angina and non-Q wave myocardial infarction: results of the TIMI III Registry ECG Ancillary Study. Thrombolysis in Myocardial Ischemia. *J Am Coll Cardiol* 1997;**30**(1):133–40.

10 Kudenchuk PJ, Maynard C, Cobb LA, Wirkus M, Martin JS, Kennedy JW, Weaver WD, for the MITI Investigators. Utility of the prehospital electrocardiogram in diagnosing acute coronary syndromes: the Myocardial Infarction Triage and Intervention (MITI) project. *J Am Coll Cardiol* 1998;**32**(1):17–27.

11 McGinn S, White PD. Acute cor pulmonale resulting from pulmonary embolism. *JAMA* 1935;**104**:1473.

12 Stein PD, Dalen JE, McIntyre KM, Sasahara AA, Wenger NK, Willis PW, 3rd. The electrocardiogram in acute pulmonary embolism. *Prog Cardiovasc Dis* 1975;**17**:247–57.

13 Sinha N, Yalamanchili K, Sukhija R, Aronow WS, Fleisher AG, Maguire GP, Lehrman SG. Role of the 12-lead electrocardiogram in diagnosing pulmonary embolism. *Cardiol Rev* 2005;**13**(1):46–9.

14 Kosuge M, Kimura K, Ishikawa T, *et al.* Electrocardiographic differentiation between acute pulmonary embolism and acute coronary syndromes on the basis of negative T waves. *Am J Cardiol* 2007;**99**(6):817–21.

15 Ginzton L, Laks M. The differential diagnosis of acute pericarditis from the normal variant: new electrocardiographic criteria. *Circulation* 1982;**65**(5):1004–9.

16 Bruce MA, Spodick DH. Atypical electrocardiogram in acute pericarditis: characteristics and prevalence. *J Electrocardiol* 1980; **13**(1):61–6.

17 Ariyarajah V, Spodick DHDS. Acute pericarditis: diagnostic cues and common electrocardiographic manifestations. *Cardiol Rev* 2007;**15**(1):24–30.

Chapter 4 | Is the ECG indicated in stable, non-cardiac patients admitted to the hospital?

Andrew Darby, Michael Ragosta
University of Virginia, Charlottesville, VA, USA

Case presentations

Case 1: A previously healthy 50-year-old man presents to the emergency department (ED) with abdominal discomfort. He reports a 2-h history of constant, intense epigastric pain associated with nausea. His medical history is notable for current tobacco use and a history of heavy alcohol use. On examination the patient's blood pressure was 90/60 and his heart rate was 90 beats per minute (bpm). His cardiovascular and pulmonary examinations were normal and his abdomen was non-tender upon palpation. Based on his symptom complex and history, the origin of his illness was assumed to be gastrointestinal. As part of a routine evaluation, an electrocardiogram (ECG) was obtained (Figure 4.1). The ECG revealed ST segment elevation inferiorly and at that time it was realized that he was having an ST elevation myocardial infarction (STEMI).

Case 2: A 38-year-old patient with asthma presented to the ED with dyspnea and cough. His past medical history was remarkable only for asthma; medications included albuterol via inhaler. He did not use tobacco but did consume minimal alcohol regularly. On examination, the patient was in moderate distress with marked bronchospasm. The remainder of the examination was normal. He received oral prednisone and multiple albuterol treatments via nebulizer. He demonstrated improvement yet continued with the bronchospasm. A 12-lead ECG was also performed, demonstrating sinus tachycardia; the ECG was otherwise normal.

The ED ECG in the hospital admission process

Case 1 provides an example in which a routine ECG dramatically altered the diagnosis and treatment for a patient initially

Critical Decisions in Emergency and Acute Care Electrocardiography, 1st edition. Edited by W.J. Brady and J.D. Truwit. © 2009 Blackwell Publishing, ISBN: 9781405159067

diagnosed with a non-cardiac condition. However, this case also raises many important clinical questions. How often does a routine ECG impact patient care? Are there certain non-cardiac diagnoses, chief complaints or patient characteristics that would more likely yield benefit from a routine ECG? These questions have important implications not only for healthcare quality, but also for healthcare costs.

The ECG often represents one element of the routine panel of tests ordered by a physician for adult patients admitted to the hospital. This practice is rarely questioned, yet the value of the routine ECG in this setting is not well known. Importantly, for patients admitted with a non-cardiac diagnosis, how often does a routine ECG change management or diagnosis?

Value of electrocardiography

The ECG is an inexpensive and valuable diagnostic tool that can aid in the diagnosis of myocardial ischemia or infarction, detect the presence of structural heart disease, provide evidence for the diagnosis of potentially life-threatening, non-cardiac conditions such as pulmonary embolism and electrolyte abnormalities, and reveal the effects of potentially cardiotoxic drugs.

An ECG is a required part of the initial evaluation of many patients presenting with chest pain or any other symptom consistent with myocardial ischemia, and should always be considered whenever myocardial ischemia enters into the differential diagnosis of a patient's symptom complex. In addition, electrocardiography is routinely performed to evaluate other potential cardiac symptoms such as dyspnea, palpitations, syncope, or presyncope. Similarly, few would argue the value of a routine ECG in a critically ill or unstable patient. This would include patients with acute respiratory failure, profound hypoxemia, hypotension and/or shock, diabetic ketoacidosis, extensive trauma, profound metabolic disarray, or acute unresponsiveness, in order to determine if there is either a primary cardiac etiology for their illness or to detect cardiac consequences of their acute illness.

The role of the routine ECG in stable patients admitted to the hospital with an apparently non-cardiac diagnosis is less

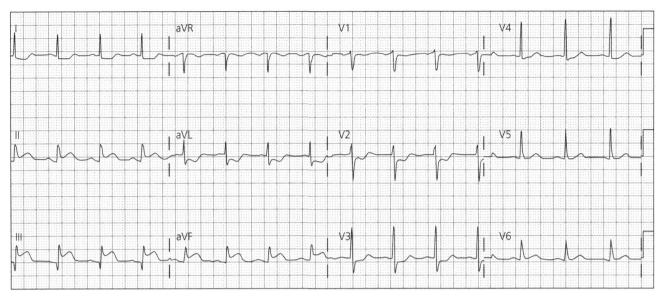

Figure 4.1 Normal sinus rhythm with ST segment elevation in the inferior leads and ST segment depression in the anterior and lateral leads. This ECG pattern suggests an acute inferior myocardial infarction with posterior involvement.

clear. Similar to other diagnostic tests, the value of an ECG in such patients depends upon the pretest probability of disease. Among patients with a low likelihood of heart disease, a routine ECG would be unlikely to provide additional useful information. In fact, a routine ECG may be more likely to produce false-positive findings and lead to additional tests and procedures resulting in significant costs and little additional benefit. Conversely, it could be reasoned that patients with a higher pretest probability of heart disease may benefit greatly from routine electrocardiography by virtue of its ability to detect unsuspected heart disease.

Relatively few studies have investigated the role of routine admission electrocardiography among stable medical patients. Moorman and colleagues prospectively evaluated the utility of the routine admission ECG in 1410 patients admitted to a general medicine service [1]. Each patient had a complete history and physical examination upon which an admission diagnosis was established. A 12-lead ECG obtained at the time of admission was analyzed separately and evaluated in the context of each patient's history and physical examination to determine whether it provided additional information. The investigators found that the admission ECG added unique information in 52 patients (3.7%), and that there were only two variables predictive of a beneficial yield of the ECG: the presence of a cardiac abnormality by history or physical examination ($P < 0.0001$) and patient age greater than 45 years ($P = 0.016$). Among patients with a cardiac abnormality identified by history or physical examination, the ECG provided additional useful information in 8.5% of patients over 45 years of age and in 2.5% of younger patients. Among these patients, the ECG was useful in diagnosing dysrhythmias such as atrial fibrillation or atrial flutter, complete heart block in a patient presenting with heart failure, and a left bundle branch block in a patient with a

paradoxically split S2. For those without an apparent cardiac abnormality by history or physical exam, however, the ECG added unique information in only 1.0% of patients (1.4% of patients over age 45, but only 0.4% of those younger). Among patients in this group, the ECG revealed unsuspected myocardial ischemia in three patients and signs of prior myocardial infarction in two, all of whom were over 45 years of age. The patients with unsuspected myocardial ischemia likely benefited from the ECG due to a change in their management, including admission to a coronary unit and administration of anti-coagulants. Moorman and colleagues concluded that the admission ECG infrequently adds additional information, but, when it does, this new information can lead to a significant change in management. The patients who benefited most from the ECG were those with a higher pretest probability of cardiac disease, evidenced by the presence of a cardiac abnormality by history or examination and/or age greater than 45 years.

A more recent, retrospective study evaluated the hypothesis that routine admission ECGs could be safely avoided in selected ED patients admitted to the hospital [2]. This study involved 636 consecutive admissions to the general medicine service at a university hospital. A set of acceptable criteria for obtaining a routine admission ECG were established and included a history of heart disease (e.g., coronary artery disease, arrhythmia, heart failure); presence of palpitations or irregular pulse; syncope; any symptoms suggestive of angina or heart failure; or the presence of hyper- or hypotension. The investigators reviewed the patient records and determined, based upon their previously established criteria, whether an ECG was indicated, which patients in each category had an ECG performed, and whether the ECG changed management or patient outcome. Interestingly, 82% of the 247 patients with no identifiable indication for an admission

ECG by pre-established criteria had one performed; the ECG changed management in only three patients (1.5%) and changed outcome in none. The change in management among these three patients consisted of obtaining additional ECGs, measurement of serial cardiac enzyme assays, and/or admission to a telemetry unit. Based upon their findings, the authors concluded that a routine admission ECG could have been safely avoided in a large subset of patients admitted to a university general medicine service with a low likelihood of cardiac disease.

Based on the available data, guidelines have been proposed for performing an ECG at the time of general hospital admission [3]. These guidelines are in agreement with the two previously mentioned studies, and do not recommend a routine ECG solely because of hospital admission. Rather, the guidelines recommend a more judicious and select use of ECGs, reserving them for patients with cardiac disease confirmed by history or physical examination, patients with systemic diseases or conditions with the potential for clinically important cardiac involvement (e.g., diabetes mellitus), patients taking medications potentially influencing the ECG (such as anti-arrhythmic drugs, anti-depressants, calcium channel blockers, digoxin, and antibiotics affecting the QT interval; see Table 4.1), and patients at risk for major electrolyte abnormalities (e.g., hypo- or hyperkalemia). It should be emphasized that guidelines are not meant to replace clinical judgment, and the physician's estimation of the pretest likelihood of cardiac disease should be the ultimate determinant as to whether or not an ECG is performed.

A routine admission ECG among stable patients presenting with an apparent non-cardiac diagnosis is not always indicated, as the likelihood of identifying an unsuspected cardiac diagnosis is very low and electrocardiographic findings rarely change management. A selective approach appears more appropriate. As exemplified in the patient case presented earlier, patients with an intermediate to high likelihood of cardiac disease are more likely to benefit from a routine ECG, particularly if their symptoms, while not classically attributed to cardiac disease, are still potentially explainable by a cardiac cause. A summary of common indications for obtaining a routine ECG in stable patients with a non-cardiac diagnosis is presented in Table 4.2.

Table 4.2 Indications for an ECG in stable, non-cardiac patients

Clinical variables
  Age > 45
  History of coronary artery disease
  History of heart failure
  History of diabetes mellitus
  Chronic kidney disease

Clinical variables
  Medications known to affect the ECG (see Table 4.1)
    Anti-arrhythmics
    Anti-depressants
    Antibiotics
  Presence of electrolyte disorder
    Hyperkalemia
    Hypokalemia
    Hypocalcemia

Symptoms/signs
  Syncope or presyncope
  Palpitations or irregular pulse
  Severe hypertension (systolic BP > 180, diastolic BP > 120)
  Abdominal complaints (discomfort, pain, nausea, vomiting)
  Unexplained dyspnea
  Confusional state in an elderly patient
  Hypothermia

Table 4.1 Commonly prescribed medications which may affect the electrocardiogram

Anti-arrhythmics
  Class IA: quinidine; procainamide; disopyramide
  Class III: sotalol; amiodarone; ibutilide; dofetilide

Anti-microbials
  Antibiotics: erythromycin; TMP/SMX
  Anti-fungals: itraconazole; ketoconazole
  Anti-malarials: chloroquine
  Anti-virals: amantadine

Anti-histamines
  Terfenadine; astemizole

Psychotropics and anti-depressants
  Tricyclics; haloperidol; phenothiazines

Miscellaneous
  Cisapride
  Organophosphate poisoning

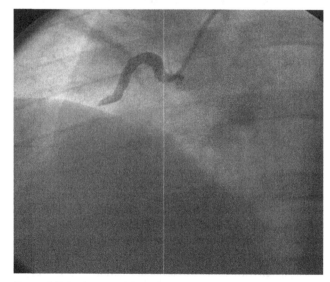

Figure 4.2 Angiogram of the right coronary artery demonstrating total occlusion of the artery in its proximal portion.

Case conclusions

The patient in Case 1 was taken emergently to the cardiac catheterization laboratory, where the right coronary artery was found to be proximally occluded and percutaneous coronary intervention was performed, with prompt restoration of flow and resolution of the patient's symptoms and electrocardiographic changes (Figure 4.2). The patient in Case 2 was admitted to the hospital for continued therapy. Prior to admission to the ED, a chest radiograph was performed and was normal, as was the ECG. During the admission, he received continued therapy including albuterol, prednisone, and azithromycin. The patient experienced no cardiac problems during this admission. The patient was discharged on hospital day 3 with bronchitis and asthma exacerbation.

References

1 Moorman JR, Hlatky MA, Eddy DM. *et al.* The yield of the routine admission electrocardiogram: A study in a general medicine service. *Ann Intern Med* 1985;**103**:590–5.

2 Garland JL, Wolfson AB. Routine admission electrocardiography in ED patients. *Ann Emerg Med* 1994;**23**(2):275–80.

3 Goldberger AL, O'Konski M. Utility of the routine electrocardiogram before surgery and on general hospital admission. *Ann Intern Med* 1986;**105**:552–7.

Chapter 5

What is the use of the ECG in preoperative assessment and cardiovascular risk stratification?

Peter M. Pollak, Ellen C. Keeley
University of Virginia, Charlottesville, VA, USA

Case presentation

A 57-year-old man presents to the emergency department (ED) after a ground-level fall, sustaining a trimalleolar ankle fracture. No other injuries are noted – this patient has an isolated, distal lower extremity injury. Preoperative "clearance" is requested by the orthopedic surgeon prior to surgery. The patient has not seen a doctor in 30 years, leads a sedentary life, and takes no medications. A routine electrocardiogram (ECG) is performed (Figure 5.1). The ECG reveals normal sinus rhythm, evidence of left ventricular hypertrophy with "strain pattern," and poor precordial R wave progression.

The ECG in preoperative evaluation

The patient, though stable, has some degree of cardiovascular risk during his planned surgery. Should he undergo further cardiac testing prior to his elective surgery? The American College of Cardiology (ACC)/American Heart Association (AHA) guidelines regarding the utility of a preoperative ECG stratifies patients and procedures according to the relative risk of cardiovascular events (Figure 5.1) [1]. Patients with active cardiac conditions (e.g., unstable angina, recent myocardial infarction (MI), severe aortic stenosis, or significant arrhythmias) are considered at highest risk. Patients without active cardiac conditions are stratified by the number of clinical risk factors they have, including ischemic heart disease, compensated or prior heart failure, diabetes mellitus, renal insufficiency, and cerebrovascular disease. Procedures are stratified as low risk (e.g., cataract surgery), intermediate risk (e.g., orthopedic or minor abdominal operations), and high risk (vascular surgery). Cardiac surgery is considered separately as it is generally performed on patients with active cardiac conditions.

Critical Decisions in Emergency and Acute Care Electrocardiography, 1st edition. Edited by W.J. Brady and J.D. Truwit. © 2009 Blackwell Publishing. ISBN: 9781405159067

Who needs an ECG prior to surgery?

According to the ACC/AHA guidelines, an ECG is a class I recommendation for patients with at least one risk factor undergoing vascular surgery or patients with known coronary disease, peripheral arterial disease, or cerebrovascular disease undergoing an intermediate-risk procedure. In patients without known coronary risk factors undergoing vascular surgery, and in patients with a single risk factor undergoing intermediate risk surgery, an ECG is a class II recommendation. A preoperative ECG is not recommended for patients without risk factors undergoing a low-risk procedure.

What does the ECG indicate about cardiovascular risk?

The ECG is a useful screening tool that frequently directs subsequent cardiovascular risk stratification. Although the ECG does not specifically assess cardiac function, it does provide information regarding potential structural and electrical abnormalities and prior MI. An ECG is non-invasive, readily available, and relatively inexpensive, thus serving as an important adjunct to preoperative evaluation. It is perhaps best viewed as both a screening tool for underlying cardiac pathology as well as a baseline against which postoperative changes can be compared.

What does the ECG indicate about the presence of structural heart disease?

Left and right ventricular hypertrophy: Many criteria have been published that correlate ECG voltage with left ventricular mass, i.e., left ventricular hypertrophy (LVH). All are limited by poor sensitivity, but have good specificity

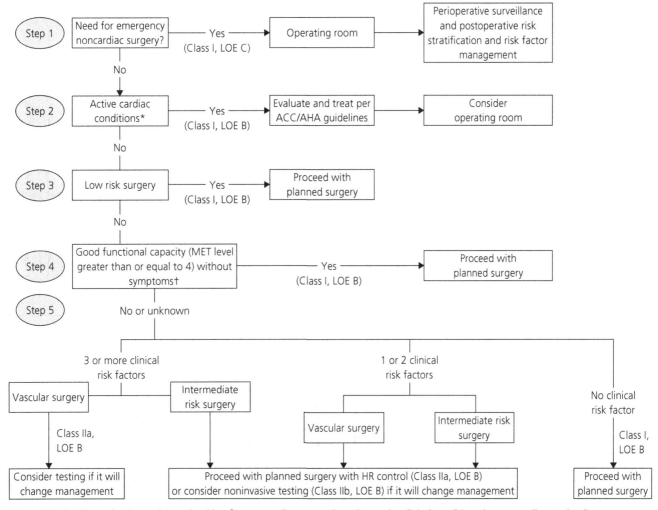

Figure 5.1 Cardiac evaluation and care algorithm for non-cardiac surgery based on active clinical conditions, known cardiovascular disease, or cardiac risk factors for patients 50 years of age or greater. ACC/AHA indicates American College of Cardiology/American Heart Association; HR, heart rate; LOE, level of evidence; MET, metabolic equivalent.

Figure reprinted with permission from Fleisher LA, Beckman JA, Brown KA, *et al.* ACC/AHA 2007 Guidelines on Perioperative Cardiovascular Evaluation and Care for Noncardiac Surgery: Executive Summary. A Report of the American College of Cardiology/American Heart Association Task Force on Practice Guidelines (Writing Committee to Revise the 2002 Guidelines on Perioperative Cardiovascular Evaluation for Noncardiac Surgery), *J Am Coll Cardiol* 2007;**50**:1707–32. Copyright Elsevier 2007.

(> 90%). A simple, accurate, and commonly accepted ECG voltage criteria is the Cornell Criteria (R wave in aVL + S wave in V3 > 24 mm in men, or > 20 mm in women) [2]. Left atrial enlargement and left axis deviation are also frequently seen with LVH [3] (Figure 5.2). Left ventricular hypertrophy on the ECG increases perioperative risk of death and MI in major vascular surgery, and is most often due to increased afterload such as in chronic hypertension, but it can also suggest a dilated cardiomyopathy and aortic stenosis [4]. Evidence of a "strain pattern" (defined as a downsloping convex ST segment with inverted asymmetrical T wave opposite the QRS axis in leads V5 or V6 or both) is secondary to subendocardial ischemia (Figure 5.2). The presence of this

pattern is more predictive of adverse outcomes than LVH voltage criteria alone [5].

Specific criteria are lacking for right ventricular hypertrophy (RVH), but it is suggested by any of the following: (1) rightward axis > +100, (2) R in V1 > 7 mm, (3) right atrial enlargement, and (4) qR in V1. Importantly, RVH can only be diagnosed when the following are excluded: (1) posterior MI, (2) right bundle branch block, (3) Wolff-Parkinson-White syndrome, (4) dextrocardia, and (5) left posterior fascicular block. Right ventricular hypertrophy is a normal variant in children. Although RVH is not associated with the same level of cardiovascular risk as LVH, it is often a marker of significant pulmonary pathology, especially those

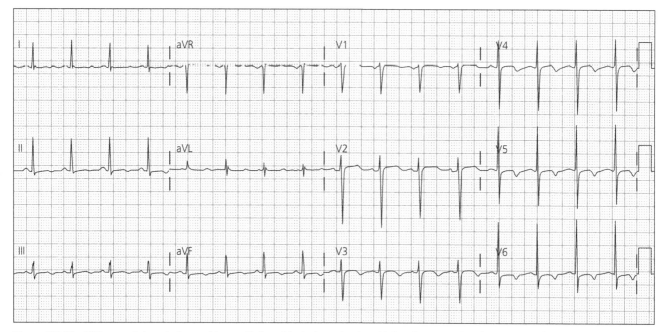

Figure 5.2 The ECG normal sinus rhythm, evidence of left ventricular hypertrophy with "strain pattern," and poor precordial R wave progression.

which increase right ventricular afterload (i.e., pulmonary hypertension).

Left and right atrial enlargement: Left atrial enlargement can be diagnosed on an ECG as a downward terminal deflection of the P wave in V1 with a negative amplitude of 1 mm (one small box deep) and duration of 0.04 s (two small boxes wide) or biphasic P wave in V1. The ECG finding of "P-mitrale" is defined by notched P waves in inferior leads (II, III, or aVF) with a duration > 0.12 s. It is the result of significant left atrial enlargement and is classically associated with mitral valve regurgitation. Left atrial enlargement is not an independent predictor of perioperative risk but is associated with hypertension, left ventricular hypertrophy, and mitral valve disease. Patients with large left atria have increased risk of atrial fibrillation, stroke, and death [6,7]. Right atrial enlargement, aka P pulmonale, is diagnosed on an ECG as a P wave amplitude > 2.5 mm in the inferior leads (II, III, aVF) with a normal axis. It is associated with systemic or pulmonary hypertension as well as tricuspid regurgitation. Impact on intra-operative risk assessment and clinical implications have not been well established.

Low voltage: Low voltage is defined as the amplitude of the entire QRS complex (R + S) < 5 mm in all limb leads and < 10 mm in each precordial lead. It is commonly seen with anything which puts "distance" between the heart and the surface leads, such as chronic lung disease, obesity, pleural or pericardial effusion, and anasarca. Low voltage may also be due to disorders of decreased cardiac voltage generation, such as adrenal insufficiency, myxedema, and infiltrative heart disease such as amyloid.

What does the ECG indicate about the presence of ischemic heart disease?

Several changes are notable on the resting ECG that suggest a history of ischemic heart disease and may lead to the recommendation of perioperative beta-blockade or preoperative non-invasive testing prior to intermediate risk or vascular surgery.

Presence of Q waves: Q waves are the first downward deflection from the isoelectric line after the P wave in sinus rhythm. The classic instance in which Q waves are found is following transmural MI. Nonetheless, not all infarctions lead to persistent Q waves. Electrocardiogram changes associated with prior MI include: (1) any Q wave in leads V2–V3 ≥ 2 ms or QS complex in leads V2 and V3, (2) Q wave ≥ 0.03 s and ≥ 0.1 mV deep or QS complex in leads I, II, aVL, aVF, or V4–V6 in any two leads of a contiguous lead grouping, and (3) R wave ≥ 0.04 in V1–V2 and R/S ≥ 1 with concordant positive T wave in the absence of a conduction defect [8].

Prominent R waves: Prominent R waves in V1 and V2 as well as "early transition," or R > S in V2, can be the result of a transmural posterior wall infarction. The R waves in this case could be more accurately described as "inverted" Q waves.

Loss of precordial R wave progression: This is a finding often thought to be associated with anterior MI [14]. The normal progression of the R wave is to progress from absent in V1, to present in V2, to greater than the S wave in V4. It is important to remember that changes in placement of the precordial surface leads will affect this transition. Additionally, poor R wave progression cannot be determined in the presence of LVH. If the R wave remains smaller than the S wave through V3, the normal R wave progression is said to be lost. A review of the predictive value of poor R wave progression for anterior MI, using nuclear imaging, found it to be no better than chance alone [9,10] (Figure 5.1).

What does the ECG indicate about the presence of conduction system abnormalities?

Left bundle branch block (LBBB): Complete LBBB requires all of the following to be present: (1) QRS duration > 0.12 s, (2) delayed instrinsicoid deflection in left precordial leads and lead I > 0.05 s, and (3) broad monophasic R waves in I, V5, V6 usually notched or slurred. Importantly, the presence of LBBB makes determination of axis, LVH, and ST changes of ischemia impossible by typical criteria. Criteria for the diagnosis of myocardial ischemia in the context of LBBB have been suggested [11]. The presence of LBBB has been linked to lower life expectancy; however, in patients undergoing non-cardiac surgery, the presence of a LBBB does not increase postoperative cardiac complications [12].

Right bundle branch block (RBBB): A RBBB is suggested by the following on ECG: (1) QRS > 0.12 s, (2) rSR' pattern in right precordial leads, and (3) wide S wave in leads I, V5, V6. It can be idiopathic (i.e., Lenegre's or Lev's disease), and can suggest chronic increase in right ventricular pressure (as in cor pulmonale) or an acute increase in right heart pressure (as in pulmonary embolus). Right bundle branch block develops acutely during right heart catheterizations in approximately 5% of cases due to mechanical irritation of the right ventricular outflow tract.

Brugada syndrome: Brugada syndrome is diagnosed on ECG as an RBBB with ST elevation in leads V1–3 with a normal QT interval. It is usually seen in young men and has been associated with increased risk of sudden cardiac death [13]. It was first described in 1992 and has been associated with a specific polymorphism in the SCN5A sodium channel. Specific perioperative strategies have been proposed to limit adverse events in these patients [14].

What does the ECG indicate about risk of intra-operative arrhythmias?

Though data directly correlating ECG findings with risk of intra-operative arrhythmia are limited, evidence of structural heart disease or previous MI has been associated with increased risk of arrhythmias [15]. The following ECG findings may also place the patient at increased risk for arrhythmia in the perioperative period.

Prolongation of the QT interval: The QT interval varies naturally with heart rate, thus, the corrected QT interval (QTc) should be used in assessing the QT interval. This is derived by dividing the QT interval by the square root of the RR interval. Normal values are < 440 ms in men and < 460 ms in women. The QT interval should be less than half of the RR (i.e., the end of the T wave should come before the halfway point between consecutive R waves). Prolongation of the QT interval can be familial, but is most often due to medications. The longer it becomes, the greater the risk of arrhythmias, specifically, torsade de pointes. Prolongation of the QTc early in the course of acute MI has been shown to predict those patients more likely to develop ventricular arrhythmias.

Electrolyte abnormalities: Electrolyte abnormalities can be diagnosed on ECG and should be corrected prior to surgery. Patients with chronic kidney disease and patients taking diuretics are at the highest risk for significant electrolyte disturbances. Two important abnormalities include peaked T waves consistent with hyperkalemia and prolonged QT interval with preserved T wave morphology consistent with hypocalcemia.

Wolff-Parkinson-White syndrome: This is a congenital disorder of electrical conduction in which an accessory pathway allows for conduction of electrical impulses from the atria to the ventricle without going through the atrioventricular (AV) node. The following ECG findings are consistent with the diagnosis: (1) normal P wave axis and morphology, (2) PR interval < 0.12 s, (3) presence of a delta wave (initial slurring of the QRS), and (4) a constant PJ interval that is < 0.26 s [16]. Wolff-Parkinson-White syndrome is important to recognize prior to surgery because use of AV nodal blocking agents in the setting of postoperative atrial fibrillation in these patients can drive electrical impulses through the accessory pathway and precipitate a ventricular rate > 300, resulting in cardiovascular collapse.

Rhythms other than sinus may place the patient into one of the ACC/AHA categories of active cardiac conditions requiring investigation prior to non-cardiac surgery. These include: high grade AV block, Mobitz II AV block, third-degree AV block, symptomatic bradycardia, symptomatic ventricular arrhythmias, supraventricular arrhythmias (including atrial fibrillation with a rapid ventricular response).

Paced rhythms: While the history, physical and chest radiograph can screen for the presence of a pacemaker or a defibrillator, the ECG helps the clinician determine whether the device is functioning prior to surgery. Every patient with a pacemaker should have a screening ECG prior to surgery

[24]. Although the risk of interference by electrocautery is minimal, pacemakers should be programmed into VOO/DOO mode for the duration of the operation [17]. Patients with a pacemaker or a defibrillator should be evaluated by their cardiologist prior to surgery.

Case conclusion

The patient was evaluated by the cardiologist prior to surgery. A perioperative beta-blocker was recommended. The patient underwent surgical correction of his complex ankle fracture without complication. He was discharged to a rehabilitation facility on hospital day 3 without consequence.

References

1 ACC/AHA. 2007 Guidelines on Perioperative Cardiovascular Evaluation and Care for Noncardiac Surgery *J Am Coll Cardiol* 2007;**50**:1707–32.

2 Casale PN, Devereux RB, Alonso DR, Campo E, Kligfield P. Improved sex-specific criteria of left ventricular hypertrophy for clinical and computer electrocardiogram interpretation. *Circulation* 1987;**75**:565–72.

3 Dahöl B, Devereux RB, Julius S, *et al.* Characteristics of 9194 patients with left ventricular hypertrophy: the LIFE Study. *Hypertension* 1998;**32**:989–97.

4 Landesberg G, Einar S, Christopherson R, *et al.* Perioperative Ischemia and cardiac complications in major vascular surgery: Importance of the preoperative twelve-lead electrocardiogram. *J Vasc Surg* 1997;**26**:570–8.

5 Okin PM, Devereux RB, Nieminen RS, *et al.* Relationship of the electrocardiographic strain pattern to left ventricular structure and function in hypertensive patients: the LIFE Study. *JACC* 2001;**38**(2):514–20.

6 Henry WL, Morganroth J, Pearlman AS, *et al.* Relation between echocardiographically determined left atrial size and atrial fibrillation. The Framingham Study. *Circulation* 1976;**53**:273–9.

7 Benjamin EJ, D'Agostino RB, Belanger AJ, *et al.* Left atrial size and risk of stroke and death. *Circulation* 1995;**92**:835–41.

8 Thygesen K, Alpert J, White H. Universal definition of myocardial infarction. ESC/ACCF/AHA/WHF Task Force for the Redinition of Myocardial Infarction. *J Am Coll Cardiol* 2007 Nov 27;**50**(22):2173–95.

9 Zema MJ, Collins M, Alonso DR, Kligfield P. Electrocardiographic poor R-wave progression. Correlation with postmortem findings. *Chest* 1981;**79**:195–200.

10 Gami AS, Holly T, Rosenthal J. Electrocardiographic poor R-wave progression: Analysis of multiple criteria reveals little usefulness. *Am Heart J* 2004;**148**:80–5.

11 Sgarbossa EB, Pinski SL, Barbagelata A, *et al.* Electrocardiographic diagnosis of evolving acute myocardial infarction in the presence of left bundle-branch block. *NEJM* 1996;**334**(8):481–7.

12 Dorman T, Breslow MJ, Pronovost PJ, *et al.* Bundle-branch block as a risk factor in non-cardiac surgery. *Arch Int Med* 2000;**160**:1149–52.

13 Brugada P, Brugada J. Right bundle branch block, persistent ST segment elevation and sudden cardiac death: a distinct clinical and electrocardiographic syndrome. A multicenter report. *J Am Coll Cardiol* 1992;**20**:1391–6.

14 Candiotti K, Mehta V. Perioperative approach to a patient with Brugada syndrome. *J Clin Anesthesia* 2004;**16**:529–32.

15 Polanczyk CA, Goldman L, Marcantonio ER, *et al.* Supraventricular arrhythmia in patients having noncardiac surgery: clinical correlates and effect on length of stay. *Ann Intern Med* 1998;**129**(4):279–85.

16 O'Keefe JH, Hammill S, Freed M. *The Complete Guide to ECGs.* Birmingham, Mass: Physicians Press, 1997.

17 Peters R, Gold M. Reversible prolonged pacemaker failure due to electrocautery. *J Int Cardiac Electrophysiol* 1998;**2**:343–4.

Chapter 6 | Which patients benefit from continuous electrocardiographic monitoring during hospitalization?

Adam Helms, John Ferguson
University of Virginia, Charlottesville, VA, USA

Case presentations

Case 1: A 62-year-old woman with a history of hypertension presents to the emergency department (ED) with intermittent exertional chest pain over the prior 2 days. She describes the pain as sharp, with no radiation and no associated symptoms. Her blood pressure is 140/88 mmHg and her heart rate is 95 beats per minute (bpm). An electrocardiogram (ECG) demonstrates 1 mm ST depression inferiorly consistent with ischemia.

Case 2: A 35-year-old man presents to the ED following an episode of syncope. He developed syncope while walking. No seizure activity was witnessed. He has no prior history of syncope but his family history is significant for his father dying suddenly at a young age. His blood pressure on exam is 124/78 mmHg and his heart rate is 62 bpm. His exam is normal except for an abrasion on his forehead. His ECG shows an RSR' pattern in V1–2 with coved ST segment elevations consistent with Brugada syndrome.

Continuous electrocardiographic monitoring for the admitted patient

In clinical practice, telemetry is often used for indications for which minimal benefit has been shown [1]. Over-utilization of telemetry results in increased cost and overcrowding of the ED while patients wait to be admitted to telemetry beds. Thus, appropriate use of telemetry is important. This chapter will explore the indications for continuous telemetry with a focus on the common indications that arise in an acute care setting, such as ischemic syndromes, arrhythmias, syncope, and heart failure.

Basic set-up and monitoring of telemetry

Several options are available for specific telemetry systems, varying by the leads monitored and the sophistication of the software that performs rhythm and ischemia monitoring. The decision of whether or not to have dedicated monitor "watchers," however, is controversial [2]. Dedicated monitor "watchers" are able to attain a higher level of expertise in electrocardiographic interpretation and are more likely to identify arrhythmias correctly. Monitor watchers and nurses should receive formal training in basic electrophysiology principles and in the interpretation of arrhythmia and ischemia, as outlined in the American Heart Association (AHA) electrocardiographic monitoring guidelines [2]. They should be aware of the spectrum of diagnoses admitted to telemetry units and understand the significance of telemetry for those diagnoses: they should be knowledgeable about how to set limits on heart rate (e.g., the upper threshold should be below the rate of an expected tachycardia), and how to set the baseline ST segment parameters to avoid false-positives or negatives. Nurses also have the responsibility of deciding which changes on telemetry require chart documentation. Together, physicians and nurses identify changes requiring direct notification of the physician and emergent call to the resuscitation team.

Critical Decisions in Emergency and Acute Care Electrocardiography, 1st edition. Edited by W.J. Brady and J.D. Truwit. © 2009 Blackwell Publishing, ISBN: 9781405159067

Role of telemetry in clinical practice

Continuous electrocardiographic recording of hospitalized patients has traditionally been used to detect life-threatening brady- or tachyarrhythmias. The widespread availability of telemetry in most hospitals has been accompanied by the development of acute resuscitation teams available for immediate response. Early defibrillation and effective basic life support has led to a significant reduction in the mortality of inhospital cardiac arrest [3,4]. The automatic detection and recording of brady- and tachyarrhythmias allows subsequent analysis and accurate diagnosis. This technology is particularly helpful in clinching the primary diagnosis in patients presenting with syncope or palpitations. Arrhythmias are also noted incidentally in patients who undergo telemetry for other reasons, such as acute coronary syndromes or heart failure. Detection of these abnormalities may significantly affect treatment. Heart rate trends over extended periods are useful in selected patients (those receiving rate control for atrial fibrillation). Changes in heart rate and rhythm can also facilitate the diagnosis of non-cardiac diseases: changes in heart rate variability can precede other clinical indicators of sepsis in neonates, allowing for the early introduction of potentially life-saving antibiotics [5]. While the benefit of admitting patients to the hospital with continuous telemetry may seem self-evident based on clinical experience, definitive indications have not been established by randomized studies.

Refer to Table 6.1 for a listing of the indications for cardiac monitoring for dysrhythmia.

Ischemic syndromes

The most common indication for continuous cardiac monitoring is myocardial ischemia or suspicion of myocardial ischemia [1]. Acute coronary syndromes have a class I indication for both arrhythmia and ST segment monitoring, while chest pain syndromes without positive biomarkers and a non-specific ECG have a class II indication for arrhythmia and ST segment monitoring [2]. When an acute coronary syndrome is diagnosed, patients should be monitored for both arrhythmias and ischemia for at least 24 h. In the GUSTO-III trial, patients presenting with ST elevation myocardial infarction (STEMI) had an incidence of ventricular arrhythmia of 7.5% [5]. Rapid detection of arrhythmias in this setting is crucial.

The duration of ECG monitoring for patients with acute coronary syndromes is variable. If reperfusion is successful and no complications arise, monitoring can be stopped at 24 h. However, in cases in which reperfusion is not successful or with complications such as recurrent ischemia, cardiogenic shock, or arrhythmias requiring cardiac pacing, defibrillation,

Table 6.1 Indications for cardiac monitoring for arrhythmia

Class I indications
    Following resuscitation from cardiac arrest
    Early phase of an acute coronary syndrome
    Unstable coronary syndromes and high-risk coronary lesions
    Following cardiac surgery
    Following non-urgent PCI with complications
    Pacemaker lead implantation in patients who are pacemaker dependent
    Patients with a temporary pacemaker or transcutaneous pacing pads
    AV block
    WPW with rapid anterograde conduction over an accessory pathway
    Long QT syndrome and associated ventricular arrhythmias
    Intra-aortic balloon counterpulsation
    Acute heart failure
    Patients in the ICU
    Diagnostic/therapeutic procedures requiring conscious sedation
Class II indications
    Postacute MI (beyond the first 24–48 h)
    Chest pain syndromes
    Non-urgent PCI without complications (stent: 6–8 h, angioplasty: 12–24 h)
    Anti-arrhythmic drug or rate control adjustment for atrial tachyarrhythmias
    Pacemaker lead implantation in patients who are not pacemaker-dependent
    Uncomplicated ablation of an arrhythmia
    Routine coronary angiography
    Subacute heart failure
    Syncope w/suspected arrhythmia
Class III (not indicated)
    Postoperative patients who are at low risk for arrhythmia
    Obstetric patients
    Permanent, rate-controlled atrial fibrillation
    Patients undergoing hemodialysis
    Stable patients with chronic PVCs

AV, atrioventricular; ICU, intensive care unit; PCI, percutaneous coronary intervention; Wolff-Parkinson-White; PVC, premature ventricular contractions.

or anti-arrhythmic drugs, monitoring should continue for 24 h past the resolution of all complications. Further monitoring is not recommended.

Patients admitted with chest pain are often not at significant risk of arrhythmia, thus prompting a change in guidelines [7]. As chest pain represents one of the most common admission diagnoses, proper risk stratification is important to preserve the limited resource of telemetry for those who really need it. To better risk-stratify chest pain patients, Goldman and colleagues developed a risk score that uses the following clinical variables: ECG suggestive of acute myocardial infarction (MI) (ST elevations or Q waves not known to be old), ECG suggestive of acute ischemia (ST depression or T wave inversions not known to be old), systolic blood pressure < 100 mmHg, rales heard above the bases bilaterally, or history of known unstable ischemic heart disease [8]. When applied prospectively, this scoring system identifies patients who are at low risk of arrhythmia and who, therefore, would not benefit from continuous ECG monitoring. Durairaj and colleagues prospectively used the Goldman risk score in a population of 1033 consecutive patients admitted to an inpatient telemetry unit [9]. In 318 patients with chest pain who were classified by the Goldman score to be very low risk (i.e., absence of all of the above risk factors), no major complications were observed. These 318 low-risk individuals comprised 31% of telemetry admissions. Hollander and colleagues also evaluated the Goldman score prospectively in 1029 patients admitted from the ED with chest pain [10]. They found that patients with a low Goldman score combined with negative initial biomarkers suffered no incidence of cardiac death or life-threatening ventricular arrhythmia, and this sample of patients comprised 59% of chest pain patients admitted for telemetry from the ED.

These studies, however, did not include ST segment monitoring, so it is still unclear as to whether or not any benefit exists for diagnosing asymptomatic ST segment deviations in low-risk chest pain patients [2]. Pelter and colleagues showed continuous ST segment monitoring of 237 patients admitted with acute coronary syndromes and identified that 17% had transient myocardial ischemia. Of note, 71% of these events were asymptomatic; regardless of symptoms, however, patients with transient ischemia were 8.5 times more likely to develop complications.

Refer to Table 6.2 for a listing of potential indications for electrocardiographic monitoring in the patient suspected of acute coronary syndrome.

Table 6.2 Monitoring for ischemia (ST segment monitoring)

Class I indications
   Early phase of acute coronary syndromes
   Chest pain or anginal equivalent symptoms
   Following non-urgent PCI with suboptimal angiographic results
     (24 h)
   Variant angina from coronary vasospasm
Class II indications
   Postacute MI (24 h)
   Following non-urgent PCI without complication (4–8 h)
   After cardiac or non-cardiac surgery in high-risk patients
   Pediatric patients at risk of ischemia from congenital or acquired
     conditions
Class III (not indicated)
   Left bundle branch block
   Ventricular paced rhythms
   Confounding rhythms that obscure the ST segment (e.g., atrial
     fibrillation)
   Agitated patients in whom frequent false-ST alarms result

MI, myocardial infarction; PCI, percutaneous coronary intervention.

Arrhythmia

The presence of an arrhythmia is an indication for inpatient continuous ECG monitoring. For patients with atrioventricular (AV) block, monitoring should persist until either the condition resolves or a permanent pacemaker is implanted. Patients with second-degree Mobitz I AV block are more likely to have a reliable escape mechanism below the level of conduction dysfunction and, therefore, need less aggressive monitoring. However, if the Mobitz I block is new, the patient should be monitored with continuous electrocardiography until clinical stability is determined. Although monitoring patients with first-degree AV block is not recommended, up to 90% of these patients will progress to complete AV block over the subsequent 5 years. Thus, some authors recommend continuous ECG monitoring for those patients with new-onset first-degree AV block until clinical stability is observed [11].

Patients with Wolff-Parkinson-White (WPW) syndrome who have rapid antegrade conduction down the accessory pathway are at risk of sudden cardiac death and should undergo continuous monitoring [2]. Likewise, patients with a newly diagnosed long QT syndrome, whether inherited or secondary to medications, are at risk of unstable ventricular tachycardia (VT) and should be admitted with continuous ECG monitoring. A need for monitoring in these patients becomes more critical if polymorphic ventricular premature beats or ventricular bigeminy are observed, as they indicate a high risk of progression to polymorphic VT [2].

Other arrhythmia-related scenarios in which continuous ECG monitoring should be considered include patients with pacemakers or implantable cardioverter-defibrillators (ICDs), sinus bradycardia, atrial dysrhythmias, and those admitted for initiation of anti-arrhythmic therapy. Patients with a newly implanted pacemaker should be monitored (class I indication) if they are pacemaker-dependent [2]. Patients presenting after the firing of their ICD, whether appropriate or not, should be monitored until further evaluation has taken place [11]. Patients who have sinus bradycardia should be monitored if they are symptomatic, require transcutaneous or transvenous pacing, or if they present with syncope [2]. Atrial dysrhythmias do not necessarily require continuous ECG monitoring: patients with a single episode of supraVT do not need ongoing telemetry. However, if the tachycardia is resistant to initial therapy or if there are frequent recurrences, monitoring can be helpful to assess the effects of rate control or anti-arrhythmic drugs [2].

Refer to Table 6.3 for potential indications in patients with potential dysrhythmia.

Syncope

Syncope is a frequent cause of hospital admissions, and represents one of the most common admitting diagnoses for

Table 6.3 Monitoring for proarrhythmia and QT interval

Class I indications
   Administration of an anti-arrhythmic drug known to cause TdP
   Prolonged QTc > 0.50 s due to an offending drug, until the drug
      washes out
   Overdose from a potentially proarrhythmic agent
   New onset bradyarrhythmia (due to the associated risk of TdP)
   Severe hypokalemia or hypomagnesemia
Class II indications
   Treatment with drugs that are associated with a possible risk of TdP
   Acute neurological events when QTc > 0.50 s
Class III (no indication)
   Healthy patients administered drugs that pose little risk of TdP

TdP, torsade de pointes.

continuous ECG monitoring [1]. However, most patients with syncope can be safely evaluated as outpatients, and few need intensive inpatient ECG monitoring. In fact, tremendous savings in healthcare costs can be accrued by more judicious use of resources in this population [12]. In general, only patients determined to be at high risk, primarily patients whose initial evaluation is consistent with cardiac syncope, [13] should be admitted to the hospital with continuous ECG monitoring (Table 6.1).

The initial approach in the evaluation of syncope should be to distinguish true syncope from non-syncopal causes of transient loss of consciousness (e.g., seizure, intoxication, concussion), from conditions that mimic loss of consciousness (e.g., cataplexy, drop attacks, psychogenic pseudoseizures),

and from simple falls [14,15]. A thorough history and physical exam should be performed, and the syncopal event should be categorized as to the most likely etiology – neurally mediated reflex (e.g., vasovagal), orthostatic hypotensive, cardiac arrhythmia, structural cardiopulmonary disease, or cerebrovascular disease [14]. The history and exam often yield clues that lead to a diagnosis for a variety of specific etiologies within these broad categories [13]. This initial evaluation leads to a diagnosis in approximately 40% of patients [16–18]. If a specific non-cardiac diagnosis is confirmed, then most of these patients can be safely triaged to outpatient follow-up with no need for inpatient continuous ECG monitoring. However, if a specific diagnosis is not suggested, attention should be focused on historical clues suggestive of a cardiac etiology. These include history of known cardiac disease, a brief or absent presyncopal period, syncope associated with injury, syncope on exertion or while supine, family history of premature cardiac disease or sudden death, age > 70 years, brief tonic-clonic activity following syncope, or symptoms suggestive of cardiac disease such as dyspnea, chest pain, or palpitations either with the syncopal episode or at baseline [19,20].

As the final element of initial risk stratification, an ECG should be performed in all patients unless a clear cause of syncope has been determined by the history and exam. The ECG is diagnostic in only a minority of patients (2–6%), but, when an abnormality is present, it provides an immediate direction to further evaluation [20]. Electrocardiogram findings that suggest a cardiac arrhythmia or structural abnormality as a cause of syncope are shown in Table 6.4.

Table 6.4 Electrocardiogram findings suggesting a cardiac arrhythmia or structural abnormality as a cause of syncope

ECG finding	Possible cause of syncope
Bundle branch block	AV block or underlying cardiomyopathy predisposing to VT
Mobitz second-degree block	AV block
Sinus bradycardia < 50 bpm	Sinus node dysfunction
Sinus pause > 3 s	Sinus node dysfunction
Short PR interval with delta wave	Wolff-Parkinson-White syndrome
Prolonged QT interval	Long QT syndrome with torsade de pointes
RBBB pattern with ST elevation in V1–V3	Brugada syndrome
Epsilon wave, localized QRS > 110 ms in V1–V3, inverted T waves in V2–V3 without RBBB, or ventricular late potentials	Arrhythmogenic right ventricular dysplasia
Q waves	Past MI with resultant monomorphic VT
Large amplitude QRS complexes (sensitive) with deep narrow Q waves in the lateral leads (specific)	Hypertrophic obstructive cardiomyopathy or severe aortic stenosis
ST segment depression or elevation	Acute coronary syndrome
Right heart strain (i.e., incomplete RBBB, rightward axis) or S1Q3T3 (S wave in lead I, Q wave in lead III, T wave inversion in lead III) pattern	Pulmonary embolism or pulmonary hypertension

AV, atrioventricular; MI, myocardial infarction; RBBB, right bundle branch block; VT, ventricular tachycardia.

Patients who present with cardiac syncope have been demonstrated to have a significantly greater mortality (around 30% at 1 year) than patients with other types of syncope [20]. When a cardiac cause of syncope is suspected, particularly an arrhythmic cause, admission to the hospital with continuous ECG monitoring may be considered. However, clear guidelines on which patients with cardiac syncope benefit from inpatient monitoring do not exist. The European Society of Cardiology's guidelines for syncope evaluation suggest that only the patient who "has an important structural heart disease and is at risk of life-threatening arrhythmias" needs to be admitted for inpatient continuous ECG monitoring [19]. As the initial evaluation in the ED may not be conclusive for the presence of heart disease, a significant suspicion of serious cardiac disease, with concern for short-term morbidity unless immediate evaluation is performed, should be sufficient for admission with continuous monitoring. Other patients in whom an arrhythmic cause of syncope is suggested by the history or ECG can be evaluated further with outpatient holter monitoring or a loop recorder. Other patients who may benefit from inpatient monitoring are those who present with a "malignant" episode of syncope, defined in the AHA guidelines as an episode that occurs with little or no warning and results in injury or property damage [21]. Clearly, patients who have neurally mediated syncope or who have no history, exam, or ECG findings of cardiac disease should not be admitted (with or without ECG monitoring) and should be further evaluated as outpatients [19,21].

Heart failure

Patients with severe acute heart failure that requires inotropic agents should have continuous ECG monitoring until the acute heart failure resolves and no hemodynamically significant arrhythmias are observed for > 24 h [2]. The rationale for monitoring in this setting is largely due to the proven arrhythmogenic potential of inotropic agents [22,23]. Subacute heart failure not requiring inotropic agents is considered a class II recommendation [2]. Opasich and colleagues examined prospectively 711 patients admitted to a heart failure unit [24]. While telemetry guided treatment in only 17% of these patients, physicians perceived that telemetry was helpful in 70% of patients. A lack of general utility for the majority of heart failure patients has been shown in other studies of patients in general telemetry units and in community hospitals [25–28].

Other indications

Telemetry can also be considered for several other indications (Table 6.4). For example, massive blood transfusion (> 10 units) is often associated with hypocalcemia and hypomagnesemia due to binding with citrate. As these ion deficiencies lead to QT prolongation with a risk of polymorphic VT, short-term telemetry is indicated until the deficiencies are corrected [11]. Severe hypokalemia or hyperkalemia may also cause dysrhythmias and arrhythmia, and QT monitoring should be considered. Subarachnoid hemorrhage has a class I indication according to the AHA guidelines for QT monitoring. Arrhythmia monitoring of stroke patients should also be strongly considered, as a significant proportion are found to have atrial fibrillation, AV block, QT prolongation, or, rarely, VT [11]. Pulmonary disease, including pneumonia or chronic obstructive pulmonary disease (COPD) exacerbation, is a common admission diagnosis for telemetry; however, no benefit has been shown in otherwise stable patients not requiring admission to an intensive care unit [2,11].

Case conclusions

The patient in Case 1 was diagnosed with a non-ST elevation myocardial infarction (NSTEMI); the cardiac biomarkers returned positive with the "typical rise and fall" pattern indicative of MI. Thus, the patient was taken to cardiac catheterization where a right coronary artery obstruction was successfully stented. The patient experienced no dysrhythmia during her admission, though review of the case demonstrated that electrocardiographic monitoring was appropriate due to the abnormal diagnostic tests (ECG and biomarker) as well as the ultimate diagnosis (coronary artery disease with NSTEMI).

Case 2 demonstrated the appropriateness of electrocardiographic monitoring in a more dramatic fashion. This patient experienced recurrent syncope with polymorphic VT noted. He was resuscitated and, ultimately, underwent placement of an automatic ICD. He was diagnosed with Brugada syndrome and was discharged on hospital day 4. He was well at 2-year follow-up.

References

1 Curry JP, Hanson CW, 3rd, Russell MW, Hanna C, Devine G, Ochroch EA. The use and effectiveness of electrocardiographic telemetry monitoring in a community hospital general care setting. *Anesth Analg* 2003;**97**(5):1483–7.

2 Drew BJ, Califf RM, Funk M, *et al.* for the American Heart Association Councils on Cardiovascular Nursing CCaCDitY. Practice standards for electrocardiographic monitoring in hospital settings: an American Heart Association scientific statement from the Councils on Cardiovascular Nursing, Clinical Cardiology, and Cardiovascular Disease in the Young: endorsed by the International Society of Computerized Electrocardiology and the American Association of Critical-Care Nurses. *Circulation* 2004; **110**(17):2721–46.

3 Gwinnutt CL, Columb M, Harris R. Outcome after cardiac arrest in adults in UK hospitals: effect of the 1997 guidelines. *Resuscitation* 2000;**47**(2):125–35.

4 Cohn AC, Wilson WM, Yan B, *et al.* Analysis of clinical outcomes following in-hospital adult cardiac arrest. *Intern Med J* 2004; **34**(7):398–402.

5 Moorman JR, Lake DE, Griffin MP. Heart rate characteristics monitoring for neonatal sepsis. *IEEE Trans Biomed Eng* 2006; **53**(1):126–32.

6 Al-Khatib SM, Stebbins AL, Califf RM, *et al.* Sustained ventricular arrhythmias and mortality among patients with acute myocardial infarction: results from the GUSTO-III trial. *Am Heart J* 2003;**145**(3):515–21.

7 Estrada CA, Rosman HS, Prasad NK, Battilana G, Alexander M, Held AC, Young MJ. Evaluation of guidelines for the use of telemetry in the non-intensive-care setting. *J Gen Intern Med* 2000;**15**(1):51–5.

8 Goldman L, Cook EF, Johnson PA, Brand DA, Rouan GW, Lee TH. Prediction of the need for intensive care in patients who come to the emergency departments with acute chest pain. *N Engl J Med* 1996;**334**(23):1498–504.

9 Durairaj L, Reilly B, Das K, *et al.* Emergency department admissions to inpatient cardiac telemetry beds: a prospective cohort study of risk stratification and outcomes. *Am J Med* 2001; **110**(1):7–11.

10 Hollander JE, Sites FD, Pollack CV, Jr., Shofer FS. Lack of utility of telemetry monitoring for identification of cardiac death and life-threatening ventricular dysrhythmias in low-risk patients with chest pain.[see comment]. *Ann Emerg Med* 2004;**43**(1):71–6.

11 Chen EH, Hollander JE. When do patients need admission to a telemetry bed? *J Emerg Med* 2007;**33**(1):53–60.

12 Blanc JJ, L'Her C, Touiza A, Garo B, L'Her E, Mansourati J. Prospective evaluation and outcome of patients admitted for syncope over a 1 year period. *Eur Heart J* 2002;**23**(10):815–20.

13 Kapoor WN. Syncope. *N Engl J Med* 2000;**343**(25):1856–62.

14 Jhanjee R, van Dijk JG, Sakaguchi S, Benditt DG. Syncope in adults: terminology, classification, and diagnostic strategy. *Pacing Clin Electrophysiol* 2006;**29**(10):1160–9.

15 Brignole M. Distinguishing syncopal from non-syncopal causes of fall in older people. *Age Ageing* 2006;**35** Suppl 2:ii46–ii50.

16 Day SC, Cook EF, Funkenstein H, Goldman L. Evaluation and outcome of emergency room patients with transient loss of consciousness. *Am J Med* 1982;**73**(1):15–23.

17 Oh JH, Hanusa BH, Kapoor WN. Do symptoms predict cardiac arrhythmias and mortality in patients with syncope? *Arch Intern Med* 1999;**159**(4):375–80.

18 Martin TP, Hanusa BH, Kapoor WN. Risk stratification of patients with syncope.[comment]. *Ann Emerg Med* 1997;**29**(4): 459–66.

19 Brignole M, Alboni P, Benditt DG, *et al.* Task Force on Syncope ESoC. Guidelines on management (diagnosis and treatment) of syncope – update 2004. *Europace* 2004;**6**(6):467–537.

20 Reed MJ, Gray A. Collapse query cause: the management of adult syncope in the emergency department. *Emerg Med J* 2006; **23**(8):589–94.

21 Strickberger SA, Benson DW, Biaggioni I, *et al.* American Heart Association Councils on Clinical Cardiology CNCDitYaS, Quality of Care and Outcomes Research Interdisciplinary Working Group, American College of Cardiology Foundation, Heart Rhythm S. AHA/ACCF scientific statement on the evaluation of syncope: from the American Heart Association Councils on Clinical Cardiology, Cardiovascular Nursing, Cardiovascular Disease in the Young, and Stroke, and the Quality of Care and Outcomes Research Interdisciplinary Working Group; and the American College of Cardiology Foundation In Collaboration With the Heart Rhythm Society. *J Am Coll Cardiol* 2006;**47**(2): 473–84.

22 Anderson JL, Askins JC, Gilbert EM, Menlove RL, Lutz JR. Occurrence of ventricular arrhythmias in patients receiving acute and chronic infusions of milrinone. *Am Heart J* 1986; **111**(3):466–74.

23 Cuffe MS, Califf RM, Adams KF, Jr., *et al.* Outcomes of a prospective trial of intravenous milrinone for exacerbations of chronic heart failure I. Short-term intravenous milrinone for acute exacerbation of chronic heart failure: a randomized controlled trial. *JAMA* 2002;**287**(12):1541–7.

24 Opasich C, Capomolla S, Riccardi PG, Febo O, Forni G, Cobelli F, Tavazzi L. Does in-patient ECG monitoring have an impact on medical care in chronic heart failure patients? *Eur J Heart Fail* 2000;**2**(3):281–5.

25 Estrada CA, Prasad NK, Rosman HS, Young MJ. Outcomes of patients hospitalized to a telemetry unit. *Am J Cardiol* 1994; **74**(4):357–62.

26 Sivaram CA, Summers JH, Ahmed N. Telemetry outside critical care units: patterns of utilization and influence on management decisions. *Clin Cardiol* 1998;**21**(7):503–5.

27 Lipskis DJ, Dannehl KN, Silverman ME. Value of radiotelemetry in a community hospital. *Am J Cardiol* 1984;**53**(9):1284–7.

28 Estrada CA, Rosman HS, Prasad NK, Battilana G, Alexander M, Held AC, Young MJ. Role of telemetry monitoring in the non-intensive care unit. *Am J Cardiol* 1995;**76**(12):960–5.

Part 2 | **The ECG in Cardinal Presentations**

Chapter 7 | How should the ECG be used in the syncope patient?

Christopher T. Bowe
Maine Medical Center, Portland, ME, USA

Case presentations

Case 1: A 28-year-old female presents to the emergency department (ED) via emergency medical services (EMS) after passing out. She was at work at a local coffee shop when she suddenly felt dizzy and subsequently awoke on the floor. She had not noticed any chest discomfort before or after the event, but had noticed that her heart seemed to be racing earlier in the day. She reports that she has experienced symptoms of heart-racing multiple times in the past and that she often has to sit down and wait for it to pass. She has never seen a physician regarding this symptom previously, nor has she had syncope. She is not short of breath. She has no significant past medical history. Vital signs reveal a heart rate of 85, blood pressure of 110/75 mmHg, respirations of 16 and oxygen saturation of 99% on room air. Her examination is notable for normal heart sounds without murmurs, gallops or a rub. She has clear lung fields, a non-tender abdomen, a normal neurological examination and her urine tests negative for pregnancy. Her electrocardiogram (ECG) demonstrates a sinus rhythm (Figure 7.1).

Case 2: A 65-year-old male presents via EMS from the golf course. As he approached the last green he felt lightheaded. His next recollection was looking up at his playing partners and hearing the approach of sirens. He now continues to feel dizzy and notes a heavy feeling in his chest. He has never passed out before, nor has he experienced this chest discomfort. He has a past medical history significant for hypertension and elevated cholesterol. He is anxious, pale, and diaphoretic. Vital signs reveal a heart rate of 49, blood pressure of 88/64 mmHg, and respirations of 20 with an oxygen saturation of 95% on oxygen. His examination is remarkable for diaphoresis and bradycardia without murmurs, gallops or a rub. He has clear lung fields with a non-tender abdomen. Bedside ultrasound reveals a 1.5 cm abdominal aorta. His ECG reveals a sinus bradycardia (Figure 7.2).

Case 3: A 76-year-old male presents to the ED via rescue from church. He was attending services when he stood and then experienced syncope. He does not recall feeling dizzy or noting any chest discomfort before or after the event. He is without complaint while lying on the stretcher. He has a past medical history significant for osteoarthritis. He is in no apparent distress. Vital signs reveal a heart rate of 55, blood pressure of 95/58 mmHg, respirations of 16, and an oxygen saturation of 97% on 2 L oxygen. His cardiac examination is significant for an occasional extrasystole, but without murmurs, gallops or a rub. He has clear lung fields, a non-tender abdomen and guaiac-negative stool. Bedside ECG reveals no ST segment elevation (Figure 7.3).

The ECG in the patient with syncope

These three patients all present to the ED after a syncopal event. Each patient has different electrocardiographic findings suggesting the cause of syncope. The skilled clinician uses the history and physical examination combined with the ECG to thoroughly evaluate the potential etiologies. Syncope is defined as a transient loss of consciousness with loss of postural tone followed by spontaneous recovery – it is a symptom, not a specific disease process. Syncope is a common chief complaint in the ED, accounting for 1–3% of all visits and an estimated 6% of hospital admissions. Additionally, up to 50% of adults will have a syncopal event in their lifetime [1]. Patients rarely require immediate stabilization as the event is typically transient. It is a challenging complaint for the clinician, as there are myriad causes of syncope, ranging from ultimately benign to immediately life-threatening. Many common etiologies are benign and do not require extensive work-up, but there remains a subset of patients who may have a potentially life-threatening condition that must be identified. Clinical decision rules have been investigated in an effort to identify patients at higher risk for adverse outcomes [2,3]. The ECG is one of the critical variables used in each of these decision rules.

The initial evaluation of a patient presenting with syncope begins with a thorough history and physical examination. The history and physical examination combined with the ECG can lead to the diagnosis in up to 69% of patients [4].

Critical Decisions in Emergency and Acute Care Electrocardiography, 1st edition. Edited by W.J. Brady and J.D. Truwit. © 2009 Blackwell Publishing, ISBN: 9781405159067

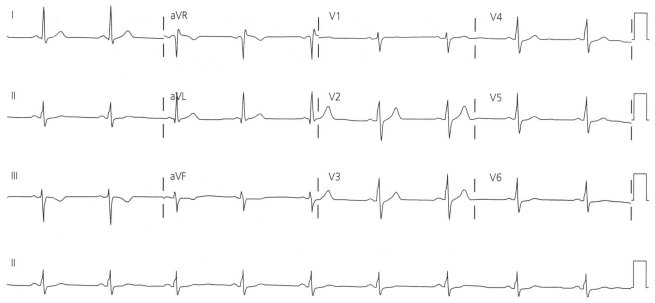

Figure 7.1 Electrocardiogram of patient #1 demonstrating Wolff-Parkinson-White syndrome. Note the classic triad of shortened PR interval, delta wave and widened QRS complex. Wolff-Parkinson-White syndrome leads to paroxysms of tachycardia, which is the likely cause of syncope in this case.

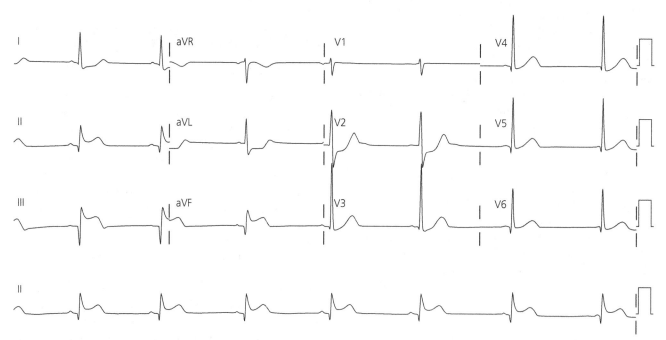

Figure 7.2 Electrocardiogram of patient #2 demonstrating an acute inferior myocardial infarction. Note the ST segment elevation in leads II, III and aVF with reciprocal ST segment depression in leads I and aVL. Also note the ST segment depression with prominent R wave in the right precordial leads, likely consistent with posterior wall infarction as well. The rhythm is a sinus bradycardia, which, combined with a low output state, is the likely cause of syncope in this case.

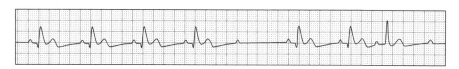

Figure 7.3 Electrocardiogram of patient #3 demonstrating Type II second-degree AV block.

Historical features can help differentiate syncope from other similar phenomena, such as seizure or mechanical fall with loss of consciousness. The history can also lead the clinician to pursue other less common but serious causes of syncope, such as abdominal pain in a female patient with ectopic pregnancy or shortness of breath in the setting of pulmonary embolism. The physical examination should include a focus on initial vital signs and any orthostatic changes. Other key features of the physical examination include both the cardiac and neurologic systems.

The American College of Cardiology states that, in addition to the history and physical examination, the 12-lead ECG is the "procedure of first choice" in the evaluation of syncope [5]. The ECG is a non-invasive, inexpensive tool for identifying many serious causes of syncope. Where the ECG does not make the diagnosis, it can still be used to help predict prognosis and risk-stratify patients.

Cardiac etiologies of syncope

Syncope can be divided into four basic diagnostic categories. These include reflex-mediated, cardiac, orthostatic, and cerebrovascular. The ECG can be helpful in the ultimate diagnosis in all subtypes, but the possibility of finding ECG abnormalities is highest in the cardiac category [6]. The cardiac subgroup can be further divided into structural cardiac disease and dysrhythmias.

Structural cardiac disease

Structural cardiac disease is an important etiology of syncope. An acute condition leading to a decrease in preload, such as physical venodilation, requires an increase in cardiac output to maintain systemic perfusion. Cardiac output is the product of stroke volume and heart rate. When the ability to increase stroke volume is limited by a structural cardiac defect, then physiologic compensation will be dependent upon an increase of the heart rate alone. This partial response may be insufficient to maintain perfusion and, subsequently, may lead to syncope. The following sections will review specific structural cardiac diseases and their ECG findings.

Cardiac tamponade: Cardiac tamponade is the result of accumulation of fluid in the pericardium. Up to 10% of cancer patients develop pericardial effusions, which can lead to tamponade [7]. If enough fluid accumulates in the pericardium at a rate faster than the ability of the parietal pericardium to accommodate it, this will lead to external compression of the heart. Compression of the right ventricle limits the return of venous blood and subsequently decreases cardiac output [7]. The classic ECG findings in cardiac tamponade include decreased voltage, tachycardia, and electrical alternans. Electrical alternans is the variation of the amplitude of the QRS voltage related to movement of the heart in the fluid-filled pericardium. Tachycardia is typically present as the autonomic regulatory center attempts to increase cardiac output, but can be limited by commonly prescribed medications.

Valvular disease: Cardiac valvular lesions can be associated with syncope. Sudden alterations of either preload or afterload secondary to acute valvular disease, can dramatically decrease cardiac output and lead to syncope. For example, a myocardial infarction (MI) causing the rupture of a papillary muscle will lead to acute mitral regurgitation and fulminant pulmonary edema. Chronic valvular disease may limit the ability of the cardiovascular system to compensate at times of stress. Aortic stenosis is the chronic valvular disease most commonly associated with syncope.

Aortic stenosis is most frequently caused by a congenital bicuspid valve, which can result in calcific degeneration of the valve or rheumatic heart disease. Left ventricular hypertrophy develops to maintain adequate stroke volume through an obstructed outflow tract. The classic symptoms of critical aortic stenosis are chest pain, dyspnea, and exertional syncope [8]. The ECG findings in patients who present with syncope secondary to aortic stenosis are non-specific. The ECG often demonstrates the signs of left ventricular hypertrophy, including ST segment T wave abnormalities, a poor R wave progression and increased QRS voltage.

Hypertrophic cardiomyopathy: Hypertrophic cardiomyopathy (HCM) is a genetic disorder that affects cardiac sarcomere proteins. It has also been referred to as idiopathic hypertrophic subaortic stenosis (IHSS) or hypertrophic obstructive cardiomyopathy (HOCM). Hypertrophic cardiomyopathy is present in approximately 1 in 500 adults [9]. This protein abnormality causes hypertrophy of the ventricular septum, leading to symptoms if the outflow tract of the left ventricle becomes partially blocked [10]. Patients may remain asymptomatic or present with complaints of exercise intolerance, dyspnea, chest pain, syncope and even sudden death. Hypertrophic cardiomyopathy is the most common cause of sudden death in young athletes [9].

Historic features and examination findings assist in uncovering the diagnosis of HCM. Patients with HCM seeking healthcare may present with exertional syncope and a family history of sudden cardiac death, though often have neither [11]. Physical examination may reveal an S4 gallop and a midsystolic murmur. This murmur will be louder with maneuvers that decrease preload, such as standing or valsalva. It will be quieter when preload is increased, as with squatting or lying supine.

The ECG in patients with HCM is abnormal in up to 90% of cases [10]. Unfortunately, the ECG abnormalities are often non-specific in adults. The most common changes include increased QRS voltage, QRS widening, ST segment and T wave changes consistent with ventricular hypertrophy, and

Q waves. However, in younger patients with the appropriate clinical history, Q waves in leads II, III, aVF, V5 and V6 are more specific for HCM and should be investigated further [6]. Patients with suspected HCM should be considered for echocardiography, which will often establish the diagnosis.

Dysrhythmias: Dysrhythmias leading to syncope follow the same final common pathway of inadequate cerebral perfusion as a result of decreased cardiac output. Tachycardic dysrhythmias decrease cardiac output by limiting the time in the diastolic portion of the cardiac cycle. The shortened diastole prevents adequate filling of the left ventricle, decreasing stroke volume and, consequently, cardiac output. Bradycardic dysrhythmias decrease cardiac output by slowing the heart rate enough that stroke volume alone cannot maintain sufficient perfusion. The following sections will review specific tachycardic and bradycardic dysrhythmias that can lead to syncope, and their ECG findings.

Sick sinus syndrome: Sick sinus syndrome refers to the presence of sinus pauses with bradycardia, as well the alternating tachycardia-bradycardia syndrome. A sinus pause is the failure of impulse generation in the sinus node. When a sinus pause occurs, there is no P wave present on the ECG. Typically, an alternate pacemaker will initiate an impulse and an escape rhythm will be result. If the pacemaker is at the level of the atrioventricular (AV) node, it will produce a narrow QRS complex at a rate ranging from 45 to 60 beats per minute (bpm). If the pacemaker is below the level of the AV node, it will result in a wide complex QRS with a rate ranging from 30 to 45 bpm. The tachycardia-bradycardia syndrome represents the fluctuation between an atrial tachycardia, often atrial fibrillation, and periods of sinus bradycardia with sinus arrest [12].

The diagnosis of sick sinus syndrome is often made with the use of telemetry monitoring in the prehospital setting, ED or inpatient telemetry units. A patient reporting syncope or presyncope placed on telemetry may demonstrate sinus pauses that did not occur while the initial ECG was obtained. It is important to recall that the normal ECG records the electrical impulses of the heart for less than 12 s. As an intermittent sinus pause may not occur at the moment the ECG was obtained, telemetry monitoring should be used to attempt to record and analyze rhythm changes and the morphology of escape rhythms if there is clinical suspicion of sinus pauses.

Atrioventricular blocks: Atrioventricular block occurs when there is an impairment of conduction through the AV node. Proper interpretation of the ECG is fundamental to correctly identifying the abnormal conduction. Atrioventricular block is divided into three different types, with the different types representing a continuum of disease.

First-degree AV block is present when conduction through the AV node is delayed but not blocked. As a result of the delay, the PR interval on the ECG, which represents the time from atrial depolarization until ventricular depolarization, is prolonged; this prolongation does not change in any fashion with subsequent beats. A PR interval of longer than 200 ms is considered abnormal. As no atrial impulses are completely blocked, however, there will be a corresponding QRS complex following each P wave (Figure 7.4a). There is often no treatment required for first-degree AV block unless evidence of additional conduction disease is present or the clinical scenario is worrisome (i.e. cardiotoxic ingestion or acute coronary syndrome, ACS).

Second-degree AV block is a progression of AV nodal disease, where one or more sinus impulses fail to conduct through the AV node and lead to ventricular depolarization. There are two subtypes of second-degree AV, which, again, represent further progression of the disease. Treatments for Type I and Type II second-degree AV block are different, so careful analysis of the ECG and correct interpretation is necessary for proper management.

Type I second-degree AV block (also referred to as Wenckebach) is present when there is a progressive delay in electrical conduction through the AV node on sequential

(a)

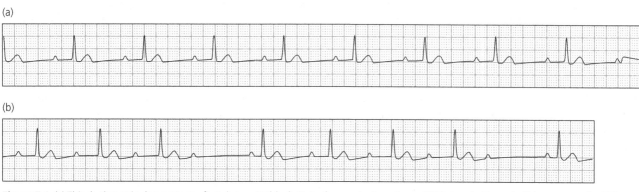

(b)

Figure 7.4 (a) This rhythm strip demonstrates first-degree AV block. Note the constant, prolonged PR interval. Also note the presence of a QRS complex following every P wave. (b) This rhythm strip demonstrates Type I second-degree AV block. Note the sequential increasing PR interval followed by a P wave without a corresponding QRS complex. The next atrial beat then resets the pattern. There is a P/QRS ratio of 5 : 4.

impulses. Eventually, an atrial impulse will not be conducted through the AV node and ventricular depolarization will not occur. The pattern then resets, usually with the same number of conducted atrial impulses before one is blocked. On the ECG, this manifests as an increasing PR interval from consecutive impulses. Each P wave has a corresponding QRS complex until one P wave is not followed by a QRS complex (Figure 7.4b). The block is further described by the ratio of P waves to QRS complexes in the repeating pattern (3 : 2, 4 : 3, etc.). As with first-degree AV block, Type I second-degree AV block does not typically require treatment unless warranted by other clinical issues.

Type II second-degree AV block (also referred to as Mobitz II) represents further progression of AV nodal conduction pathology. The atrial depolarization is followed by ventricular depolarization intermittently. The PR interval is not variable; however, not all P waves lead to QRS complexes as the AV node and infra-nodal conducting system block some impulses. There is no progressive lengthening of time for conduction through the AV node as is present in Type I second-degree AV block. On the ECG or rhythm strip, this manifests as a constant PR interval when P waves are followed by QRS complexes. However, there will not be a corresponding QRS complex for each P wave (Figure 7.5a). Type II second-degree AV block demonstrates pathology of the AV node or infra-nodal conducting system, and can deteriorate into complete heart block. Treatment in the unstable patient is with transcutaneous or transvenous pacing and management of identified underlying pathology.

Third-degree AV block (also referred to as complete heart block) represents the failure of either the AV node or the infra-nodal conduction system to conduct any impulses. The atrial depolarization is blocked and the ventricular depolarization is initiated by an escape pacemaker below the level of the AV node. This situation leads to complete electrical dissociation of the atria and the ventricles. On the ECG or rhythm strip, this manifests as both P waves and QRS complexes at a regular rate. The two rates, however, are unrelated (Figure 7.5b) with the atrial rate being greater than the ventricular rate. The QRS complex morphology will be determined by the site of the escape pacemaker. If the pacemaker is above the His bundle it will produce a narrow complex QRS, while pacemakers at or below the level of the His bundle produce a wide complex QRS [12]. Treatment of third-degree AV block is with transcutaneous or transvenous pacing and management of identified underlying pathology.

Wolff-Parkinson-White syndrome: Wolff-Parkinson-White (WPW) syndrome is a potentially serious form of ventricular pre-excitation, which was first described in 1930 [13]. Pre-excitation refers to the depolarization of the ventricles earlier than would be expected by normal conduction through the AV node. An accessory pathway is an area capable of transmitting electrical impulses between the atria and ventricles, separate from the AV node. Normally, the atria and ventricles are electrically isolated by the AV annulus. Wolff-Parkinson-White syndrome is the most common form of an accessory pathway system, occurring in 0.1–0.3% of the population. Wolff-Parkinson-White syndrome can lead to a variety of supraventricular tachycardias, syncope, and even sudden cardiac death [6].

There are three commonly noted ECG abnormalities in WPW syndrome. Each can be best understood by considering the mechanism of the accessory pathway. Secondary T wave changes also may be present [14]. First, there is a shortened PR interval (recall that the normal PR interval is 120–200 ms). The PR interval represents the normal conduction delay in the AV node. When the AV node is bypassed by the accessory pathway, which does not have an inherent delay, the conduction time to the ventricles is shortened.

Second, the QRS complex is prolonged (recall that the normal QRS duration is less than 120 ms). The QRS width represents the time of ventricular depolarization. As the ventricle is first activated by the accessory pathway, the QRS begins earlier than it would if conduction occurred via the AV node only. When the electrical stimulus does pass through the AV node and leads to ventricular activation via the His bundle, a normal QRS is formed. The summation of the two pathways results in a widened QRS complex [14].

The third abnormality of the ECG in WPW syndrome is the delta wave. The delta wave is the slurred initial upstroke of the QRS complex. This portion of the QRS complex is formed by the electrical impulse passing through the accessory pathway before the normal impulse has passed through the AV node (Figure 7.1).

Recognition of signs of WPW syndrome on the resting ECG is critical. The accessory pathway of WPW syndrome places these patients at risk for the development of various

Figure 7.5 (a) This rhythm strip demonstrates Type II second-degree AV block. Note the PR intervals do not vary in length, but there are not QRS complexes after each P wave. (b) This rhythm strip demonstrates third-degree AV block. Note the complete dissociation of the QRS complexes from P waves. Both the P waves and the QRS complexes are regular.

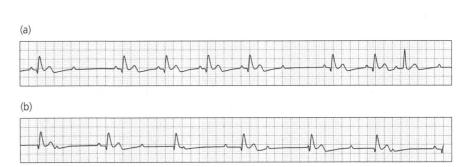

(a)

(b)

supraventricular tachycardias. Patients with WPW syndrome may have episodes of paroxysmal supraventricular tachycardia (PSVT), atrial fibrillation and atrial flutter [14]. Paroxysmal supraventricular tachycardia is the most common form of supraventricular tachycardia in patients with WPW syndrome, present in approximately 70% of cases. The abnormal accessory pathway and the AV node function as a re-entrant circuit. Patients with WPW syndrome manifest two types of PSVT, termed orthodromic and antidromic. In the orthodromic form of PSVT in WPW syndrome, the atrial stimulus proceeds to the ventricle through the AV node and returns to the atrium through the accessory pathway. This mechanism represents 90% of PSVT cases in a patient with WPW syndrome. As conduction to the ventricle is via the AV node only, the QRS complex will be narrow and regular, and the delta wave will be absent. The ventricular rate ranges from 160–220 bpm [6].

In the antidromic form of PSVT in WPW syndrome, the atrial stimulus activates the ventricle via the accessory pathway and returns to the atrium through the AV node. This mechanism is present in the remaining 10% of PSVT cases in patients with WPW. As conduction to the ventricles is via the accessory pathway only, the QRS is widened and regular. The ECG subsequently reveals a wide-complex tachycardia that appears very much like that of ventricular tachycardia [6].

Atrial fibrillation is the second most common form of supraventricular tachycardia in patients with WPW syndrome, present in approximately 25% of cases. Normally in atrial fibrillation, the AV node is able to limit the rate of ventricular depolarization by the inherent electrical delay. In the case of WPW syndrome with atrial fibrillation, electrical impulses activate the ventricle via the accessory pathway without that delay, leading to ventricular rates greater than 200 bpm. The ECG in the setting of atrial fibrillation with WPW syndrome reveals a very rapid, irregular rate with a wide QRS complex [6].

Brugada syndrome: Brugada syndrome, first described in 1992, is a particular group of ECG abnormalities associated with sudden cardiac death in previously healthy patients without structural heart disease [15]. Patients with Brugada syndrome experience recurrent episodes of ventricular tachycardia (VT) [16]. They may present for evaluation of syncope if an episode of VT is self-terminating. If the VT persists, it can degenerate into ventricular fibrillation and result in death.

Brugada syndrome has been found to result from a mutation on chromosome 3. This mutation affects the SCN5A gene responsible for cardiac voltage-gated sodium channels. The result of this mutation is a reduction in fast sodium channel currents in the right ventricular epicardium, but not those in the endocardium. The resulting voltage gradient is thought to be the cause of the ECG changes and the episodes of paroxysmal VT [17,18].

The ECG findings in Brugada syndrome are a right bundle branch block (RBBB) and ST segment elevation in V1–V3. However, the RBBB may be incomplete and the ST segment elevation may be minimal. These abnormalities may also be transient [19]. As the height and morphology of the ST segment elevation can be variable, there have been attempts to standardize the ECG findings, based upon both morphology and the amount of elevation. Type I has ST segment elevation of > 2 mm in two precordial leads followed by an inverted T wave. Type II describes a saddle-shaped ST segment elevation, while Type III demonstrates ST segment elevation of < 2 mm [17].

Patients presenting for evaluation of syncope with a family history of sudden death should lead the clinician to consider the diagnosis of Brugada syndrome. The ECG findings of a RBBB with ST segment elevation in the right precordial leads should prompt electrophysiologic testing to confirm the diagnosis. Treatment requires placement of an internal defibrillator.

Long QT syndrome: Long QT syndrome is an inherited or acquired disorder that results in prolonged repolarization of the ventricular action potential. The incidence of inherited long QT syndrome is rare, occurring in approximately 1 in 5000 patients. The genetic abnormalities affect proteins involved in transportation of sodium and potassium ions [20]. Long QT syndrome is associated with HCM and may account for up to 5% of cases of sudden cardiac death [21]. Acquired long QT syndrome may result from multiple causes including medications, electrolyte imbalance, toxins, autonomic neuropathy, acute coronary syndromes, and the human immunodeficiency virus [22].

Long QT syndrome is associated with the development of paroxysms of ventricular tachycardia (PVT). If the episode of PVT is self-limited, patients may present for evaluation of syncope. Patients with congenital long QT syndrome often report episodes of palpitations precipitated by physical or emotional stress [6].

The primary ECG abnormality in this syndrome is the prolongation of the QT interval for which the syndrome is named. Recall that the QT interval varies inversely with heart rate. Therefore, the QT interval must be corrected for the corresponding heart rate. Correction of the QT interval (QTc) can be calculated by the Bazett formula. The QTc is equal to the measured QT interval divided by the square root of the RR interval [6]. The generally accepted maximum QTc is 450 ms, though it may be normal at up to 460 ms in women [23].

Unfortunately, patients with long QT syndrome may have a normal initial ECG [23]. Yet, the ECG may demonstrate other findings suggestive of the disorder. T waves can be prolonged, biphasic, larger than normal, or demonstrate a notched appearance. T wave alternans is uncommonly found, but can be indicative of long QT syndrome. U waves may be unusually pronounced and U wave alternans has been

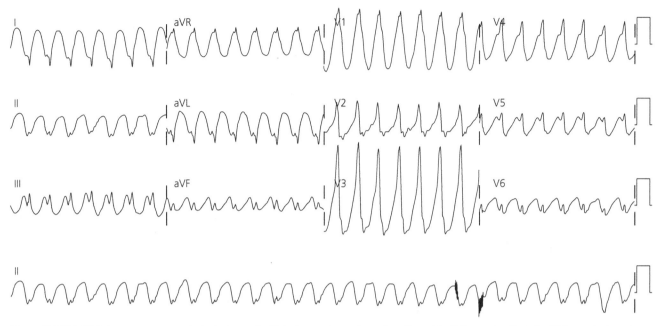

Figure 7.6 This ECG demonstrates ventricular tachycardia. Note the regular tachycardia with a wide QRS complex. Note the QRS morphology does not change.

noted. The ECG findings of a prolonged QTc and additional ECG abnormalities in the appropriate clinical setting should prompt further diagnostic testing [6].

Ventricular tachycardia: The ECG finding of a wide-complex tachycardia presents a clinical challenge. The differential diagnosis includes VT and supraventricular tachycardia (SVT) with aberrant conduction. The history and physical examination combined with careful ECG interpretation help to determine the underlying dysrhythmia. There are multiple decision tools used to help guide ECG interpretation in this clinical setting, including the Brugada criteria [24]. It is important to note that clinical stability alone does not help distinguish between VT and SVT with aberrancy. The initial assumption should be that the underlying dysrhythmia is VT until proven otherwise.

Ventricular tachycardia is a dysrhythmia where the ventricular depolarization occurs from an ectopic pacemaker below the level of the His bundle [25]. Non-sustained VT episodes are brief and self-resolving, while sustained VT denotes prolonged episodes. Ventricular tachycardia is rare in patients without underlying cardiac disease. The most common cause of VT is a re-entry mechanism. The re-entry circuit can be activated by a premature ventricular contraction (PVC). A PVC occurring during ventricular repolarization can precipitate VT. This understanding helps explain the increased risk of VT in patients who have delayed ventricular repolarization, including both Brugada and long QT syndromes.

The ECG abnormalities of VT include a wide QRS complex, tachycardic rate typically between 150 and 200 bpm, a regular rhythm, and, usually, a morphologically consistent QRS pattern (Figure 7.6). Monomorphic VT associated with underlying coronary artery disease is the most common form of VT [12].

Torsade de pointes is a paroxysmal form of VT that typically occurs in frequent, short episodes. The presence of torsades usually implies significant underlying cardiac disease. Both medications and underlying electrolyte disturbances, including hypokalemia and hypomagnesemia, are common causes of torsades [12]. The ECG findings in torsades include a rapid ventricular rate > 200 bpm and a sinusoidal variation of the amplitude and direction of the QRS complexes.

Case conclusions

In Case 1, a typical presentation of WPW syndrome is encountered. The patient is young, previously healthy and reports a history of previous palpitations. The ECG (Figure 7.1) has the classic triad of WPW syndrome with a shortened PR interval, widened QRS and delta wave. The patient was referred for electrophysiologic testing and ablative therapy.

Case 2 demonstrates syncope in the setting of an inferior myocardial infarction (IMI). Acute ischemic cardiac disease is infrequently the cause of syncope; however, a patient with risk factors and suggestive symptoms warrants further work-up. The ECG is diagnostic for acute IMI (Figure 7.2). Hypotension from both bradycardia and decreased stroke volume leads to syncope. Treatment for the IMI including thrombolytic therapy was initiated.

Case 3 demonstrates syncope from bradycardia in alternating third-degree AV block and Type II second-degree AV block (Figure 7.3). The patient was treated successfully with placement of a transvenous pacer.

References

1 Miller TH, Kruse JE. Evaluation of syncope. *Am Fam Phys* 2005;**72**:1492–500.

2 Martin TP, Hanusa BH, Kapoor WN. Risk stratification of patients with syncope. *Ann Emerg Med* 1997;**29**(4):459–66.

3 Quinn J, Stiell I, McDermott D, *et al.* Derivation of the San Francisco syncope rule to predict patients with short-term serious outcomes. *Ann Emerg Med* 2004;**43**:224–32.

4 Sarasin FP, Louis-Simonet M, Carballo D, *et al.* Prospective evaluation of patients with syncope: A population-based study. *Am J Med* 2001;**111**(3):177–84.

5 Strickberger SA, Benson DW, Biaggioni I, *et al.* AHA/ACCF Scientific statement on the evaluation of syncope. *Circulation* 2006;**113**(2):316–27.

6 Dovgalyuk J, Holstege CP, Mattu A, *et al.* The electrocardiogram in the patient with syncope. *Am J Emerg Med* 2007;**25**(6):688–701.

7 Spodick DH. Pathophysiology of cardiac tamponade. *Chest* 1998;**113**:1372–8.

8 Dunmire SM. Infective endocarditis and valvular heart disease. In: Marx JA editor. *Rosen's Emergency Medicine Concepts and Clinical Practice*. Fifth Edition. Vol 2. Mosby, Philadelphia, 2002; p. 1155.

9 Nishimura RA, Holmes DR, Jr. Clinical practice: hypertrophic obstructive cardiomyopathy. *N Engl J Med* 2004;**350**(13):1320–7.

10 Popjes ED, Sutton MS. Hypertrophic cardiomyopathy: pathophysiology, diagnosis and treatment. *Geriatrics* 2003;**58**(3):41–6.

11 Frenneaux MP. Assessing the risk of sudden cardiac death in a patient with hypertrophic cardiomyopathy. *Heart* 2004;**90**:570–5.

12 Yealy DM, Delbridge TR. Dysrhythmias. In: Marx JA editor. *Rosen's Emergency Medicine Concepts and Clinical Practice*. Fifth Edition. Vol 2. Mosby, Philadelphia, 2002; pp. 1053–98.

13 Wolff L, Parkinson J, White PD. Bundle-branch block with short PR interval in healthy young people prone to paroxysmal tachycardia. *Am Heart Journal* 1930;**5**:685–704.

14 Rosner MH, Brady WJ, Kefer MP, *et al.* Electrocardiography in the patient with the Wolff-Parkinson-White syndrome: diagnostic and initial therapeutic issues. *Am J Emerg Med* 1999;**17**:705–14.

15 Brugada P, Brugada J. Right bundle branch block persistent ST segment elevation and sudden death: a distinct clinical and electrocardiographic syndrome. A multicenter report. *J Am Coll Cardiology* 1992;**20**:1391–6.

16 Brugada P, Brugada R, Brugada J. The Brugada syndrome. *Curr Cardiology Reports* 2000;**2**:507–14.

17 Ott P, Marcus FI. Electrocardiographic markers of sudden death. *Cardiol Clin* 2006;**24**:453–69.

18 Littman L, Monroe MH, Kerns WP, *et al.* Brugada syndrome and "Brugada sign": clinical spectrum with a guide for the clinician. *Am Heart J* 2003;**145**(5):768–78.

19 Mattu A, Rogers RL, Kim H, *et al.* The Brugada syndrome. *Am J Emerg Med* 2003;**21**:146–51.

20 Hauda WE, Mayer T. Syncope and sudden death. In: Tintinalli editor. Emergency Medicine: A Comprehensive Study Guide. Sixth Edition. McGraw-Hill, New York, 2004; pp. 838–43.

21 Meyer JS, Mehdirad A, Salem BI, *et al.* Sudden arrythmia death syndrome: importance of the long QT syndrome. *Am Fam Phys* 2003;**68**:483–8.

22 Khan IA. Clinical and therapeutic aspects of congenital and acquired long QT syndrome. *Am J Med* 2002;**112**:58–66.

23 McHarg ML, Shinnar S, Rascoff H, *et al.* Syncope in childhood. *Pediatr Cardiol* 1997;**18**(36):367–71.

24 Brugada P. A new approach to the differential diagnosis of a regular tachycardia with a wide QRS complex. *Circulation* 1991;**83**:1649.

25 Wellens HJ, Bar F, Lie KI. The value of the electrocardiogram in the differential diagnosis of tachycardia with a widened QRS complex. *Am J Med* 1978;**64**(27):27–33.

Additional recommended reading

Huff JS, Decker WW, Quinn JV, *et al.* Clinical Policy: Critical Issues in the Evaluation and Management of Adult Patients Presenting to the Emergency Department with Syncope. ACEP Clinical Policy Subcommittee on Syncope. *Ann Emerg Med* 2007;**49**:431–44.

Chapter 8 | How should the ECG be used in the chest pain patient?

Jason T. Schaffer
Indiana University School of Medicine, Indianapolis, IN, USA

Case presentations

Case 1: A 61-year-old male with a past medical history significant for coronary artery disease, hypertension, and diabetes, presents to the emergency department (ED) with severe chest pain, typical for his anginal pain, which started 30 min previously. The patient took three sublingual nitroglycerin pills without relief before coming to the ED. He has associated diaphoresis, nausea, vomiting, and left-arm pain. An initial electrocardiogram (ECG) is performed (Figure 8.1), and anti-ischemic and anti-platelet treatments are started. A second ECG is completed 10 min later (Figure 8.2) demonstrating ST elevation myocardial infarction (STEMI) of the anterolateral regions.

Case 2: A 49-year-old male presents with several days of mild chest and left shoulder pain. He had noticed some dyspnea on exertion as well, and a "slight choking" sensation. His presenting vital signs are normal. The patient's symptoms, which are not relieved by nitroglycerin, are only mildly improved with morphine. An ECG is obtained (Figure 8.3), showing minimal ST segment elevation, PR segment depression, and PR segment elevation in lead aVr – consistent with acute myopericarditis. With further history, it is found that the patient has had a recent viral illness and that his dyspnea has a positional component.

Case 3: A 53-year-old male presents with groin and chest pain occurring with a syncopal episode. The patient is intoxicated and his main complaint is regarding the right groin pain radiating into the flank. An ECG is done (Figure 8.4). His ECG from 1 month prior was normal. After a liter of fluid, the patient still has a resting tachycardia of 115 beats per minute (bpm).

Case 4: A 51-year-old male present with recent onset of substernal chest pain, described as an ache. He also complains of chronic back pain and pain in his left leg when walking. The left-leg pain is new and he has had no weakness in his arms or legs. His only medical history is hypertension without medication use. His initial blood pressure is 125/48 mmHg and his heart rate is 90 bpm. An ECG is done (Figure 8.5). Leads V7, V8, and V9 are also obtained, and show no ST segment elevation. Anti-ischemic and anti-platelet therapies are initiated. The patient's pain begins to improve somewhat and a repeat ECG is done (Figure 8.6).

The ECG in the chest pain patient

The 12-lead ECG is used extensively in evaluation of a patient presenting with chest pain. The chest pain presentation is fraught with risk, pitfalls, and partially effective diagnostic tools, including the history (present history and risk factors), chest radiograph, cardiac biomarkers and other serum laboratory tests, and the 12-lead ECG. When combined with history and presentation, the 12-lead ECG is a very powerful tool. An important cautionary note is that the ECG is an imperfect tool for diagnosing all causes of chest pain, and must be interpreted in the setting of an individual patient presentation.

The ECG in suspected ACS presentations

The most frequent use of the ECG is in the adult patient presenting with chest pain with the consideration of acute coronary syndrome (ACS). As suggested by the American College of Cardiology/American Heart Association (ACC/ AHA) in this specific setting, the initial ECG should be performed within 10 min of arrival; this ECG performance is coupled with an immediate interpretation of the ECG by an experienced physician [1]. In an era where ED clinical space is at a premium and waits are long, many centers have been creative about how to accomplish time-intensive goals such as the "Door to ECG". The triage ECG may be the most effective of these strategies for low-risk chest pain patients. This assists the triage person in deciding whether to take a low-risk patient immediately to clinical space or allow them to wait in the waiting room [2]. This being the case, it often occurs that the ECG has been evaluated prior to evaluating

Critical Decisions in Emergency and Acute Care Electrocardiography,
1st edition. Edited by W.J. Brady and J.D. Truwit. © 2009 Blackwell Publishing, ISBN: 9781405159067

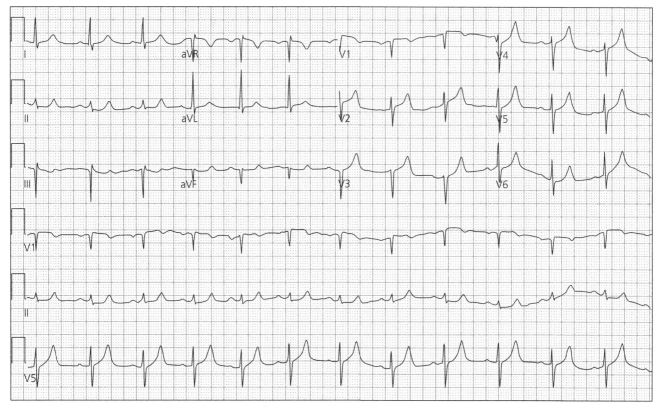

Figure 8.1 Hyperacute T waves across the precordium (leads V1 to V6) very early in the presentation of a patient with STEMI. Notice also the ST segment depression in leads II and III.

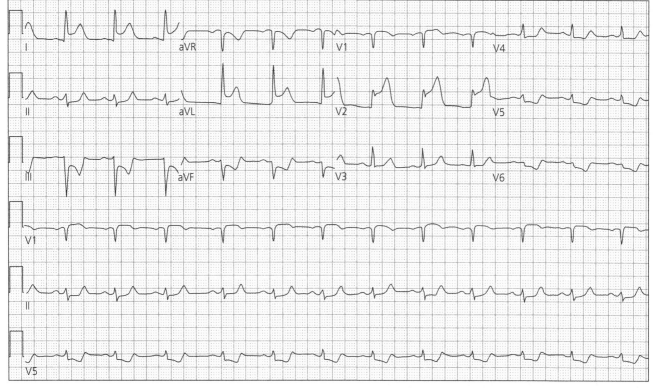

Figure 8.2 This second ECG, completed less than 15 min after the initial ECG in Figure 8.1, shows the rapid progression to STEMI in this patient. Note the distribution of ST segment elevation does not exactly match the distribution of hyperacute T waves in the previous ECG.

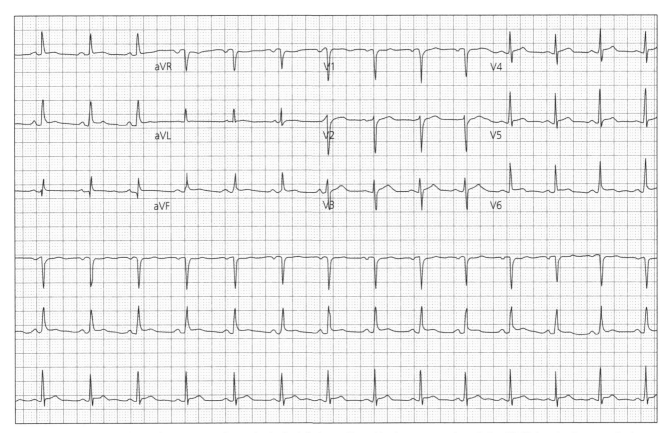

Figure 8.3 Acute pericarditis with PR segment depression in the inferior and lateral leads, most prominent in lead II. ST elevation is present in the same distribution but not as evident. Also note the PR segment elevation in lead aVr.

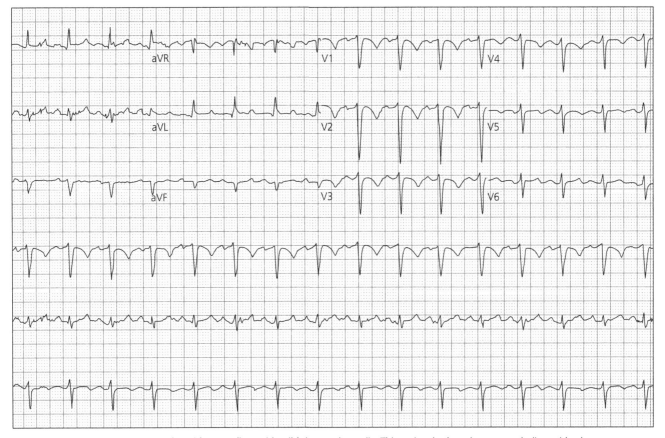

Figure 8.4 T wave inversion across the mid-precordium with mild sinus tachycardia. This patient had a pulmonary embolism with a large clot burden.

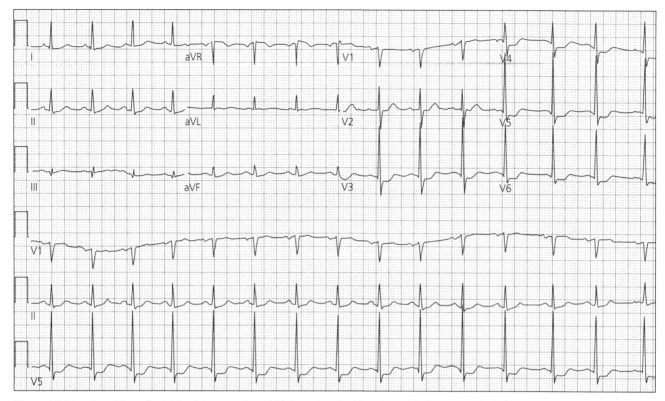

Figure 8.5 Note the evidence for LVH and the anterolateral ST depressions in this patient with chest pain, which ultimately diagnosed acute aortic dissection.

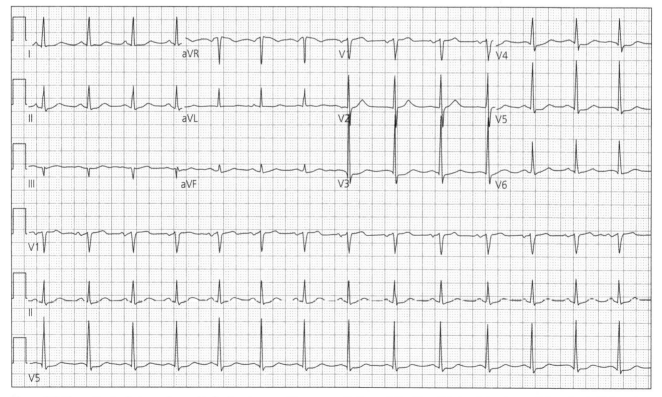

Figure 8.6 The patient's electrocardiographic findings improved (compare with Figure 8.5) with anti-ischemic treatment. This patient's ECGs and clinical presentation were more consistant with ACS and, thus, he was initially diagnosed incorrectly. Ultimately, aortic dissection was noted via echocardiography.

the patient; thus, it may be that the ECG is the first tool that is utilized for evaluation of the patient and their risk, even before the history.

Time to ECG performance: In one study focusing on the ED chest pain patient, the median time to ECG for STEMI patients was 14 min [3]. This finding is consistent with data reported from the National Hospital Ambulatory Medical Care Survey of 2004; the data, however, reported only door-to-doctor times, not door-to-ECG intervals. Median wait times for a physician in this survey were 12 min for those with ischemic chest pain, 15 min for those with other cardiac chest pain, 18 min for those with undifferentiated chest pain, and 25 min for those with non-cardiac chest pain [2]. Race and gender are still recognized as factors associated with delays in time to ECG acquisition [4–6]. In a recent study on door-to-ECG times, an association was noted between door-to-ECG performance > 10 min and adverse outcomes in the STEMI group. For patients with non-ST segment elevation acute coronary syndrome (NSTE-ACS), there was no association between this cutoff of 10 min and adverse outcomes; however, if the delay was more than 3 h the risk of an adverse event increased by sevenfold [3].

The 12-lead ECG in the diagnostic pathway: The initial presentation of the patient with chest pain may ultimately define the utility of the ECG in each case. The ECG is not a perfect tool and has its limitations, but it is at the center of the diagnostic and prognostic pathway of the patient with chest pain.

In the year 2000, the AHA/ACC redefined acute myocardial infarction (AMI) [7]. In regards to the electrocardiographic diagnosis of AMI, this redefinition was based on a more contemporary understanding of ACS as well as improved diagnostic tools and strategies. At the initiation of the evaluation, we no longer refer to "Q wave" or "non Q-wave" myocardial infarction. ST segment elevation myocardial infarction focuses on the demonstration of significant ST segment elevation in the patient with chest pain, or chest pain equivalent presentation, which is ultimately confirmed by elevations in cardiac biomarkers. Non-ST segment elevation myocardial infarction describes the patient with chest pain, or chest pain equivalent presentation, and abnormal cardiac biomarkers; the 12-lead ECG demonstrates abnormality, ranging from non-specific ST segment/T wave abnormality to pathologic ST segment depression. This change in definition better describes the approach to such patients and their potential for ACS in the ED [8].

Despite the recommendations and the time-intensive need to establish the diagnosis of STEMI, it should be noted that literature suggests that STEMI is not the most common cause of electrocardiographic ST segment elevation among chest pain patients. In fact, the two most common causes of ST segment elevation in several studies [9–11] were left ventricular hypertrophy (LVH) and left bundle branch block (LBBB).

Other ST segment elevation diagnoses in the chest pain patient include benign early repolarization, right bundle branch block (RBBB), non-specific intraventricular conduction delay, left ventricular aneurism, ventricular paced rhythm, and pericarditis. Although not all of these syndromes are acute in nature, many patients with these underlying disease processes will present with acute chest pain. Not only must the clinician be adept at evaluating the ECG for ST segment elevation, but also he/she must be proficient at distinguishing these non-AMI ECG patterns from STEMI. The steps for distinguishing non-AMI ST segment elevation syndromes from STEMI include evaluating for bundle branch blocks, anatomical distributions, morphology of the elevated ST segment, reciprocal ST segment depression, and other ECG findings supporting alternative diagnoses (i.e. PR segment depression in pericarditis).

Reciprocal ST segment depression: Reciprocal ST segment depression, also known as reciprocal change, may be helpful in the differentiation of STEMI from other ST segment elevation electrocardiographic syndromes. ST segment depression, however, is also potentially present in ST segment elevation syndromes other than STEMI, namely bundle branch block, paced rhythms, and LVH.

ST segment elevation morphology: ST segment elevation (STE) morphology may also help determine the source of the elevation. ST segment elevation due to ischemia is most commonly convex in nature. ST segment elevation with a concave morphology is more likely to be indicative of benign early repolarization, LVH, or male gender [11]. ST segments indicative of ischemia tend to be flat (horizontal or oblique) or convex [12]. These patterns, however, are not universally true and STEMI can present, especially early in the course of AMI, with a concave ST segment.

ST segment depression: Two criteria define ischemic ST segment depression: J-point depression of at least 1 mm and an ST segment that is either downward sloping or horizontal [13]. ST segment depression in ACS is often diffuse and located in the inferior or anterior leads and is not necessarily localizing to the area of injury [14]. The differential diagnostic considerations of non-ischemic ST segment depression includes digitalis effect, repolarization changes secondary to left ventricular hypertrophy, and similar repolarization changes in LBBB.

The T wave: As compared with the ST segment, little has been written about T wave changes in acute care. The T wave, however, can provide important diagnostic data. A prominent T wave in the appropriate setting may be the earliest finding of STEMI. The hyperacute T wave is a prominent T wave that is short-lived, evolving rapidly to ST segment elevation. As in Case 1 above, it may present within 30 min of occlusion of the coronary artery – hence the term "hyperacute." It is variable in its presentation, but is typically broad-based and asymmetric. Symmetry, however, is sometimes found in this scenario. The term "hyperacute" is reserved for the prominent T wave in the setting of AMI. The differential for the prominent T wave includes systemic hyperkalemia, benign early repolarization, acute pericarditis, and LVH [15].

The primary differential diagnostic considerations of the inverted T wave include ACS (both unstable angina and NSTEMI), ventricular strain patterns, myocarditis, digitalis effect, central nervous system (CNS) events, pulmonary embolism, and normal variants such as persistent juvenile T wave pattern or early repolarization [16]. The morphology of the inversion may determine the source of T wave abnormality, but, as with any electrocardiographic finding, the clinical picture must be considered. The classic ischemic inversion pattern is a narrow and symmetric T wave that is typically accompanied by an isoelectric ST segment. These T wave inversions are typically moderate in depth as opposed to the T wave inversions associated with CNS events – such as subarachnoid hemorrhage. Central nervous system-related T wave inversions tend to be large in amplitude and significantly asymmetric with a slower upstroke. T wave inversions can also be seen in pulmonary embolism. These may occur in the inferior leads as part of the classic S1-Q3-T3 pattern, or may present as shallow T wave inversions in the inferior leads or, as in Case 3, may present as deeper T wave inversions across the mid-precordial leads.

Wellens' syndrome represents a particular T wave inversion pattern; Wellens' syndrome is an association of peculiar anterior T wave inversions with proximal left anterior descending coronary artery (LAD) stenosis. The Wellens' T wave was first described in 1982 and presents as two distinct patterns that both indicate significant LAD disease [17]. The more common pattern consists of a deep symmetric T wave in the precordial leads V1 to V4, most commonly in leads V2 to V3. The less common pattern is a biphasic T wave in leads V2 to V3. The potential difficulty with the Wellens' T wave is that it typically is present during pain-free periods and may even *normalize* during periods of pain. This pattern is extremely important to recognize because these patients present an opportunity for early intervention for a group at very high risk of developing a complete LAD occlusion – with large anterior wall STEMI as the natural history. These patients will initially respond well to medical management, but, ultimately, have a poor prognosis without aggressive treatment including percutaneous coronary intervention (PCI).

Left bundle branch block: Any new bundle branch block (BBB) is significant. Specifically, new LBBB meets the criteria for reperfusion. It is often difficult to determine whether a LBBB is "new." Often in this time-intensive circumstance, it is difficult or impossible to discover prior ECGs to determine whether a BBB is new, and, when one does find an old ECG

that confirms the LBBB is new, the old ECG is from more than a few years earlier. Intensifying this dilemma, AMI patients that present with LBBB are at extreme risk with significant benefit from an aggressive approach and very high risk of poor outcome if not appropriately managed [18].

The normal/minimally abnormal ECG: Often in the evaluation of a chest pain patient, the presenting ECG is normal or minimally abnormal. How likely is it that this patient is having an acute coronary event? As previously noted, the ECG is a powerful tool in diagnosing acute coronary events. However, it is most powerful in conjunction with a supporting clinical presentation. One to six percent of patients with a normal ECG will eventually be proven to have had an AMI, and at least 4% will be found to have non-AMI ACS events [1,19–21]. In patients with non-specific ST segment/T wave changes, the percentage of patients with ACS is markedly higher – yet the clinician must interpret the ECG within the context of the clinical presentation [22].

There has been some question of whether a normal ECG may be diagnostic depending on clinical circumstances during which it is obtained. A symptomatic patient with a normal or minimally abnormal ECG has an adverse event rate similar to patients that had no symptoms at the time of their normal to near-normal ECG [23]. The previous teaching was that a normal or non-specific ECG obtained while a patient was experiencing symptoms suggestive of ACS should argue against the presentation being ACS-related. Further, the negative predictive value of the ECG does not appear to improve with a longer duration of symptoms of at least up to 12 h [24].

There are few data to evaluate the use of comparison ECGs. However, available data suggest that an unchanged ECG from a previous ECG improves the patient's prognosis and decreases the likelihood that the current presentation is ischemic in nature [25–28]. In one study, patients with a change in their ECG compared to a previous ECG had a 2.9 times greater risk of having an AMI. This group included patients with both normal and abnormal prior ECGs [28].

ECG evaluation in specific non-ACS diagnoses

Pulmonary embolism: The pulmonary embolism patient often presents with some component of chest pain and will frequently have an ECG. The classic right-sided strain pattern, the S1Q3T3, is frequently discussed and occasionally seen. However, this pattern is likely to be seen more often in the non-PE patient. This is a very non-specific pattern seen in patients with right heart strain. Although this right heart strain may be acute from a large PE, it may more often be chronic. Some of the most common non-PE causes of this pattern are previous inferior MI, pulmonary hypertension, sleep apnea, or other lung disease.

When a patient presents with unexplained sinus tachycardia or sinus tachycardia with symptoms suggestive of PE, a PE diagnosis should be considered. Despite sinus tachycardia being the most commonly quoted electrocardiographic finding for PE, one series of confirmed PE patients showed that precordial T wave inversion, as in Case 3 above, was the most common finding, seen in 68% of patients. Precordial T wave inversions exceeded sinus tachycardia (26%) in this study [30]. The bottom line is that there are many ECG changes associated with pulmonary embolism, yet they are neither sensitive nor specific enough to use the ECG as a diagnostic tool. There are some findings, however, on ECG that may prompt the physician in the appropriate clinical setting to further consider PE.

Acute aortic dissection: The concern is that a proximal dissection may involve the coronary arteries, presenting as a STEMI with severe chest pain and electrocardiographic patterns suggestive of ACS [30–32]. Case 4 above presents just such an example of this diagnostic dilemma. The signs and symptoms of acute aortic dissection are non-specific, with the most common complaint being chest pain. In a pooled analysis of patients with aortic dissection, only 32% complained of pain radiating to the back, and only 39% complained of their pain as a tearing sensation; whereas 90% had any pain and 67% had chest pain [33].

Type A dissections, proximally oriented with respect to the coronary arteries, comprise the majority of aortic dissection patients (62%); Type B dissections (distal location) comprise the balance of cases. The electrocardiographic changes that present with aortic dissection have an unclear pathologic basis. It makes sense that a proximal Type A dissection may involve the ostia of the coronary arteries and may actually disrupt blood flow through the coronaries causing a concomitant ST segment elevation AMI [34,35]. However, it is clear from several studies that ECG abnormalities may occur in both Type A and B dissections, although electrocardiographic changes do appear to be less common in Type B dissections [30–32]. The prevalence of electrocardiographic findings in aortic dissection is noted to be somewhere between 27 and 40%.

Pericarditis: Pericarditis may also be a significant ECG confounder in the chest pain patient. The ECG in pericarditis has a variable presentation, and some of the presentations are occasionally misinterpreted as STEMI with the inappropriate administration of fibrinolytics or unnecessary catheterization. Classically, a patient with pericarditis will have a progression of ECG findings through four different stages, including: ST segment elevation (Stage 1), resolution of ST segment elevation (Stage 2), T wave inversion (Stage 3), and normalization and return to baseline ECG (Stage 4). How-

ever, as with many other diagnostic findings in medicine, "classic" is rarely common. The time course of the progression of electrocardiographic changes is variable and unpredictable, and not all patients will manifest all four phases. While the patient with pericarditis alone may present with a normal ECG, up to 90% of acute myopericarditis patients will have abnormalities on their 12-lead ECG [36,37]. The key feature of the ECG in pericarditis is the diffuse nature of the electrocardiographic changes.

PR segment depression is also an indicator of pericardial disease, rather than AMI. This finding will be noted diffusely as well, with a similar time course and progression to ST segment elevation. Where ST segment elevation signifies ventricular inflammation, PR segment depression signifies atrial inflammation [37].

Case conclusions

The patient in Case 1 was found to have a STEMI of the anterolateral region (Figure 8.2), with evolution of the ECG from Figure 8.1 with prominent T waves to obvious ST segment elevation in Figure 8.2. The patient was taken for urgent PCI, where a complete occlusion of the LAD was found and successfully stented.

The patient in Case 2, diagnosed with pericarditis via the ECG (Figure 8.3), was noted to have a large pericardial effusion via echocardiography. The patient received a pericardial window.

The patient in Case 3, a diagnostic challenge for any clinician, underwent a computed tomography (CT) scan of the chest and abdomen due to his persistent tachycardia, his multiple complaints, and alcohol intoxication. Recall that the ECG (Figure 8.4) demonstrated sinus tachycardia with anterior T wave inversion. The CT of the abdomen was unremarkable, but the CT of the chest demonstrated multiple large pulmonary emboli. An echocardiogram showed normal global left ventricular function and right ventricular overload. Cardiac markers remained normal. The patient noted continued chest pain with some resolution of the electrocardiographic findings (Figures 8.5 and 8.6). A transthoracic echocardiogram performed later that day revealed a suggestion of aortic dissection, which was confirmed via transesophageal echocardiogram. The patient underwent uneventful operative repair and was discharged home 9 days later.

References

1 Anderson JL, Adams CD, Antman EM, *et al.* ACC/AHA 2007 Guidelines for the Management of Patients With Unstable Angina/Non ST-Elevation Myocardial Infarction. *J Am Coll Cardiol* 2007;**50**(7):e1–157.
2 Brown DW, Xie J, Mensah GA. Electrocardiographic Recording and Timeliness of Clinician Evaluation in the Emergency Department in Patients Presenting With Chest Pain. *Am J Cardiol* 2007;**99**(8):1115–8.

3 Diercks DB, Kirk JD, Lindsell CJ, *et al.* Door-to-ECG time in patients with chest pain presenting to the ED. *Am J Emerg Med* 2006;**24**(1):1–7.

4 Zalenski RJ, Rydman RJ, Sloan EP, *et al.* The emergency department electrocardiogram and hospital complications in myocardial infarction patients. *Acad Emerg Med* 1996;**3**(4):318–25.

5 Takakuwa KM, Shofer FS, Hollander JE. The influence of race and gender on time to initial electrocardiogram for patients with chest pain. *Acad Emerg Med* 2006;**13**(8):867–72.

6 Chang AM, Mumma B, Sease KL, *et al.* Gender bias in cardiovascular testing persists after adjustment for presenting characteristics and cardiac risk. *Acad Emerg Med* 2007;**14**(7):599–605.

7 Alpert JS, Thygesen K, Antman E, *et al.* Myocardial infarction redefined – a consensus document of The Joint European Society of Cardiology/American College of Cardiology committee for the redefinition of myocardial infarction: The Joint European Society of Cardiology/American College of Cardiology Committee. *J Am Coll Cardiol* 2000;**36**(3):959–69.

8 Conti A, Pieralli F, Sammicheli L, *et al.* Myocardial infarction redefined: Impact on case-load and outcome of patients with suspected acute coronary syndrome and nondiagnostic ECG at presentation. *Int J Cardiol* 2006;**111**(2):195–201.

9 Brady WJ, Perron AD, Martin ML, *et al.* Cause of ST segment abnormality in ED chest pain patients. *Am J Emerg Med* 2001;**19**(1):25–8.

10 Miller DH, Kligfield P, Schreiber TL, *et al.* Relationship of prior myocardial infarction to false-positive electrocardiographic diagnosis of acute injury in patients with chest pain. *Arch Intern Med* 1987;**147**(2):257–61.

11 Otto LA, Aufderheide TP. Evaluation of ST segment elevation criteria for the prehospital electrocardiographic diagnosis for acute myocardial infarction. *Ann Emerg Med* 1994;**23**(1):17–24.

12 Brady WJ, Perron AD, Syverud SA, *et al.* Reciprocal ST segment depression: impact on the electrocardiographic diagnosis of ST segment elevation acute myocardial infarction. *Am J Emerg Med* 2002;**20**(1):35–8.

13 Wang K, Asinger RW, Marriott HJL. ST-segment elevation in conditions other than acute myocardial infarction. *N Engl J Med* 2003;**349**(22):2128–35.

14 Brady WJ, Perron AD, Ullman EA, *et al.* Electrocardiographic ST segment elevation: A comparison of AMI and non-AMI ECG syndromes. *Am J Emerg Med* 2002;**20**(7):609–12.

15 Brady WJ, Chan TC, Pollack M. Electrocardiographic manifestations: patterns that confound the EKG diagnosis of acute myocardial infarction-left bundle branch block, ventricular paced rhythm, and left ventricular hypertrophy. *J Emerg Med* 2000;**18**(1):71–8.

16 Pollehn T, Brady WJ, Perron AD, *et al.* The electrocardiographic differential diagnosis of ST segment depression. *Emerg Med J* 2002;**19**(2):129–35.

17 Pollehn T, Brady WJ, Perron AD. Electrocardiographic ST segment depression. *Am J Emerg Med* 2001;**19**(4):303–9.

18 Savonitto S, Cohen MG, Politi A, *et al.* Extent of ST-segment depression and cardiac events in non-ST-segment elevation acute coronary syndromes. *Eur Heart J* 2005;**26**(20):2106–13.

19 Savonitto S, Ardissino D, Granger CB, *et al.* Prognostic value of the admission electrocardiogram in acute coronary syndromes. *JAMA* 1999;**281**(8):707–13.

20 Boden WE, Kleiger RE, Gibson RS, *et al.* Electrocardiographic evolution of posterior acute myocardial infarction: Importance of early precordial ST-segment depression. *Am J Cardiol* 1987;**59**(8):782–7.

21 Somers MP, Brady WJ, Perron AD, *et al.* The prominant T wave: electrocardiographic differential diagnosis. *Am J Emerg Med* 2002;**20**(3):243–51.

22 Hayden GE, Brady WJ, Perron AD, *et al.* Electrocardiographic T wave inversion: Differential diagnosis in the chest pain patient. *Am J Emerg Med* 2002;**20**(3):252–62.

23 de Zwaan C, Bar FW, Wellens HJ. Characteristic electrocardiographic pattern indicating a critical stenosis high in left anterior descending coronary artery in patients admitted because of impending myocardial infarction. *Am Heart J* 1982;**103**(4 Pt 2):730–6.

24 Antman EM, Anbe DT, Armstrong PW, *et al.* ACC/AHA Guidelines for the Management of Patients With ST-Elevation Myocardial Infarction: A Report of the American College of Cardiology/American Heart Association Task Force on Practice Guidelines (Committee to Revise the 1999 Guidelines for the Management of Patients With Acute Myocardial Infarction). *J Am Coll Cardiol* 2004;**44**(3):E1–E211.

25 Rodriguez RM, Tabas J. A meta-analysis of the Sgarbossa Criteria for acute myocardial infarction in the presence of left bundle branch block. *Acad Emerg Med* 2006;**13**(5 Suppl 1):S33-b-4.

26 Gula LJ, Dick A, Massel D. Diagnosing acute myocardial infarction in the setting of left bundle branch block: prevalence and observer variability from a large community study. *Coron Artery Dis* 2003;**14**(5):387–93.

27 Rouan GW, Lee TH, Cook EF, *et al.* Clinical characteristics and outcome of acute myocardial infarction in patients with initially normal or nonspecific electrocardiograms (a report from the Multicenter Chest Pain Study). *Am J Cardiol* 1989;**64**(18):1087–92.

28 McCarthy B, Wong J, Selker H, Detecting acute cardiac ischemia in the emergency department: a review of the literature. *J Gen Intern Med* 1990;**5**:365–73.

29 Slater D, Hlatky M, Mark D, *et al.* Outcome in suspected acute myocardial infarction with normal or minimally abnormal admission electrocardiographic findings. *Am J Cardiol* 1987;**60**:766–70.

30 Gibler BW, Young GP, Hedges JR, *et al.* Acute myocardial infarction in chest pain patients with nondiagnostic ECGs: Serial CK-MB sampling in the emergency department. *Ann Emerg Med* 1992;**21**(5):504–12.

31 Pope JH, Aufderheide TP, Ruthazer R, *et al.* Missed diagnoses of acute cardiac ischemia in the emergency department. *N Engl J Med* 2000;**342**(16):1163–70.

32 Brady WJ, Roberts D, Morris F. The nondiagnostic ECG in the chest pain patient: normal and nonspecific initial ECG presentations of acute MI. *Am J Emerg Med* 1999;**17**(4):394–7.

33 Chase M, Brown AM, Robey JL, *et al.* Prognostic value of symptoms during a normal or nonspecific electrocardiogram in emergency department patients with potential acute coronary syndrome. *Acad Emerg Med* 2006;**13**(10):1034–9.

34 Singer AJ, Brogan GX, Valentine SM, *et al.* Effect of duration from symptom onset on the negative predictive value of a normal ECG for exclusion of acute myocardial infarction. *Ann Emerg Med* 1997;**29**(5):575–9.

35 Brush JE, Brand DA, Acampora D, *et al.* Use of the initial

electrocardiogram to predict in-hospital complications of acute myocardial infarction. *N Engl J Med* 1985;**312**(18):1137–41.

36 Lee TH, Cook EF, Weisberg MC, *et al.* Impact of the availability of a prior electrocardiogram on the triage of the patient with acute chest pain. *J Gen Intern Med* 1990;**5**(5):381–8.

37 Fesmire FM, Percy RF, Wears RL, *et al.* Risk stratification according to the initial electrocardiogram in patients with suspected acute myocardial infarction. *Arch Intern Med* 1989;**149**(6):1294–7.

Chapter 9 | How should the ECG be used in the dyspneic patient?

Carl A. Germann
Maine Medical Center, Portland, ME, USA

Case presentations

Case 1: A 32-year-old male presents to the emergency department (ED) having had substernal chest pain and progressive dyspnea over the past 5 days. He has now noticed shortness of breath after walking up one flight of stairs. He has no medical history. He is appears well; vital signs are significant for a blood pressure of 110/60 mmHg, a pulse of 120 beats per minute (bpm), respirations of 26/minute, and oxygen saturation of 98%. The first and second heart sounds are normal, and there are no clicks or gallops. A superficial scratchy systolic sound is heard intermittently over the left lower sternal region. His examination is otherwise significant for a normal mental status and clear lung fields. The electrocardiogram (ECG) (Figure 9.1) is provided.

Case 2: A 65-year-old with chronic obstructive pulmonary disease (COPD) reports progressive exertional dyspnea over the last 6 months. He has been treated for his COPD. He states that his symptoms were relatively well controlled with these medications until recently, when his shortness of breath became progressively worse. He has no cough, fever chills, or diaphoresis. He has noticed weight loss with relative anorexia. He is anxious and has increased respiratory effort; vital signs are significant for a blood pressure of 145/80 mmHg, a pulse of 110 bpm, respirations of 30/minute, and oxygen saturation of 90%. His examination is otherwise significant for a normal mental status and scattered wheeze in the lungs bilaterally. The ECG (Figure 9.2) is provided.

The ECG in the patient with dyspnea

The differential diagnosis of dyspnea is quite broad, including diseases involving cardiac, pulmonary, neuromuscular, rheumatologic, hematologic, and psychiatric systems. A comprehensive medical history and physical examination

Critical Decisions in Emergency and Acute Care Electrocardiography, 1st edition. Edited by W.J. Brady and J.D. Truwit. © 2009 Blackwell Publishing, ISBN: 9781405159067

is the most important diagnostic tool in identifying an individual diagnosis. Often, on the basis of history alone, it may be possible to determine the cause of dyspnea. However, in up to one-third of patients with a chief complaint of dyspnea more than one etiology is present [1].

Initial diagnostic studies of patients presenting with dyspnea often include chest radiography and ECG. While the yield of routine ECG may be low, it can help identify unsuspected cardiac, coronary, or pericardial disease, or provide clues to non-cardiac causes of dyspnea such as pulmonary artery hypertension or pulmonary embolism. If the diagnosis of dyspnea remains unclear, additional testing should be pursued.

Cardiac causes of dyspnea

Any process challenging cardiac function and efficiency may impede pulmonary blood flow and produce dyspnea. Cardiac-related causes of dyspnea may be separated into electrical (dysrthymia), structural (cardiomyopathy, valvular disease), vascular, or pericardial disease. Overlap may exist regarding the etiology for a patient presenting with dyspnea.

Valvular heart disease: Aortic stenosis accounts for one-quarter of all patients with chronic valvular heart disease [2]. Signs and symptoms of disease usually progress as a result of increasing outflow obstruction. The cardiac response to this obstruction is left ventricular hypertrophy (LVH). Patients with aortic stenosis have been found to show evidence of LVH on ECG 85% of the time [3]. Left atrial enlargement also may be apparent in patients who have isolated aortic valve disease, demonstrated by an increase P wave duration (> 0.12 s) in lead II, or more commonly by a biphasic P wave in lead V1 with a negative terminal portion [3]. Additionally, a pseudo-infarction pattern of loss of R wave in the precordial leads is occasionally evident [3].

Aortic regurgitation occurs when the aortic valve leaflets fail to close effectively during diastole, allowing for the backward flow of blood from the aorta into the left ventricle [2]. Because of the increased volume, the left ventricle will typically dilate and hypertrophy over time. Associated left atrial dilatation and hypertrophy also may occur. Left axis deviation is typical of chronic aortic regurgitation and may be

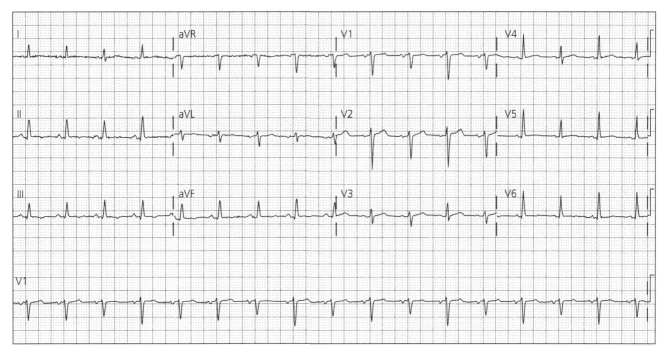

Figure 9.1 Electrical alternans. Note the intervening large QRS complex alternating with the smaller complexes – best seen in the rhythm strip.

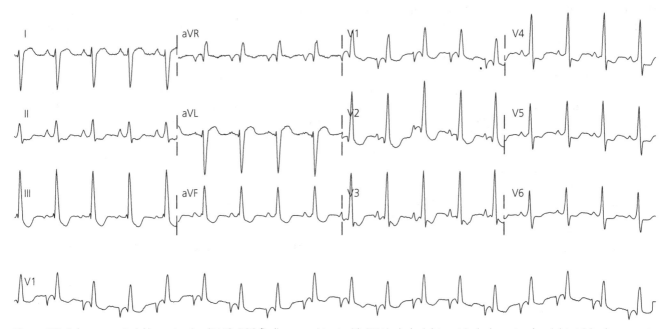

Figure 9.2 Pulmonary arterial hypertension (PAH). ECG findings consistent with PAH include right ventricular hypertrophy, right atrial enlargement, and right axis deviation.

recognized easily on ECG by a prominent R wave in lead I, deep S wave in lead III, and a biphasic RS complex in lead II with the amplitude of the S component greater than the amplitude of the R component [3,4]. Left ventricular hypertrophy with or without a strain pattern is also frequently present [3,5]. Late in the disease course, intraventricular conduction abnormalities may become manifest [3].

Mitral stenosis is most frequently due to rheumatic fever [2]. A diminished mitral valve orifice obstructs flow from the

left atrium into the left ventricle. The left atrium may dilate as the pulmonary venous pressures elevate and pulmonary compliance decreases. Progressive pulmonary hypertension may eventually lead to right-sided heart failure [2,3]. With mild disease, few changes are apparent in the ECG [3]. As left atrial pressure increases, left atrial enlargement is evidenced by P wave duration > 0.12 s in lead II, or shift of the P wave axis to between +45 and −30 degrees (Figure 9.1). Pulmonary hypertension may also cause right ventricular hypertrophy (RVH) as suggested by right axis deviation, tall R waves in the right precordium, deep S waves in the left precordium, and a slightly prolonged QRS duration. However, the unusual combination of left atrial enlargement and RVH on ECG should promote consideration of advanced mitral stenosis [6]. Longstanding mitral stenosis is associated with atrial arrhythmias, such as atrial fibrillation and flutter, premature atrial contractions, and tachydysrhythmias, caused by the dilatation, fibrosis, and disorganization of muscular architecture of the left atrium [3,7].

Hypertrophic cardiomyopathy: Hypertrophic cardiomyopathy (HCM) is a genetic disorder affecting the cardiac sarcomere and is seen in 1 of every 500 adults in the general population [8]. Many patients with HCM remain asymptomatic; however, this disorder can cause dyspnea, exercise intolerance, angina, syncope, and sudden death. These symptoms occur as the hypertrophied basal septum partially blocks the outflow tract of the left ventricle creating a functional obstruction [8,9].

The ECG is abnormal in approximately 90% of patients with HCM [9]. The most common ECG changes include increased QRS complex voltage, QRS complex widening, Q waves, and ST segment/T wave changes consistent with ventricular hypertrophy (Figure 9.2) [9]. In HCM, giant T wave inversions are typical as well [9].

The most common cause of sudden cardiac death in young athletes is HCM [8]. In these younger patients, the ECG findings are more specific for the diagnosis and should be cause for concern especially in those with a history of unexplained syncope or a family history of sudden cardiac death [10]. In the older patient, the ECG must be differentiated from those occurring in chronic hypertension, acute coronary syndrome, ischemic heart disease, and various conduction abnormalities [9].

Perhaps the most specific electrocardiographic finding in young patients with HCM is the appearance of Q waves in leads II, III, aVF, V5, and V6 in the early teenage years [11]. A recent study suggests that this finding is the earliest electrocardiographic manifestation of certain patients with HCM, preceding both wall hypertrophy and other echocardiographic abnormalities [12]. This LVH pattern increased with age, whereas conduction abnormalities were primarily seen after age 40 years [12]. The appearance of these abnormal Q waves in the teens studied had a reported sensitivity of 67%, specificity of 100%, positive-predictive value of 100%, and negative-predictive value of 78% for the diagnosis of HCM [12].

Pericardial disease: Normally, the pericardial space contains up to 50 mL of pericardial fluid. Accumulation of a greater amount of transudate, exudate, or blood in the space produces an effusion. Pericardial effusions are reported to be associated in patients presenting with heart failure, valvular disease, and myocardial infarction with respective rates of 14%, 21%, and 15% [13].

As intrapericardial volume and pressure rises, venous pressures increase to maintain cardiac filling and prevent collapse of the cardiac chambers. Cardiac tamponade is characterized by an equal elevation of atrial and pericardial pressures, an exaggerated inspiratory decrease in arterial systolic pressure (pulsus paradoxus), and arterial hypotension. Mild tamponade may be asymptomatic, while moderate tamponade can produce precordial discomfort and dyspnea. Unrelieved tamponade becomes fatal when venous return cannot increase to equal the pericardial pressure and maintain circulation.

The two ECG findings classically associated with pericardial effusion and tamponade are low voltage and electrical alternans. The generally accepted ECG requirements for low voltage are: QRS amplitude < 0.5 mV (5 mm) in all limb leads and < 1.0 mV (10 mm) in the precordial leads (P,Q,R,S). Kudo and colleagues describe low voltage on ECG in only 26% of patients who had asymptomatic pericardial effusion [14]. Larger effusions likely have a higher incidence of low voltage [14,15]. As pericardial effusion and tamponade frequently are associated with pericarditis, additional ECG findings of pericarditis also may be evident [14].

Electrical alternans occurs in the setting of large pericardial effusions or tamponade (Figure 9.3). Usually, the complexes progress between electrical axes over a few cardiac cycles, rather than true alternans that would vary beat to beat [7]. This variability in the complexes occurs as the position of the heart changes during its cycle in a swinging or rotational manner within the fluid-filled sac [16].

The ECG is by no means a confirmatory study and echocardiography remains the procedure of choice for the diagnosis of pericardial effusion. The use of echocardiography for the evaluation of all patients with suspected pericardial disease was given a class I recommendation by a 2003 task force of the American College of Cardiology, the American Heart Association, and the American Society of Echocardiography [17].

Pulmonary causes of dyspnea

Pulmonary arterial hypertension: Pulmonary arterial hypertension (PAH) is often defined as a resting mean pulmonary artery pressure (PAP) greater than 20 mmHg. Pulmonary arterial hypertension may be idiopathic, familial, or relate to specific etiologies, such as collagen vascular disease or a toxic insult. Idiopathic PAH is rare, and most prevalent in young adults who are genetically predisposed to the disorder. Elevated PAP due to pulmonary disorders is termed cor pulmonale. Primary causes of cor pulmonale include COPD, pulmonary fibrosis, interstitial lung disease, pulmonary embolism, myasthenia gravis, Guillian-Barré syndrome, primary central hypoventilation, and sleep apnea syndromes.

The diagnosis of PAH can be challenging as symptoms may be non-specific and invasive testing is required to confirm

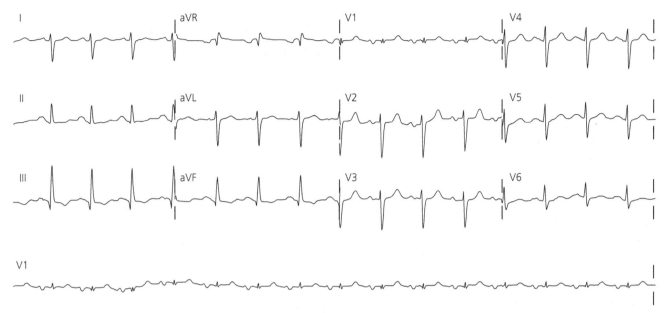

Figure 9.3 Left atrial enlargement due to mitral stenosis. This finding is demonstrated by P wave duration greater than 0.12 s in lead II.

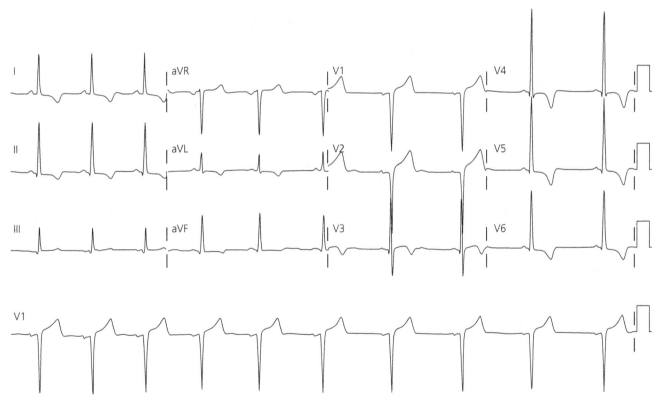

Figure 9.4 Hypertrophic cardiomyopathy. This ECG contains increased QRS voltage with ST segment/T wave changes consistent with ventricular hypertrophy.

the diagnosis. Likewise, mild and moderate PAH can exist for years without becoming clinically evident. In a study of 187 patients with PAH, dyspnea was the most common initial complaint (60%), followed by fatigue (19%), syncope (8%), chest pain (7%), near syncope (5%), palpitations (5%), and

leg edema (3%) [18]. The diagnosis is confirmed by right, and often concomitant left, heart catheterization.

Electrocardiography provides diagnostic and prognostic information regarding this diagnosis (Figure 9.4). These findings are most often attributed to the chronic effects of

PAH leading to increased right ventricular workload and/or right ventricular failure. The study of 187 patients mentioned previously found RVH and right axis deviation on ECG 87% and 79% of the time, respectively [18]. Pulmonary arterial hypertension-associated RVH may demonstrate a tall R wave and a small S wave (R/S > 1) in lead V1, a large S wave and a small R wave (R/S < 1) in lead V5 or V6, a qR complex in V1, or a rSR pattern in V1 [19,20].

The magnitude and morbidity of PAH may be implied by certain ECG findings. As the left ventricular mass normally is three times that of the right ventricle, a doubling or tripling of right ventricular mass is required to pull the electrical forces anteriorly and to the right to produce recognizable ECG changes [21]. In one study of 47 patients with PAH, the amplitude of the R wave in V1 of more than 1.2 mV or an R/S in V1 of greater than seven indicated a pulmonary artery systolic pressure of more than 90 mmHg with a sensitivity or 94% and specificity of 47% [22]. The presence of right atrial enlargement in PAH has been associated with a 2.8-fold greater risk of death over a 6-year period, while RVH correlated with a 4.3-fold greater risk of death [23]. Another retrospective study of patients with PAH found decreased survival was associated with greater degrees of right axis deviation and S1Q3 pattern [24].

The ECG has a high degree of sensitivity for the detection of abnormalities in symptomatic patients who have PAH [25]. However, ECG lacks the sensitivity and specificity to be an effective screening study [18,19,20,26]. For example, one study of 61 patients found 8 who had normal ECGs despite severe PAH by catheterization [20].

Pneumothorax: Pneumothorax is a collapse of the lung due to air within the pleural space. Symptoms may be based upon the degree and location of collapse, as well as the presence of tension. An ECG is often obtained in these patients as chest pain is almost always present. Proposed mechanisms for ECG findings of pneumothorax include the interposition of air between the heart and ECG electrodes, interposition of the collapsed lung between the heart and the ECG electrodes, and alteration in cardiac position [21]. These ECG changes should resolve with re-expansion of the lung.

While a pneumothorax cannot be diagnosed by ECG, a right and left pneumothorax may cause various changes on ECG [27,28,29]. The findings in a left pneumothorax include decreased voltage in the precordial leads and QRS axis shift. The ECG findings in right pneumothorax are often more ambiguous and less specific, but may also include a reduced voltage and QRS axis changes [27,28]. Electrocardiogram findings during pneumothorax may also include ST segment changes suggestive of cardiac ischemia or infarction, electrical alternans, and precordial T wave inversions. The extent of changes may also correlate with the size of the pneumothorax and whether tension is present [30]. However, it is important to note that any ST segment and T wave changes during this injury are not necessarily due to cardiac ischemia.

Other non-cardiac causes of dyspnea

Sarcoidosis: Sarcoidosis is a systemic granulomatous disease that results in diffuse fibrotic changes causing end-organ damage. The etiology is unknown; however, virtually any organ can be involved. Pulmonary involvement occurs in 90% of patients, whereas cardiac involvement may occur in 27% of patients with sarcoidosis [31]. A wide range of ECG findings may be present depending on the degree of pulmonary disease and whether there is co-existing cardiac involvement.

ECG abnormalities are likely due to the pulmonary fibrosis, cor pulmonale, and/or granulomatous changes of the heart wall. Electrocardiogram findings include varying degrees of atrioventricular block, bundle branch block, and ventricular arrhythmias. [32] Therapy with steroids may halt progression of left ventricular dysfunction, whereas arrhythmias warrant implantation of a cardioverter-defibrillator device [21].

Case conclusions

Case 1 represents a large pericardial effusion. This patient's ECG (Figure 9.1) demonstrates electrical alternans. Remember, electrical alternans occurs in a minority of patients with pericardial effusion. Pericardiocentesis was performed and the patient's symptoms resolved; no etiology was identified as the cause of effusion. The effusion may be due to an infectious agent. Viral infections, especially coxsackie B virus and echovirus 8, may cause pericarditis with pericardial effusion.

The patient in Case 2 presents with ECG findings suggestive of cor pulmonale related to COPD. His ECG (Figure 9.2) findings consistent with PAH include evidence of RVH, right atrial enlargement, and right axis deviation. Right heart and pulmonary artery catheterization confirmed the diagnosis of PAH in this patient.

References

1 Michelson E, Hollrah S. Evaluation of the patient with shortness of breath: an evidence based approach. *Emerg Med Clin North Am* 1999;**17**:221–37.

2 Braunwald E. Valvular heart disease. In: Wilson JD, Braunwald E, Isselbacher KJ, *et al.* editors. *Harrison's Principles of Internal Medicine*. 12th edition. New York: McGraw-Hill, 1991: 938–52.

3 Braunwald E. Valvular heart disease. In: Braunwald E, Zipes DP, Libby P, editors. *Heart Disease: a Textbook of Cardiovascular Medicine*. 6th edition. Philadelphia: WB Saunders, 2001:1643–722.

4 Goldberger AL. Electrical axis and axis deviation. In: Goldberger AL, editor. Clinical Electrocardiography: a Simplified Approach. 6th edition. St. Louis: Mosby, 1999: 44–55.

5 Surawicz B, Knilans T. Diseases of the heart and lungs. In: Surawicz B, Knilans T, editors. *Chou's Electrocardiography in Clinical Practice*. Philadelphia: WB Saunders, 2001: 256–309.

6 Surawicz B, Knilans T. Ventricular enlargement. In: Surawicz B, Knilans T, editors. *Chou's Electrocardiography in Clinical Practice.* Philadelphia: WB Saunders, 2001: 44–74.

7 Demangone D. ECG Manifestations: Noncoronary Heart Disease. *Emerg Med Clin N Am* 2006;**24**:113–31.

8 Nishimura RA, Holmes DR, Jr. Hypertrophic obstructive cardiomyopathy. *N Engl J Med* 2004;**350**:1320–7.

9 Popjes ED, Sutton MSJ. Hypertrophic cardiomyopathy: pathophysiology, diagnosis, and treatment (The heart). *Geriatrics* 2003; **58**(3):41–50.

10 Frenneaux MP. Assessing the risk of sudden cardiac death in a patient with hypertrophic cardiomyopathy. *Heart* 2004;**90**:570–5.

11 Dovalyuk J, Holstege CP, Mattu A, *et al.* The electrocardiogram in the patient with syncope. *Am J Emerg Med* 2007;**25**:688–701.

12 Shimizu M, Ino H, Yamaguchi M, *et al.* Chronological electrocardiographic changes in patients with hypertrophic cardiomyopathy associated with cardiac troponin I mutation. *Am Heart J* 2002;**143**(2):289–93.

13 Maisch B. Pericardial diseases, with a focus on etiology, pathogenesis, pathophysiology, new diagnostic imaging methods, and treatment. *Curr Opin Cardiol* 1994;**9**:379–88.

14 Kudo Y, Yamasaki F, Doi T, *et al.* Clinical significance of low voltage in asymptomatic patients with pericardial effusion free of heart disease. *Chest* 2003;**124**:2064–7.

15 Eisenberg MJ, de Romeral LM, Heidenreich PA, *et al.* The diagnosis of pericardial effusion and cardiac tamponade by 12 lead ECG. *Chest* 1996;**110**:318–24.

16 Surawicz B, Knilans T. Pericarditis and cardiac surgery. In: Surawicz B, Knilans T, editors. *Chou's Electrocardiography in Clinical Practice.* Philadelphia: WB Saunders, 2001: 239–55.

17 Cheitlen MD, Armstrong WF, Aurigemma GP, *et al.* ACC/AHA/ASE 2003 Guideline Update for the Clinical Application of Echocardiography: Summary article. A report of the American College of Cardiology/American Heart Association Task Force on Practice Guidelines (ACC/AHA/ASE Committee to Update the 1997 Guidelines for the Clinical Application of Echocardiography). *J Am Soc Echocardiogr* 2003;**16**:1091–110.

18 Rich S, Dantzker DR, Ayres SM, *et al.* Primary pulmonary hypertension. A national prospective study. *Ann Intern Med* 1987; **107**(2):216–23.

19 McGoon M, Gutterman D, Steen V, *et al.* Screening, early detection, and diagnosis of pulmonary arterial hypertension. ACCP evidence-based clinical practice guidelines. *Chest* 2004;**126**(1): 14S–34S.

20 Ahern GS, Tapson VF, Rebetz A, *et al.* Electrocardiography to define clinical status of primary pulmonary hypertension and pulmonary arterial hypertension secondary to collagen vascular disease. *Chest* 2002;**122**(2):524–7.

21 Pollack ML. ECG Manifestations of Selected Extracardiac Diseases. *Emerg Med Clin N Am* 2006;**24**:133–43.

22 Kanemoto N. Electrocardiographic and hemodynamic correlations in primary pulmonary hypertension. *Angiology* 1988;**39**(9): 781–7.

23 Bossone E, Pacioco G, Iarussi D, *et al.* The role prognostic role of the ECG in primary pulmonary hypertension. *Chest* 2002;**121**(2): 513–8.

24 Kanemoto N. Electrocardiogram in primary pulmonary hypertension. *Eur J Cardiol* 1980;**12**:181–93.

25 Bossone E, Buter G, Bodini BD, *et al.* The interpretation of the electrocardiogram in patients with pulmonary hypertension: the need for clinical correlation. *Ital Heart J* 2003;**4**:850–4.

26 Alegro S, Morrison D, Ovitt T, *et al.* Noninvasive detection of pulmonary hypertension. *Clin Cardiol* 1984;**7**:148–56.

27 Alikhan M, Biddison JH. Electrocardiographic changes with right-sided pneumothorax. *South Med J* 1998;**91**:677–80.

28 Harrington RA, McNeil BK. Pneumothorax. In: Chan TC, Brady W, Harrigan R, Ornato J, Rosen P, editors. *ECG in Emergency Medicine and Acute Care.* Philadelphia: Elsevier Mosby, 2005: 300–2.

29 Ortego-Carnicer J, Ruiz-Lorenzo F, Zarca MA, *et al.* Electrocardiographic changes in occult pneumothorax. *Resuscitation* 2002;**52**:306–7.

30 Strizik B, Forman R. New ECG changes associated with tension pneumothorax: a case report. *Chest* 1999;**115**:1742–4.

31 Shammas RL, Movahed A. Sarcoidosis of the heart. *Clin Cardiol* 1993;**16**:462–72.

32 Syed J, Myers R. Sarcoid heart disease. *Can J Cardiol* 2004;**20**: 89–93.

Chapter 10 | How should the ECG be used in the patient with altered mentation?

Tamas R. Peredy
Maine Medical Center, Portland, ME, USA

Case presentations

Case 1: A 17-year-old male presents via police transport for agitation that began hours ago. The patient is unable to provide an account of recent events but his girlfriend states that he may have ingested some seeds in an effort "to get high." Vital signs are normal except for a regular tachycardia of 125 beats per minute (bpm). The patient is calm but delirious with flushed, dry skin and large pupils. The exam also reveals some spontaneous jerky movements and a bladder filled with over 600 mL of urine. The initial electrocardiogram (ECG) reveals a sinus tachycardia (Figure 10.1).

Case 2: A 68-year-old taxi driver becomes dizzy while driving his cab. He has a history of hypertension but is on no medication. There is no history of prior central nervous system (CNS) or cardiovascular adverse health events. On physical examination, vital signs are conspicuous for hypertension (195/95) and bradycardia (45 bpm); further examination reveals rales in the lung bases and a non-focal neurological examination. A 12-lead ECG demonstrates sinus bradycardia with borderline first-degree atrioventricular (AV) block (Figure 10.2).

The ECG in the patient with altered mental status

Altered mental status (AMS) is a non-specific descriptor of cognitive dysfunction and/or level of awareness produced by a broad range of agents and conditions occurring in up to 10% of all emergency department (ED) patients and 30% in elderly ED patients [1,2]. Patients with diminished compensatory reserve such as the elderly and chronically infirm are at increased likelihood to present with AMS. In patients over 85 years of age, an initial delirium may be the presenting

complaint in up to 20% of individuals with acute myocardial infarction (AMI), rather than more standard focused symptoms of chest pain and shortness of breath. Innumerable events such as syncope, seizure, and intoxication can transiently affect mental status and are discussed elsewhere.

Altered mental status is often categorized as either changes of alertness, thought processing or both. The simple AVPU scale (single letter score with A > V > P > U; Alert, responsive to Voice, responsive to Pain, Unresponsive) avoids imprecise terms such as stupor or lethargy, and provides clinicians with rough benchmarks to follow serially. The reduced ability to understand one's self, time, place, and circumstance is commonly referred to as confusion or delirium. Alterations in motor activity that may accompany AMS manifest as agitation, withdrawal, or both fluctuating over time. Broad diagnostic possibilities coupled with difficulty in obtaining health information often force a clinician to perform large batteries of tests. Surrogate sources of information such as care-givers, family and friends, co-workers and emergency medical services (EMS) provide potentially important clues. Ideally, old records should contain recent events resulting in heathcare contacts, lists of chronic conditions, medications, current living conditions, and any relevant social habits and occupational experiences. The time course, prior similar events, and any accompanying signs and symptoms may help narrow the diagnostic possibilities and allow the clinician to tailor a more specific work-up. The ECG is often included in this broad work-up along with evaluation for primary cardiac problems.

While all disease processes can eventually manifest as brain dysfunction, the most common categories involved in AMS are neurologic, toxicologic, traumatic, and infectious [1]. Focal neurologic abnormalities, such as stroke, most often result in remarkably well-preserved overall cognitive function.

During the initial contact the clinician should confirm the presence of adequate tissue oxygen, systemic perfusion, and serum glucose. The application of continuous cardiac monitoring can quickly aid in the detection of a rhythm disturbance that may impact brain perfusion. Efforts to immediately correct non-perfusing rhythm disturbances should be performed before continuing with the diagnostic

Critical Decisions in Emergency and Acute Care Electrocardiography, 1st edition. Edited by W.J. Brady and J.D. Truwit. © 2009 Blackwell Publishing. ISBN: 9781405159067

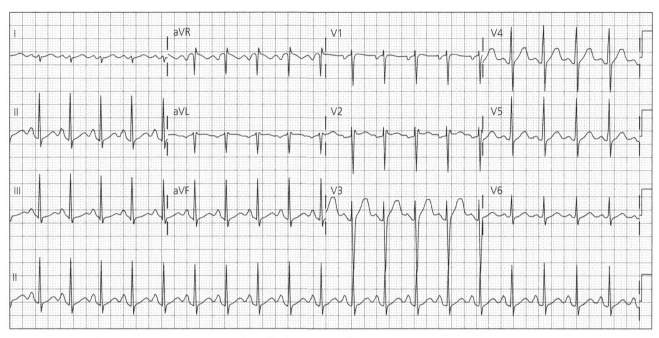

Figure 10.1 ECG of patient 1 demonstrates sinus tachycardia characteristic of anti-cholinergic syndrome.

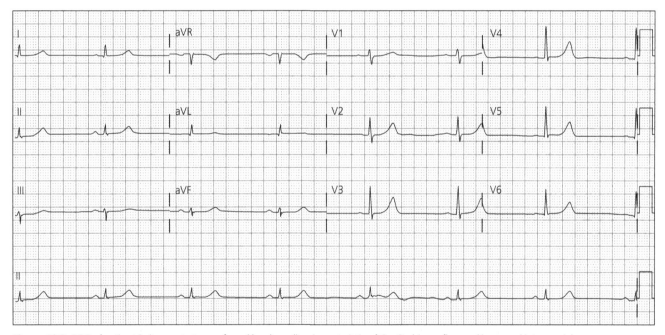

Figure 10.2 ECG of patient 2 demonstrates profound bradycardia, characteristic of the Cushing reflex, and increased intracranial pressure.

evaluation. Monitor display and rhythm strip printout generally obviates the need for a 12-lead ECG during the initial resuscitation. Entirely normal rhythm strips coupled with a normal cardiopulmonary examination should steer the clinician away from a primary cardiorespiratory problem in unresponsive patients. Electrocardiogram abnormalities can, however, provide some insight into causes of subtle or gradual behavioral changes – with both cardiovascular and non-cardiovascular etiologies.

The standard 12-lead ECG is one of a battery of ED tests, is widely available, has rapid turnaround, is non-invasive, and is inexpensive; it can assist in the possible identification of AMS etiology. In isolation, the ECG is rarely able to specifically identify the cause of AMS. Yet, the ECG, when interpreted within the context of the clinical presentation, can suggest the diagnosis or at least provide important clues leading to the diagnosis. Bradycardia, tachycardia, or conduction abnormalities can affect CNS perfusion, thus impacting the mental status. QRS complex widening, for example, may be a component of a toxidrome, impaired impulse conduction from ischemia, or an unrelated pre-existing condition. Various morphologic issues, ranging from the predominant R' wave in leads aVr (tricyclic anti-depressant poisoning) to prolonged QT interval (long QT syndrome status post VT arrest), can suggest the diagnosis. Prior ECGs and serial repeat tracings can further narrow the diagnostic possibilities.

At times it may not be possible to obtain quality tracings due to unco-operativeness in the AMS patient. Improper lead placement or inadequate skin contact may hamper quality in the AMS patient with gross chemical contamination, thoracic burns, or profuse sweating. Electrolyte disturbances may (calcium) or may not (magnesium, potassium) typically cause CNS dysfunction and produce electrocardiographic changes.

The ECG and coma

While all organ systems are subject to dysfunction with hypoxia, the brain is amongst the most oxygen-dependent end-organ; when deprived of adequate oxygen, numerous corrective reflexes are activated. Acute hypoxia produces a catecholamine surge that leads to increased chronotropy, dromotropy, and inotropy, which is overwhelmed or exhausted if hypoxemia worsens or continues. Tachycardia is also caused by direct sympathetic stimuli to the sinoatrial (SA) node – cardiac "fight or flight" response. The ventricular myocardium becomes increasingly electrically irritable during anaerobic conditions. Persistently high CNS catecholamine output states lead to a lower threshold for development of dysrhythmia and myocardial necrosis even in the absence of significant coronary atherosclerotic disease.

The ECG and primary CNS disorders

Changes on the ECG during acute CNS events such as sub-arachnoid hemorrhage (SAH) have been appreciated for nearly a century [3]. Rhythm disturbances are seen in more than 75% of stroke patients, most commonly atrial fibrillation (up to one-third), and are frequently thought to be a source of thromboemboli [4,5]. While some of morphologic electrocardiographic changes rarely may mimic AMI, a large proportion of stroke victims have non-specific changes of questionable clinical importance [6]. ST segment elevation can be seen in both cardiac (infarction, vasospasm, aneurysm, and myocarditis) and non-cardiac (pulmonary embolism [PE] hypothermia, and acute CNS pathology) conditions [6]. The therapeutic implications are disastrous if the CNS hemorrhage patient is incorrectly diagnosed with ST elevation myocardial infarction (STEMI) and managed with fibrinolysis [6]. The incidence of a simultaneous CNS event

and myocardial infarction is reported to be up to 5–10%, particularly among the elderly [4].

Neurocardiac reflexes can produce dramatic electrocardiographic changes if autonomic centers are affected [1]. Persistent sympathetic and parasympathetic outflow has been demonstrated to cause cellular injury (contraction band necrosis) despite the absence of acute coronary thrombus or significant wall narrowing [7]. These dramatic repolarization abnormalities suggest a poor prognosis.

The incidence of non-specific electrocardiographic changes is high and varies with acute brain pathology [8]. In order of frequency (from most to least frequent), distinctive electrocardiographic changes include prolonged QT interval (27%), U waves (9%), ischemic morphology (5%), and deeply inverted T waves (3%, the so-called CNS T waves) [7,8]. Central nervous system T waves are large, diffuse, deeply asymmetric inversions [7]. Other causes of giant inverted T waves include Wellens' syndrome, AMI, hypertrophic cardiomyopathy, Stokes-Adams attack, right heart strain, and sympathomimetic excess [9]. The classic neurological Cushing reflex is apnea, hypertension, and a conspicuous bradycardia (Figure 10.2) in response to elevated intracranial pressure from compressive forces upon the brainstem [7,10]. In addition to the bradycardia, other electrocardiographic findings include prolonged QT and U waves.

A predominance of sympathetic influence can sometimes produce dramatic electrocardiographic repolarization abnormalities, including tall upright T waves, and global deep T wave inversions [7]. Typically, these electrocardiographic abnormalities are globally distributed, less often they occur along a discrete vascular territory. Other less common findings include PR desegment pression, Q waves, ventricular repolarization abnormalities, prolongation of the QT interval and the presence of U waves [2,4,11]. These findings can occur with or without myocardial damage. It is likely that electrocardiographic abnormalities are most noticeable shortly after the acute event, but may normalize over time.

Neurologic conditions that can cause inverted T waves include most commonly intracranial hemorrhage. Electrocardiographic findings associated with poor outcomes in patients with acute CNS events include rhythm disturbances, conduction abnormalities, ST segment elevation, prolonged QT interval, and increased QT dispersion (wider variation in the length of the QT interval among the 12 leads) [12]. The significance of these changes includes a poor overall prognosis, as well as an increased risk for simultaneous myocardial injury. Dysrhythmias associated with acute CNS pathology include sinus bradycardia, premature ventricular contractions (PVCs), atrial fibrillation, left bundle branch block (LBBB), nodal rhythms, and heart block [3]. Central nervous system events and related pathology associated with electrocardiographic changes include seizures, cerebral tumors, intracranial hemorrhage, cerebral contusion, thromboembolic stroke, brain injury, meningeoencephalitis, intracranial and carotid surgery, and myelography [13,14].

The ECG in toxic delirium

A multitude of agents can simultaneously impact the heart and CNS causing AMS and electrocardiographic abnormalities. These potential toxins can be divided into those with direct effects on cardiac impulse conduction and muscle function, and those whose indirect effects impact global function via hypoxia, hypoglycemia, and shock.

Chemical agents may impact nerve conduction via sodium-potassium exchange pump inhibition and sodium, calcium, and potassium channel blockade. Signal initiation at the SA node is governed by the slow influx of calcium, but is influenced directly via parasympathetic and sympathetic nerve fibers as well as circulating hormones. The rapid influx of current from sodium channel opening results in speedy impulse propagation and synchronous muscular contraction. Retardation of sodium influx results in slower or asynchronous depolarization, widened depolarization interval and predisposition to arrhythmia. Generally, calcium and potassium channel blockade do not cause AMS until hypotension or dysrhythmia occurs. Lipophilic beta-blockers (propranolol) cause sedation in overdose (OD) likely from central adrenergic antagonism. Digoxin is the prototypical sodium-potassium exchange pump blocker with a narrow therapeutic to toxic window. In excess, digoxin causes a vagotonic effect, intracellular hypercalcemia resulting in bradydysrhythmias with variable blocks, and ectopy (delayed after depolarizations, DADs). Digoxin above therapeutic target levels will cause delirium, visual apparitions, and coma in up to 65% of OD patients [15].

Opioid analgesics are amongst the most commonly used and abused drugs. The well-known opioid toxidrome includes a cardiovascular depressant effect. Opioids modulate circulating catecholamines and central sympathetic outflow, reducing tachycardia and autonomic vasomotor tone. Respiratory failure from bradypnea results in progressive myocardial acidosis, irritability, and cardiorespiratory arrest with progressive bradycardia. Several opioids possess sodium channel blockade (propxyphene) with wide QRS complex rhythms; heroin can be mixed or "cut" with cardioactive adulterants such as lidocaine (sodium blockade) or clenbuterol (beta-agonism) with both wide QRS complex and tachycardic rhythms.

While opioids are widely abused, stimulants are a far more likely cause of cardiac complications requiring medical attention. Stimulants (e.g. amphetamines) induce endogenous catecholamine release or inhibit its recycling resulting in sympathomimetic CNS hypervigilance, euphoria, many forms of tachycardia, and ventricular ectopy. Cocaine has the greatest risk of fatal complication because, in addition to its adrenergic properties, it is also atherogenic (serotonergic) and arrhythmogenic (sodium channel blockade). Volatile hydrocarbons abused by huffing sensitize the myocardium to the effects of catecholamines, predisposing the heart to tachydysrhythmias and sudden death. Methylxanthines (theophylline, caffeine) are adenosine antagonists and nonspecific beta-agonists that predispose to ventricular tachydysrhythmias and seizures.

Central nervous system depressants, such as benzodiazepines, are rarely acutely deleterious to the heart. Indeed, benzodiazepines are the drug of choice in the management of stimulant or chloroquine cardiotoxicity, acting to reduce central sympathetic outflow and ventricular irritability. Ethanol in massive overdose can cause hypotension and reflex tachycardia from fluid losses: vomiting, dieresis, and vasodilatation. Chronically, ethanol is a myotoxin and is associated with higher long-term cardiovascular mortality. Central nervous system depressant withdrawal states can cause rebound autonomic hyperreactivity resulting in tremor, agitation, and seizure, but are rarely associated with cardiac effects beyond tachycardia. These various sedative agents can produce both tachycardia, due to the vasodilation and hypoperfusion, and bradycardia resulting from hypoxia.

Psychotropic medications used to treat depression, mood lability and psychosis can have obvious therapeutic behavioral effects but also potential adverse cardiac side effects. Tricyclic anti-depressants cause anti-cholinergic and alpha-antagonism reflex-induced tachycardia, sodium channel blockade and rightward-deviated vector forces, in addition to profound anti-histaminic sedation. Serotonin reuptake inhibitors can cause QT interval prolongation (citalopram) but are rarely associated with dysrhythmias. Anti-convulsants, often used for mood stabilization, possess sodium channel blockade (phenytoin, carbamazepine, oxcarbazepine). Lithium can cause bradycardia and mimics mild hypokalemia with depressed ST segments and T wave flattening.

Environmental toxins can cause electrocardiographic changes in addition to CNS pathology. Heavy metals are associated with progressive CNS injury particularly early in development. Arsenic, in particular, is also associated with ventricular dysrhythmias, QTc prolongation, ST segment changes, and T wave flattening. Direct myotoxins rarely cause CNS abnormalities until cardiac output is affected.

Case conclusions

The patient in Case 1 continued to struggle against physical restraints. The ECG (Figure 10.1) demonstrates sinus tachycardia characteristic of anti-cholinergic syndrome. The patient was given 2 mg of physostigmine with gradual improvement in his sensorium and temporary resolution of his toxidrome. He was watched overnight in the intensive care area. He was discharged home with resolution of his delirium despite lingering tachycardia.

In Case 2, a computed tomography (CT) scan revealed a large posterior fossa hemorrhage. The ECG (Figure 10.2) demonstrated profound bradycardia, characteristic of the Cushing reflex, and increased intracranial pressure. The patient underwent emergent neurosurgical decompression. The bradycardia resolved over several days postoperatively.

References

1 Kanich W, Brady WJ, Huff JS, *et al.* Altered mental status: Evaluation and etiology in the ED. *Am J Emerg Med* 2002;**20**:613–7.

2 Pickard T. Getting past the obvious in an ED case of altered mental status and ECG changes. *JAAPA* 2000;**13**:54–8.

3 Vaisrub S. Editorial: Brain and heart – the automatic connection. *JAMA* 1975;**234**:959.

4 Valeriano J, Elson J. Electrocardiographic changes in central nervous system disease. *Neurologic Clinics* 1993;**11**:257–72.

5 Van Mieghem C, Sabbe M, Knockaert D. The clinical value of the ECG in noncardiac conditions. *Chest* 2004;**125**:1561–76.

6 de Marchena E, Pittaluga JM, Ferreira AC, *et al.* Subarachnoid hemorrhage simulating myocardial infarction. *Cathet Cardiovasc Diag* 1996;**37**:170–3.

7 Perron AD, Brady WJ. Electrocardiographic manifestations of CNS events. *Am J Emerg Med* 2000;**18**:715–20.

8 Povoa R, Cavichio L, de Almeida AL, *et al.* Electrocardiographic abnormalities in neurological diseases. *Arquiv Brasil Cardiol* 2003; **80**:351–8.

9 Velasquez EM, Glancy DL. ECG of the month global t-wave inversion in a woman with altered mental status. Cerebrovascular accident. *J La State Med Soc* 2005;**157**:73–4.

10 Kalmar AF, Van Aken J, Caemaert J, *et al.* Value of Cushing reflex as warning sign for brain ischaemia during neuroendoscopy. *Brit J Anaesth* 2005;**94**:791–9.

11 Cohen JA, Abraham E. Neurogenic pulmonary edema: A sequella of non-hemorrhagic cerebrovascular accidents. *Angiology* 1976;**27**:280–92.

12 Huang CH, Chen WJ, Chang WT, *et al.* Qtc dispersion as a prognostic factor in intracerebral hemorrhage. *Am J Emerg Med* 2004;**22**:141–4.

13 Duren R, Wellens HJ. [ECG changes in intracranial disorders]. *Nederlands Tijdschrift voor Geneeskunde* 1975;**119**:1628–31.

14 Spencer RG, Cox TS, Kaplan PW. Global t-wave inversion associated with nonconvulsive status epilepticus. *Ann Int Med* 1998;**129**:163–4.

15 Smith H, Janz TG, Erker M. Digoxin toxicity presenting as altered mental status in a patient with severe chronic obstructive lung disease. *Heart Lung* 1992;**21**:78–80.

Chapter 11 | How should the ECG be used in the patient during and following cardiac arrest?

John R. Saucier
University of Vermont, College of Medicine, Burlington, VT, USA

Case presentations

Case 1: A 71-year-old white male without any known cardiac history experiences shortness of breath at home. Emergency medical services (EMS) finds a minimally responsive patient in a wide complex tachycardia with a heart rate of 140 beats per minute (bpm) and a blood pressure of 80 mmHg systolic. They attempt cardioversion but the patient develops ventricular fibrillation (VF). During the 25-min transport to the emergency department (ED) the patient remains in persistent VF despite appropriate therapy. In the ED, the initial electrocardiogram (ECG) monitor strip demonstrates asystole followed by a wide complex tachycardia with resulting carotid and femoral pulses. Ventricular fibrillation quickly returns (Figure 11.1) and is unresponsive to epinephrine, repeated counter shocks, and amiodarone. An agonal rhythm ensues (Figure 11.2) that is unresponsive to atropine. With this rhythm there are no peripheral pulses or evidence of cardiac activity on bedside ultrasound. The patient expired after 40 min of continued resuscitation in the ED.

Case 2: An 81-year-old white female suffers a low velocity motor vehicle crash. When rescue arrives they find the patient to be unresponsive, pulseless, and apneic. Response time to the scene is less than 5 min. The EMS monitor indicates VF. The patient is rapidly extricated from the vehicle and defibrillated twice. A peripheral IV and an endotracheal tube (ETT) are inserted, and epinephrine and atropine are given. The patient has a return of peripheral pulses during the 25-min transport to the ED. In the ED the patient has a Glasgow Coma scale of 3. She has good breath sounds bilaterally. Her pulse is 100 bpm and irregular, and her blood pressure is 110/76 mmHg. She is given amiodarone and converts to a regular sinus rhythm with a rate of 70 bpm and a blood pressure of 100/70 mmHg. Her 12-lead ECG shows changes consistent with an acute myocardial infarction (AMI). A computed tomography (CT) scan of chest, abdomen, and pelvis

shows a laceration of her liver. She is deemed too unstable for a cardiac catheterization. The ST segment changes on her ECG that were consistent with the AMI improve over several hours with conservative measures only. Her neurologic exam, however, does not improve over the next 48 h and life support is withdrawn.

The ECG in the patient with cardiac arrest

Cardiac arrest may occur in any location – the home, business, public area, ED, or hospital, both with and without medical personnel in attendance. Just as the setting of a cardiac event may influence the patient's outcome, so also may an ECG recorded immediately pre-event be used as a predictive instrument. Post-event, the ECG becomes vital in management of rapidly changing cardiac rhythms. Recurrent cycles of cardiac arrest and return of circulation with varying rhythm disturbances may occur before the patient either stabilizes or expires.

The most common ECG findings associated with cardiac arrest are: (1) ventricular tachycardia (VT), (2) VF, (3) asystole, and (4) pulseless electrical activity (PEA). Ventricular tachycardia may present as three forms: monomorphic ventricular tachycardia (MVT), polymorphic ventricular tachycardia (PVT) and torsade de pointes (TdP). Ventricular fibrillation is described as fine to coarse depending on the electrical amplitude, and asystole has no discernible ventricular activity. Pulseless electrical activity is defined by an idioventricular, bradyasystole, or a ventricular escape rhythm without discernible blood pressure or organ perfusion [1]. The 2005 American Heart Association (AHA) guidelines include useful algorithms for the administration of electrical countershock and/or medications for each of the above rhythms.

Pitfalls in interpreting ECG rhythms during cardiac arrest: As in more controlled situations, the interpretation of life-threatening ECG rhythms should be correlated with the patient's current clinical condition. Loose electrodes, motion artifacts, ongoing cardiopulmonary resuscitation (CPR), and concurrent procedures such as central line placement

Critical Decisions in Emergency and Acute Care Electrocardiography,
1st edition. Edited by W.J. Brady and J.D. Truwit. © 2009 Blackwell Publishing, ISBN: 9781405159067

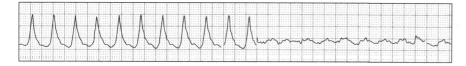

Figure 11.1 This rhythm strip illustrates a wide complex rhythm with a pulse suddenly degenerating to ventricular fibrillation without a pulse.

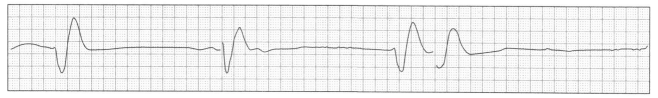

Figure 11.2 This rhythm strip illustrates an idioventricular rhythm synonymous with ventricular escape beats. Note the extremely slow rate but also the appearance of a premature ventricular beat followed by a very long pause.

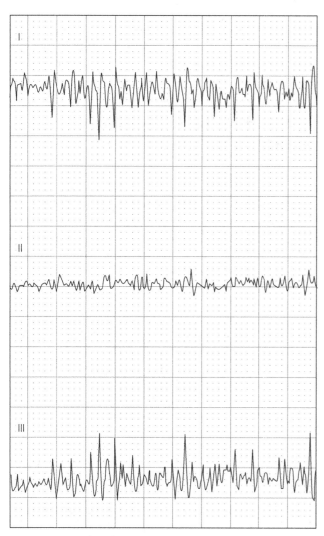

Figure 11.3 This fragment of a 12-lead ECG shows 60 cycle interference that could be mistaken for ventricular fibrillation. This patient has a normal pulse and blood pressure during this episode.

that result in patient movement, may all produce rhythm strips resembling VT or VF [2,3] (Figure 11.3). In the sometimes rapidly changing rhythms of the peri-arrest period, interpretation of an artifact as a ventricular arrhythmia may not only be common [4], but also may result in medication treatment error or even cessation of CPR when the artifact is diagnosed as refractory VF [5].

Electrocardiographic rhythm strips versus 12-lead ECGs: The interpretation of the ECG in the cardiac arrest situation is also made more complex by the difficulty of obtaining a 12-lead ECG without interrupting CPR or displacing defibrillator/pacing pads. Much of the data come in the form of rhythm strips from lead II or V1. Identifying ventricular arrythmias with a rhythm strip alone has a high rate of accuracy among tested medical students and emergency medical technicians, while diagnosing AMIs with rhythm strip alone proved more challenging [6,7]. The diagnosis of AMI and hyperkalemia, and distinguishing ventricular tachycardia from an aberrant supraventricular rhythm will most often require 12-lead ECG analysis (Figures 11.4 and 11.5). Leaving the ECG leads in place and the ECG machine in the resuscitation suite may be helpful in securing a rapid 12-lead tracing. Continuous monitoring of the 12-lead ECG is possible, but remains difficult to interpret when CPR is in progress.

ECG rhythms seen in cardiac arrest

Prognosis based on presenting cardiac arrest rhythm: The incidence of the three presenting rhythms in adult cardiac arrest varies with the population studied. In three recent surveys, VF/VT presented in 30–43%, and PEA/asystole in 57–70% of cardiac arrest victims [8–10]. Survival after VF as an initial rhythm in these same papers was 1.7%, while PEA/asystole on initial ECG was 7% in one series [9] and just the reverse at 9.5% in VF/VT and 1.7% in PEA/asystole in another [8]. Brady and colleagues [11] looked at the characteristics of VT and patient outcome in a retrospective review of 190 out-of-hospital cardiac arrests. They found that there were no differences in outcome between the three forms of VT: MVT, PVT and TdP. However, independent of the type of VT, a prolonged corrected QT interval (QTc) was associated with a significant decrease in those patients able to survive to hospital discharge from

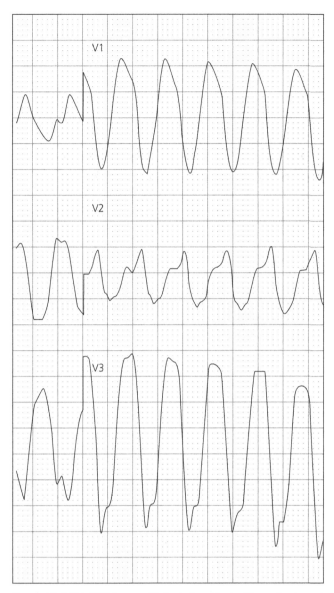

Figure 11.4 This ECG fragment is that of a patient with a potassium of 7.9. Note the wide complex ventricular tachycardia.

37.6 to 19.6% ($P = 0.01$). Other factors, such as a witnessed arrest, shorter times to defibrillation, bystander CPR, and co-morbidities have also played a significant role in survival. The use of the initial prehospital ECG rhythm, in isolation of other clinical features, should not be used as the sole determinant to initiate or continue advanced cardiac life support (ACLS) but can be helpful as a prognostic indicator.

Initial management of ECG rhythms

Ventricular fibrillation and pulseless ventricular tachycardia: The initial therapeutic decision-making in cardiac arrest will be based on the ECG, the evidence of peripheral perfusion, and the availability of a cardiac defibrillator. According to the AHA, ACLS guidelines published in

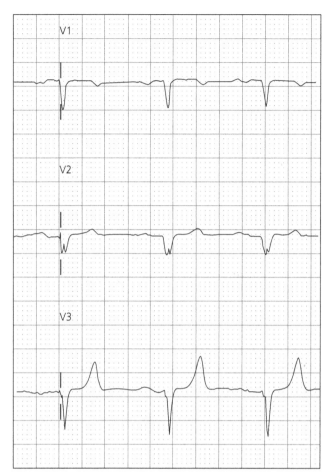

Figure 11.5 This ECG fragment is the result of the cardioversion of the patient in Figure 11.4. Calcium chloride was also given. Note the bradycardic rhythm with prominently peaked T waves.

2005 [1], if the ECG rhythm strip shows VF or VT without evidence of peripheral perfusion after 10 s of pulse palpation then one countershock is administered at 120 to 200 J if the defibrillating device is a manual biphasic defibrillator. Cardiopulmonary resuscitation is then resumed immediately for five cycles (30 compressions and two breaths for approximately 2 min). At that point a shockable rhythm as above would prompt one additional defibrillation attempt at 200 J and immediate resumption of CPR. This sequence would continue with the addition of 1 mg of epinephrine every 3– 5 min. Vasopressin 40 U may replace the first or second dose of epinephrine. After the third sequence an anti-arrhythmic such as amiodarone, or lidocaine if amiodarone is not available, may be given. Magnesium sulfate is recommended for TdP or a prolonged QTc ventricular tachycardia.

Ventricular fibrillation and concerns over the timing of countershock: The availability of automated external defibrillators (AED) has facilitated improved care in the prehospital setting through the early diagnosis and defibrillation of those cardiac arrest victims with an initial rhythm of VF or VT. The protocol under which an AED administers its fixed energy shocks has been under investigation to determine the most efficacious intervals of CPR, counter-shock, and repeated shock. Russell and colleagues address the issue of the VF waveform and its significance in the timing of initial defibrillation and in refibrillation management [12]. Correlation with the amplitude of the fibrillation waves and ultimate survival was noted in the prehospital setting, with the use of AEDs. Russell was able to document a steady decrease in what he termed the vRhythm score, an indicator of the likelihood of successful defibrillation, during the respiratory pauses of the CPR cycle to a level at which defibrillation would be less likely to occur. The current 2005 AHA guidelines recommend an initial countershock followed by approximately 2 min (five cycles of CPR) and then repeat countershock if needed. If there has been a prolonged (> 4 min) response time before CPR then the AHA recommendations are for 2 min of CPR first and then counter-shock if required [13]. Russell expresses concern that this protocol may delay beneficial countershock unnecessarily and that the fibrillation amplitude rather than the "down" time should determine initial and subsequent countershocks.

Asystole/pulseless electrical activity

Asystole and PEA are lumped together into those rhythms associated with cardiac arrest that are non-ventricular. Perhaps a more useful definition is rhythms that do not respond to countershock. These rhythms include idioventricular rhythm (also known as a ventricular escape rhythm when P waves are seen and complete atrioventricular block is suspected) that produces a wide QRS complex with a rate of 40 bps or less, and true ventricular asystole with or without P waves. If ECGs immediately preceding the cardiac arrest are available then telltale signs of hyperkalemia or hypothermia (Figure 11.6) may be seen progressing to PEA/asystole, and specific therapies directed at these etiologies can be initiated.

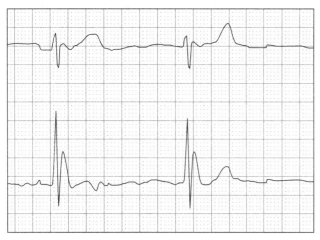

Figure 11.6 This patient had severe hypothermia with a core temperature of 27.8 °C. Note the prominent J point elevation on the ECG. These are called Osborne waves in this clinical setting.

Distinguishing between true asystole and a fine or low ampli-tude VF can be difficult in the artifact-producing milieu of CPR. Initial brief CPR and then defibrillation may be appro-priate when unable to distinguish, as initial countershock for asystole is associated with a higher mortality rate than those receiving initial CPR medical management without immedi-ate countershock [14].

How should the ECG be used following cardiac arrest?

Continuous ECG monitoring following successful resuscita-tion from cardiac arrest will help guide treatment of rhythm disturbances as they occur. As in the immediate period pre-ceding cardiac arrest, ECG findings should also be sought that suggest specific arrest etiologies and resultant management strategies. For instance, a QRS wider than 0.10 s in associ-ation with a rightward shift in the terminal 40 ms in leads III and aVf might indicate a tricyclic anti-depressant overdose in which sodium bicarbonate therapy could be therapeutic [15]. Evidence of an AMI either contributing to the cardiac arrest or resulting from the hypoxia might also prompt another treatment pathway.

Rhythm disturbances following cardiac arrest: Tachycardia and bradycardia are commonly found in close proximity on rhythm strips taken during resuscitation from a cardiac arrest as well as in the post arrest period (Figure 11.7). These fluctuating disturbances present a difficult manage-ment problem as non-treatment may result in degeneration of these rhythms to VF or asystole. Over-aggressive treat-ment may more commonly result in PEA that can be refract-ory to other treatment modalities. The incidence of VF and VT may be reduced with the administration of a beta-blocker if the cardiac arrest event was the result of an AMI. The data derived from the incidence of VF following an AMI, but not necessarily those with an associated cardiac arrest, show a reduction from 4.35 to 0.35% attributed to the use of beta-blockers and correction of hypokalemia to levels greater than 4.0 mEq/L [16]. The prophylactic use of lidocaine and mag-nesium in the AMI setting to prevent VF is associated with an *increase* in mortality rate but its effect in the general post-cardiac arrest population is not known [17]. Watchful waiting is appropriate if recombinant plasminogen activator (rt-PA) is given, as ventricular ectopy and VT are commonly seen about 20–45 min after successful reperfusion with the drug. Attention should be directed at correcting hypoxia, acidosis, hypokalemia, and volume status. It is usually prudent to avoid the pitfall of "chasing" the chaotic rhythms seen in the post-arrest period with pharmaceutical interventions.

Significance of ECG evidence of AMI surrounding cardiac arrest: An AMI and resultant lethal arrhythmia is the etiology of up to 80% of sudden cardiac deaths in adults. This leads to the question of whether rt-Pa or percutaneous

Figure 11.7 This ECG shows the chaotic rhythm that can be seen immediately after a cardiac arrest. There was a pulse with this rhythm but it is difficult to tell which QRS appearing complex is the electrical representation of that pulse.

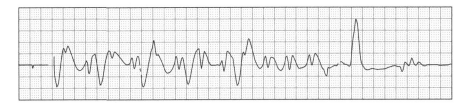

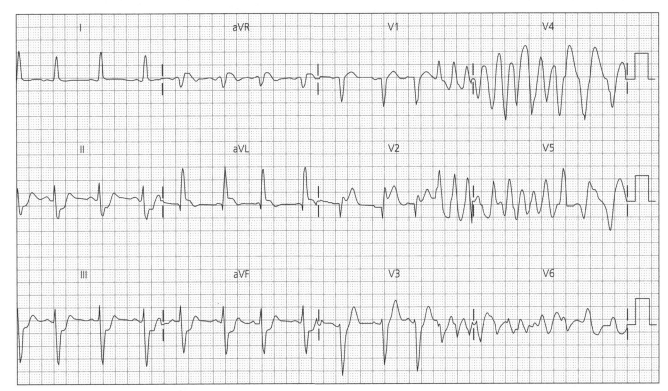

Figure 11.8 This ECG shows ST elevation in V1, V2, and aVL, as well as ST depression in leads II, III, and aVf. These findings are consistent with anterior lateral myocardial infarction. Note also the sudden degeneration to ventricular fibrillation in V 4, 5, and 6.

coronary intervention (PCI) would improve survival in patients suffering cardiac arrest. Lederer and colleagues answer in the affirmative for rt-PA in their group of 108 patients given the drug versus 210 control subjects receiving standard therapy. The rt-PA group had a significant early survival improvement over the control group (48 versus 33%). The treatment group was treated during CPR solely on the basis of a cardiac arrest regardless of the ECG findings [18]. The presence of ST elevation either before (Figure 11.8) or after cardiac arrest (Figure 11.9) has also been studied. Those with return of circulation who receive PCI and successful coronary intervention have survival without neurologic deficit rates of up to 100%. Unfortunately, of those patients who present comatose to the catheterization lab only 29% survive with no neurologic deficit [19,20].

Case conclusions

Case 1: This patient illustrates the all-too common scenario of a progressive downhill course from unstable VT through VF and finally PEA. The ECG was helpful in directing therapy

for the various rhythm disturbances and, as a result, a brief return of spontaneous circulation occurred. The prehospital phase focused on treatment of the VF, while the ED treatment was directed towards the PEA. Note the sudden change of high amplitude VT to low amplitude VF in Figure 11.1. This should prompt rapid reassessment of lead placement, ventilation, and perfusion, as well as preparing for defibrillation. Figure 11.2 shows the wide slow complexes of PEA prompting a search for common causes including the development of pneumothorax, tamponade, and hyperkalemia. Unfortunately, in this case, directed therapy proved to be futile.

Case 2: This patient was successfully resuscitated from her episode of VF. Her ECG in the ED following stabilization is shown in Figure 11.9 demonstrating changes consistent with an AMI in the inferior and posterior aspects of the heart. She exhibited rises in both troponin T and CK MB fractions. These ECG and biomarker changes may also have occurred secondary to a severe hypoxic brain injury in a manner similar to Takotsubo cardiomyopathy [21]. Unfortunately, the patient never regained consciousness and was taken off life support after 48 h.

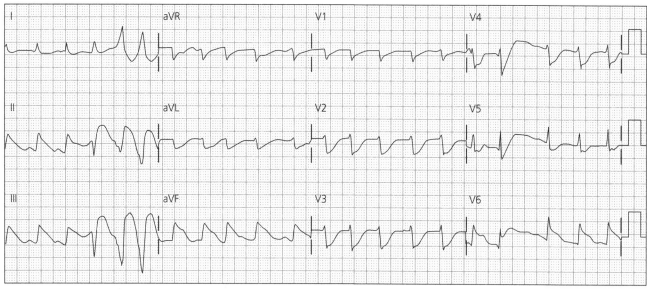

Figure 11.9 This ECG was taken shortly after resuscitating a patient from a cardiac arrest. Note the short run of ventricular tachycardia in leads I, II, and III, which is self-limited. There is ST elevation in leads II, III and aVf and depression in leads V2, V3, and V4, indicating widespread ischemia in the inferior and posterior distribution.

References

1 AHA Workgroup. Management of cardiac arrest. *Circulation* 2005;**112**:IV-58-IV-66.

2 Stevenson WG, Maisel WH. Electrocardiography artifact: what you do not know, you do not recognize. *Am J Med* 2001;**110**(5): 402–3.

3 Chase C, Brady WJ. Artifactual electrocardiographic change mimicking clinical abnormality on the ECG. *Am J Emerg Med* 2000;**18**(3):312–6.

4 Knight BP, Pelosi F, Michaud GF, *et al.* Physician interpretation of electrocardiographic artifact that mimics ventricular tachycardia. *Am J Med* 2001;**110**(5):335–8.

5 Knight BP, Pelosi F, Michaud GF, *et al.* Clinical consequences of electrocardiographic artifact mimicking ventricular tachycardia. *New Engl J Med* 1999;**341**(17):1270–4.

6 Little B, Mainie I, Ho KJ, *et al.* Electrocardiogram and rhythm strip interpretation by final year medical students. *Ulster Med J* 2001;**70**(2):108–10.

7 Brown LH, Gough JE, Hawley CR. Accuracy of rural EMS provider interpretation of three-lead ECG rhythm strips. *Prehosp Emerg Care* 1997;**1**(4):259–62.

8 Holmberg M, Holmberg S, Herlitz J. Incidence, duration and survival of ventricular fibrillation in out-of-hospital cardiac arrest patients in Sweden. *Resuscitation* 2000;**44**(1):7–17.

9 Stratton SJ, Niemann JT. Outcome from out-of-hospital cardiac arrest caused by nonventricular arrhythmias: contribution of successful resuscitation to overall survivorship supports the current practice of initiating out-of-hospital ACLS. *Acad Emerg Med* 1998;**32**(4):448–45.

10 Wang HE, Min A, Hostler D, *et al.* Differential effects of out-of-hospital interventions on short and long-term survival after cardiopulmonary arrest. *Resuscitation* 2005;**67**(1):69–74.

11 Brady WJ, DeBehnke DJ, Laundrie D. Prevalence, therapeutic response, and outcome of ventricular tachycardia in the out-of-hospital setting: a comparison of monomorphic ventricular tachycardia, polymorphic ventricular tachycardia, and torsades de pointes. *Acad Emerg Med* 1999;**6**(6):609–17.

12 Russell JK, White RD, Crone WE. Analysis of ventricular fibrillation waveform in refibrillation. *Crit Care Med* 2006;**34**(12): S432–437.

13 AHA Workgroup. Electrical therapies: AEDs, defibrillation, cardioversion, and pacing. *Circulation* 2005;**112**:IV-35-IV-46.

14 Martin DR, Gavin T, Bianco J, *et al.* Initial countershock in the treatment of asystole. *Resuscitation* 1993;**26**(1):63–8.

15 Harrigan RA, Brady WJ. ECG abnormalities in tricyclic antidepressant ingestion. *Am J Emerg Med* 1999;**17**(4):387–93.

16 Antman EM, Berlin JA. Declining incidence of ventricular fibrillation in myocardial infarction; implications for the prophylactic use of lidocaine. *Circulation* 1992;**86**:764–73.

17 MacMahon S, Collins R, Peto R, *et al.* Effects of prophylactic lidocaine in suspected acute myocardial infarction. An overview of results from the randomized controlled trials. *JAMA* 1988; **260**(3):1910–6.

18 Lederer W, Lichtengberger C, Pechlaner C, *et al.* Recombinant tissue plasminogen activator during cardiopulmonary resuscitation in 108 patients with out-of-hospital cardiac arrest. *Resuscitation* 2001;**50**(1):71–6.

19 Gorjup V, Radsel P, Ploj T, *et al.* Acute ST-elevation myocardial infarction after successful cardiopulmonary resuscitation. *Resuscitation* 2007;**72**(3):379–85.

20 Garot P, Lefevre T, Eltchaninoff H, *et al.* Six-month outcome of emergency percutaneous coronary intervention in resuscitated patients after cardiac arrest complicating ST-elevation myocardial infarction. *Circulation* 2007;**115**(11):1354–62.

21 Inoko M, Nakashima J, Haruna T, *et al.* Images in cardiovascular medicine. Serial changes of the electrocardiogram during the progression of subarachnoidal hemorrhage. *Circulation* 2005; **112**(21):e331–332.

Chapter 12 | What is the impact/proper role of the ECG in the undifferentiated cardiorespiratory failure patient?

Michael Osmundson
Mercer University School of Medicine, Savannah, GA, USA

Case Presentations

Case 1: A 24-year-old female with sudden onset of severe respiratory distress and syncope presents to the emergency department (ED). She reports chest pain across the right precordium, worse with inspiration. She is markedly diaphoretic and confused, with cyanosis noted around the mouth and nailbeds. She reports dizziness prior to the syncopal episode. She has had brief periods of palpitations and dizziness in the remote past and several episodes of syncope in her life. She smokes and is on oral contraceptives. Vital signs include temperature 37.5 °C, pulse 282 beats per minute (bpm), respirations 42, blood pressure 82/40 mmHg, oxygen saturation 100% (on oxygen) (Figure 12.1).

Case 2: A 24-year-old female presents with sudden onset of severe respiratory distress and syncope. She reports chest pain across the right precordium, worse with inspiration. She is coarsely diaphoretic and confused with cyanosis noted around the mouth and nailbeds. She reports no previous episodes and has no significant past medical history. She smokes and is on oral contraceptives. Vital signs include temperature 38.2 °C, pulse 185 bpm, respirations 42, blood pressure 82/40 mmHg, oxygen saturation 88% (on oxygen) (Figure 12.2).

Case 3: A 71-year-old male with a history of hypertension complains of severe respiratory distress and dizziness that has gradually worsened over the last 2 h, ultimately culminating in syncope. Vital signs include temperature 37.5 °C, pulse 42 bpm, respirations 42, blood pressure 82/40 mmHg, oxygen saturation 100% (on oxygen) (Figure 12.3).

Case 4: A 71-year-old male with a history of hypertension complains of severe respiratory distress and dizziness that has gradually worsened over the last 2 h, ultimately culminating in syncope. Vital signs include temperature 37.5 °C, pulse 162 bpm, respirations 42, blood pressure 82/40 mmHg, oxygen saturation 100% (on oxygen) (Figure 12.4).

Case 5: A 62-year-old female presents with a gradual progression of altered mental status and tachypnea over the last 6 h. She is now obtunded and cyanotic. Vital signs include temperature 39.5 °C, pulse 132 bpm, respirations 42, blood pressure 82/40 mmHg, oxygen saturation 88% (on oxygen) (Figure 12.5).

Case 6: A 62-year-old female presents with gradual progression of altered mental status and tachypnea over the last 6 h. Her family states that she has been very depressed and they have found a suicide note. She is now obtunded and cyanotic. Vital signs include temperature 37.5 °C, pulse 136 bpm, respirations 36, blood pressure 82/40 mmHg, oxygen saturation 88% (on oxygen) (Figure 12.6).

The ECG in undifferentiated cardiorespiratory failure

In the patient presenting with undifferentiated cardiopulmonary failure, the clinician is frequently forced to make a series of immediate critical decisions based on limited clinical data. Besides the history (if available) and physical examination, the electrocardiogram (ECG) can be a key bedside test that is available immediately and can focus the differential diagnosis in a particular direction. While the complete differential for cardiopulmonary failure is exceedingly broad, there are a limited number of life-threats that must be identified quickly and only a limited number of real-time tests that can be utilized in uncovering the etiology. The ECG is one such test.

Critical Decisions in Emergency and Acute Care Electrocardiography,
1st edition. Edited by W.J. Brady and J.D. Truwit. © 2009 Blackwell Publishing, ISBN: 9781405159067

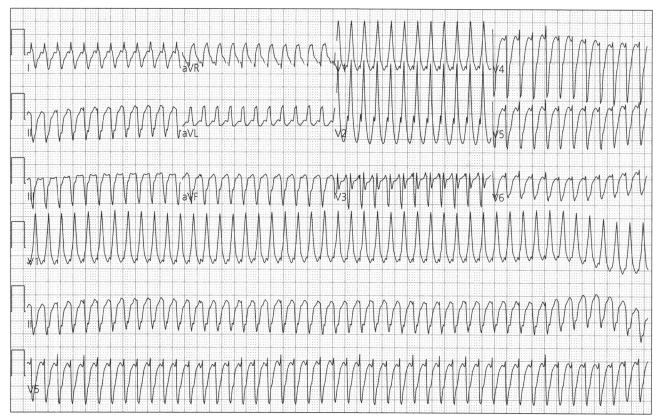

Figure 12.1 ECG demonstrating WPW syndrome findings. Note the shortened PR interval and the widened QRS complex. The QRS is much wider in the initial phase and narrower at its terminal phase demonstrating the classic delta wave.

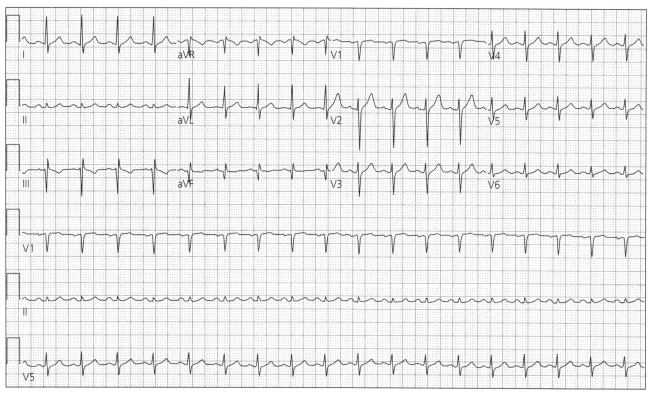

Figure 12.2 ECG demonstrating PE findings. Note sinus tachycardia and the elements of right ventricular strain: S wave in lead I, Q wave in lead III and flipped T wave in lead III ($S_1Q_3T_3$).

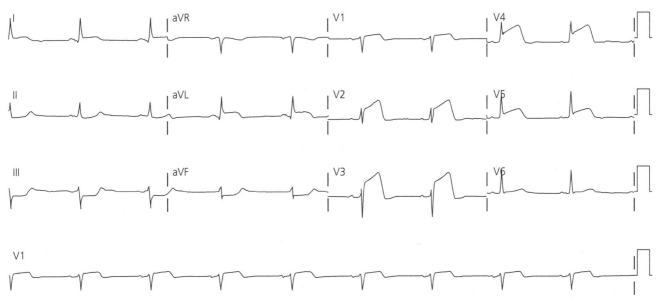

Figure 12.3 ECG demonstrating AMI with bradycardia. Note ST elevation in leads V1–4, aVL and I, with reciprocal ST depression in leads II, III, and aVF. This is a pattern classic for LAD occlusion and is an illustration of an acute anterolateral MI.

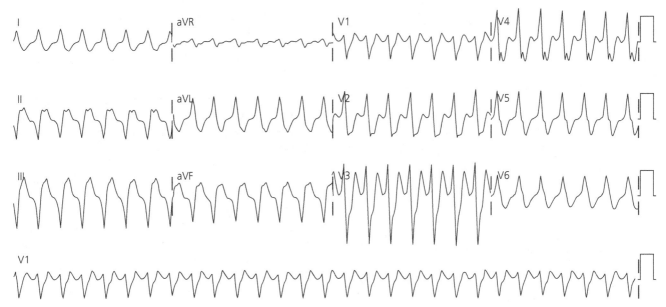

Figure 12.4 ECG demonstrating VT. Note the widened QRS complex and the P waves that are visible following the QRS complex especially apparent in leads V2 and V4. These may represent AV disassociation or retrograde P waves. In this clinical setting, a wide complex tachycardia should first be assumed to be VT.

The differential diagnosis of cardiorespiratory failure

Cardiopulmonary failure is the final common pathway for a large number of pathologic processes that can impact a patient. At the bedside of the hypotensive and/or hypoxic patient, it is most helpful initially to differentiate primary cardiac etiologies from other reasons for clinical decompensation (e.g. toxic/metabolic, thromboembolic, etc.). The primary role of the clinician in this setting is to quickly identify what organ system has failed the patient while simultaneously directing resuscitation towards the most likely etiologies. If recognizable patterns are identified on the ECG (e.g. ST elevated myocardial infarction, STEMI) specific therapies can be initiated to treat the primary pathophysiologic process (e.g. cath. lab. or fibrinolysis).

On many occasions, however, a specific recognizable pattern such as STEMI may not be readily apparent in the patient with undifferentiated cardiorespiratory failure. In

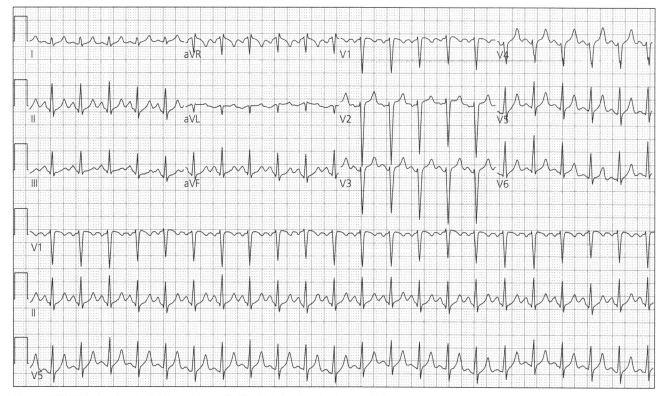

Figure 12.5 ECG showing classic sinus tachycardia. The QRS duration is normal as is the PR segment length. Every QRS complex is preceded by a P wave.

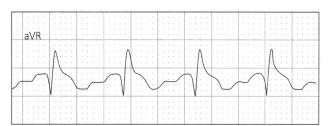

Figure 12.6 ECG showing TCA overdose wide complex with terminal R in aVR. The R wave seen in aVR has been associated with poor outcome and an increased risk of seizures and cardiac instability.

these situations, an alternative strategy is to initially stratify patients presenting with bradydysrhythmias from those with tachydysrhythmias, and then attempt to differentiate possible etiologies within classifications. In any case, the ECG offers many important clues to the cause of the patient's disease process.

Electrocardiographic features of syndromes contributing to cardiorespiratory failure

Acute myocardial infarction (AMI) is clearly a high-priority diagnosis that must be entertained in the evaluation of this patient population. The clinician needs to keep in mind that,

particularly in the elderly patient population, this can be difficult diagnosis with atypical presentation being the norm. Discussion of STEMI and other acute coronary syndromes (ACS) appears elsewhere in this text.

When reviewing the ECG of the patient with undifferentiated cardiorespiratory failure, the clinician needs to search for specific ECG findings that will lead towards the underlying pathology. Key disease processes that *may* be apparent on the ECG include hyperkalemia, acidosis, hypoxia, hypothermia, hypothyroidism, decompensated atrial fibrillation/ flutter and other tachydysrhythmias, pulmonary embolus, medication overdose (e.g. tricyclic anti-depressant, TCA), pericarditis and myocarditis. Many other ECG findings (e.g. ventricular tachycardia) are simply final common pathways of numerous disease processes and do not point towards a specific etiology [1–3].

Hyperkalemia is manifested by tall, narrow, and peaked T waves as the serum potassium concentration rises above 5.5 mEq/L. P wave flattening and PR interval prolongation usually will occur before widening of the QRS complex as the atrial tissue is more sensitive to rising potassium levels than the ventricular tissue. Widening of the QRS complex is typically uniform across the 12-lead ECG when serum potassium exceeds 6.5 mEq/L, unlike that seen with a bundle branch block. With extreme hyperkalemia (serum values over 10 mEq/L.), the QRS complex widens to merge with the T wave resulting in the characteristic sine-wave pattern [4,5].

The ECG manifestations of acidosis and hypoxia are similar, and include myocardial irritation manifested by ectopic beats, prolongation of the PR interval, and, ultimately, profound bradycardia [6]. Hypothermia is manifested by tremor artifact (due to shivering), Osborne J waves and profound sinus bradycardia. Osborne waves are usually present when the core body temperature falls to less than 32 °C. The PR and QT intervals will prolong with progressive hypothermia. Slow atrial fibrillation is also seen in significant hypothermia [7].

Severe decompensated hypothyroidism can present with sinus bradycardia, prolonged PR and QT intervals, and flattened or inverted T waves. Low voltage complexes are frequently encountered, but may also be due to pericardial effusions which are present in up to 30% of these cases. Conduction disturbances (various degrees of atrioventricular [AV] blocks) are seen three times more often in myxedema patients than in the general population [8,9].

A number of distinct disease processes can present with tachydysrhythmias. Profound hyperthyroidism and thyrotoxicosis can present with refractory sinus tachycardia, with a reported incidence of 40%. Atrial fibrillation is seen in 10–22% of cases, yet is rare in patients younger than 40 years old. Conduction disturbances can also be seen with hyperthyroidism, most commonly a left anterior fascicular block or right bundle branch block (RBBB) occur in 15% of patients without heart disease. Non-specific ST segment/T wave abnormalities are seen in 25% of thyrotoxic patients. PR prolongation is often seen as well [8–10].

The diagnosis of pulmonary embolism (PE) should always enter the clinician's mind when faced with a patient with undifferentiated cardiopulmonary decompensation. While the ECG can aid in the diagnosis, the findings are usually non-specific. The presenting ECG rhythm may be *normal* in up to 27% of patients with PE; the "classic" appearance of S1Q3T3 is seen in less than half of patients with this disease (11–50%) and is unreliable. Many other ECG changes are commonly seen: sinus tachycardia (8–69%), premature beats (4–23%), atrial fibrillation or flutter (0–35%), and axis changes (8–80%) may all be identified. Identifying right ventricular dysfunction is an important finding in PE as it correlates with severity of disease and outcomes. RV dysfunction can be demonstrated if three or more of the following ECG findings are present: (1) RBBB, (2) S waves in lead I and aVL > 1.5 mm, (3) R wave transition zone shifted to V5, (4) Q waves in leads III and aVF but not in lead II, (5) QRS axis > 90°, (6) low limb lead voltage < 5 mm, or (7) T wave inversion in leads III and aVF or in leads V1–V4 [4,11,12].

Decompensated primary tachycardias can also lead to the clinical syndrome of cardiopulmonary failure. The appearance of paroxysmal supraventricular tachycardia (PSVT) can vary from a narrow complex to a wide complex tachycardia (PSVT with aberrancy) that can closely mimic the appearance of ventricular tachycardia (VT). A regular, narrow complex tachycardia without definable P waves (or, more specifically, anterograde P waves) suggests PSVT. Patients older than 35 years (and those with pre-existing cardiac disease) suggest VT and those younger than 35 years suggest PSVT with aberrancy. Additional clues to the presence of VT include capture beats, fusion beats, and AV dissociation [12,13].

Wolff-Parkinson-White (WPW) and other pre-excitation syndromes are caused by atrial impulses bypassing the AV node and entering the ventricular myocardium directly (thus arriving at the ventricle before the normally conducted impulse through the AV node and via the His-Purkinje system). This can result in a narrow complex tachycardia (with the classic shortened P-R interval and the delta wave) or the (more worrisome appearing) classic wide complex tachycardia. Supraventricular tachycardia (SVT) is often seen, with ventricular rates exceedingly fast (> 220 bpm). Atrial fibrillation is also a common finding in WPW syndrome (usually with extremely fast ventricular rates, even exceeding 300 bpm) [14].

While there are myriad toxidromes that can present with cardiopulmonary failure, TCA overdose bears special mention as it has distinct ECG findings and important therapeutic interventions. Although TCAs are no longer a frequently used medication for anti-depressant therapy, they are still prescribed extensively for therapy of migraine headaches and insomnia. Tricyclic anti-depressants block several key transmitters, such as norepinephrine, serotonin, and dopamine. They have profound anti-cholinergic effects and act as both Class I and Class III anti-arrhythmics. In TCA overdose, a common presenting rhythm is sinus tachycardia, which is largely a result of their anti-cholinergic properties. Other effects include P-R prolongation, QRS widening, QTC prolongation, and heart block. They also have notable negative inotropic effects, which can result in profound, refractory hypotension. Major cardiac effects tend to follow a progression of findings: first comes widening of QRS > 100 ms followed by a positive deflection in the terminal portion of the QRS in lead aVR (commonly described as a prominent R wave in lead AVR). The effects of TCAs are more likely in patients with pre-existing cardiac disease and those patients already on certain anti-arrhythmic agents [2,3,15].

While it is rare for pericarditis itself to cause decompensation, when accompanied by either myocarditis or large pericardial effusion it may manifest with cardiopulmonary failure. The ECG patterns in pericarditis follow a typical progression: the inflammation produces a classic myocardial injury pattern (concave ST elevation). However, as it typically involves a large portion of the heart, it is seen diffusely throughout the ECG, not in a classic, single vessel distribution (e.g. right coronary artery [RCA], left anterior descending [LAD] coronary artery, or circumflex) as is typical for myocardial infarction (MI). PR depression below the baseline is pathognomic for pericarditis [8]. As noted above, it is unusual for pericarditis to result in significant cardiopulmonary depression unless it is associated with hemodynamically significant pericardial effusion.

The ECG manifestations of myocarditis can be highly variable. Classically, prolongation of QRS and QT intervals

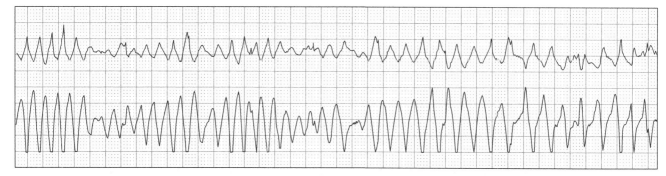

Figure 12.7 Rhythm strip demonstrating torsade de pointes or PVT. This is a finding suggesting underlying QT prolongation as a primary etiology.

and diffuse T wave inversions (without ST abnormalities) are described. However, if occurring in association with pericarditis, the ECG may also show the more typical ST elevation associated with that process [8,16].

As noted above, ventricular dysrhythmias are a final common pathway for a number of disease processes. Their presence will only rarely point to a distinct etiology for the patient's cardiopulmonary failure. Termination of these rhythms is a primary goal for the clinician. Ventricular tachycardia is defined as a series of more than three consecutive wide complex beats originating within the ventricular muscle or conduction system with a rate > 100 bpm. It is usually a regular rhythm. When AV nodal disassociation can be demonstrated, VT is highly likely. A good rule of thumb is the "Brady rule": a wide complex tachycardia in a patient > 35 years old without pre-existing known tachydysrhythmia is presumed to be VT. New-onset wide complex tachycardia in a patient younger than 35 years with pre-existing heart disease is also presumed to be VT. Another quick test is that morphologies that are inconsistent with RBBB are likely to be VT [8,12].

One ECG finding in ventricular dysrhythmia can point the clinician in a specific direction: this is the finding of polymorphic ventricular tachycardia (PVT, or torsade de pointes) (Figure 12.7). Torsades is seen most frequently in patients with a prolonged QT interval (prolonged qt segment syndrome). This condition can be congenital or induced with a dizzying variety of commonly prescribed medications. The ECG appearance is one of progressively varying polarity and amplitude of the QRS complex [17].

Case conclusions

Case 1 represents the classic presentation of re-entry SVT resulting in significant cardiopulmonary compromise. The ECG shows a classic wide complex, extreme tachycardia associated with WPW syndrome. Interventions in this case would include a trial of procainimide or electrical cardioversion. However, given the patient's extremis at presentation, immediate electric cardioversion is best advised.

Case 2 demonstrates a classic presentation for PE. The ECG demonstrates findings classic for PE: sinus tachycardia and findings of right heart strain (S wave in Lead I, Q wave and flipped T wave in Lead III). Interventions in this case would include heparinization and fluid resuscitation. Given the severity of the patient's condition, one should also consider fibrinolytics.

Case 3 is a classic presentation of STEMI. The ECG demonstrates marked ST segment elevation (anterior and lateral leads) with reciprocal ST depression (inferior leads) classic for LAD occlusion. Interventions include aspirin, heparin, fluid resuscitation, and urgent revascularization (percutaneous coronary intervention or fibrinolytics).

Case 4 represents a typical patient with VT. The ECG demonstrates a wide complex tachycardia with either AV disassociation or retrograde P waves. In this setting of an elderly patient in extremis, one should presume VT first. Interventions include electric cardioversion, amiodarone or lidocaine. A careful search for ischemia or other causative agent for the arrhythmia is indicated.

Case 5 is a patient with sepsis. Although the patient presents in cardiopulmonary failure, the rhythm (sinus tachycardia) represents a physiologic response to shock and no rhythm specific interventions are warranted. Interventions should include fluid resuscitation and early use of pressors if hypotension remains refractory. Case 6 represents a TCA overdose. The ECG demonstrates sinus tachycardia, a widened QRS complex, and a terminal r-wave in lead aVR. Interventions include volume resuscitation and sodium bicarbonate injections. The goal of bicarbonate therapy is to return the QRS duration to normal (< 0.12 ms). The prognostic value of the terminal R wave in aVR is notable, and may correlate with the incidence of seizures and cardiac instability.

References

1 Van Mieghem C, Sabbe M, Knockaert D. The clinical value of the ECG in noncardiac conditions. *Chest* 2004;**125**(4):1561–76.

2 Holstege CP, Eldridge DL, Rowden AK. ECG manifestations: the poisoned patient. *Emerg Med Clin North Am* 2006;**24**(1):159–77, vii.

3 Delk C, Holstege CP, Brady WJ. Electrocardiographic abnormalities associated with poisoning. *Am J Emerg Med* 2007;**25**(6):672–87.

4 Wald DA. ECG manifestations of selected metabolic and endocrine disorders. *Emerg Med Clin North Am* 2006;**24**(1):145–57, vii.

5 Mattu A, Brady WJ, Robinson DA. Electrocardiographic manifestations of hyperkalemia. *Am J Emerg Med* 2000;**18**(6):721–9.

6 Aberra A, Komukai K, Howarth FC, *et al.* The effect of acidosis on the ECG of the Rat Heart. *Exp Physiol* 2001;**86**(1):27–31.

7 Mattu A, Brady WJ, Perron AD. Electrocardiographic manifestations of hypothermia. *Am J Emerg Med* 2002;**20**(4):314–26.

8 Demangone D. ECG Manifestations: Noncoronary heart disease. *Emerg Med Clin North Am* 2006;**24**(1):113–31.

9 Ruiz-Bailen M. Reversible myocardial dysfunction in critically ill, noncardiac patients. *Crit Care Med* 2002;**30**(6):1280–90.

10 Van Mieghem C, Sabbe M, Knockaert D. The clinical value of the ECG in noncardiac conditions. *Chest* 2004;**125**(4):1561–76.

11 Chan TC, Vilke GM, Pollack M, *et al.* Electrocardiographic manifestations: pulmonary embolism. *J Emerg Med* 2001;**21**(3): 263–70.

12 Brady WJ, Skiles J. Wide QRS complex tachycardia: ECG differential diagnosis. *Am J Emerg Med* 1999;**17**(4):376–81.

13 Kumar UN, Rao RK, Scheinman MM. The 12-lead electrocardiogram in supraventricular tachycardia. *Cardiol Clin* 2006;**24**(3): 427–3.

14 Rosner MH, Brady WJ, Kefer MP, *et al.* Electrocardiography in the Patient with the Wolff-Parkinson-White Syndrome: Diagnostic and Initial Therapeutic Issues. *Am J Emerg Med* 1999;**17**(7): 705–14.

15 Harrigan RA, Brady WJ. ECG abnormalities in tricyclic antidepressant ingestion. *Am J Emerg Med* 1999;**17**(4):387–93.

16 Brady WJ, Ferguson JD, Ullman EA, *et al.* Myocarditis: emergency department recognition and management. *Emerg Med Clin North Am* 2004;**22**(4):865–85.

17 Miller JM, Das MK, Yadav AV, *et al.* Value of the 12-lead ECG in wide QRS tachycardia. *Cardiol Clin* 2006;**24**(3):439–51.

Part 3 | **The ECG in ACS**

Chapter 13 | **What is the role of the ECG in ACS?**

Samuel J. Stellpflug[1], Joel S. Holger[1], Stephen W. Smith[2]

[1]University of Minnesota and Regions, St Paul, Minneapolis, MN, USA
[2]University of Minnesota and Hennepin County Medical Center, Minneapolis, MN, USA

Case presentations

Case 1: A 50-year-old male presents to the emergency department (ED) from home complaining of dyspnea and minimal chest pain. Figure 13.1a is the initial ED electrocardiogram (ECG). Over the course of the next 45 min, the chest pain increases. Figure 13.1b shows the repeat ECG.

Case 2: A 74-year-old male presents to the ED complaining of chest pain for the past 2 h; he is hypertensive. He is given aspirin and nitroglycerin, after which his blood pressure (BP) drops to the normal range. His initial ED ECGs are shown in Figure 13.2a (standard left-sided ECG) and 13.2b (right-sided ECG).

Case 3: A 56-year-old male presents via emergency medical services (EMS) with hand numbness and no other symptoms. Neurologic exam is normal, and the ECG in Figure 13.3 is recorded.

The role of the ECG in the ACS patient

Acute coronary syndrome (ACS) encompasses a spectrum of three less than distinct entities known as ST elevation myocardial infarction (STEMI), non-ST elevation myocardial infarction (NSTEMI), and unstable angina (UA). Acute coronary syndrome is the syndrome of symptoms, ECG findings, and biomarker results that stem from a ruptured atherosclerotic plaque with epicardial coronary occlusion and/or downstream embolization of platelet-rich thrombi. Even with continued technologic improvements of adjunctive testing, the 12-lead ECG remains the first test performed after the initial clinical evaluation of suspected ACS. It is inexpensive, quickly performed, and readily available. Initial plasma cardiac troponin indicating myocardial damage is not adequately sensitive for rapid diagnosis. Furthermore, troponin does not distinguish between MI from acute complete persistent epicardial coronary occlusion (STEMI, which needs emergent reperfusion in order to salvage myocardium) and NSTEMI (MI that does not represent a significant quantity of myocardium at imminent risk of loss). This is especially true early in the process. The ECG is used initially in cases of ACS to make the first important clinical decision, which is whether or not the patient will benefit from immediate coronary artery reperfusion therapy. Early reperfusion of occluded coronary arteries in patients with STEMI improves survival and decreases complications [1,2]. The standard of care for "door-to-needle-time" is < 30 min for fibrinolysis or < 90 min for percutaneous coronary intervention (PCI). On the other hand, fibrinolytics are not indicated for UA/NSTEMI. Percutaneous coronary intervention, though it clearly reduces both morbidity and mortality of UA/NSTEMI if done within 48 h of arrival, only needs to be done emergently for persistent uncontrollable ischemia or hemodynamic instability [3].

ST elevation myocardial infarction

Acute MI is a broad continuum, such that STEMI and NSTEMI have an arbitrary ECG distinction. ST elevation (STE) is the single best immediately available surrogate marker for detecting acute complete coronary occlusion without collateral circulation, signifying a significant region of injured myocardium at imminent risk of irreversible infarction, requiring immediate reperfusion therapy for salvage.

However, many patients without "diagnostic" STE, but with MI diagnosed later by biomarkers, have complete occlusion that was not detected by the ECG, either because the ECG was not sensitive enough (often, but not always, due to occlusion of a branch artery, or of the circumflex artery, see Chapter 22) or because the interpreter was not skilled enough. ST elevation may be < 1–2 mm, or in one lead only, even in anterior MI, but especially in leads with a small QRS such as aVL. Amongst other considerations, proportionality of the ST segment and T wave to the QRS is critical; a small QRS cannot be followed by the "necessary" 1–2 mm of STE

Critical Decisions in Emergency and Acute Care Electrocardiography,
1st edition. Edited by W.J. Brady and J.D. Truwit. © 2009 Blackwell
Publishing, ISBN: 9781405159067

(a)

(b)

(c)

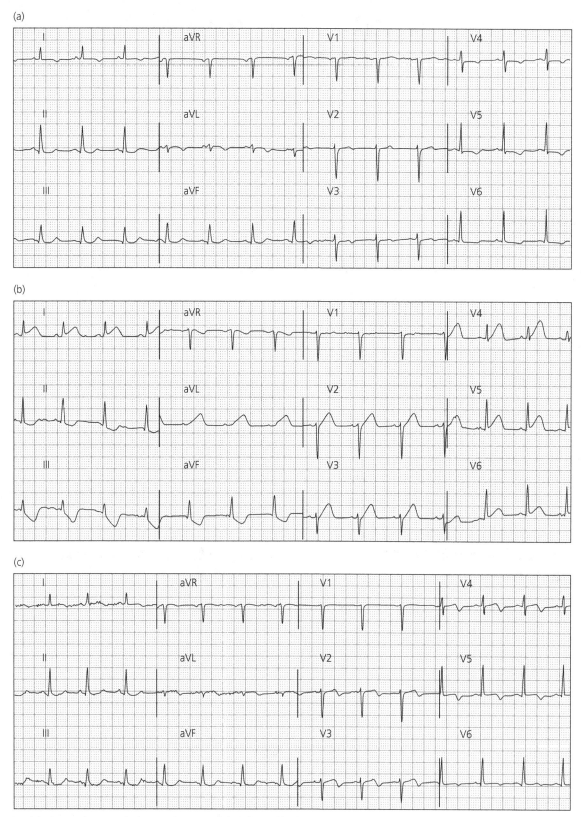

Figure 13.1 (a) Abnormal T waves in the anterior precordial and lateral leads, and minimal ST elevation, in the presence of a low voltage QRS, in lead aVL. There are abnormal ST segments in inferior leads (non-specific). (b) Straightening of the ST segments in most leads and STE in lateral leads with reciprocal ST depression in II, III, and aVF. Also notable is the enlargement of the T waves in V2–V6, and I and aVL (hyperacute T-waves). (c) was recorded 20 min after fibrinolytic therapy, with the patient pain-free. ST resolution with terminal T wave inversion in V2–V6, I, and aVL is diagnostic of reperfusion, and is identical to Wellens' syndrome, which occurs after spontaneous reperfusion (see Chapter 15).

(a)

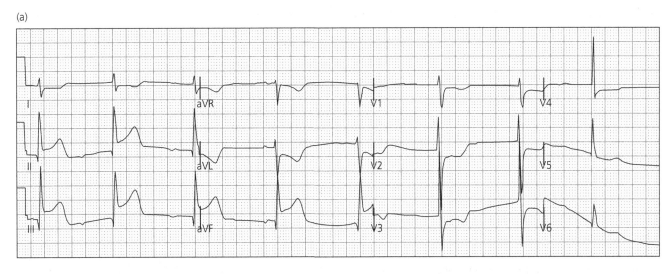

(b)

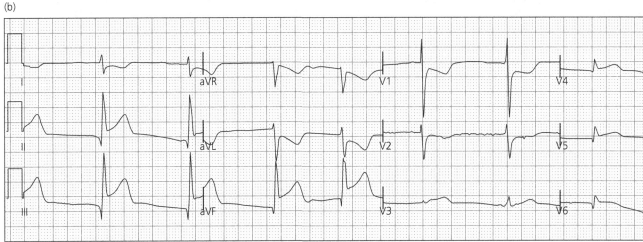

Figure 13.2 (a) ST elevation in II, III, aVF, with reciprocal ST depression in I and aVL, as well as ST depression in the anterior precordial leads, diagnostic of inferoposterior infarction. A right-sided ECG was performed and is shown in (b), in which the inferior changes are essentially identical to the initial ECG, as expected. In RV4, RV5, and RV6 there is 1 mm of ST elevation, diagnostic of RV involvement.

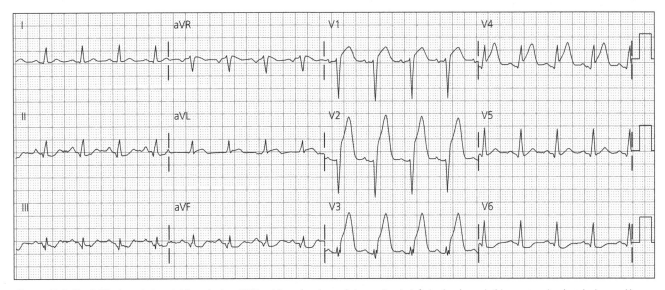

Figure 13.3 The ECG of an obvious LAD occlusion. STE in aVL and reciprocal depression in inferior leads mark this as a proximal occlusion and large anterior MI.

suggested in diagnostic criteria. Patients with such borderline ECGs who do not get the benefit of immediate reperfusion therapy permanently lose myocardium if they are not fortunate enough to have spontaneous reperfusion, or reperfusion due to anti-platelet or anti-thrombotic therapy. Conversely, most STE is not a result of coronary occlusion, but rather a result of pseudo-infarction patterns (see Chapters 14, 21, and 24) [4–6]. Even among patients with clearly diagnostic ECGs, but especially among those with borderline ECGs, reperfusion therapy is under-utilized or frequently delayed [7]. Physician uncertainty or error in ECG misinterpretation is one of the leading contributors to this under-utilization [7]. More recent literature still shows that 30% of eligible patients do not undergo reperfusion [8]. Unfortunately, computer ECG algorithms, though reasonably specific for STEMI, are not adequately sensitive (60–80%) [7].

Furthermore, atypical presentations contribute to under-utilization of reperfusion therapy. Many patients do not undergo an ECG recording in a timely manner, or not at all, because of atypical symptoms. Approximately one-third of patients with acute MI present to the ED with symptom complexes that do not include chest pain; women and the elderly in particular may present with dyspnea, weakness, or arm, hand, back, abdominal, or jaw pain [9]. Frequently, when the ECG is recorded in these patients, its findings may be ignored because the clinical presentation is so atypical. Some STE is subtle and must be interpreted in the light of the clinical situation; some is so obviously diagnostic of coronary occlusion that it must be acted upon in spite of the clinical presentation (see Figure 13.3).

This underscores the need to record an ECG promptly for any discomfort above the umbilicus that could be due to myocardial ischemia, to understand how to interpret the ECG in the context of the clinical symptoms, and to seek adjunctive means of determining whether subtle ECG findings are a result of coronary occlusion.

ST elevation and the indications for reperfusion are discussed in Chapter 24, pseudo-infarction patterns and abnormal QRS in Chapter 21, diagnostic adjuncts in Chapter 19, the electrocardiographically silent ECG, and the normal and non-diagnostic ECG in Chapter 22. The evolution of STEMI is discussed in chapters 17 and 16. Risk profiles of the ECG, including STE, STD, and T inversion are discussed in chapters 27 and 15. Some essential observations on STE, ST depression, and T wave inversion are included here.

ST segment elevation

Acute high-grade occlusion (> 90%) of coronary arteries alters the electric surface potential of the epicardium, which typically manifests itself on the ECG as STE, usually in two or more adjacent leads. This STE can be minimal, even < 1 mm, or it can be very large, sometimes greater than 10 mm. This is the injury pattern that represents a myocardial region at risk for irreversible cell death, or infarction. ST elevation represents "injury" (viable myocardium at risk, not yet necrosed), not infarction (irreversible cell death) [10].

Many recommendations have evolved over the years regarding the definition of STE criteria for reperfusion therapy (see Chapter 24). The differences involve the magnitude of the STE and the number of contiguous ECG leads required. In 2000, a joint effort between the European Society of Cardiology (ESC) and the American College of Cardiology (ACC) defined STE in the setting of acute MI as STE at the J point ≥ 0.2 mV (2 mm) in two or more contiguous leads V1, V2, or V3, or ≥ 0.1 mV (1 mm) in other leads [11]. Another more recent joint effort by the ESC and ACC Foundation (ACCF) along with the American Heart Association (AHA) and the World Heart Federation (WHF) in 2007 made some small changes, requiring at least 2 mm (0.2 mV) only in leads V2 and V3, and requiring only 0.15 mV of STE in women (see Figure 13.4). Contiguity is defined as V1–V6 in the anterior plane, and leads III, aVF, II, inverted aVR, I, and aVL (see Figure 13.4) [12]. See Figure 13.4 for a summary of these STEMI recommendations.

ST elevation should be measured from the PR segment to the upper edge of the ST segment at the J point. The amplitude of the STE differs based on where the measurements are made in the tracing. Results differ based on the measurement at the J point versus 60 ms or 80 ms after the J point [10]. The latter two measurements will result in significantly higher STE measurements. Defining these measurements is much more important in their use as research tools than for diagnosing patients in the clinical setting. A knowledgeable subjective interpretation of the ST segment appearance is more accurate than using measured criteria [13].

Evolution of STEMI

Figure 13.5 shows the classic ECG progression with persistent coronary occlusion, from a normal ECG to the changes at minutes, hours, days, and then months after the initial infarct. If the first minutes after acute coronary occlusion could be captured on an ECG, the first change that may be evident would be prolonging of the QT interval, then the

ST Elevation:
    New ST elevation at the J point in two contiguous leads with the
    cut off points:
        ≥ 0.2 mV in men or ≥ 0.15 mV in women in leads V2–V3
        and/or ≥ 0.1 mV in men and women in other leads

Lead Contiguity:
    Anterior: V1–V6
    Inferior: II, III, aVF
    Lateral: I, aVL
    Frontal: aVL, I, aVR, II, III, aVF

Figure 13.4 2007 Recommendations for ST elevation and contiguity in STEMI [12].

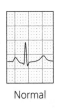 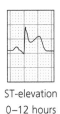 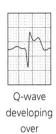 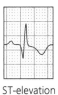

| Normal | Hyperacute T-wave minutes-hours | ST-elevation 0–12 hours | Q-wave developing over 1–12 hours | ST-elevation with T-wave inversion 2–5 days | T-wave recovery weeks-months |

Figure 13.5 Courtesy of K. Wang. *Atlas of Electrocardiography*.

appearance of hyperacute T waves, followed by STE that occurs within the first 0–12 h. Development of the Q wave can begin in the first hour after occlusion, and is typically completed approximately 8–12 h post-occlusion, if there is persistent occlusion without collateral circulation. The presence of enlarged T waves (in some cases referred to as "hyperacute"), even in the presence of STE or developing abnormal Q waves, indicates that the myocardium is salvageable. A scoring system utilizing the height of the T wave and the presence of Q waves and T wave inversion, has been developed. A high score (associated with tall T waves) indicates high acuteness, and, thus, significant benefit from reperfusion [14]. A subsequent study demonstrated that reperfusion therapy in patients with high acuteness scores, even after 2 h of delay from symptom onset, resulted in smaller infarction size in both inferior and anterior MIs [15].

In non-reperfused MI, resolution of STE and T wave inversion should occur within 2–5 days after the event, with ultimate T wave recovery and Q wave persistence over the following weeks to months. Persistent T wave inversion may last indefinitely. ST elevation completely resolves within 2 weeks after 95% of inferior MIs and 40% of anterior MIs. Approximately 60% of patients who have MI with persistent ST segment displacement have an anatomic ventricular aneurysm [10].

The evolution of the ST segment itself from normal to peak elevation occurs over a much shorter timeframe than the evolution of the entire QRS/ST/T wave complex, though this depends on the extent of the ischemia: with some flow through the artery, or with significant collateral circulation, myocardium can remain viable, with continued STE and upright T waves, for many hours. Figure 13.6 demonstrates

0713   0726   0739   0756

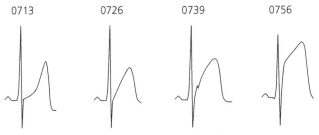

Figure 13.6 Classic evolution of ST segment morphology and hyperacute T wave during STEMI. Reprinted with permission from Chan TC, Brady WJ. *et al. ECG in Emergency Medicine and Acute Care.* Elsevier, 2005.

the changes during a STEMI from a normal, upwardly concave ST segment, to a straight, then to a convex, ST segment with a tall and wide T wave, diagnostic of STEMI. The times at which the tracings were taken are noted above each PQRST complex.

Non-ST elevation MI and unstable angina

Along with STEMI, the two other entities that make up ACS are NSTEMI and UA. Non-ST elevation myocardial infarction is an acute MI, as diagnosed by the appropriate clinical scenario plus elevated serum biomarkers of myocardial necrosis, but without sufficient, or diagnostic, or recorded STE (though many of these patients would have had transient STE at some point if the ECG had been recorded at the right time). The ECG in NSTEMI usually demonstrates minimal STE, ST depression and/or T wave changes (see Chapter 15), but may have entirely non-specific findings in about 20% of patients. Even 0.5 mm of ST depression is an independent predictor of decreased 4-year survival rate in patients with ACS [16]. The ST depression and T wave changes seen in NSTEMI and UA may be transient, often representing reversible ischemia. Higher magnitude of ST depression correlates with higher risk. Martin and colleagues found that the "STEMI equivalent" of ST depression ≥ 0.1 mV in two or more anatomically contiguous leads, in addition to the standard STEMI criteria, increased the sensitivity of diagnosing MI from 50 to 84%, while decreasing specificity only slightly from 97 to 93% [17].

Normal T waves on a normal ECG are usually upright in leads I, II, V3–V6; inverted in aVR; and variable in leads III, aVL, aVF, and V1 [10]. If T waves are abnormally inverted, especially in the presence of symptoms consistent with ACS, the cause should be assumed to be ischemia. Minimal T wave inversions of < 1 mm, however, have not been shown to be associated with adverse outcomes compared with patients who have ACS and an otherwise normal ECG [18]. T wave inversions associated with ACS that are > 1 mm in magnitude or are present in two or more leads are associated with a higher risk of complications, especially if they are of the Wellens' pattern type [19,20]. In general, evolving T wave inversion in ACS is caused by either: (1) acute ischemia, (2) spontaneous or therapeutic reperfusion, or (3) in the presence of QS waves, prolonged occlusion [10]. The depth of the T inversion correlates with the amount of viable myocardium after reperfusion (see chapters 15 and 27).

The diagnosis of NSTEMI is confirmed in the appropriate clinical setting with the elevation of serum cardiac biomarkers of cellular damage. Unstable angina refers to the symptoms and ECG changes consistent with fully reversible ischemia, and may be initially indistinguishable from NSTEMI based on ECG findings. By definition, biomarkers are not elevated in UA, and the ischemia is reversible. The ECG has been used within this spectrum to stratify for the likelihood of presence or absence of ACS in patients presenting with suspicious symptoms. A normal ECG, flat T waves, or T waves inverted less than 0.5 mm in leads with dominant R waves places the patient in the "low likelihood" category. ST depression of 0.5 to 1 mm or T wave inversion > 0.5 mm in leads with dominant R waves confers an "intermediate likelihood" of ACS. ST deviation > 1 mm, or "marked" T wave inversion in multiple leads confers a "high likelihood" of ACS [21]. Longer duration of symptoms is more likely to be NSTEMI versus UA; however, clinical differentiation of these two entities without the use of biomarkers is entirely uncertain. Non-ST elevation myocardial infarction/unstable angina, in contrast to STEMI, result from non-occlusive thrombus, small risk area, brief occlusion, and/or an occlusion that maintains good collateral circulation [10]. If the patient is in a high-risk group with ST depression and/or elevated biomarkers, and/or recurrent symptoms, "early" PCI (typically within 48 h), along with appropriate medical therapy, reduces morbidity and mortality [3].

Conclusion

The ECG is the first and most important diagnostic tool in ACS. Accurate and timely interpretation is essential for the reperfusion decision. Recognizing the various ECG manifestations of ACS, from normal to subtle ST and T wave abnormalities, to obvious changes of persistent ischemia, to changes that fulfill STEMI criteria, is critical. Clinical judgment, along with ECG expertise, will help to avoid the pitfalls of ECG insensitivity and pseudo-infarction patterns that mimic ischemic changes. Timely reperfusion of occluded coronaries will reduce both morbidity and mortality.

Case conclusions

In Case 1, a lateral STEMI was diagnosed, the patient was treated with a fibrinolytic agent; approximately 20 min later, he was pain-free with a repeat ECG confirming reperfusion. The proximal LAD was the infarct-related artery. In Case 2, the patient went to angiography and had a stent placed in a proximal portion of his RCA. Lastly, in Case 3, the patient's absence of typical symptoms were ignored because there is only one explanation for the ECG: acute STEMI. He went to the catheterization laboratory but died before the occluded LAD could be opened.

References

1 Keeley EC, Hillis LD. Primary PCI for myocardial infarction with ST-segment elevation. *N Engl J Med* 2007;**356**:47–54.
2 Fibrinolytic Therapy Trialists' (FTT) Collaborative Group. Indications for fibrinolytic therapy in suspected acute myocardial infarction: collaborative overview of early mortality and major morbidity results from all randomised trials of more than 1000 patients. *Lancet* 1994;**343**:311–22.
3 Cannon CP, Weintraub WS, Demopoulos LA, *et al.* Comparison of early invasive and conservative strategies in patients with unstable coronary syndromes treated with the glycoprotein IIb/IIIa inhibitor tirofiban. (TACTICS)-TIMI 18. *N Engl J Med* 2001;**344**:1879–87.
4 Sharkey SW, Berger CR, Brunette DD, Henry TD. Impact of the electrocardiogram on the delivery of thrombolytic therapy for acute myocardial infarction. *Am J Cardiol* 1994;**73**:550–3.
5 Wang K, Asinger RW, Marriott HJ. ST-segment elevation in conditions other than acute myocardial infarction. *N Engl J Med* 2003;**349**:2128–35.
6 Larson DM, Menssen KM, Sharkey SW, *et al.* "False-Positive" Cardiac Catheterization Laboratory Activation Among Patients with Suspected ST-Segment Elevation Myocardial Infarction. *JAMA* 2007;**298**:2754–60.
7 Smith SW, Zvosec DL, Henry TD, Sharkey SW. The ECG in Acute MI: an Evidence-Based Manual of Reperfusion Therapy. Philadelphia: Lippincott, Williams, and Wilkins, 2002:358.
8 Eagle KA, Goodman SG, Avezum A, *et al.* Practice variation and missed opportunities for reperfusion in ST-segment-elevation myocardial infarction: findings from the Global Registry of Acute Coronary Events (GRACE). *Lancet* 2002;**359**:373–7.
9 Canto JG, Shlipak MG, Roger WJ, *et al.* Prevalence, clinical characteristics, and mortality among patients with myocardial infarction presenting without chest pain. *JAMA* 2000;**283**:3223–9.
10 Smith SW, Whitwam W. Acute Coronary Syndromes. *Emerg Med Clin North Am* 2006;**24**:53–89.
11 Joint European Society of Cardiology/American College of Cardiology Committee. Myocardial infarction redefined: A consensus document of the Joint European Society of Cardiology/American College of Cardiology committee for the redefinition of myocardial infarction. *J Am Coll Cardiol* 2000;**36**:959–69.
12 Thygesen K, Alpert JS, White HD, *et al.* Universal Definition of Myocardial Infarction. *Circulation* 2007;**116**:2634–53.
13 Massel D, Dawdy JA, Melendez LJ. Strict reliance on a computer algorithm or measurable ST segment criteria may lead to errors in thrombolytic therapy eligibility. *Am Heart J* 2000;**140**:221–6.
14 Wilkins ML, Pryor AD, Maynard C, *et al.* An electrocardiographic acuteness score for quantifying the timing of a myocardial infarction to guide decisions regarding reperfusion therapy. *Am J Cardiol* 1995;**75**:617–20.
15 Corey KE, Maynard C, Pahlm O, *et al.* Combined historical and electrocardiographic timing of acute anterior and inferior myocardial infarcts for prediction of reperfusion achievable size limitation. *Am J Cardiol* 1999;**83**:826–31.
16 Hyde TA, French JK, Wong CK, *et al.* Four-year survival of patients with acute coronary syndromes without ST-segment

elevation and prognostic significance of 0.5-mm ST-segment depression. *Am J Cardiol* 1999;**84**:379–85.

17 Martin TN, Groenning BA, Murray HM, *et al.* ST-Segment Deviation Analysis of the Admission 12-Lead Electrocardiogram as an Aid to Early Diagnosis of Acute Myocardial Infarction With a Cardiac Magnetic Resonance Imaging Gold Standard. *J Am Coll Cardiol* 2007;**50**:1021–8.

18 Diderholm E, Andren B, Frostfeldt G, *et al.* ST depression in ECG at entry indicates severe coronary lesions and large benefits of an early invasive treatment strategy in unstable coronary artery disease; the FRISC II ECG substudy. The fast revascularisation during instability in coronary artery disease. *Eur Heart J* 2002;**23**:41–9.

19 de Zwaan C, Bar FW, Janssen JHA, *et al.* Angiographic and clinical characteristics of patients with unstable angina showing an ECG pattern indicating critical narrowing of the proximal LAD coronary artery. *Am Heart J* 1989;**117**:657–65.

20 de Zwaan C, Bar FW, Wellens HJJ. Characteristic electrocardiographic pattern indicating a critical stenosis high in left anterior descending coronary artery in patients admitted because of impending myocardial infarction. *Am Heart J* 1982;**103**:730–6.

21 Braunwald E, Jones RH, Mark DB, *et al.* Diagnosing and managing unstable angina. Agency for Health Care Policy and Research. *Circulation* 1994; **90**:613–22.

Chapter 14 | What pseudoinfarction patterns mimic ST elevation myocardial infarction?

Stephen W. Smith[1], David M. Larson[2]

[1]University of Minnesota, Hennepin County Medical Center, Minneapolis, MN, USA
[2]University of Minnesota Medical School, St Paul, MN, USA

Case presentations

Case 1: A 35-year-old male comes to the emergency department (ED) after awakening with substernal intermittent chest pain. His cardiac risk factors include a history of dyslipidemia and a family history of coronary disease. Vital signs are normal. He is moderately overweight. The ECG (Figure 14.1) shows ST elevation (STE) in leads I, aVL and V1–V4. The initial troponin is negative.

Case 2: A 48-year-old male presents to the ED complaining of anterior chest pain intermittently for about 8 h. Upon arrival, the pain is constant, non-radiating and sometimes worse with taking a deep breath. He has a history of smoking and hypertension treated with a diuretic. He has had 2 weeks of cough. He appears anxious and in obvious pain. Vital signs and exam are unremarkable. The ECG demonstrates STE in I, II, III, AVF, V1–6 (Figure 14.2). The initial troponin is normal.

Case 3: A 71-year-old female develops chest pain and shortness of breath after an emotionally stressful event. She has a history of hypertension and hyperlipidemia. Vital signs are blood pressure (BP) 100/60, heart rate (HR) 100. She appears diaphoretic and dyspneic. Chest is clear to auscultation. Heart sounds reveal an S3 gallop. Her initial ECG (Figure 14.3) demonstrates STE diagnostic of ischemia in leads I, II, AVL, and V4–6.

Mimics of acute myocardial infarction

These three cases are examples of patients with symptoms and ECG findings suggestive of an acute ST elevation

Critical Decisions in Emergency and Acute Care Electrocardiography,
1st edition. Edited by W.J. Brady and J.D. Truwit. © 2009 Blackwell Publishing, ISBN: 9781405159067

myocardial infarction (STEMI) who do not, however, have angiographic evidence of coronary artery occlusion. In up to 85% of patients with chest pain (CP) and STE, the STE is due to a non-AMI diagnosis, with up to 25% due to left ventricular hypertrophy (LVH) [1–3,4]. Larson and colleagues found that, of 1335 patients taken for emergency angiography based on the ECG and clinical findings of probable STEMI, 16.0% had either no culprit artery or negative biomarkers, and 9.2% had both no culprit and negative biomarkers [5]. The most frequent STEMI mimics, in decreasing order, were: (1) myo- or pericarditis (2.6%), (2) prior MI with persistent STE (2.2%), (3) benign early repolarization (BER, 1.9%), (4) "non-diagnostic" ECG, (5) stress cardiomyopathy (1.3%), and (6) and left bundle branch block (1.1%).

Pseudo-infarction patterns

1 Due to abnormal QRS (see Chapter 5)
  a. Bundle branch block
  b. LVH
  c. Wolff-Parkinson-White (WPW) syndrome
2 BER (normal ST elevation or normal variant)
3 Pericarditis/myocarditis
4 Stress cardiomyopathy
5 Left ventricular aneurysm (persistent ST elevation after previous MI)
6 Brugada syndrome (is really an abnormal QRS, but very subtly so)
7 Hyperkalemia
8 Pulmonary embolism
9 Subarachnoid hemorrhage or other stroke

Left ventricular hypertrophy, bundle branch block, WPW syndrome, and Brugada syndrome have an abnormal QRS (abnormal depolarization), which is the cause of the abnormal repolarization (ST segment and T wave abnormalities). Thus, in the presence of abnormal repolarization (ST elevation or depression, or T wave inversion), it is crucial to scrutinize the QRS; if the QRS is abnormal, then the ST T

(a)

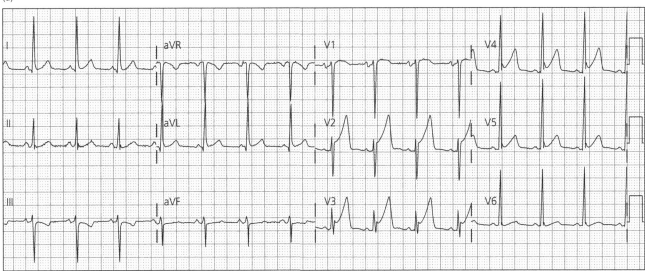

(b)

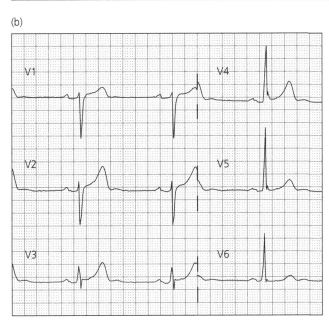

Figure 14.1 Benign early repolarization. (a) ECG characteristics favoring BER: There is no terminal QRS distortion (normal S waves in V2 and V3), the ST segment has upward concavity, there is no reciprocal ST depression. Although the T wave does "tower" over the R wave in V2, the mean R wave amplitude from V2 to V4 is large (= 12 mm). A mean R wave of > 10 mm is unusual in LAD occlusion. However, the decision rule favors acute anterior MI, because the mean STE in V2–V4 is > 2 mm. Furthermore, the regression equation, (1.553 × mean STEJ) + (0.0546 × QTc-B) – (0.3813 × mean RA), with QTc-B of 420 ms, yields a value of 22.55 (> 21), which would indicate LAD occlusion. Moreover, the STE was increased from a previous tracing, even though the heart rate was previously slower (Figure 14.1b, V1–V6 only). Usually, STE of BER diminishes with increasing heart rate. Angiography was appropriately undertaken, but the coronaries were normal and troponins negative.

abnormalities may be "secondary" to this abnormal QRS, not "primarily" due to ischemia.

Serial ECGs/echocardiography/angiography

Many entities associated with pseudo-infarction patterns can be distinguished from acute MI by an absence of rapid evolution on the ECG. Much more immediately reliable, however, is the absence of a regional wall motion abnormality on echocardiogram. When in doubt, emergent echocardiogram or angiography is indicated (see Chapter 6).

Normal variant or benign early repolarization

STE of up to 3.5 mm in one or more precordial leads may be a normal finding, especially in younger men, and is referred to as benign early repolarization (BER) [6]. BER is a normal variant that may mimic STEMI. Benign early repolarization has been observed to have a higher prevalence in males, of age less than 40, black race and in those more athletically active [7]. In fact, STE in precordial leads is so common that BER can be considered to be simply "normal" rather that a normal variant [6]. In only 2% of cases is the STE ≥ 5 mm

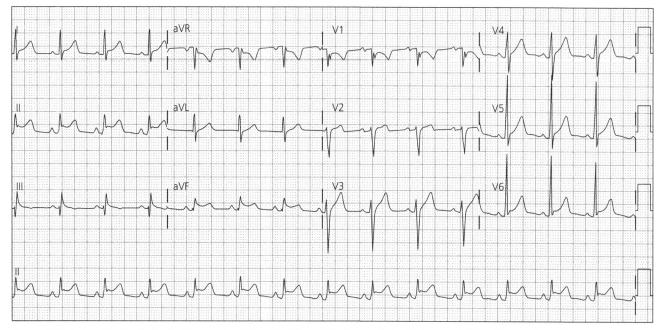

Figure 14.2 Pericarditis. This is classic diffuse pericarditis, with diffuse STE in limb leads II > III, also I, and aVF, *without* reciprocal ST depression in aVL, and STE in precordial leads V6 and V5 > V4 > V3 > V2. There is significant PR depression in leads II and V3–V6. The STE is upwardly concave, as it must be to diagnose pericarditis.

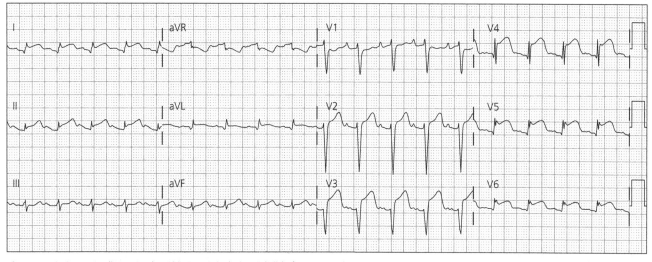

Figure 14.3 Stress cardiomyopathy. This ECG is indistinguishable from anterolateral MI, except that there is also STE in lead II, and unless the clinical scenario is inconsistent with MI, angiography must be undertaken.

[1]. T waves in BER are prominent, as in STEMI, and R waves are much more pronounced than in STEMI. In a large study comparing 167 cases of BER to 250 left anterior descending (LAD) occlusions (anterior STEMI), but analyzing only the 125 STEMI which were difficult to differentiate from BER, BER had a mean T wave amplitude, in V2–V4, of 6.2 mm (versus 6.8 mm) and a mean R amplitude of 11.3 mm (versus 4.6 mm) [8,9]. Mean STE at the J point, and at 60 ms after the J point, was 1.3 mm and 1.9 mm, respectively, significantly

lower than the means for LAD occlusion (2.0 mm and 2.9 mm). Mean QTc-B was 390 ± 27 ms versus 420 ± 28 ms [8].

As the term implies, BER is not associated with immediate adverse clinical outcomes. However, in patients who present with typical symptoms of ACS it is frequently challenging for physicians to distinguish BER from AMI [10]. Some of these patients may be appropriately referred for emergent cardiac catheterization or receive fibrinolytic therapy, even in the absence of MI [5].

Electrocardiographic features of BER, in contrast to STEMI

(1) Concave upward STE in all limb leads and all of leads V2–V6: "Like a cord suspended from the descending R limb at one end and the apex of the T wave at the other end" [11]. Upward concavity does not exclude anterior MI from LAD occlusion and is, in fact, very common in early LAD occlusion [12]; absence of upward concavity does not absolutely exclude BER (Figure 14.11).

(2) Notching or slurring of the J point: Often resulting in a nearly pathognomonic "J-wave" (Figures 14.1 and 14.11); however, the J wave may occasionally be seen in STEMI.

(3) Large concordant, asymmetric T waves: These waves have a more gradual upstroke than downstroke.

(4) Temporal stability: This is more likely to be present on previous ECGs; there are exceptions to this, however (Figure 14.1). Lead placement can affect amount of STE. Isoproterenol and exercise are known to decrease STE.

(5) Absence of reciprocal ST depression: Especially absent in aVL with inferior BER.

(6) Occasionally associated "benign T wave inversion": This consists of biphasic T waves, especially in leads V3–V5. T wave inversion in anterior MI is more likely in leads V2–V4 (see Figure 15.6).

(7) Short QT interval compared with AMI: Only 4% of subtle LAD occlusion, versus 40% of BER, has a QTc-B < 380 ms (Smith SW, *et al.*, unpublished data).

(8) Presence of S waves, or J waves, in V2 and V3: That is, absence of "terminal QRS distortion".

(9) High R wave amplitude: Mean R wave amplitude from V2 to V4 is > 5 mm in only 34% of subtle LAD occlusion (sensitivity 66%) and in 94% of BER (specificity 94%), and is ≥ 10 mm in 10% of subtle LAD occlusion versus 59% of BER (Smith SW, *et al.*, unpublished data).

(10) Rarely present in inferior leads when not present in precordial leads: Also, inferior STE due to BER is always < 1 mm. Isolated STE in inferior leads should not be assumed to be due to BER. However, STE in inferior leads without reciprocal STD in aVL is likely not due to STEMI.

Summary and decision rule: With precordial ST elevation in V2–V4, if any one of the following is present, BER is very unlikely and a provisional diagnosis of STEMI may be made (Smith SW *et al.*, unpublished data):

(a) Single lead with > 5 mm of STE.

(b) Anterior or inferior reciprocal ST depression.

(c) Terminal QRS distortion (loss of S wave in V2 or V3, without a J-wave, see Chapter 3 and Figure 14.10(a).

(d) A single lead of V2–V6 with a straight or convex (non-concave) ST segment.

(e) Mean STE (V2–V4) of ≥ 2 mm.

(f) Mean R wave (V2–V4) of ≤ 5 mm.

Furthermore, a multivariate decision rule was developed for those ECGs in which the decision between BER and LAD occlusion is difficult (no lead with > 5 mm STE, no ST depression, no terminal QRS distortion, concavity in all leads). If the value of the equation $(1.553 \times \text{mean STEJ}) + (0.0546 \times \text{QTc-B}) - (0.3813 \times \text{mean RA}) \leq 21$, it favors BER; if > 21 it favors LAD occlusion, with a sensitivity, specificity, and accuracy of 91%, 87%, 88% [9].

Pericarditis/myocarditis

Myo-pericarditis (Figures 14.4 and 14.5) may present with symptoms and ECG abnormalities, primarily STE, suggestive of acute MI. Most pericarditis is a diffuse inflammation of the entire pericardial surface and has an ST vector pointing anterior, leftward, and inferior, towards the apex of the heart (towards leads II and V5 and away from aVR). This results in diffuse STE, including lead aVL. In pericarditis, lead II thus has higher STE than lead III (contrasting with most inferior MI); the highest STE is in V3–V6 and in the inferior leads, with reciprocal depression *only* in aVR. Inferolateral STEMI, then, frequently appears identical to pericarditis, with one usual difference: at least a minimal amount of reciprocal ST depression is nearly always present in aVL in MI, but appears in pericarditis only if the pericarditis is localized to the inferior wall (diffuse pericarditis is far more common).

Patients with pericarditis often have a preceding acute viral infection, including a fever. The chest pain may be pleuritic, and worse with swallowing or positional changes such as reclining. A pericardial friction rub may be heard. Bedside echocardiography may show pericardial effusion. However, the absence of any of these clinical findings does not rule out pericarditis. Urgent echocardiogram, by presence of regional wall motion abnormality (RWMA), is the best means of distinguishing pericarditis (absent) from STEMI (present); however, there may be RWMA in localized myocarditis (Figure 14.5).

ECG features of myo-pericarditis [13]: (see Figures 14.4 and 14.5)

(1) Diffuse concave upward STE involving more than one vascular territory. ST elevation rarely exceeds 5 mm and is greatest in leads II and V5. Typically, STE in lead II > lead III, whereas in AMI, due to occlusion of the right coronary artery, STE in lead III > lead II. ST elevation in the lateral precordial leads (V5–V6) is usually greater than the anterior precordial leads (V1–V4).

(2) Reciprocal ST depression in aVR.

(3) Depression of the PR segment relative to the TP segment resulting from atrial repolarization abnormalities, best observed in leads II, III, AVF, and V5–V6. This may be one of the earliest ECG manifestations of acute pericarditis [14]. Although some PR depression is normal due to the normal

(a)

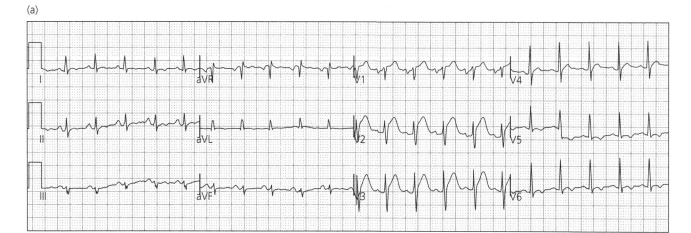

(b)

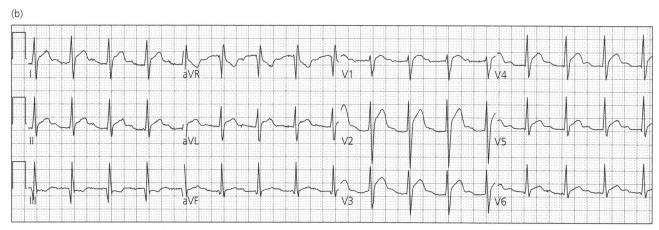

Figure 14.4 Myo-pericarditis. (a) Myocarditis that is nearly indistinguishable from STEMI. The STE is 3 mm or more in lead V2, the ST segments are almost straight, and all STE is limited to one coronary distribution, the LAD. Furthermore, the QTc-B is 440 ms, and there is non-specific T-inversion in V5 and V6. Only the R waves (mean = 8 mm) argue against acute MI. The initial troponin was elevated. He underwent emergent cath. and had normal coronary arteries, but an ejection fraction of 20%. (b) Pericarditis. A 27-year-old male presented with chest pain. The STE is 3 mm or more in lead V2, and the ST segments are straight. The QTc-B is 457 ms, also suggestive of MI. However, the distribution of ST elevation is unusual for MI, with the ST vector left and anterior, towards leads I and V2, resulting in STE in inferior leads II, but not III or aVL. The tall R waves (mean > 10 mm) argue against acute MI. Troponins and angiogram were normal.

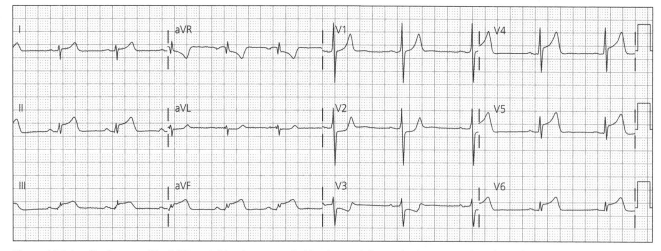

Figure 14.5 Localized myocarditis. A 30-year-old male presented with substernal chest pain, dyspnea, and an elevated troponin. His ECG shows STE in leads II, III, and aVF and V4–V6, with minimal reciprocal depression in aVL, and profound STD in V2–V3, indistinguishable from inferoposterolateral MI. Immediate coronary angiography revealed normal coronaries; cardiac MRI demonstrated myo-pericarditis of the inferoposterolateral wall.

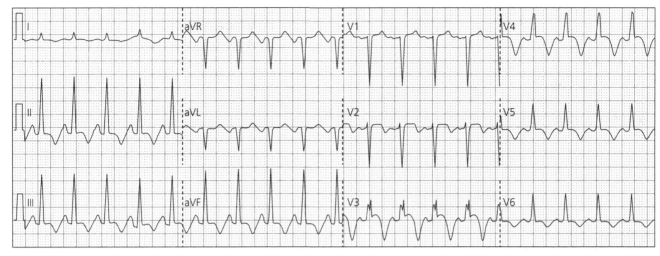

Figure 14.6 Stress cardiomyopathy with upwardly convex ST elevation and deep T wave inversion. If an ECG had been recorded earlier, would there have been STE with upright T waves? The electrocardiographic natural history of this disorder is uncertain.

atrial repolarization wave, PR depression > 0.8 mm is specific, but not sensitive, for pericarditis. Reciprocal PR segment elevation in aVR is also strongly suggestive of pericarditis [15].

(4) Absence of reciprocal ST depression in AVL with STE in lead III and vice versa. This may be the only feature that clearly distinguishes pericarditis from acute MI.

(5) Absence of acute pathological Q waves.

Localized myo-pericarditis (Figure 14.5) presents exceptions to the above rules. When the inflammation is limited to only one wall of the heart (e.g. inferior), there may be STE in a regional distribution similar to acute MI (e.g. lead III, with reciprocal STD in lead aVL). Conversely, an acute inferior and anterolateral STEMI, due to an occlusion of a wraparound LAD, may present with diffuse STE of more than one vascular territory. Unlike pericarditis, these usually have reciprocal STD in lead aVL (see Figure 9.1).

The ECG in pericarditis evolves variably over days to weeks; there are four ECG stages: Stage 1: diffuse STE with PR depression; Stage 2: ST segment normalization; Stage 3: T wave inversion; Stage 4: normalization. Generally, pericarditis has more prominent STE, with a less prominent T wave, than BER; a ST/T ratio in lead V6 of > 0.25 favors pericarditis and a ratio < 0.25 favors BER [16]. Of course, like BER, acute MI also has prominent T waves.

Myocarditis is most readily confused with acute MI because of elevations of cardiac biomarkers (Figures 14.4a and 14.5) [17]. When there is localized inflammation, myocarditis may mimic STEMI not only by ECG and biomarkers, but also with a regional wall motion abnormality. The diagnosis is often presumed to be acute MI until angiography reveals open and normal vessels. Cardiac magnetic resonance imaging (MRI) has a sensitivity and specificity of 90% in histologically proven myocarditis and has become the study of choice to confirm suspected myocarditis [18].

Stress cardiomyopathy

Stress cardiomyopathy (SCM), also know as Tako-tsubo cardiomyopathy, apical ballooning syndrome, or "broken heart syndrome," is characterized by acute and reversible left ventricular systolic dysfunction (LVSD) without obstructive coronary disease, which is often preceded by severe psychologic or physical stress occurring predominantly in postmenopausal women [19]. The cause of this syndrome is unknown, but some speculate that there may be catecholamine-mediated direct myocardial injury or microvascular spasm [20]. In a series of 1335 patients from Minnesota with suspected STEMI, SCM was diagnosed in 16 of 372 (4.3%) female patients with STE diagnostic of MI (Figure 14.3) [5]. The ECG shows precordial acute STE (1–3 mm) with evolutionary T wave inversion in the subacute phase, identical to STEMI; this T wave inversion may be the first ECG abnormality recorded (Figure 14.6). The left ventriculogram from this patient demonstrates the characteristic apical ballooning that looks similar to the Japanese octopus trap or Tako-tsubo (Figure 14.7). In 286 SCM patients, STE was present in 82% and T wave abnormalities in 64% [21]. There are slight elevations of cardiac biomarkers, and one-third present with hemodynamic compromise requiring vasopressors or intra-aortic balloon counterpulsation [19]. The diagnosis is usually made retrospectively after cath. reveals normal coronary arteries and the typical apical ballooning; cardiac MRI is also helpful. The LVSD is reversible and the prognosis is generally good. This syndrome should be suspected when a postmenopausal female with relatively few cardiac risk factors presents after a recent severe emotional or physical stress; in such cases, urgent angiography, if quickly available, should be preferred to fibrinolysis. Emergency echocardiography showing typical apical ballooning may also be helpful.

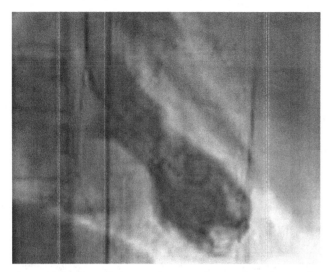

Figure 14.7 Left ventriculogram of stress cardiomyopathy patient. Notice that the base constricts while the apex, to the lower right, balloons out.

Prior myocardial infarction/ left ventricular aneurysm

Patients with a previous transmural myocardial infarction, with or without a left ventricular aneurysm (LVA), may have persistent STE (Figure 14.8a–c). In one series of patients with a prior MI presenting with chest pain and STE, only 50% proved to have an acute MI [22]. Left ventricular aneurysm most commonly involves the anterior wall resulting in persistent STE, with QS waves, in V1–V4. Inferior LVA presents more commonly with STE and QR waves.

In contrast to acute MI, which has tall T waves (see Chapter 16), in LVA the T waves may be flattened or inverted. Thus, the best discriminator of LVA versus acute MI is the T wave amplitude/QRS amplitude ratio. If the ratio: (sum of the T wave amplitude) to (sum of QRS amplitude)

(a)

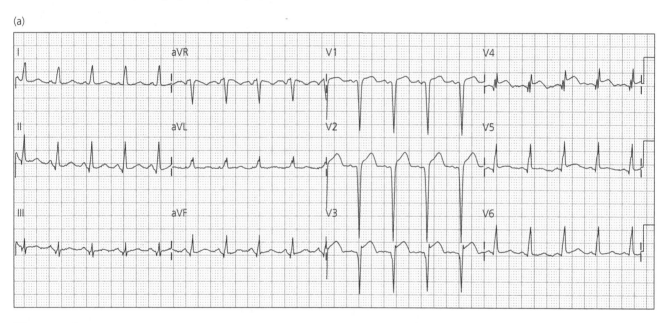

(b)

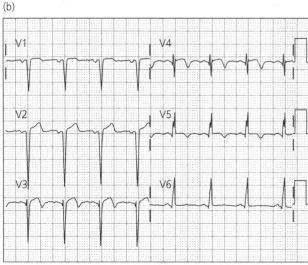

Figure 14.8 LVA (prior MI with persistent STE). QS waves with STE in V2 and V3 can be due to LVH or cardiomyopathy, but when extending to V4, especially with a QR wave, it is a result of MI (either acute or old). Previous ECGs had QS waves with some T inversion (Figure 14.8b, V1–V6 only). Thus, one might suspect T wave pseudonormalization on the new ECG, with possible acute MI superimposed on old MI. However, *acute MI has larger T waves*. The ratio of T(V1–V4)/QRS(V1–V4) = $(1 + 2 + 2 + 2)/(19 + 28 + 15 + 7) = 7/69 = 0.10$. A value < 0.22 is very unusual for acute LAD occlusion; this low value, especially with a QS wave, is usually associated with LVA, as in this case. Bedside ED echo showed anterior wall motion abnormality with anterior wall thinning and diastolic dysfunction (dyskinesis). The patient ruled out by serial negative troponins. (c) A second case of prior MI with persistent STE; note anterior QS waves with T inversion and low T/QRS ratio.

(c)

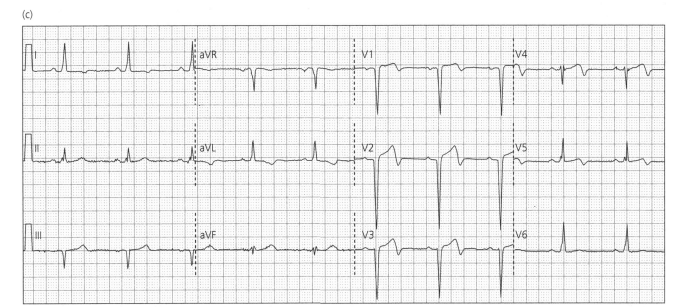

Figure 14.8 (cont'd)

in V1–V4 is > 0.22, it favors AMI whereas a ratio < 0.22 favors LVA with a sensitivity and specificity of 95% and 91%, respectively [23]. Even more useful is comparison with an index ECG (prior ECG), but these are not always available. Echocardiography may also be useful if it shows dyskinesis (diastolic dysfunction), which is the anatomic definition of aneurysm. Unfortunately, persistent STE after old MI also occurs without anatomic aneurysm. Regional wall motion abnormality without dyskinesis (akinesis or hypokinesis) is present in both acute MI and old MI. In some cases, coronary angiography will be required to make the diagnosis. New STEMI in the same location as previous Q wave MI may also have deep QS waves, but has tall T waves.

Brugada syndrome

Brugada syndrome is characterized by: (1) persistent STE in V1–V3 accompanied by a right bundle branch block (complete or incomplete), 2) no apparent structural heart disease, and 3) propensity for life-threatening ventricular tachyarrhythmias, due to gene mutations causing an ion channel defect [24]. There appear to be electrophysiologic similarities to early repolarization and hypothermia. There is an association between Brugada syndrome and sudden, unexpected death in Southeast Asian men. The ECG in Brugada syndrome shows one of two peculiar forms of STE in the right precordial leads. In the first, the terminal portion of the QRS complex in lead V1 is elevated as an R′ with the ST segment elevated and downsloping and usually ending in a negative T wave; V2 and V3 may appear similar but with a more horizontal ST segment (Figure 14.9). The second morpho-

logy has an upwardly concave saddle-type configuration [1]. Neither manifests reciprocal ST depression in inferior leads nor a long QT interval [25]. Transient forms of disease have been described in which the ECG may normalize, as happened in the case in Figure 14.9 (but not shown). Hyperpyrexia may unmask Brugada syndrome, as some of the abnormal sodium channels are temperature-sensitive [26].

Hyperkalemia

Severe hyperkalemia may result in STE with peaked T waves that mimic an AMI. The earliest ECG sign of hyperkalemia typically involves a tall, narrow, peaked, or tented T wave with a short QT interval (in contrast to STEMI). This has a narrower base than the peaked T wave of AMI. Further progression of hyperkalemia will demonstrate PR and QRS prolongation and flattening or absence of the P wave (Figure 14.10). As the QRS interval widens, the ST segment may appear elevated. In contrast to AMI, the ST segment in hyperkalemia is downsloping [6]. See also Figure 16.2.

Pulmonary embolism

Pulmonary embolism (PE) will occasionally manifest a pseudo-infarction pattern, with precordial T-wave inversion (see Figure 15.5). The classical description includes the $S_1Q_3T_3$ pattern. However, STE, as well as T wave inversion, may be seen in the anterior and inferior leads. Among patients with precordial T inversions, T wave inversion in both V1 and III was highly sensitive and specific for PE [27].

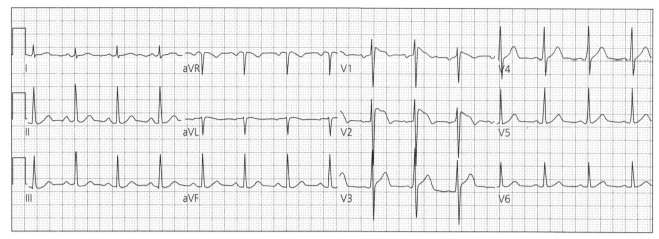

Figure 14.9 Brugada syndrome. A 41-year-old male with chest pain. He was taken for angiography based upon the STE in V1 and V2. Later, it was noticed that this represents Brugada syndrome. He underwent electrophysiologic (EP) study and a cardioverter-defibrillator was implanted. A later ECG was normal, showing no evidence of Brugada syndrome (intermittent).

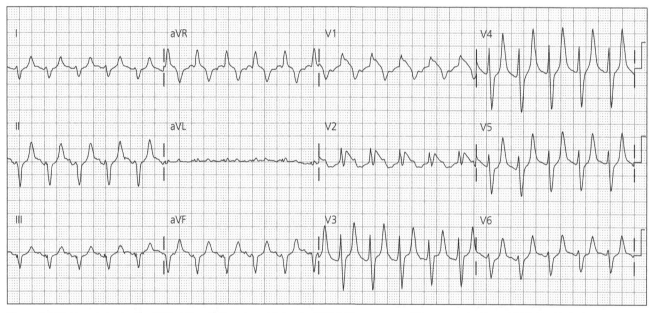

Figure 14.10 Hyperkalemia. The STE in V1 and V2 can be mistaken for STEMI. The very tented T waves and widened QRS should alert to hyperkalemia. K was 8.4 mEq/L.

General strategies for differentiating pseudo-infarction from STEMI

(1) Evaluate the QRS. Is it LBBB, RBBB, LVH, WPW, paced rhythm, or intraventricular conduction delay (see Chapter 21)? If so, are the ST-T abnormalities consistent with the abnormal QRS? Or are the ST-T abnormalities superimposed on the expected ST-T abnormalities? Look especially for *proportionality* and *concordance*.

(2) Look for reciprocal ST depression. If not due to abnormal QRS, reciprocal depression is highly likely to represent ACS.

This is especially true for inferior MI: if there is no ST depression in aVL, it is unlikely to be MI; if ST depression is present, MI is very likely. When considering anterior MI, if there is inferior or anterior ST depression, then AMI is highly likely (with or without STE in I and aVL) [28].

(3) Look for convex or straight ST segments; although concavity is frequently found in anterior MI, non-concave ST segments are infrequently normal.

(4) If the STE is borderline, the differential is between normal versus BER versus STEMI: use the decision rule above to make the distinction (see Figure 14.11).

(5) Widespread STE involving more than one vascular territory is unlikely to be acute MI unless there is a wraparound LAD or inferolateral MI. In both cases, there will almost

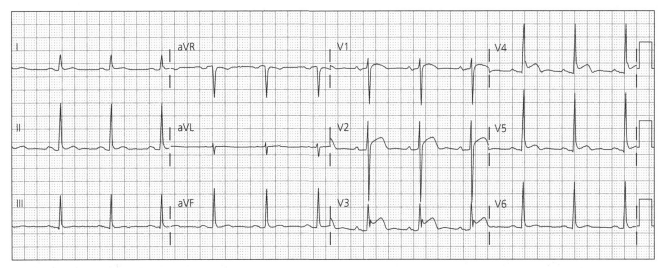

Figure 14.11 Early repolarization. There is STE in leads V2–V5, with convexity in V2, strongly suggesting anterior STEMI. The mean STE in V2–V4 is 2 mm; although there is loss of the S wave in V3, there is a J wave. The QTc is 317 ms, which is extremely unusual in anterior MI. The mean R amplitude in V2–V4 is 14 mm, also very unusual in anterior MI. To an experienced ECG interpreter, acute MI is unlikely because of the short QT, tall R waves, and prominent J waves. The logistic regression value is $(1.553 \times 2) + (0.0546 \times 317) - (0.3813 \times 14) = 15.1$ (< 21 greatly favors BER). However, no physician could be faulted, in the right clinical situation, for administering fibrinolytics to a patient with this ECG.

always be reciprocal STD in aVL. Isolated inferior STE, without precordial STE, is more often than not due to AMI, but there should be associate reciprocal STD in aVL.

(6) Acute STEMI has high T wave voltage. This contrasts with low T wave voltage in LVA.

Distinguishing AMI from pseudo-infarction can be challenging [29]. The physician at the bedside must balance the risk and cost of fibrinolysis or emergency coronary angiography against the consequences of delaying reperfusion. The AHA/ACC STEMI guidelines [30] acknowledge that using the diagnostic criteria of 0.1 mV (1 mm) of STE in precordial leads may decrease the specificity for STEMI. Using stricter criteria to increase the specificity of the ECG in AMI will result in decreasing the sensitivity [31]. In any case, the subjective interpretation of an experienced interpreter is more sensitive and specific than any mm STE criteria [32]. In most borderline cases, an emergent echocardiogram can differentiate; in some cases, transfer for cath., rather than fibrinolysis, is the wisest strategy.

Case conclusions

In Case 1, a comparison with a previous ECG (Figure 14.1b) showed increase in STE. The decision is made by the ED physician to send him for emergency coronary angiography; this was normal. The STE was due to BER. In Case 2, the ED physician sent the patient for angiography; the coronary arteries were normal. An erythrocyte sedimentation rate was elevated and a pericardial friction rub was later heard. The

diagnosis was acute pericarditis. The patient in Case 3 was sent for angiography, which showed normal coronaries. There was severe LVSD with an ejection fraction (EF) of 30% and apical hypokinesis. Cardiac MRI was consistent with SCM. A repeat echocardiogram 2 weeks later showed resolution, with an EF of 55%.

References

1 Brady WJ. ST segment and T wave abnormalities not caused by acute coronary syndromes. *Emerg Med Clin North Am* 2006;**24**: 91–111, vi.

2 Brady WJ. ST segment elevation in ED adult chest pain patients: etiology and diagnostic accuracy for AMI. *J Emerg Med* 1998; **16**:797–8.

3 Otto LA, Aufderheide TP. Evaluation of ST segment elevation criteria for the prehospital electrocardiographic diagnosis of acute myocardial infarction. *Ann Emerg Med* 1994;**23**:17–24.

4 Brady WJ, Perron AD, Martin ML, *et al.* Cause of ST segment abnormality in ED chest pain patients. *Am J Emerg Med* 2001;**19**:25–8.

5 Larson DM, Menssen KM, Sharkey SW, *et al.* "False-Positive" Cardiac Catheterization Laboratory Activation Among Patients with Suspected ST-Segment Elevation Myocardial Infarction. *JAMA* 2007;**298**:2754–60.

6 Wang K, Asinger RW, Marriott HJ. ST-segment elevation in conditions other than acute myocardial infarction. *N Engl J Med* 2003;**349**:2128–35.

7 Klatsky AL, Oehm R, Cooper R, *et al.* The Early Repolarization Normal Variant Electrocardiogram: Correlates and Consequences. *Am J Med* 2003;**115**:171–7.

8 Smith SW, Khalil A. Corrected QT Interval Distinguishes Early Repolarization from Subtle Anterior STEMI: Derivation of a Rule (abstract, presentation). *Acad Emerg Med* 2007;**14**:S125.

9 Smith SW, Khalil A, Henry TD. *Validation of an Electrocardiographic Decision Rule to Differentiate Early Repolarization from Subtle Anterior Myocardial Infarction due to Proven Left Anterior Descending Artery Occlusion*. Chicago, IL: Society for Academic Emergency Medicine, 2008.

10 Turnipseed SD, Bair AE, Kirk JD, *et al.* Electrocardiogram differentiation of benign early repolarization versus acute myocardial infarction by emergency physicians and cardiologists. *Acad Emerg Med* 2006;**13**:961–6.

11 Fenichel NN. A long term study of concave RS-T elevation – a normal variant of the electrocardiogram. *Angiology* 1962;**13**:360–6.

12 Smith SW. Upwardly concave ST segment morphology is common in acute left anterior descending coronary occlusion. *J Emerg Med* 2006;**31**:69–77.

13 Smith SW, Zvosec DL, Henry TD, Sharkey SW. *The ECG in Acute MI: an Evidence-Based Manual of Reperfusion Therapy*. Philadelphia: Lippincott, Williams, and Wilkins, 2002:358.

14 Baljepally R, Spodick DH. PR-segment deviation as the initial electrocardiographic response in acute pericarditis. *Am J Cardiol* 1998;**81**:1505–6.

15 Spodick DH. The electrocardiogram in acute pericarditis: distributions of morphologic and axial changes in stages. *Prog Cardiovasc Dis* 1974;**33**:470–4.

16 Chan TC, Brady WJ, Pollack M. Electrocardiographic manifestations: acute myopericarditis. *J Emerg Med* 1999;**17**:865–72.

17 Sarda L, Colin P, Boccara F, *et al.* Myocarditis in patients with clinical presentation of myocardial infarction and normal coronary arteries. *J Am Coll Cardiol* 2001;**37**:786–92.

18 Mahrholdt H, Goedecke C, Wagner A, *et al.* Cardiovascular magnetic resonance assessment of human myocarditis: a comparison to histology and molecular pathology. *Circulation* 2004;**109**:1250–8.

19 Sharkey SW, Lesser JR, Zenovich AG, *et al.* Acute and reversible cardiomyopathy provoked by stress in women from the United States. *Circulation* 2005;**111**:472–9.

20 Wittstein IS, Thiemann DR, Lima JA, *et al.* Neurohumoral features of myocardial stunning due to sudden emotional stress. *N Engl J Med* 2005;**352**:539–48.

21 Gianni M, Dentali F, Grandi AM, *et al.* Apical ballooning syndrome or takotsubo cardiomyopathy: a systematic review. *Eur Heart J* 2006;**27**:1523–9.

22 Miller DH, Kligfield P, Schreiber TL, Borer JS. Relationship of prior myocardial infarction to false-positive electrocardiographic diagnosis of acute injury in patients with chest pain. *Arch Intern Med* 1987;**147**:257–61.

23 Smith SW. T/QRS amplitude ratio best distinguishes the ST elevation of anterior left ventricular aneurysm from anterior acute myocardial infarction. *Am J Emerg Med* 2005;**23**:279–87.

24 Brugada P, Brugada J. Right bundle branch block, persistent ST segment elevation and sudden cardiac death: a distinct clinical and electrocardiographic syndrome. A multicenter report. *J Am Coll Cardiol* 1992;**20**:1391–6.

25 Gussak I, Antzelevitch C, Bjerregaard P, *et al.* The Brugada syndrome: clinical, electrophysiologic and genetic aspects. *J Am Coll Cardiol* 1999;**33**:5–15.

26 Unlu M, Bengi F, Amasyali B, Kose S. Brugada-like electrocardiographic changes induced by fever. *Emerg Med J* 2007;**24**:e4.

27 Kosuge M, Kimura K, Ishikawa T, *et al.* Electrocardiographic differentiation between acute pulmonary embolism and acute coronary syndromes on the basis of negative T waves. *Am J Cardiol* 2007;**99**:817–21.

28 Tamura A, Kataoka H, Mikuriya Y, Nasu M. Inferior ST segment depression as a useful marker for identifying proximal left anterior descending artery occlusion during acute anterior myocardial infarction. *Eur Heart J* 1995b;**16**:1795–9.

29 Brady WJ, Perron AD, Chan T. Electrocardiographic ST segment elevation: Correct identification of AMI and non-AMI syndromes by emergency physicians. *Acad Emerg Med* 2001;**8**:349–60.

30 Antman EM, Anbe DT, Armstrong PW, *et al.* ACC/AHA guidelines for the management of patients with ST-elevation myocardial infarction – executive summary. A report of the American College of Cardiology/American Heart Association Task Force on Practice Guidelines (Writing Committee to revise the 1999 guidelines for the management of patients with acute myocardial infarction). *J Am Coll Cardiol* 2004;**44**:671–719.

31 Menown IB, Mackenzie G, Adgey AA. Optimizing the initial 12-lead electrocardiographic diagnosis of acute myocardial infarction. *Eur Heart J* 2000;**21**:275–83.

32 Massel D, Dawdy JA, Melendez LJ. Strict reliance on a computer algorithm or measurable ST segment criteria may lead to errors in thrombolytic therapy eligibility. *Am Heart J* 2000;**140**:221–6.

Chapter 15 | What ECG changes might myocardial ischemia cause other than ST segment elevation or Q waves, and what are the differential diagnoses of these changes?

Stefan C. Bertog[2,3], Stephen W. Smith[1,3]

[1]University of Minnesota, Hennepin County Medical Center, Minneapolis, MN, USA
[2]University of Minnesota School of Medicine, Minneapolis, MN, USA
[3]Veterans Administration Medical Center, Minneapolis, MN, USA

Case presentations

Case 1: A 51-year-old man presents with 2 h of substernal and epigastric pain. He had an inferior myocardial infarction (MI) 6 months previously, at which time an angiogram revealed diffuse left anterior descending (LAD) and circumflex disease. The circumflex artery was previously stented. Figure 15.1(a) shows the electrocardiogram (ECG) after resolution of pain, which demonstrates Wellens' type T waves, the importance of which was not appreciated in the early evaluation. Serial troponin I was measurable at 0.37, 0.4, and 0.35 ng/mL, but below the 99% reference value (erroneously considered "negative").

Case 2: A 71-year-old male presents with progressive left chest pain radiating to his left arm for over 2 weeks. Figure 15.2(a) is the first ECG, showing Wellens' pattern A T waves, recorded at 4:33 pm with pain that was only slightly relieved after nitroglycerine. Acetylsalicylic acid (ASA), heparin, and eptifibatide are given and the patient is taken to the catheterization laboratory because of continuing pain.

Case 3: A 39-year-old male with a history of cocaine abuse and several other risk factors presents to the emergency department (ED) with chest pain lasting 4 h, accompanied by upper extremity numbness and tingling, dyspnea, and diaphoresis. He had had similar pain on and off for 2 years approximately once every 2–3 months, sometimes with exertion, lasting minutes to hours, but never this long. There

is no relief with nitroglycerine in the ED. Figure 15.3 is his initial ECG (previous baseline ECG was normal).

General discussion of ST and T wave, and U wave abnormalities in ischemia

When confronted with ST segment depression or T wave abnormalities, it is useful to classify a primary from secondary ST depression. With primary ST depression, the T wave abnormalities are accompanied by a normal QRS, and likely reflect myocardial ischemia. In secondary ST depression, the T wave abnormalities are in response to QRS complex abnormalities and do *not* reflect ischemia. These repolarization changes are seen in left ventricular hypertrophy, left bundle branch block, Wolff-Parkinson-White (WPW), and other processes. Secondary repolarization changes are discussed in Chapter 21.

T wave abnormalities

T wave inversion: The normal T wave vector is oriented inferior, lateral to the left, and usually anterior (in some cases posterior instead of anterior, especially in young adults). For this reason, T waves should always be upright in aVL and II and inverted in aVR. They are occasionally inverted in III and less commonly in aVF. In the precordial leads, T waves are always upright in V4–V6. They are usually upright in the right precordial leads but may be inverted in V1 and/or V2, especially in the younger and female population. In young healthy persons, the T wave is rarely inverted in V3 and

Critical Decisions in Emergency and Acute Care Electrocardiography, 1st edition. Edited by W.J. Brady and J.D. Truwit. © 2009 Blackwell Publishing, ISBN: 9781405159067

(a)

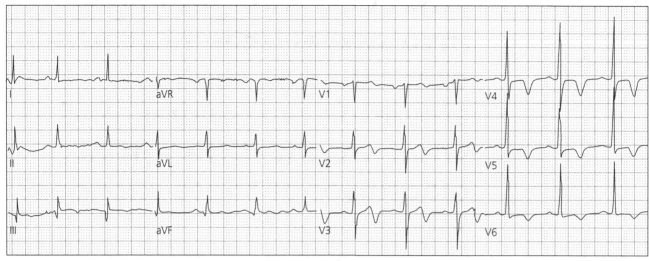

(b)

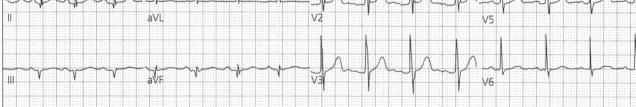

Figure 15.1 Wellens' T waves, pattern A. (a) Terminal T wave inversions in V2–V6 (Wellens' type A). (b) Baseline ECG, with old Q waves inferiorly.

exceptionally rarely in V4 ("persistent" juvenile T wave pattern), in which there is right ventricular prominence as a leftover from fetal circulation. The upslope of the T wave is usually more gradual than the downslope, and the T wave amplitude is usually > 10% of the R wave amplitude.

What is the significance of abnormally inverted T waves? In the right clinical context (e.g. chest pain or anginal equivalent), dynamic or new T inversions (other than in leads III, aVF and aVR), especially when in conjunction with ST segment depression and QT prolongation (> 425 ms), should raise suspicion for myocardial ischemia (see Figures 15.1, 15.2, and 15.4). T inversions are particularly worrisome and associated with worse outcomes if > 1 mm, and in > 1 lead in a coronary distribution. Isolated or minimally inverted non-dynamic T waves (< 1 mm) may be a result of acute coronary syndrome (ACS), but have not been definitely shown to portend worse outcomes compared

with patients who have ACS and a normal ECG [1]. However, in the undifferentiated chest pain patient, such T waves do confer a higher probability of ACS.

T inversions located predominantly in anterior precordial leads (Wellens' T waves) should raise the suspicion of a significant (frequently proximal) LAD stenosis (Figures 15.1 and 15.2). De Zwann and Wellens were the first to describe this typical pattern of pronounced symmetric or biphasic T wave inversions in the precordial leads in a cohort of patients with unstable angina or non-ST segment elevation myocardial infarction (UA/NSTEMI); thus, in the right clinical context, the condition is now frequently called Wellens' syndrome with Wellens' T waves [2]. In this cohort, this T wave pattern was very specific for a significant LAD lesion that was usually proximal [3]; some were, however, in the mid-LAD [4].

Wellens' T inversions are identical to anterior T inversions frequently seen after spontaneous or therapeutic reperfusion of an occluded LAD [5,6], and presumably represent

(a)

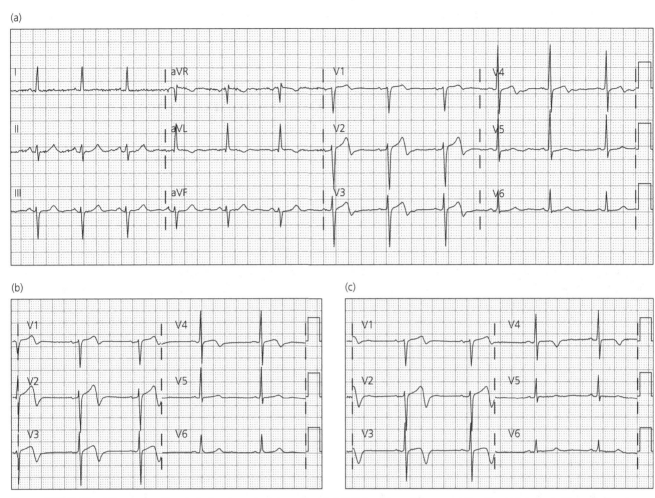

Figure 15.2 Wellens' T waves, pattern A starting to evolve into pattern B. (a) Wellens' type A T waves at time 0, which in the setting of ischemic symptoms is diagnostic of unstable LAD plaque. (b) and (c) (V1–V6 only), recorded at t = 1 h and 4 h, respectively, show the typical T wave evolution from Type A towards Type B, with T wave inversion becoming symmetric only in lead V4; thus, (c) cannot be called pattern B. However, later still, all T waves will be typically symmetrically inverted (pattern B). For a classic fully developed pattern B, see Figure 19.1.

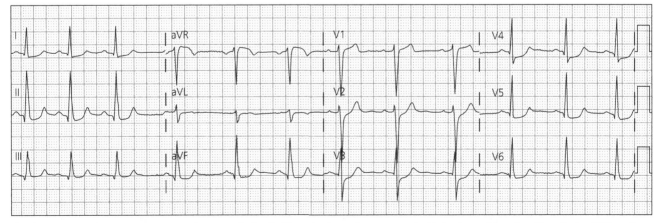

Figure 15.3 Dynamic ST depression. I, II, III, aVF, and V2–V6 all have ST depression compared with the (normal) baseline. There is also STE in aVR, which is associated with three-vessel and left main disease. The ST depression on the ECG probably represents subendocardial ischemia (*not* transient posterior STEMI).

the aftermath of spontaneous reperfusion of transient LAD occlusion of which the ST elevation (STE) was never recorded. The reperfusion may be from collateral circulation or from a recanalized or reperfused infarct-related artery. When untreated, these cases frequently progress to extensive anterior Q wave MI because of subsequent complete and persistent occlusion.

In the original description [2], the typical precordial T wave inversions are more commonly symmetric deep T inversions (pattern B, see Chapter 19, Figure 1c) and less commonly biphasic T inversions, also called "terminal T wave inversion – because the terminal portion of the T wave is inverted (pattern I, Figures 15.1a and 15.2a). They were always present in V2 and V3, but also occasionally in V1 and in V4–V6; furthermore, they occurred in the setting of minimal (< 1 mm) convex or concave STE (pattern A) or an isoelectric ST segment (pattern B). Most commonly, this finding was seen in patients who presented with a recent chest pain history but at the time of the ECG were pain-free. This supports the idea that what Wellens was witnessing was the aftermath of spontaneously reperfused LAD occlusion. Importantly, after the first description, the association of the ECG findings with an LAD lesion were validated in a prospective study of 180 patients [3]. The mean LAD stenosis was 85% and all 33 patients with complete obstruction had collateral circulation. The majority (91%) of individuals with UA/NSTEMI who develop the characteristic Wellens' pattern do so on admission, or within 24 h [3]. Finally, the changes may be transient, resolve with treatment, or persist for months [2,3,7].

T inversions have also been described in inferior and lateral leads (Figure 15.4) [4]. Given that identical T inversions occur after reperfusion of inferior lateral MI, it is supposed that these represent the same pathologic process (spontaneous reperfusion of previously injured myocardium). Additionally, ischemia from cocaine abuse, with or without LAD stenosis, can result in Wellens' T waves [8].

Finally, after prolonged coronary occlusion and complete QS wave infarction, there is shallow T wave inversion. Deep T inversion is associated with reperfusion; the amount of myocardium infarcted is best reflected by the QRS. If there is no Q wave, much myocardium is preserved; QR waves generally indicate some preservation, and QS waves indicate profound myocardial loss.

Differential diagnosis of T wave inversion

Conditions with a normal QRS: Pulmonary embolism deserves special mention as this condition can cause T wave inversions in the precordial leads very similar to the Wellens' pattern seen in the setting of ACS and severe LAD stenosis (Figure 15.5). Moreover, these two conditions may be very difficult to distinguish from one another on clinical grounds. However, simultaneous T inversions in lead V1 as well as lead III are rarely seen in the setting of precordial T inversions caused by acute coronary syndromes, but suggest pulmonary embolism [9].

Intracerebral event, especially hemorrhage, may present with precordial or diffuse T inversions due to global small vessel ischemia [10,11]. Although some suggest the QT interval is particularly prolonged in these cases, there is no proven way to differentiate this from ACS on the ECG.

Benign T wave inversion (Figure 15.6), a T wave pattern sometimes seen in young healthy African American males and a variant of early repolarization, is frequently associated with subtle STE in the anterior leads, as well a prominent J wave [12]. It may help to distinguish benign T wave inversion from Wellens' T waves by a shorter QT interval, taller R waves, and extension of the T inversion to V5 and V6.

Persistent juvenile T waves, especially in right precordial leads (see T wave inversion section).

Myocarditis may present with diffuse T inversions [13], as may the later stages of pericarditis (frequently in all leads except aVR and V1) [13]. The absence of a single coronary distribution may differentiate the two entities (see Chapter 14).

"Memory" T inversion after electronic ventricular pacing, in which T waves that are appropriately inverted during pacing

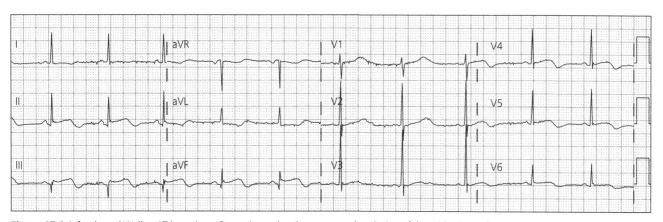

Figure 15.4 Inferolateral Wellens' T inversions. On angiography, there was total occlusion of the mid-RCA, a dominant vessel, with large visible clot. Thrombectomy and stent were performed.

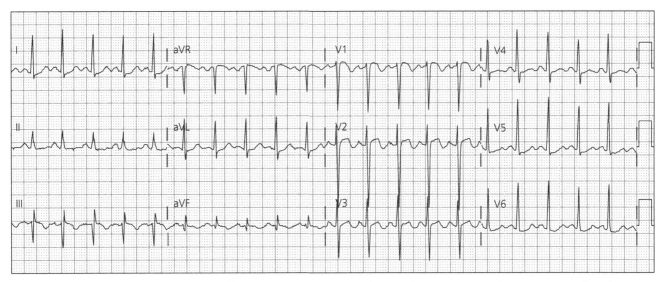

Figure 15.5 Pulmonary embolism (PE). A patient with severe chest pain and dyspnea. There are T inversions, with some STE, across the right precordium. Emergency physician-performed bedside cardiac echo revealed a greatly enlarged right ventricle. Pulmonary embolism was diagnosed with computed tomography (CT) angiogram. Note that there is T inversion in III and V1, a very specific finding for PE.

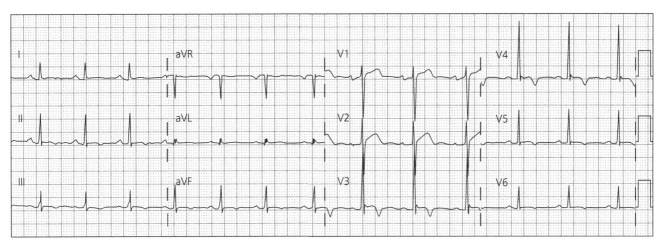

Figure 15.6 Benign T wave inversion. This looks like Wellens' syndrome. However, there are distinct J waves typical of early repolarization, the QT interval is short (387 ms), there is very high R wave amplitude, and the T inversion extends to V6, all supporting benign T inversion.

remain inverted for up to 20 min after cessation of even brief pacing and can remain inverted longer after prolonged pacing [14–16]. A positive T in aVL, positive or isoelectric T in lead I and a maximal precordial T inversion > T inversion in lead III was 92% sensitive and 100% specific for cardiac "memory" T waves versus ischemic T waves, regardless of the coronary distribution [17].

Stress cardiomyopathy (see Figures 15.4–15.6) and discussion in Chapter 4. Profound emotional or physical distress may result in dyspnea, chest pain, pulmonary edema, and STE indistinguishable from STEMI, or diffuse T wave inversions indistinguishable from NSTEMI.

Conditions with an abnormal QRS resulting in secondary T inversions

Left ventricular hypertrophy (LVH): (See chapter 21.) The T inversions of LVH are usually non-symmetrical (preterminal, with gradual downslope and abrupt upslope). T inversions are in leads with downsloping ST depression, in the lateral and anterolateral (aVL, I, V4–V6) leads, not in V1–V3. They should be in the opposite direction ("discordant")

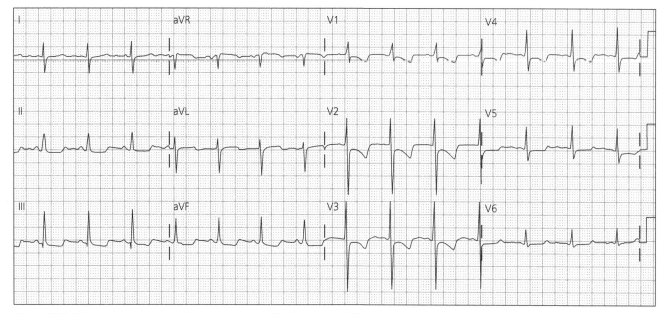

Figure 15.7 Right ventricular hypertrophy, with secondary ST depression and T inversion in right precordial leads. Criteria for RVH are met with S wave in lead I and R > S in V1. **Need permission**. Reprinted with permission from Smith SW, Zvosec DL, Sharkey SW, Henry TD. *The ECG in Acute MI: An Evidence-Based Manual of Reperfusion Therapy.* 1st Edition. Philadelphia: Lippincott, Williams, and Wilkins, 2002:54.

from the major portion of the QRS, which is positive in V4–V6 (and thus the T wave is negative). There must be voltage criteria for LVH. There is usually no QT prolongation. There is frequently STE in leads V1–V3 that is opposite (discordant) to deep S waves.

Right ventricular hypertrophy (RVH): This should be suspected in the presence of prominent R forces and width in the right precordial leads, S waves in V5, V6, or I, or incomplete or complete right bundle branch block, and right axis deviation. Right ventricular hypertrophy may manifest T wave inversion, with or without ST depression, in right precordial leads. In the setting of RVH, right precordial T inversion should be expected (see Figure 15.7).

Hypertrophic cardiomyopathy: ST segment and T wave changes can be found in any lead in addition to voltage criteria for LVH. One subtype of hypertrophic cardiomyopathy, the isolated apical variant, deserves special mention as it can be indistinguishable from the ECG findings seen with anterior wall ischemia due to an LAD lesion [18,19].

Wolff-Parkinson-White syndrome: This has an abnormal early depolarization through a bypass tract (pre-excitation). This may result in secondary repolarization abnormalities with ST depression and/or T wave inversion as well as STE and Q -waves (see Chapter 21, Figures 17, 18). It is recognized by the slurred upstroke of the QRS (delta wave) and a short PR interval.

Left and right bundle branch block, intraventricular conduction delay, and ventricular paced rhythm are discussed in Chapter 5.

Peaked or enlarged T waves are discussed in Chapter 16.

T wave flattening

This is a frequent and non-specific finding. If it is new or dynamic and occurs in the setting of chest pain it may be secondary to myocardial ischemia.

U wave

A U wave is a low amplitude, positive or negative, usually monophasic deflection after the T wave, usually with the same vector as the T wave. Therefore, it is usually positive in II, isoelectric in aVL and aVR and may be, less commonly, inverted in III and aVF. When inverted in the precordial leads, it implies structural or ischemic heart disease. The cause of the U wave has been debated and is uncertain.

A negative U wave, other than in lead aVR, III, or aVF, implies ischemic heart disease. It has been described during variant (vasospastic) angina attacks [20] and during stress testing, under which circumstances it has high specificity (though low sensitivity) for the presence of a significant LAD stenosis [21]. It may also be seen with uncontrolled hypertension [22,23], under which circumstances the U wave is usually negative-positive (biphasic), whereas in acute ischemia it is more likely to be positive-negative [24]. In a patient with chest pain, a negative U wave in the precordial leads represents a significant LAD lesion until proven otherwise (Figure 15.8a–c). Interestingly, patients with an anterior wall MI and negative U waves in the precordial leads have smaller infarcts, less STE, better collateral circulation, and a larger amount of stunned but viable myocardium [25]. Similarly, a prominent negative U wave

(a)

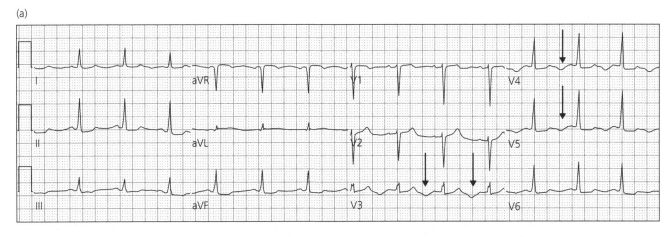

(b)

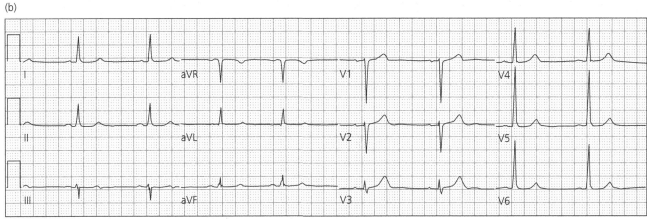

(c)

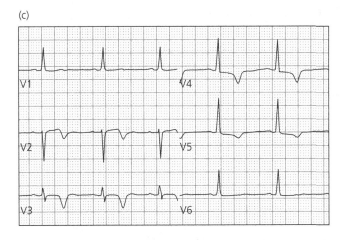

Figure 15.8 (a) Negative U waves (arrows). This 89-year-old had an episode of unresponsiveness. The ECG shows slight ST depression in inferior and lateral leads, and profound negative U waves in V3–V5. (b) Baseline of V1–V6, with none of these abnormalities. The troponin was positive. Angiogram showed severe subtotal LAD stenosis with TIMI II flow. (c) Reperfusion T waves after percutaneous coronary intervention. (V1–V6 only).

in all inferior leads in the presence of chest pain may be due to inferior ischemia [26]. This negative U wave may indeed, as with terminal T wave inversion, signify spontaneous reperfusion.

In the appropriate clinical context, an increase in U wave amplitude in the precordial leads should raise suspicion of posterior ischemia (due to a right coronary artery [RCA] or left circumflex [LCX] lesion) [27]. This could be considered the mirror image of a negative U wave.

ST segment depression

What are the diagnostic, prognostic and therapeutic implications of ST segment depression in the setting of chest pain? (see also Chapter 27)

Primary ST depression (Figures 15.3, 15.9, and 15.10) may be due to subendocardial ischemia or, if limited to right precordial leads, may be due to posterior epicardial or transmural

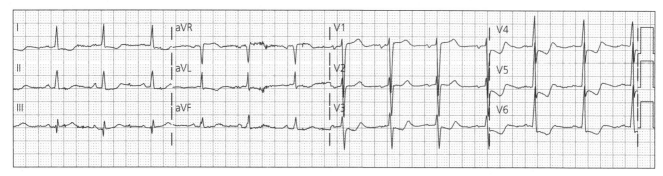

Figure 15.9 Subendocardial ischemia with lateral ST depression, misinterpreted as LVH with secondary repolarization abnormalities. The ST depression is out of proportion to the QRS, and is concordant in lead V3. Echocardiography revealed acute lateral and apical WMA, but no LVH. Troponins were elevated and there was a new 90% stenosis of the first diagonal and of the obtuse marginal arteries. The patient underwent three-vessel CABG. An ECG on day #4 showed resolution of ST depression and the WMA. Reprinted with permission from Smith SW, Zvosec DL, Sharkey SW, Henry TD. *The ECG in Acute MI: An Evidence-Based Manual of Reperfusion Therapy.* 1st Edition. Philadelphia: Lippincott, Williams, and Wilkins, 2002:57.

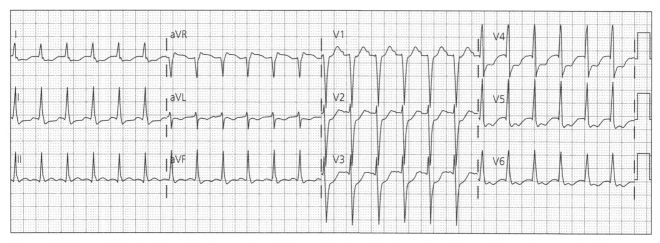

Figure 15.10 Pure posterior MI with anterior ST depression. A 50-year-old patient with chest pain and dyspnea followed by ventricular fibrillation. Angiogram confirmed a hazy mid-circumflex 90% culprit lesion, with decreased perfusion to the posterior wall. Though on ECG it appears to be a small MI, the maximum troponin was 135 ng/mL, with CK-MB of 126 IU/L. Echo later that day showed posterolateral akinesis, anterior hypokinesis, and concentric LVH, with moderately severe decreased ejection fraction at 35%.

ischemia with or without infarction (reciprocal to posterior STE, signifying complete coronary occlusion with epicardial or transmural ischemia of the posterior wall). In either case, ST depression of just 0.5 mm is associated with increased mortality and, when ≥ 1.0 mm, especially if present in ≥ two consecutive leads, is associated with high mortality [28,29].

ST depression due to subendocardial ischemia

Horizontal or downsloping ST depression of dynamic character is very specific for subendocardial ischemia. Concurrent T wave inversion may or may not be present. If previous ECGs demonstrate no ST segment shifts and subsequently develop horizontal or downsloping ST depression (≥ 0.05 mV), it is even more suspicious for myocardial ischemia, especially if it resolves spontaneously or after anti-ischemic therapy.

Therefore, a previous ECG is invaluable in the assessment of a patient with chest pain [30]. The more pronounced the ST depression and the more leads involved, the greater the likelihood of MI as defined by biomarkers. Lloyd-Jones and colleagues demonstrated that, in patients with chest discomfort suggestive of myocardial ischemia, the odds ratio for a non-STEMI, as diagnosed by CK-MB (not troponin) was 3.3 (1.6–6.9) if ST depression involved at least three leads and was 5.1 (2.2–11.6) if the ST depression was also ≥ 0.2 mV (2 mm) [31]. Furthermore, the more pronounced and the more leads involved, the more likely multivessel disease was present. Gorgels and colleagues found that ST depression in I, II, AVL and V4–V6 in conjunction with STE in aVR was associated with left main stenosis or three-vessel disease (see Figure 27.4) [32]. Likewise, the sum of the ST deviation (STE + ST depression in all leads, "ST segment score") of > 12 mm is associated with multivessel or left main coronary disease [32], as is ST depression that is most prominent in lead V4 [33]. Finally, the presence, extent, and severity of ST depression have important prognostic implications and may help in therapeutic decision-making. Several studies have shown the prognostic importance of ST depression on the admission ECG in patients with both non-STEMI and UA [1,28,34–36]. ST depression at admission was related to poor outcome with a rate of death and MI twice as high in patients with major ST depression compared with patients with only minor ST depression [34]. In addition, an ST segment score predicted the magnitude of benefit with early invasive treatment independent of age, sex, or troponin status. ST depression, independent of troponin, predicted benefit from an early invasive management of ACS [37].

Anterior ST depression representing posterior MI

As described below, ST depression in the right precordial leads may represent epicardial or transmural posterior ischemia with or without MI (Figure 15.10). However, in general, ECG lead-specific ST depression does not localize the territory of subendocardial ischemia or the vessel involved. This is true even if typical in morphology and with dynamic character. In exercise testing, it has been repeatedly shown that there is no correlation between ST depression on the ECG and the location of the ischemic territory or vessel involved [38–45]. It is unknown whether such a correlation exists in UA/NSTEMI, but there is no evidence that it does.

ST depression does localize the area of ischemia in posterior epicardial or transmural ischemia with or without MI: in the anteroseptal leads (V1–V3), ST depression may represent transmural (epicardial) posterior ischemia and is really a mirror image of STE that goes unrecorded unless there are posterior leads. Frequently, if concomitant MI (in addition to injury) has already developed, the ST depression is associated with an increase in the R force in the right precordial leads, with an increase in the R/S ratio. Transmural posterior ischemia or MI is infrequently isolated; it is more commonly associated with an inferior wall or lateral wall MI and, hence, is frequently accompanied by STE in the inferior and/or lateral leads. If one is uncertain about the etiology of ST depression in the right precordial leads it is helpful to apply posterior leads (V7–V9), which will show STE if the ST depression represents a true posterior wall MI (see Chapter 18).

Differential diagnosis of ST segment depression

Abnormal QRS

Left ventricular hypertrophy: See above under T inversion.

Right ventricular hypertrophy: See above under T inversion. One should be cautious to interpret isolated ST depression

in the right precordial leads as secondary to RVH unless it occurs in the presence of typical findings suggestive of RVH and preferably in the right clinical context (see Figure 15.7).

Right bundle branch block (RBBB): Typically, the ST depression in the setting of RBBB is in right precordial leads (V1/V2 sometimes V3) and almost never elsewhere (refer to Chapter 21).

Left bundle branch block (LBBB): See Chapter 21.

Non-specific intraventricular conduction delay: As a general rule, these are similar to the ST segment changes seen in LBBB; the ST segment shifts almost always occur discordant to the dominant QRS force.

Ventricular pacing: These are analogous to LBBB (refer to Chapter 21).

Hypokalemia: Typical features of progressive hypokalemia are a decrease in the T amplitude or T inversion, followed by ST depression which is usually subtle and can be horizontal or downsloping (Figure 15.11). With more severe hypokalemia, a positive U wave can be seen, especially in the anterior precordial leads. With correction of the potassium level the ST segment will normalize, and it may be impossible to rule out ischemia until this is done. ST depression is unlikely unless serum potassium is < 3.0 mmol/L.

Digitalis: Characteristic ST segment/T wave changes suggestive of digitalis effect are the following: (1) downsloping or scooped ST depression, (2) flattened, biphasic, or inverted T waves, (3) positive U wave, and (4) shortening of the QT interval (refer to Figure 15.12 for a representative example of the digitalis effect). It is frequently impossible to distinguish these findings from ST depression related to ischemia. Importantly, the magnitude of these changes do not reflect the digoxin level: the ECG may have pronounced ST T changes with a subtherapeutic digoxin level, but no significant changes with a toxic digoxin level. QT prolongation may help in the detection of ischemia in the presence of digoxin because it is never seen from digitalis alone.

Pre-excitation or Wolff-Parkinson-White pattern: See discussion above in T inversion and Chapter 14.

General evaluation issues with respect to ST segment depression and T/U wave abnormalities

(1) Unexplained ST segment and T wave abnormalities are simply "non-specific ST/T changes." One must interpret them within the clinical context.
(2) It is most helpful if ST segment and T wave abnormalities are dynamic. A comparison ECG is invaluable: even subtle ST depression or T inversion, if new, or if they resolve with

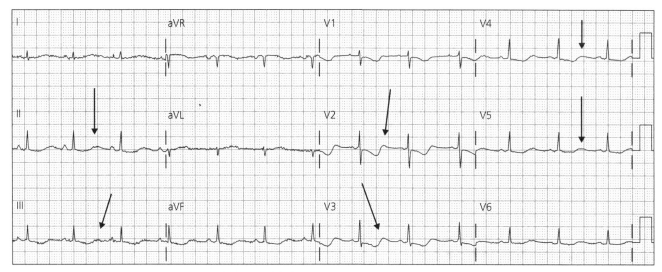

Figure 15.11 Hypokalemia (K = 2.3 mEq/L). Note scooped ST depression in inferior leads, as well as downsloping ST depression and T inversion in precordial leads. All these leads also have large positive U waves (arrows).

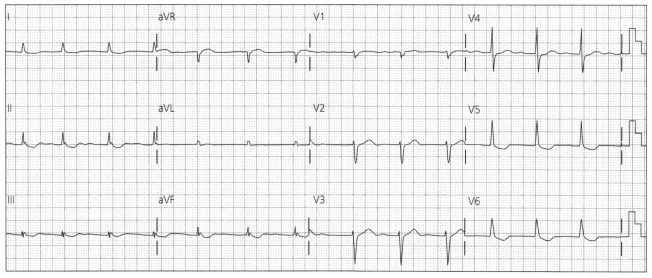

Figure 15.12 Digitalis. See the scooped ST depression in II, III, aVF, V5, and V6. There is a positive U wave and a short QT interval (QTc = 376 in leads with scooped ST depression). Courtesy of K. Wang. *Atlas of Electrocardiography.*

anti-ischemic therapy, are much more specific for ischemia than non-dynamic abnormalities.

(3) ST depression that is marked, or that is horizontal or downsloping, raises suspicion for myocardial ischemia.

(4) A few subtle but specific changes are associated with a high likelihood of ischemia in the setting of chest pain or anginal-equivalent symptoms:

    a New negative U waves.

    b New symmetric or biphasic T inversions in the anterior leads especially in conjunction with an isoelectric ST segment or subtle ST segment elevation.

    c Pronounced horizontal or downsloping ST segment depression.

    d Horizontal ST segment depression in the anteroseptal leads V1–V3.

Case conclusions

The patient in Case 1 was admitted and "ruled out" with serial troponins that were measurable, but below the laboratory reference. He underwent upper gastrointestinal (GI) scope (negative). He died 1 week later, with LAD occlusion on autopsy.

Catheterization in Case 2 revealed a 60% LAD stenosis at the takeoff, and then throughout its proximal and mid portions there were a series of subtotal stenoses. There was TIMI 1 flow at the apical LAD. This was stented; maximum troponin was 2.57 ng/mL. An initial anterior wall motion (WMA) abnormality completely recovered and the ECG normalized.

In Case 3, the patient was taken for immediate angiogram, where he was found to have 60% LAD, 90% first diagonal

(D1), and 60% circumflex stenosis. The RCA was occluded, with left to right collateral filling. Ejection fraction was 40% and maximum troponin I was 10.25 ng/mL. The patient went for coronary bypass surgery.

References

1 Diderholm E, Andren B, Frostfeldt G, *et al.* ST depression in ECG at entry indicates severe coronary lesions and large benefits of an early invasive treatment strategy in unstable coronary artery disease; the FRISC II ECG substudy. The fast revascularisation during instability in coronary artery disease. *Eur Heart J* 2002; **23**:41–9.

2 de Zwaan C, Bar FW, Wellens HJJ. Characteristic electrocardiographic pattern indicating a critical stenosis high in left anterior descending coronary artery in patients admitted because of impending myocardial infarction. *Am Heart J* 1982;**103**:730–6.

3 de Zwaan C, Bar FW, Janssen JHA, *et al.* Angiographic and clinical characteristics of patients with unstable angina showing an ECG pattern indicating critical narrowing of the proximal LAD coronary artery. *Am Heart J* 1989;**117**:657–65.

4 Kardesoglu E, Celik T, Cebeci BS, *et al.* Wellens' syndrome: a case report. *J Int Med Res* 2003;**31**:585–90.

5 Doevendans PA, Gorgels AP, van der Zee R, *et al.* Electrocardiographic diagnosis of reperfusion during thrombolytic therapy in acute myocardial infarction. *Am J Cardiol* 1995;**75**:1206–10.

6 Wehrens XH, Doevendans PA, Ophuis TJ, Wellens HJ. A comparison of electrocardiographic changes during reperfusion of acute myocardial infarction by thrombolysis or percutaneous transluminal coronary angioplasty. *Am Heart J* 2000;**139**:430–6.

7 Tandy TK, Bottomy DP, Lewis J. Wellens' syndrome. *Ann Emerg Med* 1999;**33**:347–51.

8 Langston W, Pollack M. Pseudo-Wellens syndrome in a cocaine user. *Am J Emerg Med* 2006;**24**:122–3.

9 Kosuge M, Kimura K, Ishikawa T, *et al.* Electrocardiographic differentiation between acute pulmonary embolism and acute coronary syndromes on the basis of negative T waves. *Am J Cardiol* 2007;**99**:817–21.

10 Kono T, Morita H, Kuroiwa T, *et al.* Left ventricular wall motion abnormalities in patients with subarachnoid hemorrhage: neurogenic stunned myocardium. *J Am Coll Cardiol* 1994;**24**:636–640.

11 Perron AD, Brady WJ. Electrocardiographic manifestations of CNS events. *Am J Emerg Med* 2000;**18**:715–20.

12 Wang K, Asinger RW, Marriott HJ. ST-segment elevation in conditions other than acute myocardial infarction. *N Engl J Med* 2003;**349**:2128–35.

13 Surawicz B, Knilans T. *Chou's Electrocardiography in Clinical Practice. Adult and Pediatric.* Philadelphia, PA: Saunders, 2001.

14 Rosenbaum MB, Blanco HH, Elizari MV, *et al.* Electrotonic modulation of the T wave and cardiac memory. *Am J Cardiol* 1982;**50**:213–22.

15 del Balzo U, Rosen MR. T wave changes persisting after ventricular pacing in canine heart are altered by 4-aminopyridine but not by lidocaine. Implications with respect to phenomenon of cardiac "memory". *Circulation* 1992;**85**:1464–72.

16 Shvilkin A, Danilo P, Jr., Wang J, *et al.* Evolution and resolution of long-term cardiac memory. *Circulation* 1998;**97**:1810–7.

17 Shvilkin A, Ho KK, Rosen MR, Josephson ME. T-vector direction differentiates postpacing from ischemic T-wave inversion in precordial leads. *Circulation* 2005;**111**:969–74.

18 Maron BJ, Bonow RO, Seshagiri TN, *et al.* Hypertrophic cardiomyopathy with ventricular septal hypertrophy localized to the apical region of the left ventricle (apical hypertrophic cardiomyopathy). *Am J Cardiol* 1982;**49**:1838–48.

19 Yamaguchi H, Ishimura T, Nishiyama S, *et al.* Hypertrophic nonobstructive cardiomyopathy with giant negative T waves (apical hypertrophy): ventriculographic and echocardiographic features in 30 patients. *Am J Cardiol* 1979;**44**:401–12.

20 Miwa K, Murakami T, Kambara H, Kawai C. U wave inversion during attacks of variant angina. *Br Heart J* 1983;**50**:378–82.

21 Gerson MC, Phillips JF, Morris SN, McHenry PL. Exercise-induced U-wave inversion as a marker of stenosis of the left anterior descending coronary artery. *Circulation* 1979;**60**:1014–20.

22 Gerson MC, McHenry PL. Resting U wave inversion as a marker of stenosis of the left anterior descending coronary artery. *Am J Med* 1980;**69**:545–50.

23 Kishida H, Cole JS, Surawicz B. Negative U wave: a highly specific but poorly understood sign of heart disease. *Am J Cardiol* 1982;**49**:2030–6.

24 Miwa K, Miyagi Y, Fujita M, *et al.* Transient terminal U wave inversion as a more specific marker for myocardial ischemia. *Am Heart J* 1993;**125**:981–6.

25 Tamura A, Nagase K, Mikuriya Y, Nasu M. Relation between negative U waves in precordial leads on the admission electrocardiogram and time course of left ventricular wall motion in anterior wall acute myocardial infarction. *Am J Cardiol* 1999;**84**: 332–4, A8.

26 Miyakoda H, Endo A, Kato M, *et al.* Exercise-induced U-wave changes in patients with coronary artery disease – correlation with tomographic thallium-201 myocardial imaging. *Jpn Circ J* 1996;**60**:641–51.

27 Chikamori T, Takata J, Seo H, *et al.* Diagnostic significance of an exercise-induced prominent U wave in acute myocardial infarction. *Am J Cardiol* 1996;**78**:1277–81.

28 Hyde TA, French JK, Wong CK, *et al.* Four-year survival of patients with acute coronary syndromes without ST-segment elevation and prognostic significance of 0.5-mm ST-segment depression. *Am J Cardiol* 1999;**84**:379–85.

29 Cannon CP, McCabe CH, Stone PH, *et al.* The electrocardiogram predicts one-year outcome of patients with unstable angina and non-Q wave myocardial infarction: results of the TIMI III Registry ECG Ancillary Study. Thrombolysis in Myocardial Ischemia. *J Am Coll Cardiol* 1997;**30**:133–40.

30 Lee TH, Cook EF, Weisberg MC, *et al.* Impact of the availability of a prior electrocardiogram on the triage of the patient with acute chest pain. *J Gen Intern Med* 1990;**5**:381–8.

31 Lloyd-Jones DM, Camargo CA, Jr., Lapuerta P, *et al.* Electrocardiographic and clinical predictors of acute myocardial infarction in patients with unstable angina pectoris. *Am J Cardiol* 1998;**81**:1182–6.

32 Gorgels AP, Vos MA, Mulleneers R, *et al.* Value of the electrocardiogram in diagnosing the number of severely narrowed coronary arteries in rest angina pectoris. *Am J Cardiol* 1993;**72**: 999–1003.

33 Atie J, Brugada P, Brugada J, *et al.* Clinical presentation and prognosis of left main coronary artery disease in the 1980s. *Eur Heart J* 1991;**12**:495–502.

34 Holmvang L, Clemmensen P, Lindahl B, *et al.* Quantitative analysis of the admission electrocardiogram identifies patients with

unstable coronary artery disease who benefit the most from early invasive treatment. *J Am Coll Cardiol* 2003;**41**:905–15.

35 Holmvang L, Luscher MS, Clemmensen P, *et al*. Very early risk stratification using combined ECG and biochemical assessment in patients with unstable coronary artery disease (A thrombin inhibition in myocardial ischemia [TRIM] substudy). The TRIM Study Group. *Circulation* 1998;**98**:2004–9.

36 Kaul P, Fu Y, Chang WC, *et al*. Prognostic value of ST segment depression in acute coronary syndromes: insights from PARAGON-A applied to GUSTO-IIb. PARAGON-A and GUSTO IIb Investigators. Platelet IIb/IIIa Antagonism for the Reduction of Acute Global Organization Network. *J Am Coll Cardiol* 2001;**38**:64–71.

37 Cannon CP, Weintraub WS, Demopoulos LA, *et al*. Comparison of early invasive and conservative strategies in patients with unstable coronary syndromes treated with the glycoprotein IIb/IIIa inhibitor tirofiban. (TACTICS)-TIMI 18. *N Engl J Med* 2001;**344**:1879–87.

38 Abouantoun S, Ahnve S, Savvides M, *et al*. Can areas of myocardial ischemia be localized by the exercise electrocardiogram? A correlative study with thallium-201 scintigraphy. *Am Heart J* 1984;**108**:933–41.

39 Dunn RF, Freedman B, Bailey IK, *et al*. Localization of coronary artery disease with exercise electrocardiography: correlation wit thallium-201 myocardial perfusion scanning. *Am J Cardiol* 1981;**48**:837–43.

40 Fox RM, Hakki AH, Iskandrian AS. Relation between electrocardiographic and scintigraphic location of myocardial ischemia during exercise in one-vessel coronary artery disease. *Am J Cardiol* 1984;**53**:1529–31.

41 Fuchs RM, Achuff SC, Grunwald L, *et al*. Electrocardiographic localization of coronary artery narrowings: studies during myocardial ischemia and infarction in patients with one-vessel disease. *Circulation* 1982;**66**:1168–76.

42 Hosoya Y, Ikeda K, Yamaki M, *et al*. The clinical significance of exercise-induced ST segment changes in patients with previous inferior myocardial infarction. *Am Heart J* 1990;**120**: 554–61.

43 Kang X, Berman DS, Lewin HC, *et al*. Comparative localization of myocardial ischemia by exercise electrocardiography and myocardial perfusion SPECT. *J Nucl Cardiol* 2000;**7**:140–5.

44 Kubota I, Ikeda K, Ohyama T, *et al*. Body surface distributions of ST segment changes after exercise in effort angina pectoris without myocardial infarction. *Am Heart J* 1985;**110**: 949–55.

45 Kurata C, Tawarahara K, Okayama K, *et al*. Localization of exercise-induced myocardial ischemia with ST depression. *Intern Med* 1992;**31**:583–8.

Chapter 16 | **What is a hyperacute T wave?**

Mark D. Connelly[1], Joel S. Holger[1], Stephen W. Smith[2]
[1]Regions Hospital, St Paul, MN, USA
[2]University of Minnesota, Hennegin County Medical Center, Minneapolis, MN, USA

Case presentations

Case 1: A 63-year-old male presents to the emergency department (ED) with 2 h of recurrent bilateral shoulder pain, now also with chest discomfort, and radiating to the arms. Immediately upon arrival, the nurse places the patient on a cardiac monitor and notices prominent T waves. An urgent electrocardiogram (ECG) (Figure 16.1) and metabolic panel are ordered to rule out ST elevation myocardial infarction (STEMI) and/or hyperkalemia.

Case 2: A 54-year-old female with end-stage kidney disease presents to the ED with shortness of breath and anxiety, increasing over the past 2 days since her last dialysis treatment. Past medical history includes type II diabetes, hypertension, and coronary artery disease. She denies chest pain, fevers, cough, or productive sputum. The patient is placed on a cardiac monitor, has an IV inserted, and receives oxygen. An ECG (Figure 16.2) and portable chest x-ray are ordered. Chest x-ray demonstrates pulmonary vascular congestion indicative of congestive heart failure (CHF).

The hyperacute T wave

After QT prolongation [1], the hyperacute T wave is the earliest described sign of acute ischemia, preceding ST elevation (STE). Hyperacute T waves are bulky, wide-based, and symmetrical, usually with increased amplitude, and often associated with a depressed ST takeoff [2,3]. Proportionality is critical: a hyperacute T wave need not have any absolute measurements; rather, it needs to be large in proportion to the preceding QRS (Figure 16.3a, lead V3). The different morphologies that may characterize hyperacute T waves can be seen in Figure 16.4.

Studies have shown progressive ECG changes from the hyperacute and acute settings, to the subacute and chronic phases of acute MI [4–6]. These changes involve the T wave,

Critical Decisions in Emergency and Acute Care Electrocardiography,
1st edition. Edited by W.J. Brady and J.D. Truwit. © 2009 Blackwell Publishing, ISBN: 9781405159067

ST segment, and QRS complexes. The T wave in STEMI may remain enlarged even as the ST segment elevates, and even after development of Q waves. The classic ECG progression in coronary occlusion is demonstrated in Figure 16.5.

Hyperacute T waves have been demonstrated to occur as early as 1–2 min after injury in experimental models [7]. However, the first change in the ECG after coronary occlusion is prolongation of the QT interval, occurring within < 1 min of experimental (balloon) occlusion [1]. Hyperacute T waves are seen within 30 min of coronary occlusion, and appear in leads that correspond to the area of injury on the ECG [8–10]. Thus, these findings may be seen in all the typical leads for anterior (Figures 16.3 and 16.6), inferior, and lateral (Figure 16.1) MI, respectively. In clinical practice, hyperacute T waves are not often seen as they diminish over time and are, thus, less prominent by the time the first ECG is recorded. The hyperacute T wave usually becomes less visually prominent as the ST segment becomes more elevated. Hence, the physician is more likely to find STE as the most apparent first ECG finding. If there is reperfusion of the infarct artery, the STE may diminish or resolve first, leaving a hyperacute T wave as a residual sign, which then disappears with continued perfusion (Figure 16.3; see Figure 20.2a–d for an excellent example of this).

The prominent T wave has long been described as one of the earliest ECG changes of acute ischemia [4,7,11–14]. Pardee was one of the first to note these changes in humans. He described this T wave as being a "larger size than customary and shows a somewhat sharper peak" [13]. In other early literature these changes were referred to as "upright coronary T waves" [15]. Currently, accentuated T waves in the beginning phase of STEMI are labeled *hyperacute T waves* [9,12,15–17]. These hyperacute T waves are prominent, symmetric T waves with increased amplitude, and the specificity for MI is higher if they appear in two contiguous leads [18].

Hyperacute T waves are thought to be associated with transmural ischemia or infarction. When ischemia is limited to the subendocardial layer alone, the cells are unable to maintain prolonged activation, and, thus, the axis change from positive to negative is directed away from the involved area of the left ventricle, and the T wave is negative. However, when the ischemic defect extends transmurally,

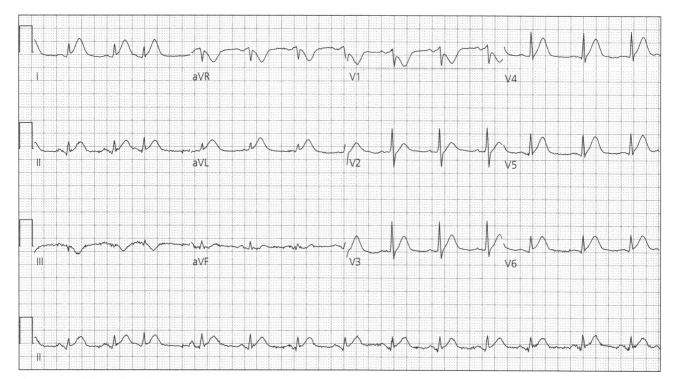

Figure 16.1 This ECG shows hyperacute T waves and ST segment changes in leads V4–V6, I, II, and aVL, which suggest an acute inferolateral MI. There is also possible posterior involvement as seen in lead V1. ST and T wave abnormalities resolved after reperfusion.

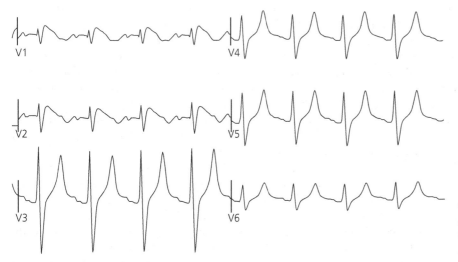

Figure 16.2 Hyperkalemia (K = 6.4 mEq/L) with tall symmetric T waves and QRS complex widening. There is also ST elevation in V1 and V2 that is typical for hyperkalemia and frequently mistaken for STEMI.

through all layers of the myocardium, the ischemia directs the T wave axis toward the area of infarction, becoming hyperacute and positive [19,20].

In posterolateral and posterior transmural injury, hyperacute T waves in V1 and V2 have been described after reperfusion, but not during acute occlusion. These could be called "pseudohyperacute T waves" (Figure 16.7) [21,22]. They are apparently a result of recording the inverted T waves of reperfusion from the opposite (anterior) wall.

Recent research has found that the hyperacute T wave, even after the development of STE and Q waves, may repres-

ent ongoing ischemia of viable myocardium, with significant potential for salvage [10,23,24]. Reperfusion therapy performed when T waves are still enlarged has resulted in decreased morbidity and mortality, in spite of prolonged symptoms or the presence of Q waves [6,12,25]. In a substudy of the thrombolytic GUSTO-1 trial, patients who were treated while the T wave amplitude was high, defined as > 98th percentile of the upper limit of normal, had significantly lower 30-day mortality (5.2% versus 8.6%), and were less likely to develop cardiogenic shock (6.1% versus 8.6%) and congestive heart failure (15% versus 24%) [12]. In this

(a)

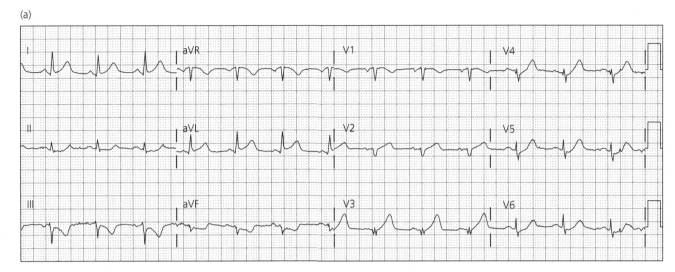

(b)

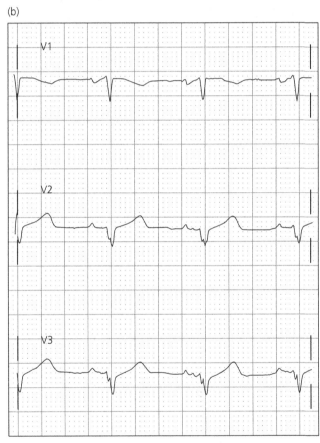

Figure 16.3 (a) From a 50-year-old with chest pain, this ECG shows STE in I and aVL, with reciprocal ST depression in inferior leads. The T wave in V3 is very large in proportion with the QRS. This was an acute LAD occlusion. (b) (V1–V3 only) Pain is resolved 20 min later, and hyperacute T wave has resolved without any intervening ST elevation.

trial, inferior infarctions were much more likely to have hyperacute T waves on their initial ECG than anterior infarctions. A proposed reason for the improved outcome is that these patients had an earlier time to treatment, and that this finding is a reliable marker of ischemia of viable myocardium, probably more reliable than the time of onset of symptoms [24].

Reperfusion therapy has been shown to benefit patients in terms of reduction of infarct size after thrombolytic therapy,

even after the appearance of abnormal Q waves, typically a late finding. This demonstrates that reperfusion therapy may benefit all phases of AMI [26]. However, if the *hyperacute* phase can be appreciated and acted upon, there may be less overall cardiac ischemia time and more salvageable myocardium. Sclarovsky introduced a grading scale to assess the severity of acute ischemia in order to correlate protection against ischemia provided by either collateral flow or metabolic "preconditioning" developed in response to prior

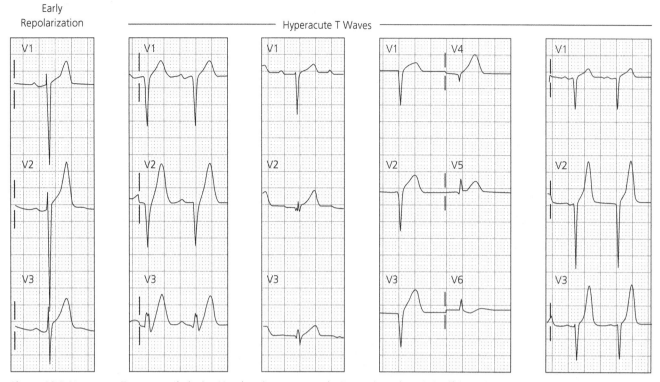

Figure 16.4 Hyperacute T wave morphologies. Note how in many cases the T wave is not large in itself, but is large in *proportion* to the QRS or the R wave. In contrast, early repolarization has large T waves, but also a well-formed R wave.

Figure 16.5 Typical evolution of T wave, ST segment, and Q wave in acute inferior myocardial infarction. Reprinted with permission from Wang K. *Atlas of Electrocardiography*.

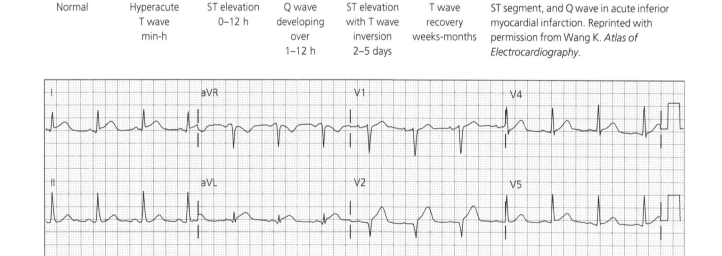

Figure 16.6 Hyperacute T waves in acute anterior infarction in leads V2 and V3. Note the poor R wave amplitude. In spite of minimal ST elevation, this is diagnostic of LAD occlusion.

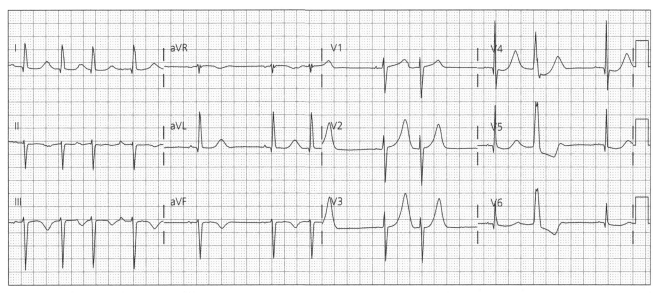

Figure 16.7 "Pseudohyperacute" T waves in leads V1 and V2. The first ECG had shown anterior ST depression of posterior MI, as proven by inferior and posterior regional wall motion abnormality. This ECG is after reperfusion. Posterior leads would presumably show T wave inversion of reperfusion, but these anterior leads show the reciprocal of this T wave inversion, and it manifests as large T waves. Thus, these are reperfusion T waves of the posterior wall, as seen from anterior leads.

ischemia: Grade I = hyperacute T waves only; Grade II = STE with or without hyperacute T waves, but with preserved appearance of the QRS complex; and Grade III = distortion of the terminal portion of the QRS complex by disappearance of the S wave. The more protection, the longer the time that can elapse before infarction occurs (Grade I = most protected and Grade III = least protected) [19].

Limited data exist regarding the definition of these T waves by measurement of their amplitude. Macfarlane studied almost 2000 normal subjects in Scotland to define the percentiles in the above noted GUSTO-1 substudy [27]. In general, the normal upper limits of T wave amplitude are > 10 mm in leads V2–V4, > 7.5 mm in lead V5, > 5 mm in leads I, II, aVF, V1 and V6, and > 2.5 mm in leads aVL and III [12]. These limits are generally somewhat higher in males; normal in benign early repolarization (BER) is 6 mm [28]. Smith

found that the mean T amplitude from V2 to V4 was greater in proven LAD occlusion (6.95 mm) versus early repolarization (6.01 mm), but this had a P value of 0.06. However, the T wave to R wave ratio was significantly greater because of the smaller R-wave in acute MI. (Unpublished data, Smith SW).

Differential diagnosis: In the precordium, an increase in T wave voltage can also be seen in hyperkalemia, angina, left ventricular hypertrophy, anemia, and early repolarization (BER, a normal "variant", Figure 16.8) [4,11,29,30]. Prominent T waves can also be seen in acute pericarditis, bundle branch block, pre-excitation syndromes, and short QT syndrome [31]. Peaked T wave as a result of hyperkalemia can be seen in Case 2, Figure 16.2. These T waves are usually tall, narrow-based, and often have a symmetric appearance

Hyperkalemia   Hyperacute Ischemia   Normal Variant

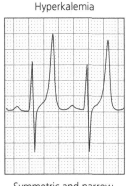
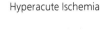
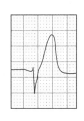
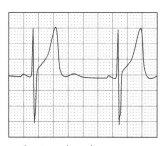

Figure 16.8 From left to right, typical large T waves of hyperkalemia, ischemia (hyperacute T waves), and benign early repolarization. Note that in ischemia, there is a low R wave amplitude and a long QT interval. Reprinted with permission from Wang K. *Atlas of Electrocardiography*.

Symmetric and narrow. Tends to have a short QT interval.

Broad and not pointed. Tends to have a long QT interval.

Asymmetric and not narrow

(Figures 16.2 and 16.8) [32]. Normal T waves of BER appear asymmetric with a somewhat gradual upslope and a more precipitous downslope, and are associated with high R wave voltage, whereas hyperacute T waves are usually associated with relatively low R wave voltage, such that the T wave appears to "tower" over the R wave; this is also true as the ST segment begins to elevate. In one study, T to QRS amplitude > 0.75, J point amplitude > 3 mm, and J point to T amplitude > 0.25 were associated with MI versus BER [33]. Furthermore, the QTc-B (Bazett-corrected QT) is longer in patients with hyperacute T waves, and shorter in BER or hyperkalemia [1,34].

Conclusion

It is important to recognize hyperacute T waves and to differentiate them from normal and other conditions with large T waves. It is equally important to understand that hyperacute T waves both precede and are concurrent with STE, and that, regardless of time since symptom onset, they are associated with myocardial salvage because they represent viable, but ischemic, myocardium.

Case conclusions

In Case 1, the serum potassium returned at 3.7 mEq/L. After administration of appropriate adjunctive medications, he was taken for percutaneous coronary intervention of an occluded proximal and mid right coronary artery (RCA), as well as a distal segment, and the posterior descending limb, of the RCA. In Case 2, the serum potassium was found to be 6.7 mEq/L. The patient was treated with calcium, bicarbonate, dextrose and insulin, and binding resin, and referred for immediate hemodialysis. Immediately after the medications, the QRS complex narrowed and the T waves normalized.

References

1 Kenigsberg DN, Khanal S, Kowalski M, *et al.* Prolongation of the QTc interval is seen uniformly during early transmural ischemia. *J Am Coll Cardiol* 2007;**49**(12):1299–305.

2 Smith SW, Zvosec DL, Henry TD, *et al.* editors. *The ECG in Acute MI: an Evidence-Based Manual of Reperfusion Therapy.* 1st edition. Philadelphia: Lippincott, Williams, and Wilkins, 2002: 358.

3 Soo CS. Tall precordial T waves with depressed ST take-off: an early sign of acute myocardial infarction? *Singapore Med J* 1995;**36**(2):236–7.

4 Dressler W, Roesler H. High T waves in the earliest stage of myocardial infarction. *Am Heart J* 1947;**34**:627–45.

5 Wiggers HC, Wiggers CJ. The interpretation of monophasic action potentials from the mammalian ventricle indicated by changes following coronary occlusion. *Am J Physiol* 1935;**113**: 683–9.

6 Wilkins ML, Pryor AD, Maynard C. An electrocardiographic acuteness score for quantifying the timing of a myocardial

infarction to guide decisions regarding reperfusion therapy. *Am J Cardiol* 1995;**75**(8):617–20.

7 Smith FM. The ligation of coronary arteries with electrocardiographic study. *Arch Intern Med* 1918;**5**:1–27.

8 Bayley RH, LaDue JS, York DJ. Electrocardiographic changes (local ventricular ischemia and injury) produced in the dog by temporary occlusion of a coronary artery, showing a new stage in the evolution of myocardial infarction. *Am Heart J* 1944;27:164–9.

9 Graham GK, Laforet EG. An electrocardiographic and morphologic study of changes following ligation of the left coronary artery in human beings: a report of two cases. *Am Heart J* 1952;**43**:42–52.

10 Smith SW, Whitwam W. Acute Coronary Syndromes. *Emerg Med Clin North Am* 2006;**24**(1):53–89.

11 Freundlich J. The diagnostic significance of tall upright T waves in the chest leads. *Am Heart J* 1956;**52**:749–67.

12 Hochrein J, Sun F, Pieper KS, *et al.* Higher T wave amplitude associated with better prognosis in patients receiving thrombolytic therapy for acute myocardial infarction (a GUSTO-1 substudy). Global Utilization of Streptokinase and Tissue plasminogen activator for Occluded Coronary Arteries. *Am J Cardiol* 1998; **81**(9):1078–84.

13 Pardee HEB. An electrocardiographic sign of coronary artery obstruction. Arch Intern Med 1920;**26**:244–57.

14 Wasserburger RH, Corliss RJ. Prominent precordial T waves as an expression of coronary insufficiency. *Am J Cardiol* 1965;**16**: 195–205.

15 Bohning A, Katz LN. Unusual changes in the electrocardiograms of patients with recent coronary occlusion. *Am J Med Sci* 1933; **186**:39–52.

16 Wachtel FW, Teich EM. Tall precordial T waves as the earliest sign in diaphragmatic wall infarction. *Am Heart J* 1956;**51**:917–20.

17 Wood F, Wolferth C. Huge T waves in precordial leads in cardiac infarction. *Am Heart J* 1934;**9**:706–21.

18 Thygesen K, Alpert JS, White HD, *et al.* Universal Definition of Myocardial Infarction. *Circulation* 2007;**116**:2634–53.

19 Sclarovsky S, (ed.). *Electrocardiography of Acute Myocardial Ischemic Syndromes.* London: Martin Dunitz, 1999.

20 Wagner GS. *Marriott's Practical Electrocardiography.* 10th edition. Philadelphia: Lippincott, Williams, and Wilkins, 2001.

21 Jaffe HL. Typical and atypical electrocardiograms in myocardial infarction caused by acute coronary occlusion and coronary insufficiency. *Dis Chest* 1955;**27**:243–54.

22 Tulloch JA. The electrocardiographic features of high myocardial infarction. *Br Heart J* 1952;**14**:379.

23 Blomkalns AL, Lindsell CJ, Chandra A, *et al.* Can electrocardiographic criteria predict adverse cardiac events and positive cardiac markers? *Acad Emerg Med* 2003;**10**(3):205–10.

24 Engblom H, Heden B, Hedstrom E, *et al.* ECG Estimate Of Ischemic Acuteness and Time from Pain Onset for Predicting Myocardial Salvage in Patients Undergoing Primary Percutaneous Coronary Intervention. AHA Abstract 2404. *Circulation* 2007;**116**(Suppl 2):II_528.

25 Corey KE, Maynard C, Pahlm O, *et al.* Combined historical and electrocardiographic timing of acute anterior and inferior myocardial infarcts for prediction of reperfusion achievable size limitation. *Am J Cardiol* 1999;**83**(6):826–31.

26 Raitt MH, Maynard C, Wagner GS, *et al.* Appearance of abnormal Q waves early in the course of acute myocardial infarction:

implications for efficacy of thrombolytic therapy. *J Am Coll Cardiol* 1995;**25**(5):1084–8.

27 Macfarlane PW, Lawrie TDV. Appendix 1: Normal limits. In: *Comprehensive Electrocardiography*. Pergamon Press: New York, 1989: 1446–57.

28 Brady WJ. ST segment and T wave abnormalities not caused by acute coronary syndromes. *Emerg Med Clin North Am* 2006; **24**(1):91–111, vi.

29 Epstein FH, Pollack AA, Ostrander LDJ. Electrocardiographic survey in Peru. *Am J Med Sci* 1964;**247**:687–93.

30 Pinto IJ, Nanda NC, Biswas AK, *et al.* Tall upright T waves in the precordial leads. *Circulation* 1967;**36**:708–16.

31 Mattu AW, Brady WJ. *ECG's for the Emergency Physician*. London: BMJ Publishing Group, 2003.

32 Braun HA, Surawicz B, Bellet S. T waves in hyperpotassemia. *Am J Med Sci* 1955;**2**:147–56.

33 Collins MS, Carter JE, Dougherty JM, *et al.* Hyperacute T wave criteria using computer ECG analysis. *Ann Emerg Med* 1990; **19**(2):114–20.

34 Smith SW, Khalil A. Corrected QT Interval Distinguishes Early Repolarization from Subtle Anterior STEMI: Derivation of a Rule (abstract, presentation). *Acad Emerg Med* 2007;**14**(Suppl 5):S125.

Chapter 17 | What is the significance of Q waves?

Wayne Whitwam[1], Vipin Khetarpal[2]
[1]University of California, San Diego, CA, USA
[2]Harper Hospital Wayne State University School of Medicine , Detroit, MI, USA

Case presentations

Case 1: A 53-year-old male with history of inferior myocardial infarction (MI) presents with 1 h of chest pain. The electrocardiogram (ECG) is shown in Figure 17.1. After review of the ECG, the physician confirms that the patient's discomfort has only been present for 1 h. He is emergently taken for percutaneous coronary intervention (PCI).

Case 2: A 55-year-old male with a medical history of hypertension, diabetes and tobacco use presents to the emergency department (ED) with a 2-day history of intermittent squeezing pain with mild exertion that radiates to the left shoulder and arm, consistent with accelerated angina. The physical examination is unremarkable. An ECG obtained at presentation manifests both inferior and lateral acute MI, with ST elevation (STE) in leads I, II, AVF, V5 and V6, and ST segment depression in AVR (Figure 17.2). R waves were seen in leads V1 and V2 suggesting a chronic persistent occlusion of a lateral vessel. The first troponin I was elevated (> 50 ng/mL).

The significance of Q waves

The initial downward deflection of ventricular depolarization on the ECG is called a Q wave. This vector, normally of short duration and low amplitude, represents the rapid depolarization of the thin septal wall between the two ventricles, and may be found on most leads. In addition to physiologic and position effects, the Q wave may represent myocardial injury, ventricular enlargement or altered ventricular conduction [1]. QS waves are Q waves without a succeeding R wave (Figure 17.1, lead III). QR waves have an R wave after the Q wave (Figure 17.1, lead V4, Figure 17.2, lead II). qR and Qr, respectively, reflect the size of the accompanying Q or R wave.

Pathologic Q waves are usually wider and deeper, ≥ 30 ms in duration or > 25% of following R wave in amplitude. Leads III and aVR can have Q waves that are deep or ≥ 30 ms in duration, without any underlying pathology [1]. However, Q waves seen in leads I, II, aVL, aVF, or V4–V6 are considered abnormal.

With MI, tissue that was previously generating voltage for the overlying lead (resulting in an R-wave) is now infarcted and that voltage is lost. The new resultant electrical vector is generated by tissue on the opposite side of the heart, and, thus, is directed away from the area of tissue loss and its overlying ECG lead, creating a negative deflection. Hence, an abnormal Q wave is recorded in leads facing the area of myocardial necrosis. Electrically dead or necrotic tissue acts as an "electrical window," transmitting the depolarizing forces (R wave) as recorded from the opposite position of the heart [2]. Q waves of MI are usually present in any two contiguous leads and are ≥ 1 mm in depth. These criteria are limited and may lead to false-negative and false-positive diagnoses. For example, Q waves in V1 and V2 may be normal (see Figure 17.3) [3].

Electrocardiogram changes other than Q waves may denote MI, referred to as *Q wave equivalents*. In the precordial leads, these are observed: (1) R wave diminution, or poor R wave progression, (2) reverse R wave progression, in which R waves increase then decrease in amplitude across the precordial leads (although this must be distinguished from precordial electrode misconnection), and (3) tall R waves in leads V1 and V2, representing "Q waves" of "posterior infarction" (now considered "lateral," see below). With R wave loss there is a rough correlation between the sum of R wave voltages in all 12 ECG leads and the left ventricular ejection fraction, such that patients with total R wave voltage less than 4 mm in leads aVL, aVF, and V1–V6 have significantly reduced left ventricular dysfunction and a worse prognosis [4].

Q waves commonly, but erroneously, are considered markers of irreversible infarction. Thus, reperfusion therapy often is denied to patients with Q waves. Within 1 h of onset of anterior MI, QR waves (but not usually QS waves) occur in the right precordial leads in approximately half of patients (see Figure 25.4); these frequently disappear after reperfusion. Such QR waves are caused by ischemia of the conducting system, supplied by the left anterior descending (LAD)

Critical Decisions in Emergency and Acute Care Electrocardiography,
1st edition. Edited by W.J. Brady and J.D. Truwit. © 2009 Blackwell Publishing, ISBN: 9781405159067

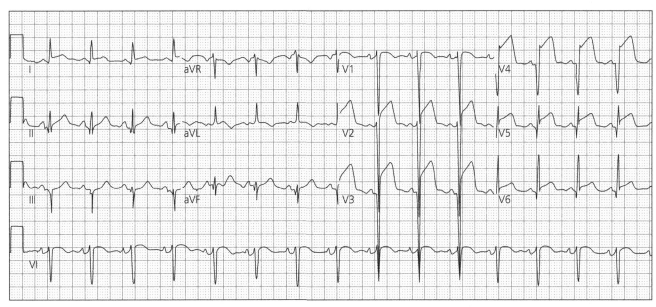

Figure 17.1 Early anterior MI with Q waves already present. There is profound ST elevation in leads V2–V6, and also STE in I and aVL (proximal). There are Q waves in V3 and V4, but they are QR (not QS) waves, as can be seen by the spike just before the ST segment in V4. These early Q waves are present in 50% of anterior MI and do not represent early infarction, rather ischemia and injury of the conduction system. They will disappear with successful reperfusion. Q waves in inferior leads represent his previous inferior MI.

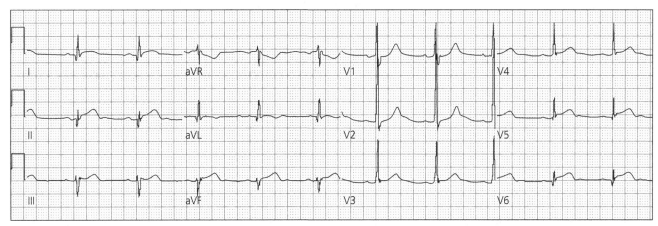

Figure 17.2 Inferolateral injury due to occlusion of a large first obtuse marginal of the dominant left circumflex artery, manifested by subtle STE in leads I, II, aVF, and V5–V6. The RS pattern in leads V1–V2 suggests old lateral MI (formerly misnamed *posterior* MI). There were no other occluded vessels. The septal R waves persisted on a follow-up ECG 2 years later. The ST segment depression in aVR (-aVR) is highly diagnostic for an acute lateral STEMI, but is often missed, as it was in this case.

coronary artery, and not necessarily by irreversible infarction [5]. The presence of abnormal Q waves in the leads with STE on the admission ECG is associated with larger infarct size and increased in-hospital mortality (see Figure 27.3) [6]. Patients with high ST segments and absence of Q waves have the greatest benefit from thrombolytic therapy, but those who have persistent high STE in the presence of QR waves also receive significant benefit [7]. Q waves develop in relation to the duration of occlusion, the extent to which collateral vessels maintain myocardial viability during occlusion, the size of the infarction, and the occurrence of reinfarction. Q waves signifying necrosis should be developed completely

within 8–12 h of onset of persistent occlusion [2,8]. In the era before invasive treatment of non-ST elevation myocardial infarction (NSTEMI), approximately 14% of those without Q waves after 48 h developed them later, and this was highly associated with reinfarction [9].

Myocardial infarction resulting in a QS pattern indicates large irreversible myocardial loss (see Figure 25.4), with no net depolarization towards the overlying lead. In most patients, these Q waves persist indefinitely, but in up to 30% of those patients who do not receive reperfusion therapy the Q waves eventually disappear within months to years, particularly in inferior wall MI [10,11]. In contrast, Q waves

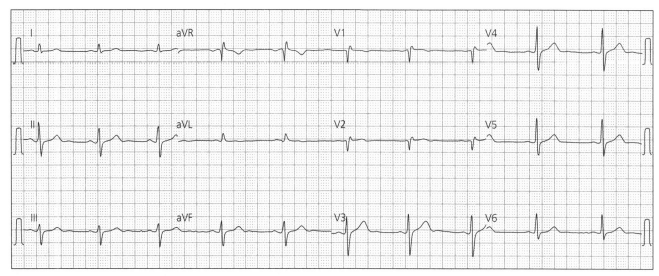

Figure 17.3 Normal septal Q waves in leads V1–V2 in a 36-year-old male with confirmed normal myocardium.

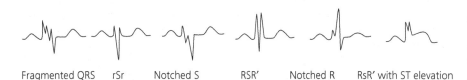

Fragmented QRS   rSr   Notched S   RSR′   Notched R   RsR′ with ST elevation

Figure 17.4 Different morphologies of a "fragmented QRS" on a 12-lead ECG. Reprinted with permission from Das MK, et al. *Circulation* 2006;**113**:2495–501. ©Copyright 2006 American Heart Association [13].

in patients who receive early reperfusion therapy disappear within a few days to weeks [8,12]. The sensitivity of Q waves in detecting a myocardial scar is 36% with a specificity of 99% and negative predictive value of 71% [13].

The presence of a fragmented QRS complex may supplement the analysis of Q waves in detection of myocardial scar on the ECG. The fragmented QRS pattern is defined as an RSR′ without evidence of a typical bundle branch pattern (Figure 17.4). When used along with Q waves, this increases the sensitivity for old MI detection to 91%, without any significant decrease in specificity [13].

The presence of Q waves following MI (QWMI) has shown a decreasing trend from 66.6 to 37.5% in the last two decades, while the incidence of non-Q wave MI (NQWMI) has increased reciprocally. Rapid use of reperfusion therapy in patients with STEMI probably accounts for this decrease, but the expanded definition of MI using the more sensitive troponin standard also contributes significantly [14]. Compared with NQWMI, in-hospital mortality rate for QWMI is significantly higher. However, post-discharge prognosis when followed up to 10 years is comparable in the two groups. In a population based 20-year study, the long-term survival rates for patients with QWMI were 91, 86, 75, and 56% at 1, 2, 5 and 10 years after hospital discharge, respectively. Corresponding survival rates were 85, 80, 65, and 47% for patients with NQWMI [14]. Such outcomes may be different in the future because of invasive therapy for NQWMI used today.

Anatomic correlates of infarction

Until recently, autopsy findings have been the basis of the correlation between Q wave and myocardial scar. Cardiovascular magnetic resonance (CMR) imaging with late gadolinium enhancement allows precise *in vivo* detection of location and transmural extent of MI, detecting an MI down to 1% of the total myocardial mass [15]. Cardiovascular magnetic resonance-generated data show that 30% of transmural infarcts may not show a Q wave on ECG, while 28% of subendocardial infarcts may manifest Q waves. The primary determinant of the presence of a Q wave is the total size of infarct rather than its transmural extent. Thus, with a larger MI, there is more likely to be a Q wave on the ECG [16].

For purposes of convention, new correlations have been established for identifying Q wave infarction based on CMR imaging (Figure 17.5). Q waves in V1–V2 are associated with *septal* wall MI, but may also appear in anterior wall infarctions. A septal MI follows occlusion of either the septal branches of the LAD distal to the diagonal branches. See Figure 17.5 for the new classification of cardiac segments [17].

Under historic definitions, a Q wave in lead aVL, without a Q in V6, is a "high lateral wall MI" following a left circumflex (LCX) occlusion. In the new convention, a Q wave in aVL corresponds with a *mid-anterior* MI (diagonal branch occlusion) [18].

(a)

Left Ventricular Segmentation

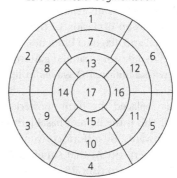

1. basal anterior
2. basal anteroseptal
3. basal inferoseptal
4. basal inferior
5. basal inferolateral
6. basal anterolateral

7. mid anterior
8. mid anteroseptal
9. mid inferoseptal
10. mid inferior
11. mid inferolateral
12. mid anterolateral

13. apical anterior
14. apical septal
15. apical inferior
16. apical lateral
17. apex

(b)

Name	ECG pattern	Infarction area (CMR)
Septal	Q in V1–V2	
Mid-anterior	Q (qs or qr) in aVL and sometimes in I and/or V2–V3	
Apical-anterior	Q in V1–V2 to V3–V6	
Extensive anterior	Q in V1–V2 to V4–V6, aVL and sometimes I	
Lateral	RS in V1–V2 and/or Q wave in leads I, aVL, V6 and/or diminished R wave in V6	
Inferior	Q in II, III, aVF	

Figure 17.5 (a) The 17 segments of the heart, as seen by MRI (looking from the feet up, so that the right side of the figure is the left side of the heart, the center (17) is the apex of the heart, and the outer ring (1–6) are the six most posterior-superior (or "basal") segments. Segment 4 is no longer called "posterior," but rather "inferobasal." Reproduced with permission from Cerqueira MD, *et al. Circulation* 2002;**105**:539–42. ©Copyright 2002 American Heart Association [17]. (b) The new proposed terminology for ECG patterns of Q wave MI or Q wave equivalents with the names given to MI and related infarction area documented by cardiac magnetic resonance. An RS pattern seen in leads V1–V2 is now described as a lateral rather than posterior infarct. Reprinted with permission from Bayés de Luna A, *et al. Circulation* 2006;**114**:1755–60. ©Copyright 2006 American Heart Association [18].

Following a mid-LAD occlusion, Q waves that appear in leads V1–V2 to V3–V6 will manifest as an *apical-anterior* MI by the new convention, whereas an occlusion of the LAD, proximal to both the first septal and diagonal branches, produces an *extensive-anterior* MI, manifesting a similar pattern to a mid-LAD occlusion, but with additional Q waves in lead aVL and sometimes lead I.

The new convention has replaced the term "posterior" with "inferobasal" wall [18]. This is the high or basal part of the inferior wall that bends upwards. By historic convention, an MI of the right coronary artery (RCA) that supplies the inferior wall would produce the characteristic RS morphology seen in leads V1–V2. In fact, occlusion of the RCA produces an *inferior* MI with Q waves in leads II, III, and aVF (the presence of significant Q wave in lead III alone does not indicate MI).

On magnetic resonance imaging (MRI), it is clear that the area of the heart opposite lead I is the lateral wall. Thus, occlusion of LCX producing a tall R wave in lead V1 is, strictly speaking, an MI of the lateral wall (not "posterior"); thus, a "posterior MI" is actually a *lateral* MI. When the RCA or LCX is large and dominant, the MI will encompass elements of both the lateral and inferior MI, producing Q waves in II, III, and aVF, as well as the RS pattern in V1–V2 [18].

Differential diagnosis

Any process, acute or chronic, that causes sufficient loss of regional electromotive potentials can result in Q waves. Examples include dilated or hypertrophic cardiomyopathy, myocarditis, bundle branch block and infiltrative diseases [19]. A complete summary of ECG differential diagnosis is shown in Table 17.1. These conditions should be considered in differential diagnosis when evaluating an ECG that shows significant Q waves.

Case conclusions

The patient in Case 1 was taken for successful emergent PCI of a proximal LAD. The precordial ST segments resolved, as did the QR waves. Intraluminal clot with marked narrowing of the LAD was noted. Cardiac biomarkers were positive for cardiac injury. In Case 2, a coronary angiogram revealed a complete obstruction of the first obtuse marginal branch of the dominant LCX. Following angioplasty and stenting of this occlusion, a transthoracic echocardiogram documented inferolateral hypokinesis with reduced systolic function and an ejection fraction (EF) of 45%. The patient was started on anti-anginal therapy and discharged from the hospital a few days later in a stable condition. An adenosine cardiac perfusion stress test 2 years later showed a complete MI of the inferolateral wall. On the ECG, the R waves seen in leads V1 and V2 persisted, whereas any Q waves in the inferior leads that may have appeared had since resolved.

Table 17.1 Electrocardiographic differential diagnosis of Q wave myocardial infarction

Pseudo-infarction patterns are ECG patterns that mimic or confound the diagnosis of prior myocardial infarction.

Cardiac
Most common (QS waves in leads V1 to V3)
  Left ventricular hypertrophy
  Left bundle branch block
  Dilated cardiomyopathy
  Normal variant Q waves in leads V1, V2, III, aVL and aVF
Less common
  Right ventricular hypertrophy
  Left anterior fasicular block
  Hypertrophic cardiomyopathy
  Wolff-Parkinson-White syndrome
  Acute myocarditis
  Athlete's heart
  Dextrocardia
  Amyloidosis
  Sarcoidosis
  Scleroderma
  Duchenne's muscular dystrophy
  Friedreich's ataxia
  Chaga's disease
  Cardiac tumor
  Echinococcus cyst

Non-cardiac
  Misplacement of precordial electrode
  Chronic obstructive pulmonary disease
  Pulmonary embolism
  Pneumothorax
  Hyperkalemia
  Acute pancreatitis

References

1 Surawicz B, Knilans T. *Chou's Electrocardiography in Clinical Practice. Adult and Pediatric.* Philadelphia, PA: WB Saunders, 2001.

2 Smith SW, Whitwam W. Acute Coronary Syndromes. *Emerg Med Clin North Am* 2006;**24**:53–89.

3 Alpert JS, Thygesen K, Antman E, Bassand JP. Myocardial infarction redefined – a consensus document of The Joint European Society of Cardiology/American College of Cardiology Committee for the redefinition of myocardial infarction. *J Am Coll Cardiol* 2000;**36**:959–69.

4 Askenazi J, Parisi AF, Cohn PF, *et al.* Value of the QRS complex in assessing left ventricular ejection fraction. *Am J Cardiol* 1978; **41**:494–9.

5 Barold SS, Falkoff MD, Ong LS, Heinle RA. Significance of transient electrocardiographic Q waves in coronary artery disease. *Cardiol Clin* 1987;**5**:367–80.

6 Birnbaum Y, Chetrit A, Sclarovsky S, *et al.* Abnormal Q waves on the admission electrocardiogram of patients with first acute myocardial infarction: prognostic implications. *Clin Cardiol* 1997;**20**: 477–81.

7 Raitt MH, Maynard C, Wagner GS, *et al.* Appearance of abnormal Q waves early in the course of acute myocardial infarction:

implications for efficacy of thrombolytic therapy. *J Am Coll Cardiol* 1995;**25**:1084–8.

8 Bar FW, Volders PG, Hoppener B, *et al.* Development of ST-segment elevation and Q- and R-wave changes in acute myocardial infarction and the influence of thrombolytic therapy. *Am J Cardiol* 1996;**77**:337–43.

9 Kleiger RE, Boden WE, Schechtman KB, *et al.* Frequency and significance of late evolution of Q waves in patients with initial non-Q-wave acute myocardial infarction. Diltiazem Reinfarction Study Group. *Am J Cardiol* 1990;**65**:23–7.

10 Bergovec M, Prpic H, Zigman M, *et al.* Regression of ECG signs of myocardial infarction related to infarct size and left ventricular function. *J Electrocardiol* 1993;**26**:1–8.

11 Kaplan BM, Berkson DM. Serial electrocardiograms after myocardial infarction. *Ann Intern Med* 1964;**60**:430–5.

12 Blanke H, Scherff F, Karsch KR, *et al.* Electrocardiographic changes after streptokinase-induced recanalization in patients with acute left anterior descending artery obstruction. *Circulation* 1983;**68**:406–12.

13 Das MK, Khan B, Jacob S, *et al.* Significance of a fragmented QRS complex versus a Q wave in patients with coronary artery disease. *Circulation* 2006;**113**:2495–501.

14 Furman MI, Dauerman HL, Goldberg RJ, *et al.* Twenty-two year (1975 to 1997) trends in the incidence, in-hospital and long-term case fatality rates from initial Q-wave and non-Q-wave myocardial infarction: a multi-hospital, community-wide perspective. *J Am Coll Cardiol* 2001;**37**:1571–80.

15 Ricciardi MJ, Wu E, Davidson CJ, *et al.* Visualization of discrete microinfarction after percutaneous coronary intervention associated with mild creatine kinase-MB elevation. *Circulation* 2001; **103**:2780–3.

16 Moon JCC, De Arenaza DP, Elkington AG, *et al.* The Pathologic Basis of Q-Wave and Non-Q-Wave Myocardial Infarction. *J Am Coll Card* 2004;**44**:554–60.

17 Cerqueira MD, Weissman NJ, Dilsizian V, *et al.* Standardized myocardial segmentation and nomenclature for tomographic imaging of the heart: a statement for healthcare professionals from the Cardiac Imaging Committee of the Council on Clinical Cardiology of the American Heart Association. *Circulation* 2002; **105**:539–42.

18 Bayés de Luna A, Wagner G, Birnbaum Y, *et al.* A new terminology for left ventricular walls and location of myocardial infarcts that present Q wave based on the standard of cardiac magnetic resonance imaging: a statement for healthcare professionals from a committee appointed by the International Society for Holter and Noninvasive Electrocardiography. *Circulation* 2006;**114**:1755–60.

19 Goldberger AL. *Myocardial Infarction: Electrocardiographic Differential Diagnosis.* St. Louis: Mosby, 1991:386 pp.

Chapter 18 | What are the ECG indications for additional electrocardiographic leads (including electrocardiographic body-surface mapping) in chest pain patients?

Daniel T. O'Laughlin[1], Khaled Bachour[2], Wayne Whitwam[3]
[1]University of Minnesota School of Medicine, Minneapolis, MN, USA
[2]Wayne State University School of Medicine, Detroit, MI, USA
[3]University of California, San Diego, CA, USA

Case presentations

Case 1: A 69-year-old female presents with 1 h of chest pain and weakness to the emergency department (ED) of a small hospital without cardiac catheterization lab capabilities. Her exam is unremarkable. A standard 12-lead electrocardiogram (ECG) is obtained and, after immediate review, a posterior lead ECG is ordered (Figure 18.1). This demonstrates findings of posterior myocardial infarction (MI), with ST elevation (STE) in leads V6–V9. Due to weather conditions, the patient's transfer to a tertiary cardiac referral center will be delayed by 3 h. The patient has no absolute contraindications to fibrinolytic therapy.

Case 2: A 61-year-old male presents with 1 h of chest pain, associated with dyspnea, diaphoresis, and nausea, to the ED of a tertiary care center that has cardiac catheterization capabilities. He has no history of coronary disease, but smokes and has hypertension, though is non-compliant with therapy. He takes aspirin intermittently. He does have a history of previous stroke with some residual weakness. His first 12-lead ECG is shown in Figure 18.2a and a right-sided ECG obtained 2 min later is shown in Figure 18.2b. The first ECG demonstrates STE in leads II, III, aVF, and V3, and ST depression in I, aVL, and V2 with a complete heart block at a ventricular rate of 47 beats per minute (bpm). The right-sided ECG demonstrates significant STE across all of the right-sided leads.

ECG indications for additional electrocardiographic leads

The traditional ECG obtains a 10 s interval of cardiac electrical activity derived from 12 leads with three limb leads (leads I, II, III), three augmented limb leads (leads aVR, aVL, aVF) and six precordial leads (V1–V6). The 12-lead ECG does have certain limitations that limit the sensitivity and specificity for identifying an acute ischemic event. In addition to the difficulties encountered as a result of confounding electrical patterns, the 12-lead ECG is limited by the inadequate representation of the right ventricle [1] and of the posterior, lateral, and apical walls of the left ventricle [2].

The initial 12-lead ECG manifests diagnostic STE in approximately 45% of patients with an acute myocardial infarction (AMI) as diagnosed by CK-MB [3–6]; this may rise to 60% with use of serial ECGs [3]. If ST depression and T wave inversion are included, initial and serial ECGs are 55% and 68% sensitive for AMI (as diagnosed by CK-MB) [3]; in a study using cardiac magnetic resonance imaging (MRI) as the standard diagnosis, STE on the initial ECG had a sensitivity of 50%; adding ST depression improved sensitivity to 84% [7]. Several studies have assessed the potential improved prognostic value of adding posterior and right-sided ECG leads. The majority, but not all [8], of these studies have demonstrated significant improvements in detection of AMI in the lateral and posterior regions of the myocardium [1,8–13].

Critical Decisions in Emergency and Acute Care Electrocardiography, 1st edition. Edited by W.J. Brady and J.D. Truwit. © 2009 Blackwell Publishing, ISBN: 9781405159067

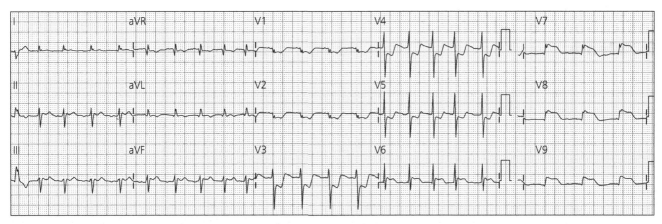

Figure 18.1 Case 1. Standard 12-lead ECG plus leads V7–V9 show posterior wall injury. Note the ST depression in leads V1–V5 and STE in V6. The addition of the V7–V9 leads demonstrates that STE continues along the posterior wall of the left ventricle, in leads V7–V9.

(a)

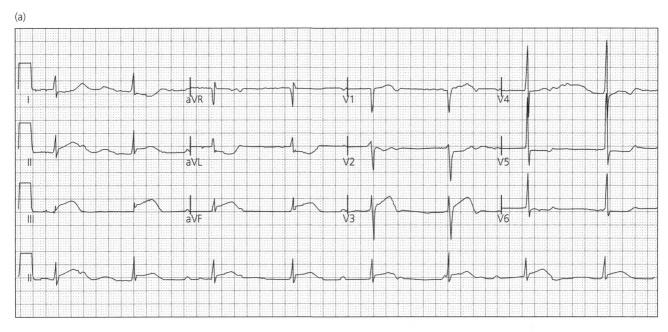

(b)

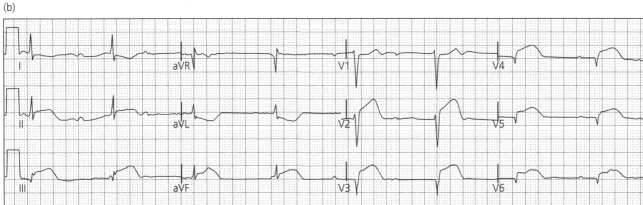

Figure 18.2 (a) Case 2. Standard 12-lead ECG shows STE in leads II, III, aVF, and V3, and ST depression in I, aVL, and V2. Complete heart block is present due to involvement of the RCA branch supplying the AV node. (b) Right-sided leads demonstrate significant STE across all of the right-sided leads consistent with extensive RV infarction.

Indications for additional ECG leads

Three clinical scenarios best identify patients that may benefit from the recording of additional leads. First, the recording of additional leads should be considered when there is right precordial ST depression suggesting posterior ST elevation myocardial infarction (STEMI); STE on posterior leads would change the diagnosis from non-ST elevation myocardial infarction (NSTEMI) to STEMI, for which the patient may qualify for reperfusion therapies (see Case 1). Second, the recording of right-sided leads is recommended for patients experiencing an acute inferior wall left ventricular infarction as involvement of the right ventricle may result in alteration of treatment (see Case 2). Third, additional leads may be considered in patients with increased suspicion for acute coronary syndrome (ACS), but with a non-specific standard 12-lead ECG. These leads may increase the detection of a subtle STEMI and allow for timely reperfusion interventions.

The use of additional right-sided and posterior leads has not been shown to provide added benefit over standard 12-lead ECG in low-risk patients presenting with chest pain [8,14,15]. The 2007 joint scientific statement regarding the standardization and interpretation of the electrocardiogram released by the American Heart Association (AHA), American College of Cardiology (ACC) and the Heart Rhythm Society does not recommend the routine recording of these leads in the absence of an acute coronary event as outlined in the first and second scenarios above [16].

Posterior precordial leads and posterior wall infarction

The posterior wall (or, by new terminology, the "inferobasal" wall) [17] of the left ventricle is supplied by the right coronary artery (RCA) and the left circumflex artery (LCX). Approximately 85% of adults have a right side dominant coronary artery anatomy, which results in the RCA supplying the atrioventricular (AV) nodal branch and the inferior wall. Occlusion of either RCA or the LCX, or the corresponding branches, may result in posterior MI (PMI), regardless of dominance. The posterior wall is involved in approximately 15–20% of AMIs. The majority of these events are associated with acute infarction of the inferior or lateral (or both) walls of the left ventricle [18]. Isolated PMIs make up anywhere from 3 to 11% of all AMIs, and generally are the result of an occlusion of a non-dominant LCX or one of the obtuse marginal branch vessels [18–21].

12-Lead ECG findings in PMI

Posterior myocardial infarction ECG patterns are most commonly missed because of the distance from the posterior wall to the anterior chest, the electrical orientation of the heart, the lack of posterior leads in the standard 12-lead ECG, and the effect from summation forces [18,22]. The diagnosis of PMI has traditionally been based on the presence of ST depression in the anterior precordial leads; however, this may be present with subendocardial ischemia as well as posterior STEMI [23,24]. In the presence of inferior STEMI, anterior ST depression is almost always a result of posterior STEMI [12,25,26]; it is infrequently the result of subendocardial ischemia [25]. Isolated anterior ST depression can be due to isolated PMI, especially if in right precordial leads V1–V4, or to subendocardial ischemia.

Posterior STEMI only manifests ≥ 1 mm of anterior ST depression in approximately three-quarters of cases [12,27]. An upsloping ST segment with an upright T wave is more likely to be posterior STEMI; a downsloping ST segment with an inverted T wave may be either posterior MI or subendocardial ischemia. The ACC/AHA guidelines allow right precordial ST depression as the only ST depression indication for fibrinolytic therapy.

Left circumflex artery occlusion may present with isolated posterior MI or associated inferior and/or lateral left ventricular wall infarction. The 12-lead ECG findings with LCX occlusion may manifest as either STE in the inferior leads (II, III, aVF) and/or the lateral leads (I, aVL, V5, V6), or ST depression in the anterior precordial leads (V1–V4), or as a normal ECG. Findings may be very subtle. Whereas RCA and left anterior descending coronary artery (LAD) occlusion manifest STE in 80–90% of occlusions [13,28], LCX occlusion manifests with STE in inferior or lateral leads in only one-third of cases, with another one-third manifesting anterior ST depression only, and the final one-third with no ST deviation at all [13,19,25,28,29]. When there is STE in lateral leads, it is rarely pronounced [30]. For this reason, newer guidelines for the diagnosis of MI use 1 mm, rather than 2 mm, of STE in leads V4–V6 as a cutoff for STEMI [17]. In a study by Schmitt and colleagues, patients with AMI involving the LCX demonstrated ≥ 2 mm STE in leads V1–V6 on a standard 12-lead ECG in 46% of cases. In a subgroup in which posterior leads were also obtained, ≥ 2 mm STE in V1–V6 or ≥ 1 mm for limb leads identified 50% of circumflex occlusions, whereas the addition of posterior leads, using a cutoff of ≥ 1 mm, improved sensitivity to 61% [13]. By comparison, extended leads (posterior and right) improved sensitivity of STE from 77 to 81% for the RCA, and 85 to 90% for the LAD [13]. These findings reinforce the difficulties in ECG evaluation of the posterior and lateral wall of the left ventricle.

The rapid recognition of posterior MI in the setting of concurrent inferior or lateral wall AMI is of significant clinical importance as these patients are experiencing a larger region of infarction and are prone to increased complications and have poorer prognosis [12,20,31–33]. The risks for dysrhythmia, left ventricular dysfunction, mitral regurgitation, and death increase proportionally with the size of the infarction [11,34].

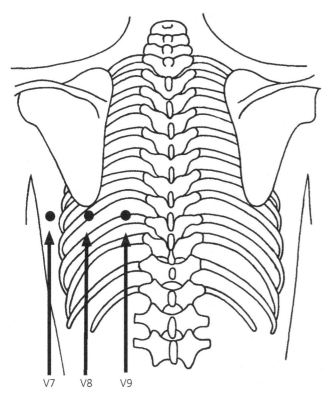

Figure 18.3 Posterior lead orientation. Leads should be placed in the same horizontal plane as V4–V6. V7 in line with the posterior axillary line. V8 inferior to the scapular tip. V9 at the paravertebral border.

Posterior lead orientation and diagnostic criterion

The posterior precordial leads are positioned in the fifth intercostal space at the same horizontal line as V6 (Figure 18.3). Lead V7 is placed at the posterior axillary line, V8 just below the tip of the scapula, and V9 at the paravertebral border [16]. ST elevation up to 0.5 mm measured at the J point relative to the PR segment in all three leads can be normal [35]. Wung and Drew evaluated the posterior ST segment changes during percutaneous transluminal coronary angioplasty (PTCA) of the LCX, and determined that utilizing a criterion of STE of ≥ 0.5 mm, rather than ≥ 1 mm, demonstrated a sensitivity of 94% for detecting LCX occlusion-related STE [27]. This is compared with a sensitivity of 49% when the criterion was ≥ 1 mm STE. Conversely, Matetzky and colleagues showed 100% specificity for posterior MI of STE ≥ 0.5 mm in at least one posterior lead. In Wung's study, 81% of patients with ≥ 1 mm STE in posterior leads also had other significant STE on the 12-lead ECG, and 96% had some ST deviation [27]. However, 22–39% of patients experiencing PMI who have ≥ 0.5 mm STE in the posterior leads do not demonstrate ST depression in V1–V3 [11,12, 27].

Right-sided ECG and right ventricular infarction

In a "right-side dominant" coronary system, which is present in approximately 85% of patients, the right ventricular "marginal" branches off of the RCA to the right ventricle, and right ventricular myocardial infarction (RVMI) is a result of RCA occlusion proximal to this branch. Alternatively, an isolated RVMI may more rarely result from occlusion of that branch itself. Additionally, the LAD supplies a small amount of the right ventricle, so that anterior (LV) MI often results in clinically insignificant, small RVMI [36,37].

Approximately 3% of RVMI occurs as an isolated event [36]. Up to 50% of patients with acute inferior STEMI will have associated RVMI [38,39]. Hemodynamic instability of clinically significant RVMI occurs in 10–15% of these patients; this is primarily volume-sensitive hypotension from right-sided failure and subsequent poor left ventricular filling pressures [39]. Evidence for RVMI should be sought in all patients with inferior STEMI as they are at substantially increased risk of major complications [40]. Although the clinical triad of hypotension, clear lung fields, and elevated jugular venous pressure in the setting of a STEMI is specific for a clinically significant RVMI, it has a sensitivity of less than 25% [39]. Other clinical findings for RVMI include right ventricular gallops, tricuspid regurgitation, and AV dissociation [38,41,42]. Right ventricular myocardial infarction has a high short-term morbidity and mortality, especially without reperfusion [40,43,44].

Right-sided ECG recording is recommended in the evaluation of all patients with ECG evidence of inferior AMI or other clinical suspicion for RVMI. This is particularly true if the inferior MI is a result of RCA occlusion, because the RV marginal branch almost always originates from the RCA. Right coronary artery occlusion can be identified by the presence or absence of reciprocal ST depression in lead I, and the relative height of the ST segment in leads II and III, with higher STE in lead III favoring the RCA [25]. The routine recording of the right-sided ECG leads is not recommended in the absence of ECG evidence of AMI or strong clinical suspicion of RVMI.

Right ventricular myocardial infarction should be suspected especially if there is STE in lead V1, which lies over the right ventricle. In very large RVMI, the STE can extend from V2 to V5, especially if right ventricular hypertrophy is present, and may mimic an anteroseptal MI ("pseudo-anteroseptal MI"); these are best differentiated by inferior STE and/or by right-sided STE. Additionally, pseudo-anteroseptal MI has the highest STE in lead V2, whereas LV anteroseptal MI is higher in V3 [25,45].

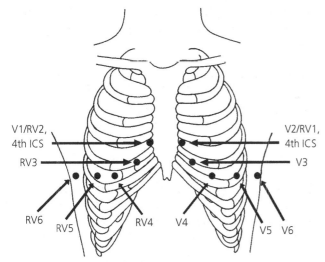

Figure 18.4 Standard and right-sided lead orientation. The right-sided leads are a mirror image of the standard leads. V1–V2/RV1–RV2 positioned in the fourth intercostal space (ICS) lateral to the sternum, V4–V6 and RV4–RV6 are positioned in the fifth ICS in the same horizontal plane. The V4/RV4 lead at the midclavicular line, V5/RV5 lead at the anterior axillary line, and V6/RV6 at the midaxillary line.

Right-sided lead orientation and diagnostic criterion

The right-sided leads are identified as V1R through V6R and are positioned across the anterior chest wall in a mirror image to the standard precordial leads (Figure 18.4). Findings on the right-sided ECG in RVMI include STE in leads V2R–V6R. V4R has been shown to provide the best single lead evidence for RVMI [43,46–49]. ST elevation ≥ 1 mm in V4R demonstrates sensitivity and specificity for diagnosis of RVMI of 90–100% and 68–95%, respectively [47–49]. The sensitivity and specificity of STE in V4R decreases in the setting of a concomitant posterior LV STEMI [50]. V4R is oriented opposite the posterior wall in the horizontal plane, and the ST segment vectors resulting from infarction of the thicker posterior left ventricle will dominate those of a RVMI and be more likely to result in a prominent R wave and flat or depressed ST segment in the right-sided leads [50].

Electrocardiographic body-surface mapping

Multi-lead body-surface mapping (BSM) uses multiple extra ECG leads applied to the anterior and posterior chest in order to achieve complete visualization of the epicardium. The number of leads varied in different studies from as few as 16 to as many as 500 or more. With computer processing, the information from multiple lead-systems is used to establish color maps that can be further analyzed to enhance the diagnosis of a variety of cardiac conditions. The potential uses of the technology include higher diagnostic yield in acute and old MI, as well as in transient ischemia and a variety of arrhythmias.

Body-surface mapping provides output tracings of all leads and also of four separate body maps, both posterior and anterior, of the "isointegrals" of the QRS, the ST-T complex, and the "isopotentials" of the ST segment at the J point (ST0), and the ST segment at 60 ms after the J point (ST60) (see Figure 18.5). Isointegrals measure voltage over a period of time and, therefore, in mV-ms; thus, the isointegral is the area under the curve. In contrast, isopotentials are the voltage at one point in time, using mV or mm units; the T-P segment is the isoelectric line. "QRS isointegral" is the area under the curve for the QRS complex and represents the ventricular depolarization. On the QRS color map, green represents an isoelectric point where the summation of the deflections of the QRS complex is neutral (R = Q + S). ST-T isointegral is the area under the ST segment and T wave representing the ventricular repolarization. The lead with the greatest (+) deflection on BSM is called the maxima. Conversely, the minima is the lead with greatest (−) deflection. The maxima and minima are variables of the electrical force direction and of the amount at a certain point (isopotential) or over an interval (isointegral).

Yellow/orange/red is increasingly positive voltage, green isoelectric, and light to dark blue increasingly negative voltage. Thus, red on the QRS, ST, and ST-T maps shows the location of the predominance of positive voltage of each of these phases of the QRS. Hyperacute T waves are seen as deep red, and red on the ST-T map > red on the ST map also indicates hyperacute T waves. A combination of red on the QRS map and blue on the ST-T map indicates T wave inversion (T axis opposite QRS axis).

A major motivation for researchers has been to increase the accuracy of diagnosing acute MI in patients who present with a non-diagnostic ECG. In fact, multi-lead BSM has been shown to increase the sensitivity for detecting acute MI compared with 12-lead ECG in a variety of clinical presentations including patients with ST segment depression [51–56].

McMechan and colleagues developed a regression algorithm that achieved a specificity of 100% and sensitivity of 96.6% for detecting acute MI [54]. In the setting of inferior MI, Menown and colleagues found that BSM was superior to the 12-lead ECG in diagnosing right ventricle and posterior wall infarction, even with the use of the additional leads V2R–V4R and V7–V9 [55]. Body-surface mapping has also been helpful in differentiating chest pain with newly diagnosed left bundle branch block (LBBB) [57]. Pure LBBB has a special pattern of depolarization-repolarization on BSM that is lost in the presence of acute MI in the standard 12-lead ECG [58,59].

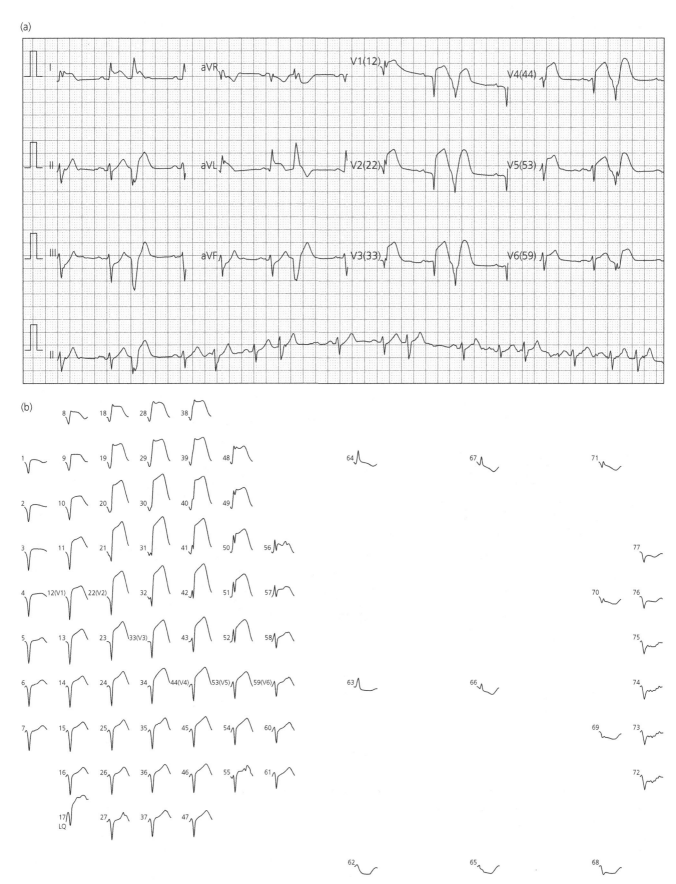

Figure 18.5 Body-surface mapping of large anterior MI. (a) Twelve-lead ECG reveals widespread STE in the precordial leads and I and aVL. (b) Similarly, 80-lead ECG shows widespread STE in the anterior and left lateral leads (with the ST0, STT, and ST60 maps showing deep red on the map in the anterior precordial region. The QRS map is also red in this region because the QRS axis is also anterior. All maps are blue posteriorly, as all vectors [QRS, ST, and STT] are away from the posterior leads).

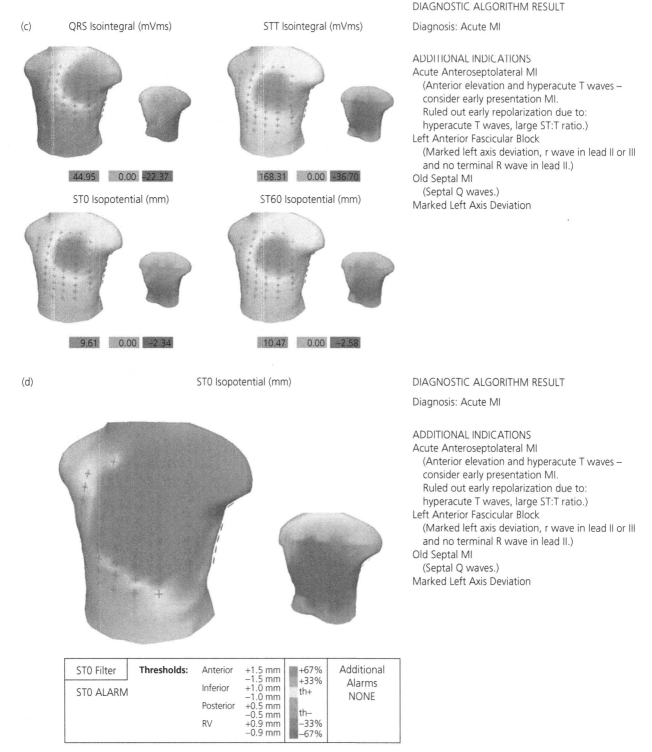

Figure 18.5 *(cont'd)* (c) ST0 and ST60 isopotential maps show a large area of STE on the anterior surface and ST depression on the posterior surface. (d) The anterior STE and posterior ST depression are > 1.5 mm and a 0.5 mm threshold, respectively, resulting in deep colors. Reprinted with permission from Elsevier, Self WH, *et al. Am J Emerg Med* 2006;**24**:87–112 [58].

The technology has not been utilized in the practice of medicine for reasons related to the size of equipment, complexity of ECG analysis, the complexity of map analysis, and the time-effectiveness of the technology in real-life situations. Moreover, the superior diagnostic and prognostic value of BSM has not been tested in large randomized therapeutic studies in cardiology, which limits the clinical impact of the technology. Nevertheless, interest in this application has been renewed, in part, as a result of the development of smaller mobile equipment and the rapid application of the leads using a plastic harness [53,60]. These systems allow for acquisition of a 12-lead ECG, as well as BSM, early in the setting of chest pain, within the 10-min time limit recommended by present guidelines [39,56,60,61]. In addition, automated algorithms have been developed that allow fast interpretation of the maps with superior sensitivity in detecting acute MI compared with a physician's interpretation of 12-lead ECG [53].

Conclusion

The number of leads in a standard ECG has remained virtually unchanged for over 50 years. The role of an expanded lead set that ranges from the addition of posterior and right-sided leads, to more extensive body-surface maps, is still open to interpretation. The routine use of extended leads is not recommended and should be reserved for those patients with evidence for ACS on a standard 12-lead ECG to assess for right ventricular infarction, or in situations where additional leads may change a patient's diagnosis from AMI with ST depression to STEMI and, thereby, indicate qualification for reperfusion strategies. In cases of high clinical suspicion for ACS and a non-specific ECG, additional leads may also be of benefit.

Case conclusions

In addition to the usual medications for an acute STEMI, a fibrinolytic agent was administered to the patient in Case 1. The patient arrived at the referral center pain-free and with resolution of STE and ST depression, consistent with reperfusion. Subsequent angiography revealed a culprit lesion in the proximal circumflex, with TIMI-3 flow. This was stented. Based on the initial ECG in Case 2, the cardiac catheterization team was activated. En route, the patient developed ventricular fibrillation; he was resuscitated with a single countershock. Subsequent dysrhythmias required treatment with amiodarone. Angiogram demonstrated right side-dominant circulation with a severe mid-right coronary artery (RCA) occlusion, proximal to the RV marginal branch; it was successfully stented. A temporary transvenous pacemaker was placed to manage the patient's third-degree heart block.

References

1 Zalenski RJ, Cooke D, Rydman R, et al. Assessing the diagnostic value of an ECG containing leads V4R, V8, and V9: the 15-lead ECG. Ann Emerg Med 1993;**22**:786–93.
2 Zimetbaum PJ, Josephson ME. Use of the electrocardiogram in acute myocardial infarction. N Engl J Med 2003;**348**:933–40.
3 Fesmire FM, Percy RF, Bardoner JB, et al. Usefulness of automated serial 12-lead ECG monitoring during the initial emergency department evaluation of patients with chest pain. Ann Emerg Med 1998;**31**:3–11.
4 Fesmire FM, Percy RF, Wears RL, MacMath TL. Initial ECG in Q wave and non-Q wave myocardial infarction. Ann Emerg Med 1989;**18**:741–6.
5 Rouan GW, Lee TH, Cook EF, et al. Clinical characteristics and outcome of acute myocardial infarction in patients with initially normal or nonspecific electrocardiograms (a report from the Multicenter Chest Pain Study). Am J Cardiol 1989;**64**:1087–92.
6 Rude RE, Poole WK, Muller J, et al. Electrocardiographic and clinical criteria for recognition of acute myocardial infarction based on analysis of 3,697 patients. Am J Cardiol 1983;**52**:936–42.
7 Martin TN, Groenning BA, Murray HM, et al. ST-segment deviation analysis of the admission 12-lead electrocardiogram as an aid to early diagnosis of acute myocardial infarction with a cardiac magnetic resonance imaging gold standard. J Am Coll Cardiol 2007;**50**:1021–8.
8 Zalenski RJ, Rydman RJ, Sloan EP, et al. Value of posterior and right ventricular leads in comparison to the standard 12-lead electrocardiogram in evaluation of ST-segment elevation in suspected acute myocardial infarction. Am J Cardiol 1997;**79**:1579–85.
9 Agarwal JB. Routine use of a 15-lead electrocardiogram for patients presenting to the emergency department with chest pain. J Electrocardiol 1998;**31**(Suppl):172–7.
10 Agarwal JB, Khaw K, Aurignac F, LoCurto A. Importance of posterior chest leads in patients with suspected myocardial infarction, but nondiagnostic, routine 12-lead electrogram. Am J Cardiol 1999;**83**:323–6.
11 Matetzky S, Friemark D, Feinberg MS, et al. Acute myocardial infarction with isolated ST-segment elevation in posterior chest leads V7–V9: "hidden" ST-segment elevations revealing acute posterior infarction. J Am Coll Cardiol 1999;**34**:748–53.
12 Matetzky S, Freimark D, Chouraqui P, et al. Significance of ST segment elevations in posterior chest leads (V7–V9) in patients with acute inferior myocardial infarction: application for thrombolytic therapy. J Am Coll Cardiol 1998;**31**:506–11.
13 Schmitt C, Lehmann G, Schmieder S, et al. Diagnosis of acute myocardial infarction in angiographically documented occluded infarct vessel: limitations of ST-segment elevation in standard and extended ECG leads. Chest 2001;**120**:1540–6.
14 Ganim RP, Lewis WR, Diercks DB, et al. Right precordial and posterior electrocardiographic leads do not increase detection of ischemia in low-risk patients presenting with chest pain. Cardiology 2004;**102**:100–3.
15 Brady WJ, Hwang V, Sullivan R. A comparison of 12- and 15-lead ECGs in ED chest pain patients: impact on diagnosis, therapy, and disposition. Am J Emerg Med 2000;**18**:239–43.
16 Kligfield P, Gettes LS, Bailey JJ, et al. Recommendations for the Standardization and Interpretation of the Electrocardiogram: Part I: The Electrocardiogram and Its Technology: A Scientific Statement From the American Heart Association Electrocardiography

and Arrhythmias Committee, Council on Clinical Cardiology; the American College of Cardiology Foundation; and the Heart Rhythm Society Endorsed by the International Society for Computerized Electrocardiology. *Circulation* 2007;**115**:1306–24.

17 Thygesen K, Alpert JS, White HD, *et al.* Universal definition of myocardial infarction. *Circulation* 2007;**116**:2634–53.

18 Brady WJ, Erling B, Pollack M, Chan TC. Electrocardiographic manifestations: Acute posterior wall myocardial infarction. *J Emerg Med* 2001;**20**:391–401.

19 O'Keefe JHJ, Sayed-Taha K, Gibson W, *et al.* Do patients with left circumflex coronary artery-related acute myocardial infarction without ST-segment elevation benefit from reperfusion therapy? (see comments). *Am J Cardiol* 1995;**75**:718–20.

20 Oraii S, Maleki I, Tavakolian AA, *et al.* Prevalence and outcome of ST-segment elevation in posterior electrocardiographic leads during acute myocardial infarction. *J Electrocardiol* 1999;**32**:275–8.

21 Roul G, Bareiss P, Germain P, *et al.* Isolated ST segment depression from V2 to V4 leads, an early electrocardiographic sign of posterior myocardial infarction. *Arch Mal Coeur Vaiss* 1991;**84**:1815–9.

22 Petrovici R, Emmett L, Lee DS, *et al.* Electrocardiographic prediction of the severity of posterior wall perfusion defects on rest technetium-99m Sestamibi myocardial perfusion imaging. *J Electrocardiol* 2005;**38**:195–203.

23 Gibson RS, Crampton RS, Watson DD, *et al.* Precordial ST-segment depression during acute inferior myocardial infarction: clinical, scintigraphic and angiographic correlations. *Circulation* 1982;**66**:732–41.

24 Goldberg HL, Borer JS, Jacobstein JG, *et al.* Anterior S-T segment depression in acute inferior myocardial infarction: indicator of posterolateral infarction. *Am J Cardiol* 1981;**48**:1009–15.

25 Smith SW, Zvosec DL, Henry TD, Sharkey SW. The ECG in Acute MI: an Evidence-Based Manual of Reperfusion Therapy. Philadelphia: Lippincott, Williams, and Wilkins, 2002:358.

26 Wong CK, Freedman SB. Usefulness of continuous ST monitoring in inferior wall acute myocardial infarction for describing the relation between precordial ST depression and inferior ST elevation. *Am J Cardiol* 1993;**72**:532–7.

27 Wung SF, Drew BJ. New electrocardiographic criteria for posterior wall acute myocardial ischemia validated by a percutaneous transluminal coronary angioplasty model of acute myocardial infarction. *Am J Cardiol* 2001;**87**:970–4; A4.

28 Berry C, Zalewsky A, Kovach R, *et al.* Surface electrocardiogram in the detection of transmural myocardial ischemia during coronary artery occlusion. *Am J Cardiol* 1989;**63**:21–6.

29 Shah A, Wagner GS, Green CL, *et al.* Electrocardiographic differentiation of the ST-segment depression of acute myocardial injury due to the left circumflex artery occlusion from that of myocardial ischemia of nonocclusive etiologies. *Am J Cardiol* 1997;**80**:512–3.

30 Veldkamp RF, Sawchak S, Pope JE, *et al.* Performance of an automated real-time ST segment analysis program to detect coronary occlusion and reperfusion. *J Electrocardiol* 1996;**29**:257–63.

31 Birnbaum Y, Herz I, Sclarovsky S, *et al.* Prognostic significance of precordial ST segment depression on admission electrocardiogram in patients with inferior wall myocardial infarction. *J Am Coll Cardiol* 1996;**28**:313–8.

32 Peterson ED, Hathaway WR, Zabel KM, *et al.* Prognostic significance of precordial ST segment depression during inferior myocardial infarction in the thrombolytic era: results in 16,521 patients. *J Am Coll Cardiol* 1996;**28**:305–12.

33 Wong CK, Freedman SB, Bautovich G, *et al.* Mechanism and significance of precordial ST-segment depression during inferior wall acute myocardial infarction associated with severe narrowing of the dominant right coronary artery. *Am J Cardiol* 1993;**71**:1025–30.

34 Somers MP, Brady WJ, Bateman DC, *et al.* Additional electrocardiographic leads in the ED chest pain patient: right ventricular and posterior leads. *Am J Emerg Med* 2003;**21**:563–73.

35 Taha B, Reddy S, Agarwal J, Khaw K. Normal limits of ST segment measurements in posterior ECG leads. *J Electrocardiol* 1998;**31**(Suppl):178–9.

36 Andersen HR, Falk E, Nielsen D. Right ventricular infarction: frequency, size and topography in coronary heart disease: a prospective study comprising 107 consecutive autopsies from a coronary care unit. *J Am Coll Cardiol* 1987;**10**:1223–32.

37 Andersen HR, Falk E, Nielsen D. Right ventricular infarction: diagnostic accuracy of electrocardiographic right chest leads V3R to V7R investigated prospectively in 43 consecutive fatal cases from a coronary care unit. *Br Heart J* 1989;**61**:514–20.

38 Kinch JW, Ryan TJ. Right ventricular infarction. [see comment]. *New Engl J Med* 1994;**330**:1211–7.

39 Antman EM, Anbe DT, Armstrong PW, *et al.* ACC/AHA guidelines for the management of patients with ST-elevation myocardial infarction – executive summary. A report of the American College of Cardiology/American Heart Association Task Force on Practice Guidelines (Writing Committee to revise the 1999 guidelines for the management of patients with acute myocardial infarction). *J Am Coll Cardiol* 2004;**44**:671–719.

40 Mehta SR, Eikelboom JW, Natarajan MK, *et al.* Impact of right ventricular involvement on mortality and morbidity in patients with inferior myocardial infarction. *J Am Coll Cardiol* 2001;**37**:37–43.

41 Braat SH, Brugada P, De Zwaan C, *et al.* Right and left ventricular ejection fraction in acute inferior wall infarction with or without ST segment elevation in lead V4R. *J Am Coll Cardiol* 1984;**4**:940–4.

42 Braat SH, de Zwaan C, Brugada P, *et al.* Right ventricular involvement with acute inferior wall myocardial infarction identifies high risk of developing atrioventricular nodal conduction disturbances. *Am Heart J* 1984;**107**:1183–7.

43 Zehender M, Kasper W, Schonthaler M, *et al.* Right ventricular infarction as an independent predictor of prognosis after acute inferior myocardial infarction. *N Engl J Med* 1993;**328**:981–8.

44 Haji SA, Movahed A. Right ventricular infarction – diagnosis and treatment. *Clin Cardiol* 2000;**23**:473–82.

45 Smith SW, Whitwam W. Acute coronary syndromes. *Emerg Med Clin North Am* 2006;**24**:53–89.

46 Robalino BD, Whitlow PL, Underwood DA, Salcedo EE. Electrocardiographic manifestations of right ventricular infarction. *Am Heart J* 1989;**118**:138–44.

47 Braat SH, Brugada P, de Zwaan C, *et al.* Value of electrocardiogram in diagnosing right ventricular involvement in patients with an acute inferior wall myocardial infarction. *Br Heart J* 1983;**49**:368–72.

48 Lopez-Sendon J, Coma-Canella I, Alcasena S, *et al.* Electrocardiographic findings in acute right ventricular infarction: sensitivity and specificity of electrocardiographic alterations in right precordial leads V4R, V3R, V1, V2, and V3. *J Am Coll Cardiol* 1985;**6**:1273–9.

49 Croft CH, Nicod P, Corbett JR, *et al.* Detection of acute right ventricular infarction by right precordial electrocardiography. *Am J Cardiol* 1982;**50**:421–7.

50 Mittal SR, Jain S. Electrocardiographic diagnosis of right ventricular infarction in the presence of left ventricular posterior infarction. *Int J Cardiol* 1999;**68**:125–8.

51 Menown IB, Allen J, Anderson JM, Adgey AA. Early diagnosis of right ventricular or posterior infarction associated with inferior wall left ventricular acute myocardial infarction. *Am J Cardiol* 2000;**85**:934–8.

52 Kornreich F, Montague TJ, Rautaharju PM. Body surface potential mapping of ST segment changes in acute myocardial infarction. Implications for ECG enrollment criteria for thrombolytic therapy. *Circulation* 1993;**87**:773–82.

53 McClelland AJ, Owens CG, Menown IB, *et al.* Comparison of the 80-lead body surface map to physician and to 12-lead electrocardiogram in detection of acute myocardial infarction. *Am J Cardiol* 2003;**92**:252–7.

54 McMechan SR, MacKenzie G, Allen J, *et al.* Body surface ECG potential maps in acute myocardial infarction. *J Electrocardiol* 1995;**28**(Suppl):184–90.

55 Menown IB, Allen J, Anderson JM, Adgey AA. ST depression only on the initial 12-lead ECG: early diagnosis of acute myocardial infarction. *Eur Heart J* 2001;**22**:218–27.

56 Menown IB, Patterson RS, MacKenzie G, Adgey AA. Body-surface map models for early diagnosis of acute myocardial infarction. *J Electrocardiol* 1998;**31**(Suppl):180–8.

57 Maynard SJ, Menown IB, Manoharan G, *et al.* Body surface mapping improves early diagnosis of acute myocardial infarction in patients with chest pain and left bundle branch block. *Heart* 2003;**89**:998–1002.

58 Self WH, Mattu A, Martin M, *et al.* Body surface mapping in the ED evaluation of the patient with chest pain: use of the 80-lead electrocardiogram system. *Am J Emerg Med* 2006;**24**:87–112.

59 Stilli D, Musso E, Macchi E, *et al.* Diagnostic value of body surface maps in left bundle-branch block. *Adv Cardiol* 1981;**28**:36–41.

60 McMechan SR, Cullen CM, MacKenzie G, *et al.* Discriminant function analysis of body surface potential maps in acute myocardial infarction. *J Electrocardiol* 1994;**27**(Suppl):117–20.

61 Fox TR, Burton JH, Strout TD, *et al.* Time to body surface map acquisition compared with ED 12-lead and right-sided ECG. *Am J Emerg Med* 2003;**21**:164–5.

Chapter 19 | What further diagnostic adjuncts to the standard 12-lead ECG may help to diagnose ACS?

Mark D. Connelly[1], Joel S. Holger[1], Stefan C. Bertog[2], Stephen W. Smith[3]
[1]Regions Hospital, St Paul, MN, USA
[2]Veterans Administration Medical Center, and University of Minnesota, Minneapolis, MN, USA
[3]University of Minnesota, Hennepin County Medical Center, Minneapolis, MN, USA

Case presentations

Case 1: A 45-year-old woman presents to the emergency department (ED) immediately after resolution of 3 h of atypical chest pain, associated with anxiety and diaphoresis, but no dyspnea, nausea, or vomiting. She has no other medical history. Vital signs are unremarkable. The electrocardiogram (ECG) reveals suggestive but non-diagnostic terminal T wave inversion in lead V2 only (Figure 19.1, V1–V3 only, remainder of ECG normal).

Case 2: A 44-year-old male presents with sharp and pleuritic chest pain. Vital signs and exam are normal. The ECG in Figure 19.2 is recorded.

Case 3: A 64-year-old male presents with syncope after taking tamsulosin, an alpha-blocker, for urinary retention; there was no chest pain or dyspnea. The exam is normal. The ECGs in Figure 19.3a and b are recorded.

Adjunctive modalities in the diagnosis of ACS

Because of non-diagnostic ST elevation (STE), or pseudo-infarction patterns, or QRS abnormalities that obscure the ST segment and T wave analysis, coronary occlusion can be difficult to assess using symptoms, exam, and an initial ECG alone.

Previous ECG comparison and serial ECG monitoring

Diagnosis of ischemia is more accurate if a prior ECG is available for comparison [1]. Changes may be subtle or obvious. In patients with symptoms of acute coronary syndrome (ACS), non-diagnostic ST segment and T wave abnormalities are associated with a higher probability of ACS if changed from a previous ECG [1,2], and patients with ACS who have a changed ECG are at higher risk of adverse outcomes if the ECG is changed [2]. Moreover, the probability that STE is a result of coronary occlusion, rather than a pseudo-infarction pattern such as early repolarization, is much higher if the STE is increased from a previous tracing.

Additionally, repeat ECG tracings, as frequently as every 15–20 min in patients at high risk with ongoing symptoms, may become diagnostic (see Chapter 20). In lower risk patients, a repeat ECG every 3–4 h, or at any time with a change in symptoms, may show evolving changes not initially apparent on the first ECG [3]. Serial 12-lead ECG monitoring (SECG) uses computer-processed data from ST segments on repeated 12-lead ECGs (typically measured 60 ms after the J point), and plots the amplitude of the ST segment against time to detect changes from the baseline ECG. Serial 12-lead ECG monitoring is more sensitive than an initial ECG for detection of acute myocardial infarction (AMI) (68.1% versus 55.4%) and of ACS (34.2% versus 27.5%), and SECG was more specific for detection of ACS (99.4% versus 97.1%) [4]. See Figure 25.1.

Cardiac biomarkers

Myocardial cell damage results in the release into the blood of cardiac proteins that are used as markers of damage ("biomarkers"). The most important biomarkers are cardiac troponin (cTn) I and T because they have absolute myocardial

Critical Decisions in Emergency and Acute Care Electrocardiography,
1st edition. Edited by W.J. Brady and J.D. Truwit. © 2009 Blackwell Publishing, ISBN: 9781405159067.

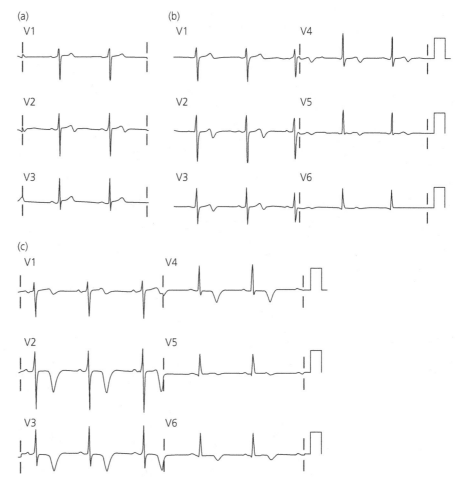

Figure 19.1 Case 1. (a) t = 0: (V1–V3 only) shows minimal T wave inversion only in V2, with a suggestion in V1 (possible Wellens' syndrome, needing confirmation by comparison with old ECG [which was normal] and/or by serial ECGs). (b) t = 2 h: biphasic T waves extend out to V5, confirming Wellens' (pattern A) syndrome. (c) t = 9 h: T waves have evolved still further and are symmetrically inverted (Wellens' pattern B). Reprinted with permission from Smith SW. Acute Coronary Syndromes. *Emerg Med Clin N Am* 2006;**24**(1):53–89.

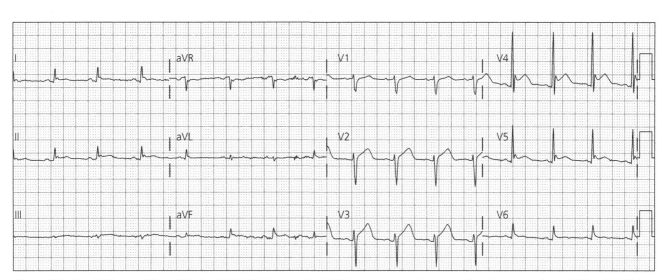

Figure 19.2 Case 2. There is diffuse STE in leads V2–V6, II, I, and aVF > III (ST vector anterior, left, and, inferior) and no reciprocal STD in aVL. ECG (and symptoms) are highly suggestive of pericarditis, but inferolateral MI is possible.

specificity and very high sensitivity for cell damage. Elevated biomarkers are part of the definition of MI; however, they do not reflect the etiology of myocardial damage, which may or may not be due to ACS. There are four new diagnostic categories for acute MI; the most relevant to the present discussion requires a rising and falling pattern of biomarkers cTnI or T (cTnI or cTnT) or, less preferably, the enzyme CK-MB, accompanied by one of the following: symptoms of ischemia, typical ECG changes, development of pathologic Q waves, or imaging evidence of new loss of viable myocardium [5].

(a)

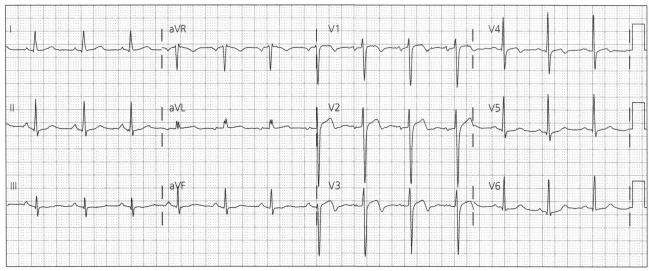

(b)

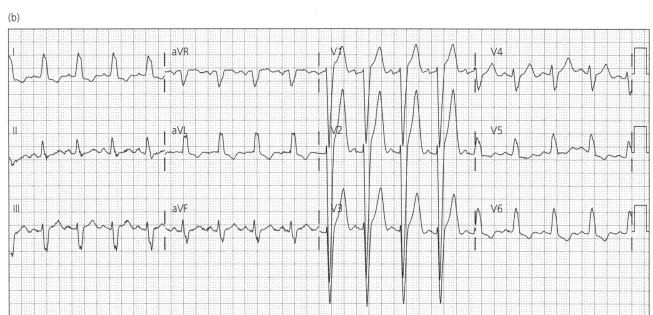

Figure 19.3 Case 3. (a) There is LVH voltage; there is T wave inversion in V2–V4, suggestive of Wellens' syndrome. (b) This repeat ECG was recorded 1 h later, and shows faster heart rate (100) with LBBB and no specific indicators of MI (see Chapter 21). This turned out to be a rate-dependent LBBB; there was no ischemia.

Cardiac Tn should not be detected in the blood of normal subjects; therefore, any value above the specific assay's upper limit of performance characteristics (above the 99th percentile reference control group) is abnormal. Assays have different sensitivity and precision; in one study, no assay was able to achieve the 10% imprecision recommendation at the 99th percentile reference limit defined by its manufacturer [6]. It is important to choose the right cTnI assay and for the physician to know his/her assay's analytical characteristics (see Case 1, Chapter 14 for the consequences of ignorance). An elevated cTn without clinical evidence of ACS should lead to other etiologies of necrosis such as myocarditis, aortic

dissection, congestive heart failure (CHF), renal failure, pulmonary embolism, or septic shock [5].

Cardiac biomarkers have characteristic release and clearance features after damage; they are typically measurable in the blood within 4 to 6 h of MI and remain elevated for 4–10 days. This is due to prolonged release, not to long half-life, which is roughly half an hour. CK-MB has a similar initial release pattern but may normalize within 24 h. Early measurements of cardiac biomarkers are not sensitive enough to rule out early ST elevation myocardial infarction (STEMI). Thus, the diagnosis of STEMI (acute decrease in epicardial coronary flow that imminently threatens significant myocardial territory) relies on the ECG. Patients at risk for ACS should have a level determined initially and repeat levels performed at least every 4 h over the next 6–9 h. These may need to be repeated at 12–24 h if they are negative and the clinical suspicion remains high. Change in biomarker level over just 90 min improves diagnostic sensitivity and specificity [7].

Studies published before 2000 refer to conditions with minimal elevations of biomarkers as consistent with ischemia or unstable angina; now, in contrast, any elevated cTn is, by definition, MI (not unstable angina). A minimal cTn elevation does not signify a large MI; however, it is a marker for an unstable thrombogenic coronary plaque that is at risk for later, larger infarct. Initial biomarker levels are directly correlated with mortality [8,9], as are serially positive markers [10]. In one study, cTnT was serially measured in 734 patients with ischemic symptoms and transient STE or ST depression. Mortality at 30 days was 10% in baseline-positive patients, 5% in patients positive only at hour 8 or 16, and 0% in TnI-negative patients. Cardiogenic shock and CHF occurred most often in baseline-positive patients and least often in cTnT-negative patients [10]. Biomarker positivity is also correlated with benefit from such therapies as GPIIb-IIIa inhibitors and early invasive management [11].

Emergent reperfusion therapy is based on the ECG, not on cTn. However, cTn may help to clarify the interpretation of a difficult ECG, one that could represent either STEMI or pseudo-infarction. It may also help to clarify ECGs with borderline STE. Angiogram and percutaneous coronary intervention (PCI) within 48 h will be necessary for most patients with a positive cTn (STEMI and NSTEMI), but is only immediately necessary in those with the ECG findings of a STEMI, indicating complete and persistent occlusion. ST elevation myocardial infarction does have higher peak cTn levels than NSTEMI (though this has never been formally documented), but the initial cTn, if positive, is not necessarily higher and does not help in differentiating STEMI from NSTEMI. Faced with STEMI versus pseudo-infarction, an even minimally elevated cTn is strong evidence that the ECG represents coronary occlusion and is a very good reason for emergent angiogram and possible PCI. Conversely, with an ECG clearly positive for STEMI, negative biomarkers are meaningless.

ECG adjuncts in left bundle branch block

In the presence of left bundle branch block (LBBB), serial ECGs, and comparison with a previous ECG, can increase the sensitivity for STEMI over a baseline ECG (Figure 19.4) [12,13]. Wackers found that serial ECG changes were observed in 67% of patients with a LBBB and AMI. Change in STE was 54% sensitive and 97% specific for AMI [14]. Stark and colleagues found that a change in the ST segments of 1 mm was 80% sensitive for angiographic balloon occlusion in LBBB

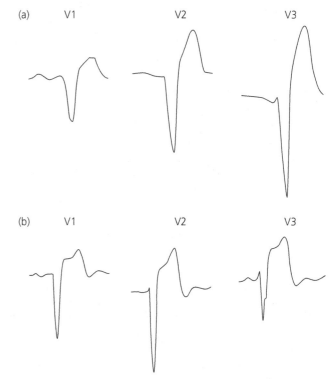

Figure 19.4 Serial ECG changes in patients with LBBB and LAD occlusion. (a) Initial recording of leads V1–V3; this is very suggestive of LAD occlusion because the ST/S ratio > 0.25. (b) Same leads recorded 2 h later confirm evolution of anterior MI. Reprinted with permission from Edhouse JA, *et al.* Suspected myocardial infarction and left bundle branch block: electrocardiographic indicators of acute ischaemia. *J Accid Emerg Med* 1999;**16**:331–5.

(mean delta ST was 2.7 mm) and 75% sensitive in those with normal conduction, supporting the notion that the ECG may be just as sensitive for STEMI in the presence of LBBB as in normal conduction [13].

Additional ECG leads

The addition of right-sided or posterior leads to the standard 12-lead ECG improves the sensitivity for STEMI, but their routine use in all chest pain patients has a low yield [15]. Isolated right ventricular MI (RVMI) is rare without concurrent inferior MI; if there is no ECG evidence of old or new inferior MI, a right-sided ECG will only rarely reveal acute RVMI. Therefore, its routine use is not recommended. Isolated posterior MI, without STE in inferior or lateral leads, is more common, estimated in approximately 3.3–8.5% of patients with AMI (see Chapters 8 and 22) [11,12]. Therefore, when there is high suspicion, and certainly when there is anterior ST depression, posterior leads are very useful. ST elevation of only 0.5 mm in leads V7–V9 is very sensitive and specific for posterior MI [16–18]. See Figure 19.5 of posterior MI

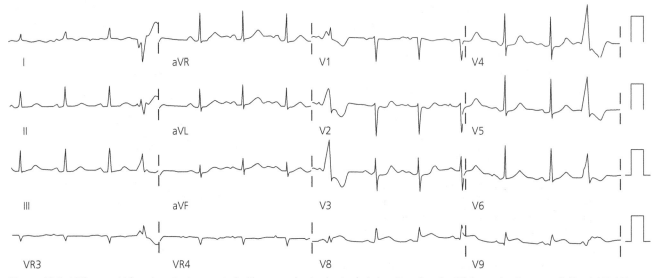

Figure 19.5 A 79-year-old female patient presented with severe chest pain at admission. Based on the ST depression in precordial leads V1–V4, the patient was diagnosed as having "anterior subendocardial ischemia." Cardiac enzyme tests showed elevated TnT (3.2) and CK-MB (135). ST elevation in leads V8 and V9 demonstrates posterior STEMI. Reprinted with permission from Zhou SH *et al. Comput Cardiol* 2006;**33**:33–6 [18].

diagnosed with posterior leads V8 and V9 (see also Figure 18.1). See Figure 8.2 for RVMI diagnosed with right-sided leads.

Non-invasive imaging

Non-invasive imaging modalities that evaluate for tissue perfusion, myocyte viability, myocardial thickening, and wall motion abnormalities, may aid the clinician in patients with suspected myocardial ischemia. These include echocardiography, radionuclide ventriculography, magnetic resonance imaging (MRI), and myocardial perfusion scintigraphy. Other, less common, imaging techniques are positron emission tomography (PET) and x-ray computed tomography (CT) [5].

The most important role of acute echocardiography or radionuclide imaging is in patients with a high degree of suspicion for AMI but a non-diagnostic ECG. A normal transthoracic echocardiogram or resting ECG-gated scintigram has a 95–98% negative predictive value for excluding acute MI of a large myocardial territory [5,19–21]. Immediate cardiac ultrasound is very useful in the setting of suspected STEMI with an equivocal ECG or clinical presentation. Additionally, these modalities may help in the diagnosis of unstable angina (non-diagnostic ECG and negative biomarkers) or if the etiology of positive cTn is uncertain (is it due to ACS or other?) [22,23].

Echocardiography

Echocardiography (echo) can be useful in ACS, especially in patients with non-specific or subtle ST-T changes suggestive of ischemia, or pseudoinfarction patterns, LBBB, and pacemakers. Regional wall motion abnormalities (RWMA) in the setting of acute chest pain can represent active ischemia, acute MI, or areas of previous MI.

Echo may confirm the diagnosis in cases where the ECG is non-diagnostic or subtle. For example, echo would have been very useful in Case 3, Chapter 22, in which subtle STE of anterior MI was missed, and also in cases of missed STEMI associated with Figures 16.3 and 16.6 (also subtle anterior MI).

Echo may also show an alternative diagnosis when there is ambiguity about the ECG diagnosis and the need for immediate reperfusion: examples include demonstration of a pericardial effusion in pericarditis (see Case 2, Figure 19.2), demonstration of a large right ventricle in pulmonary embolism (see Figure 15.5), or demonstration of posterior RWMA, distinguishing precordial ST depression due to subendocardial ischemia from that of posterior transmural ischemia (an indication for immediate reperfusion, see Figure 15.10). Echo is less useful when symptoms have resolved or in patients with wall motion abnormalities that may be pre-existing; in the latter case, old MI can often be differentiated from acute MI by the presence of wall thinning or diastolic dysfunction (dyskinesis). Also, echo is the test of choice for evaluating complications of MIs such as ventricular septal defect, ventricular free wall rupture, or acute papillary muscle rupture.

In patients at low risk for coronary occlusion who do not need immediate reperfusion, RWMA may remain after resolution of ischemia (stunned myocardium) and help in the diagnosis of non-STEMI ACS. Regional wall motion abnormality is more likely to be present if the study can be obtained during symptoms or shortly thereafter. Cheitlin and colleagues state that the absence of segmental wall motion abnormalities has a negative predictive value as high as 98% for MI, with moderate specificity (66%) [24].

Echo can also be used to help differentiate other causes of acute chest pain such as peri-myocarditis, aortic dissection, pulmonary embolism, valvular dysfunction, cardiomyopathy, or decompensated CHF [5]. Echocardiographic contrast agents may improve imaging but have not yet been validated for detection of myocardial necrosis [25]. The usefulness of echo in the acute chest pain patient can be seen in Case 2, Figure 19.2.

Finally, cardiac ultrasound can be performed by the treating physician at the bedside. However, subtle wall motion abnormality requires excellent technique in image acquisition and a very experienced interpreter.

Myocardial perfusion imaging

Myocardial perfusion imaging has no role in the decision for immediate reperfusion, but is useful in the diagnosis of ACS (unstable angina) in those with non-diagnostic ECGs ± serial negative biomarkers, or if the etiology of positive cTns is uncertain (ACS versus other critical illness). This imaging modality can be performed in either the resting mode (which may be able to be performed during the ED evaluation) or combined with a stress mode after a "wash-out" period using exercise or a biochemically induced stress phase. Radionuclide tracers, thallium-201, technetium-99m sestamibi, tetrofosmin, and [^{18}F]2-fluorodeoxyglucose (FDG) are taken up intracellularly by normal myocytes, which allows for imaging viable myocardium. Sestamibi is the most commonly used agent. These tracers may readily detect areas of infarction and inducible perfusion abnormalities by comparing stress with rest imaging, although small areas of infarction can be missed [5]. Single photon emission computed tomography (SPECT) with ECG-gated imaging provides an accurate assessment of myocardial motion, thickening, and global function [26].

Resting myocardial perfusion imaging studies have reported sensitivities of 94–100% for the detection of coronary artery disease in chest pain patients [27]. A 2001 review reported sensitivities and specificities for acute MI of 91.5 to 100% and 49.3 to 84.4%, respectively. Sensitivity was 89% and specificity 77% for detection of any ACS [28]. A large multicenter ED study enrolling 2475 patients using rest perfusion scanning in a protocol found a decrease in hospital admission of 10% [23]. In this study, the 30-day risk of an acute MI with a normal resting scan was 0.6%. The most appropriate use for this modality may be in patients deemed low risk, as the negative predictive value is very high with negative resting scans, especially if the tracer is injected during an episode of chest pain. Problems limiting their usefulness include interpretation difficulties of breast shadows and diaphragm interference of assessing the inferior wall of the left ventricle, as well as the need for 24-h technician availability and stocking of radioactive tracer.

Magnetic resonance imaging and computed tomography

Neither CT nor MRI have any role in the emergent reperfusion decision. Either or both may be useful in the diagnosis of ACS in patients with a non-diagnostic ECG and serial cTns. If there is suspicion that positive cTns are a result of non-ACS pathology, they may confirm absence of coronary disease. Magnetic resonance imaging has recently been validated for the assessment of myocardial function. However, in the acute setting there are two issues: access and acquisition time. Contrast agents with MRI have been validated for detection of chronic MI, but their assessment of myocardial perfusion is not well validated at this time [5]. One ED MRI study evaluated 161 patients with at least 30 min of chest pain and a non-diagnostic ECG within 12 h of symptoms, and found a sensitivity of 84% and a specificity of 84% for ACS [29]. At this time there is no standard protocol for the use of MR angiography, and MR can only image the proximal and mid-segments of the coronary anatomy, limiting its usefulness.

Acute MI on CT will visualize as decreased focal enhancement, eventually progressing to later imaging showing hyper-enhancement similar to contrast MRI [30]. This finding would be incidental during CT scanning to rule out other suspected etiologies of chest pain.

Coronary calcium deposits assessed by electron-beam CT scanning does correlate with atherosclerosis and findings indicate a sensitivity and negative predictive value for coronary artery disease (CAD) > 80% [31]. However, this technique has limitations for non-calcified plaques and active coronary lesions. With advances in multidetector (MD) CT and angiography (CTA), stenosis in proximal and mid-coronary arteries can readily be identified. Angiography has been tested primarily in patients in the elective setting, in which it has shown sensitivity up to 92% and specificity up to 94% in identifying coronary stenosis [32]. Initial studies of CTA in the diagnosis of ACS appear promising. Like magnetic resonance angiography, an accepted protocol for CT in this setting has not been well established.

Coronary angiography

The coronary angiogram, in conjunction with ancillary tools such as intravascular ultrasound, remains the reference standard for diagnosis of ACS and coronary stenosis. Angiography is necessary for any PCI. In the presence of symptoms suggestive of myocardial ischemia and an ECG that suggests significant active transmural or epicardial ischemia (e.g. STE in two contiguous leads, ST depression in the right precordial leads, or hyperacute T waves), coronary angiography is essential if it is immediately available *and* if there are no contraindications to percutaneous and surgical intervention (e.g. severe thrombocytopenia, life-threatening active bleeding, etc.).

There are limitations to angiography. First, the angiogram is a luminogram: one can only interpret the lumen of the vessel and, more importantly, only in limited views. Hence, a potentially flow-limiting coronary stenosis may remain undetected, especially when there is tortuous coronary anatomy, heavy coronary calcification, or overlap of vessels. Second, the mechanism of an acute coronary event is plaque rupture, which can occur in non-flow limiting lesions and is driven by the condition and composition of the vessel wall, which cannot be directly visualized angiographically. Evaluation of the vessel wall requires intravascular ultrasound or optical coherence tomography. Other clues to the presence of ruptured plaque are ulceration, fissure, or dissection, or haziness/filling defect (indicative of thrombus); however, these clues are frequently not present and are imperfect in the identification of a ruptured plaque.

The angiogram has its limitations. In spite of true ACS, the angiogram may not always show occlusion or stenosis. First, there may be dynamic coronary stenosis. This occurs with coronary spasm or with complete thrombotic occlusion and subsequent complete lysis (recanalization) of thrombus. In these cases, absence of occlusion (or of low flow [TIMI 0–2 flow]) does not rule out occlusion and STEMI at the time of the ECG and symptoms; spontaneous reperfusion between the time of the ECG and the angiogram is well known. Fortunately, even in true ACS, the prognosis is generally favorable in the absence of flow-limiting coronary lesions.

Second, in the setting of multiple ruptured plaques, it is frequently not possible to determine the location of the culprit. After successful PCI of the most severe stenosis, largest vessel, or most rewarding lesion, it is essential to remain vigilant for this possibility, as is demonstrated in the case associated with Figures 19.6a–d and 19.7a–d.

Third, angiographers have their limitations. Most experienced angiographers will admit to have missed an occluded coronary artery that was filled by faint collaterals, which they may have seen if they had been more vigilant. Thus, consultation with a second angiographer may improve the accuracy of a difficult angiogram.

Finally, coronary angiography can be used to help rule out ACS in a patient thought to have STEMI. For an example, see Case I and Figure 14.1, Chapter 14. In this case, a patient with chest pain with significant STE that was new compared with a previous ECG was sent for angiography with anticipation of PCI, but the coronaries were normal; the ECG diagnosis was early repolarization.

Summary

Because of non-diagnostic STE, or pseudo-infarction patterns, or QRS abnormalities that obscure the ST segment and T

wave analysis, coronary occlusion can be difficult to assess using an ECG alone. Fortunately, the clinician can compare the ECG with a previous one, perform serial ECGs, do emergency echo, or perform an angiogram to clarify the clinical situation. In less urgent circumstances, the diagnosis of MI is made by biomarkers, and most patients with a diagnosis of MI will undergo angiography to evaluate the need for revascularization. Those patients who are critically ill and have a positive cTn may need further evaluation to determine if the cTn elevation is from pulmonary embolism, sepsis, aortic dissection, etc., or if it is a result of ACS. Patients with ischemic symptoms and non-diagnostic ECG and negative serial cTn may require stress echo, radionuclide stress testing, CT/MR imaging, or angiography to further delineate the etiology of symptoms and rule out life-threatening coronary disease.

Case conclusions

In Case 1, a previous ECG was obtained from 1 year prior, revealing that the subtle T-inversion in V2 was new. Serial ECGs revealed progressive evolution of T wave inversion (Figures 19.1b and c), developing from Wellens' pattern A (Figure 19.1b, terminal, asymmetric inversion) to pattern B (symmetric inversion, Figure 19.1c). This confirmed the diagnosis. At angiogram, a tight LAD stenosis and culprit lesion were found and stented. In Case 2, symptoms and ECG findings (Figure 19.2) were suggestive of pericarditis. An immediate bedside echo performed by the emergency physician showed a moderate pericardial effusion and no wall motion abnormality. A formal echo confirmed this. The patient did well on anti-inflammatory medications. In the patient in Case 3, the initial ECG suggested ischemia, but a previous identical ECG was found. The second ECG, with LBBB, was again worrisome. The patient did not immediately undergo catheterization because of atypical symptoms;

(a)

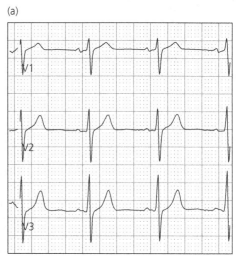

Figure 19.6 Confusing angiography case: ECGs. (a) Baseline, completely normal, ECG (V1–V3 only).

(b)

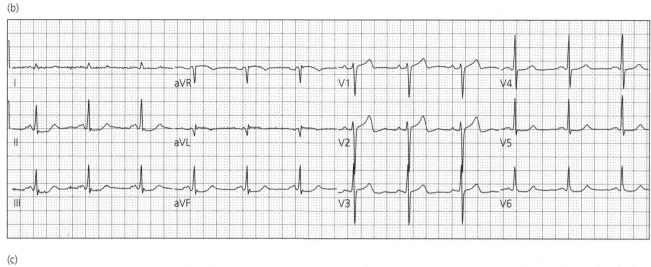

(c)

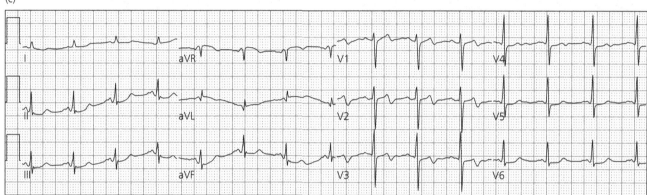

(d)

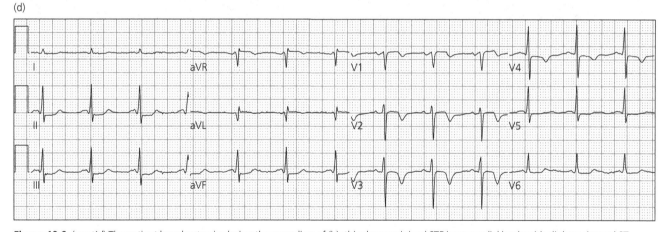

Figure 19.6 (*cont'd*) The patient has chest pain during the recording of (b); this shows minimal STE in precordial leads with slight reciprocal ST depression in inferior leads, suspicious for LAD ischemia. However, immediate angiography showed subtotal occlusion of the RCA (Figure 19.7a) with an open LAD (however, with a hazy appearance, Figure 19.7b). The RCA was thought to be the culprit and it was stented, leaving the LAD for later (Figure 19.7c). The next morning, the patient had chest pain and the ECG in (c) demonstrated Wellens' syndrome, pattern A (biphasic T waves), diagnostic of LAD ACS. Therefore, the LAD lesion was also stented (Figure 19.7d). (d) ECG the day after evolution into Wellens' pattern B (symmetrically inverted T waves).

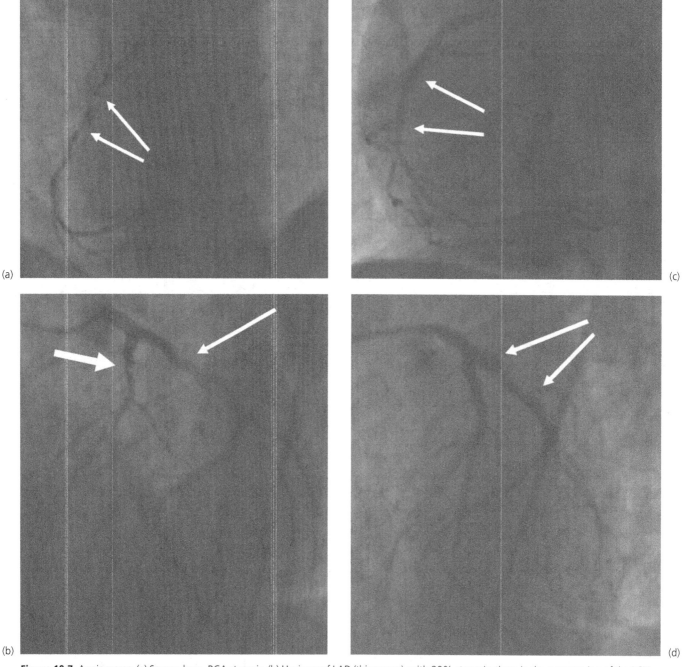

Figure 19.7 Angiograms. (a) Severe, long, RCA stenosis. (b) Haziness of LAD (thin arrow), with 90% stenosis; there is also a narrowing of the LCX (fat arrow). (c) RCA is open after stenting. (d) LAD is open after stenting.

rather, an emergency echo was done which showed concentric left ventricular hypertrophy and no wall motion abnormality. He ruled out by serial cTns and had a negative stress sestamibi. The LBBB pattern was rate-dependent.

References

1 Lee TH, Cook EF, Weisberg MC, *et al*. Impact of the availability of a prior electrocardiogram on the triage of the patient with acute chest pain. *J Gen Intern Med* 1990;**5**:381–8.

2 Fesmire FM, Percy RF, Wears RL. Diagnostic and prognostic importance of comparing the initial to the previous electrocardiogram in patients admitted for suspected acute myocardial infarction. *South Med J* 1991;**84**:841–6.

3 Cannon CP. *Management of Acute Coronary Syndromes*. 2nd Edition. New Jersey: Humana Press, 2003.

4 Fesmire FM, Percy RF, Bardoner JB, *et al*. Usefulness of automated serial 12-lead ECG monitoring during the initial emergency department evaluation of patients with chest pain. *Ann Emerg Med* 1998;**31**:3–11.

5 Thygesen K, Alpert JS, White HD, *et al.* Universal definition of myocardial infarction. *Circulation* 2007;**116**:2634–53.

6 Panteghini M, Pagani F, Yeo KT, *et al.* Evaluation of imprecision for cardiac troponin assays at low-range concentrations. *Clin Chem* 2004;**50**:327–32.

7 McCord J, Nowak RM, McCullough PA, *et al.* Ninety-minute exclusion of acute myocardial infarction by use of quantitative point-of-care testing of myoglobin and troponin I. *Circulation* 2001;**104**:1483–8.

8 Antman EM, Tanasijevic MJ, Thompson B, *et al.* Cardiac-specific troponin I levels to predict the risk of mortality in patients with acute coronary syndromes. *N Engl J Med* 1996;**335**:1342–9.

9 Ohman EM, Armstrong PW, Christenson RH, *et al.* Cardiac troponin T levels for risk stratification in acute myocardial ischemia. *N Engl J Med* 1996;**335**:1333–41.

10 Newby LK, Christenson RH, Ohman EM, *et al.* Value of serial troponin T measures for early and late risk stratification in patients with acute coronary syndromes. The GUSTO-IIA Investigators. *Circulation* 1998;**98**:1853–9.

11 Anderson JL, Adams CD, Antman EM, *et al.* ACC/AHA 2007 Guidelines for the Management of Patients With Unstable Angina/Non ST-Elevation Myocardial Infarction. A Report of the American College of Cardiology/American Heart Association Task Force on Practice Guidelines. *J Am Coll Cardiol* 2007;**50**:1–157.

12 Smith SW, Zvosec DL, Henry TD, Sharkey SW. *The ECG in Acute MI: an Evidence-Based Manual of Reperfusion Therapy.* Philadelphia: Lippincott, Williams, and Wilkins, 2002:358.

13 Stark KS, Krucoff MW, Schryver B, Kent KM. Quantification of ST-segment changes during coronary angioplasty in patients with left bundle branch block. *Am J Cardiol* 1991;**67**:1219–22.

14 Wackers FJ. Complete left bundle branch block: Is the diagnosis of myocardial infarction possible? *Int J Cardiol* 1983;**2**:521–9.

15 Schmitt C, Lehmann G, Schmieder S, *et al.* Diagnosis of acute myocardial infarction in angiographically documented occluded infarct vessel: limitations of ST-segment elevation in standard and extended ECG leads. *Chest* 2001;**120**:1540–6.

16 Taha B, Reddy S, Agarwal J, Khaw K. Normal limits of ST segment measurements in posterior ECG leads. *J Electrocardiol* 1998;**31**(Suppl):178–9.

17 Wung SF, Kahn DY. A quantitative evaluation of ST segment changes on the 18 lead electrocardiogram during acute coronary occlusions. *J Electrocardiol* 2006;**39**:275–81.

18 Zhou SH, Startt/Selvester RH, Liu X, *et al.* An automated algorithm to improve ECG detection of posterior STEMI associated with left circumflex coronary artery occlusion. *Computers in Cardiology* 2006;**33**:33–36.

19 Buda AJ. The role of echocardiography in the evaluation of mechanical complications of acute myocardial infarction. *Circulation* 1991;**84**(Suppl 1):I-109-I-121.

20 Peels CH, Visser CA, Kupper AJ, *et al.* Usefulness of two-dimensional echocardiography for immediate detection of myocardial ischemia in the emergency room. *Am J Cardiol* 1990;**65**: 687–91.

21 Tatum JL, Jesse RL, Kontos MC, *et al.* Comprehensive strategy for the evaluation and triage of the chest pain patient. *Ann Emerg Med* 1997;**29**:116–25.

22 Stowers SA, Eisenstein EL, Wackers FJT, *et al.* An economic analysis of an aggressive diagnostic strategy with single photon emission computed tomography myocardial perfusion imaging and early exercise stress testing in emergency department patients who present with chest pain but non-diagnostic electrocardiograms: results from a randomized trial. *Ann Emerg Med* 2000;**35**:17–25.

23 Udelson JE, Beshansky J, Ballin DS, *et al.* Myocardial perfusion imaging for evaluation and triage of patients with suspected acute cardiac ischemia: a randomized controlled trial. *JAMA* 2002;**288**:2693–700.

24 Cheitlin MD, Armstrong WF, Aurigemma GP, *et al.* ACC/ AHA/ASE 2003 guideline update for the clinical application of echocardiography: A report of the American College of Cardiology/American Heart Association task force on practice guidelines (ACC/AHA/ASE committee to update the 1997 guidelines for the clinical application of echocardiography). *J Am Coll Cardiol* 2003;**42**:954–70.

25 Korosoglu G, Labadze N, Hansen A, *et al.* Usefulness of real-time myocardial perfusion imaging in the evaluation of patients with first time chest pain. *Am J Cardiol* 2004;**94**:1225–31.

26 Mahmarian JJ, Moye L, Verani MSE, *et al.* Criteria for the accurate interpretation of changes in left ventricular ejection fraction and cardiac volumes as assessed by rest and exercise gated radionuclide angiography. *J Am Coll Cardiol* 1991;**18**: 112–9.

27 Barnett K, Feldman JA. Noninvasive imaging techniques to aid in the triage of patients with suspected acute coronary syndrome: A review. *Emerg Med Clin N Am* 2005;**23**:977–98.

28 Ioannidis J, Salem D, Chew PW, Lau J. Accuracy of imaging technologies in the diagnosis of acute cardiac ischemia in the emergency department. *Ann Emerg Med* 2001;**37**:471–7.

29 Kwong RY, Schussheim AE, Rekhraj S, *et al.* Detecting acute coronary syndrome in the emergency department with cardiac magnetic resonance imaging. *Circulation* 2003;**107**:531–7.

30 Mahnken AH, Koos R, Katoh M, *et al.* Assessment of myocardial viability in reperfused acute myocardial infarction using 16-slice computed tomography in comparison to magnetic resonance imaging. *J Am Coll Cardiol* 2005;**45**:2042–7.

31 Kontos MC, Tatum JL. Imaging in the evaluation of the patient with suspected acute coronary syndrome. *Semin Nucl Med* 2003;**33**:246–58.

32 Achenbach S, Moshage W, Ropers D, *et al.* Value of electron-beam computed tomography for the noninvasive detection of high-grade coronary artery stenoses and occlusions. *N Engl J Med* 1998;**339**:1964–71.

Chapter 20 | Is serial electrocardiography (serial ECGs and ST segment monitoring) of value in the ECG diagnosis of ACS?

Daniel T. O'Laughlin
University of Minnesota School of Medicine, Minneapolis, MN, USA

Case presentations

Case 1: A 48-year-old woman presents to the emergency department (ED) after onset of "burning" chest pain, with no associated symptoms, while working out on a treadmill early in the morning. Six hours later, while walking, she experienced the same chest pain and bilateral forearm pain, and called 911. On arrival of the emergency medical services (EMS), the patient was pain-free and had a normal electrocardiogram (ECG). She was transported without incident to an urban hospital with percutaneous coronary intervention (PCI) capabilities. After an aspirin, the first ECG is recorded and is non-diagnostic. (Figure 20.1a). The initial biomarkers are negative. Admission to the chest pain evaluation unit is planned, but after 90 min in the ED her pain recurs. A second ECG (Figure 20.1b) is obtained.

Case 2: A 58-year-old male smoker is transported by the EMS for severe chest pain. Paramedics obtain an ECG (Figure 20.2a), place the patient on oxygen, and administer aspirin, nitroglycerin tablets, and morphine during the 30-min transport to an urban hospital with PCI capabilities. En route, the paramedics obtain frequent ECGs (Figures 20.2a–d), which demonstrate labile ST segments. The paramedics activate the catheterization laboratory via a prehospital ST elevation myocardial infarction (STEMI) alert program.

Case 3: A 71-year-old female is transported to an urban hospital with PCI services for chest pain. En route, paramedics obtain an ECG (Figure 20.3a) and administer aspirin, oxygen, nitroglycerin, and morphine. The patient initially improves and is without pain when the paramedics obtain another ECG (Figure 20.3b). On arrival the pain is again severe, at 8/10, and a third ECG is identical to the first (Figure 20.3b).

Critical Decisions in Emergency and Acute Care Electrocardiography,
1st edition. Edited by W.J. Brady and J.D. Truwit. © 2009 Blackwell Publishing, ISBN: 9781405159067

The use of serial ECGs

A standard 12-lead ECG will record the electrical activity that is occurring in a patient during a 10 s "snapshot" of time in what is actually a dynamic process. Patients with acute coronary syndrome (ACS) frequently demonstrate instability of their ST segments due to spontaneous thrombosis and lysis, and resulting intermittent occlusion or critical stenosis (Cases 1–3) [1–4]. A single static ECG may, therefore, capture a period of time when the ECG is relatively non-diagnostic, or even normal (Figure 20.4), in a patient with evolving ACS, including STEMI.

The 12-lead ECG is the dominant tool for initial evaluation, as well as ongoing assessment of treatment interventions. In one study of ED chest pain patients, 1–4% with an "absolutely normal" ECG, and 4% of those with non-specific findings, were ultimately diagnosed with acute myocardial infarction (AMI) [5]. In this same group, unstable angina (UA) was diagnosed in 4% of those who had a normal initial ECG. Conversely, in other studies, 6–8% (and 22–35%) of patients with MI had an initially normal (or non-diagnostic) ECG (Figure 20.4) [6].

Only 45% of patients with acute MI, as diagnosed by CK-MB, demonstrate an initial ECG that is diagnostic for injury (ST elevation diagnostic of STEMI) [7]. Another 10% with AMI have abnormalities diagnostic of ischemia, but not STEMI. These numbers change to 62 and 6%, respectively, after 1 h of ST segment monitoring [7]. Specificity for STEMI versus pseudo-infarction, and ACS versus no ACS, was also improved. This led to an increase in the number of patients eligible for reperfusion, and also decreased inappropriate reperfusion.

Similarly, when the interpretation of an initial ECG is in doubt, comparison with a prehospital ECG is essential because it may reveal the diagnosis (see Figure 23.3). Comparison with recent ECGs in the patient's medical record is similarly essential, leading to the diagnosis or providing prognostic information that may help in admission decisions. Patients with a negative initial ECG that is changed from a

(a)

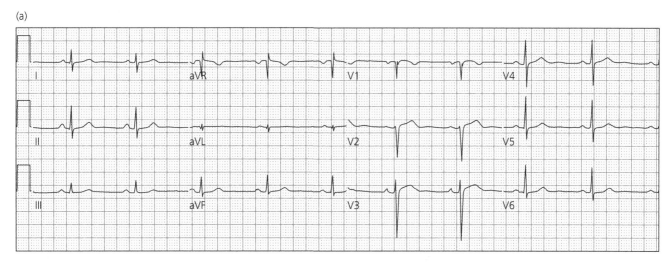

(b)

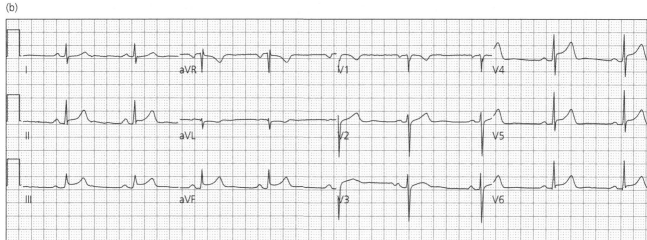

Figure 20.1 Developing inferolateral MI in Case 1, due to a "wraparound LAD." (a) Non-diagnostic first ECG. (b) Second ECG at 90 min after the first. New STE is now present in leads II, III, aVF, V4, and V5, with reciprocal STD in aVL, diagnostic of inferolateral STEMI. It was a result of a distal LAD dissecting occlusion.

(a)

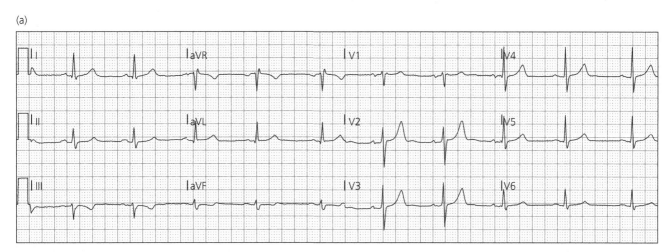

Figure 20.2 Developing anterior STEMI in Case 2. (a) First ECG (t = 0), with 10/10 pain, is non-diagnostic, but has prominent T waves in V2.

(b)

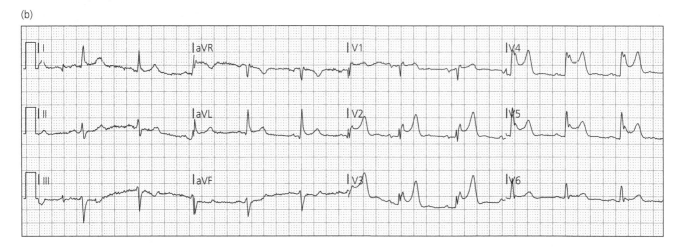

(c)

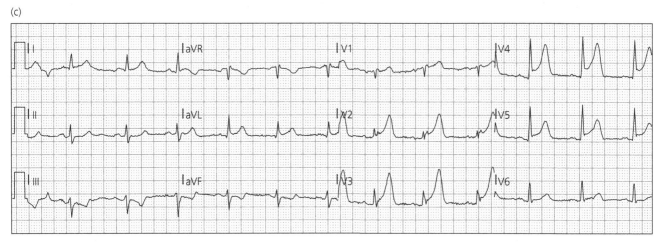

(d)

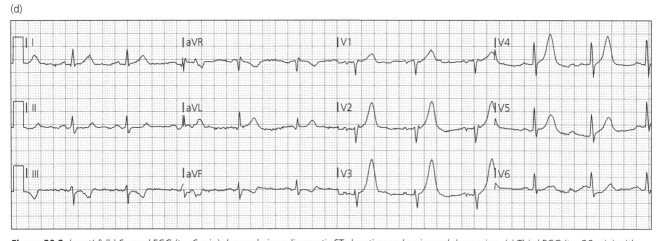

Figure 20.2 (*cont'd*) (b) Second ECG (t = 6 min) shows obvious diagnostic ST elevation and reciprocal depression. (c) Third ECG (t = 26 min) with pain at 4/10. Diagnostic ST elevation is still present, but not as marked. (d) Fourth ECG (t = 32 min) with pain at 1/10 demonstrates near complete resolution of the STE, but prominent T waves remain. Inferior ST depression is still present.

(a)

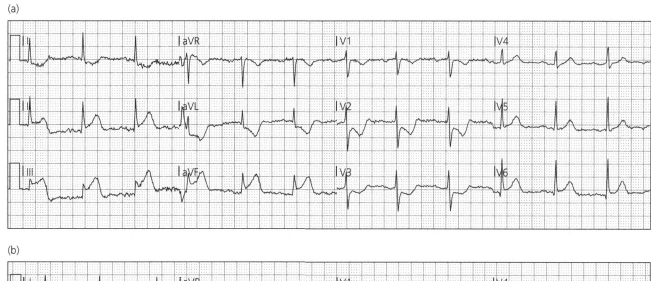

(b)

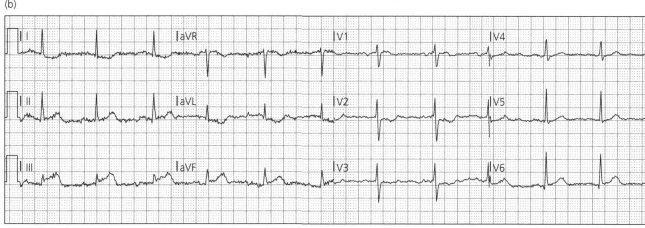

(c)

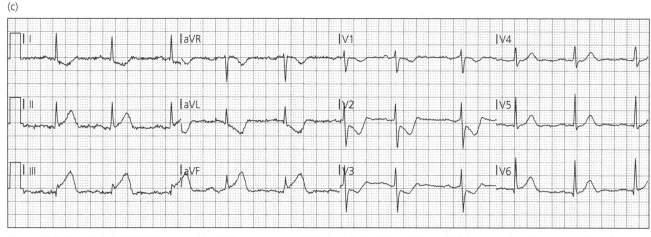

Figure 20.3 Case 3. (a) Initial ECG obtained by EMS demonstrates STE in leads II, III, aVF, and V6, and ST depression in aVL, and V2–V3. Findings are consistent with a STEMI involving the inferior and posterior and lateral regions. (b) Second ECG was obtained 4 min after the first. The ST changes are significantly improved in all leads. (c) Third ECG is obtained at the time of arrival to the ED, 11 min after the second (15 min after the first).

previous ECG had double the risk for interventions. Patients with a positive ECG that had changed from a previous ECG had four times the risk for life-threatening complications [8]. Patients with normal or non-specific ECGs have better short-term clinical outcomes, and fewer complications, if the ECG does not become positive [9–12]. Zalenski and colleagues

saw no significant differences in the rate of in-hospital complications between MI patients with negative and positive ECGs, but all complications in ECG-negative patients occurred only after development of serial ECG positivity [13].

The use of continuous ST segment monitoring in the ED has yet to become commonplace. The ability to obtain

(a)

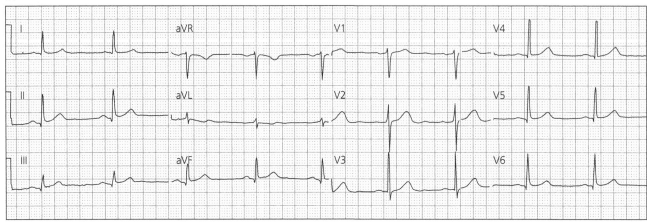

(b)

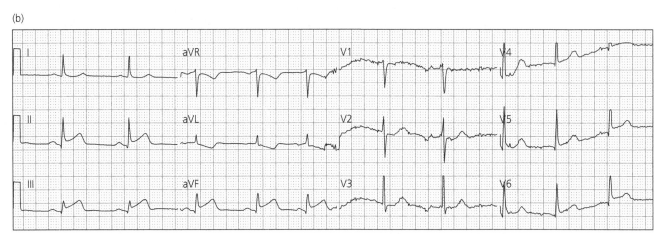

Figure 20.4 Prehospital serial ECG identifies inferior STEMI. (a) Paramedics record this prehospital ECG of a patient with chest pain; it is essentially normal, though in retrospect one can see minimal STE in II, III, and aVF, with reciprocal ST depression in aVL. (b) Only 3 min later, with continued chest pain. Now there is clear inferior STEMI. This led to early prehospital activation of the cath. lab. and a very fast reperfusion time.

serial electrocardiograms (SECGs) is much less limited. The acquisition of SECGs requires only the use of a standard 12-lead ECG machine and staff resources to obtain the studies. The optimal interval between serial studies is not well established. Fesmire and colleagues found, in their study of 1000 patients presenting with chest pain, that the average time from onset of continuous ST segment monitoring with automatic SECGs until new injury pattern developed was 13.7 min (± 18.4 min) [7]. Serial electrocardiogram evaluation intervals should therefore be short, every 5–10 min, in patients with high clinical suspicion for ACS and an initial ECG without clear findings for an ACS event [14]. Patients with a lower clinical suspicion may have study intervals ranging from every 30 to 120 min.

Serial electrocardiograms do present some challenges. Comparison of SECGs can be inaccurate if the lead placement is altered between studies. The ideal technique would include the use of the exact same lead locations and patient positioning for each study where possible. Comparisons made between a standard 12-lead ECG and a mathematically derived 12-lead ECG from a reduced lead set should be

avoided. Although derived ECGs can approximate a standard 12-lead ECG, they are not equivalent [15]. Simultaneous recordings of standard 12-lead ECG and a derived 12-lead ECG have demonstrated variations in amplitude of the ST segment, which prevents accurate comparisons [16]. Comparisons, therefore, should ideally be performed utilizing a consistent ECG technique. Serial electrocardiograms may also be subject to under-sampling errors if the interval between studies is too long and if significant unrecorded changes occur in the interval between the studies [3].

Continuous ST segment monitoring

Continuous ST segment monitoring is a dynamic tool for the monitoring of an often dynamic ischemic process that involves the intermittent vasospasm and constriction of an infarct-related artery (IRA), unstable thrombus, and/or dynamic downstream microvascular dysfunction [14,17]. Hackett and colleagues demonstrated that intermittent coronary occlusion is frequently present in the early phase of MI, and often the transient ST monitor changes are not associated with chest pain [2]. With continuous monitoring, evolving ACS that results in early changes in the ST segments can be identified, and therapeutic interventions can be rapidly initiated. Patients that demonstrate diagnostic changes while undergoing continuous 12-lead monitoring should be admitted to a cardiac intensive care unit and be assessed for reperfusion therapies [7]. See Case 25.1 and Figure 25.1.

Continuous ST segment monitoring equipment features may vary. Typical features of these monitors include the ability to sample ST segment trends in the standard 12 leads. Sampling intervals may vary from a few seconds to 1–2 min. Changes in the ST segment in either direction from the established baseline can be measured, plotted over time, and displayed, with alarms generated as appropriate. Alarm thresholds typically include a change of 200 µV in a single lead or 100 µV in two or more electrically contiguous leads. False alarms can be triggered from electrical noise, which can be minimized with careful attention to skin preparation. Patients that reposition from a supine to a side-lying position are the most common trigger of false-ST segment monitor alarms [18].

Continuous ST segment monitoring is also beneficial in the evaluation of patients with confounding patterns on the initial ECG, such as left ventricular hypertrophy (LVH) and left bundle branch block (LBBB). The detection of AMI in these conditions can be extremely difficult, if not impossible. Dynamic changes in the ST segment from an AMI will still occur with these conditions and can be detected on the 12-lead continuous ST segment monitor [1]. Absence of change helps to rule out STEMI [7].

Assessment of coronary artery patency

Reperfusion of an IRA, following the administration of thrombolytic agents, is a dynamic process with frequent instability in the IRA patency and will often occur asymptomatically [4,19,20]. Continuous ST segment monitoring has been advocated to provide up to the minute assessment for changes following reperfusion treatment [4,20–22]. Serial electrocardiogram monitoring may detect both reperfusion and reocclusion (see Chapter 25; especially Figure 25.1).

Conclusion

Serial electrocardiogram and continuous ST segment monitoring has a clear benefit in the evaluation of patients at high risk for ACS when their initial ECG is non-diagnostic. These tools also provide significant benefit in the monitoring of patients who have recently undergone reperfusion treatment, to assess for evidence of success or failure of the treatment.

Case conclusions

In Case 1, the second ED ECG demonstrates inferolateral STEMI. Repeat biomarkers were elevated. The patient was taken emergently for angiography, which demonstrated 99% stenosis of the distal left anterior descending (LAD) coronary artery, which supplied the apical inferior wall with a corresponding apical-inferior wall motion abnormality (thus, this is a "wraparound," in which distal occlusion results in inferior, not anterior, MI). Because of technical considerations, it could not be opened. She was discharged home without incident and at a 6-week follow-up was doing well and had an ejection fraction of 65% as determined by echocardiogram. In Case 2, the patient had pain of 1/10 on arrival to the ED. The patient underwent angiography, which revealed a 100% proximal LAD lesion. He had successful PCI with stenting of the LAD and was discharged home without incident. The patient in Case 3 was rapidly transferred to the catheterization lab; on arrival, heart rate was 20–30 beats per minute with hypotension. She underwent emergent pacemaker placement and aortic balloon pump, and required the use of vasopressor agents during and following the procedure. She was found to have severe stenosis of the RCA, and, despite successful stenting, demonstrated the "no-reflow" phenomenon with persistent injury pattern. She had a prolonged recovery.

References

1 Fesmire FM. ECG diagnosis of acute myocardial infarction in the presence of left bundle-branch block in patients undergoing continuous ECG monitoring. *Ann Emerg Med* 1995;**26**:69–82.

2 Hackett D, Davies G, Chierchia S, Maseri A. Intermittent coronary occlusion in acute myocardial infarction. Value of combined thrombolytic and vasodilator therapy. *N Engl J Med* 1987;**317**:1055–9.

3 Krucoff MW, Johanson P, Baeza R, *et al.* Clinical utility of serial and continuous ST-segment recovery assessment in patients with acute ST-elevation myocardial infarction: assessing the dynamics of epicardial and myocardial reperfusion. *Circulation* 2004;**110**:e533–9.

4 Kwon K, Freedman SB, Wilcox I, *et al.* The unstable ST segment early after thrombolysis for acute infarction and its usefulness as a marker of recurrent coronary occlusion. *Am J Cardiol* 1991;**67**:109–15.

5 Brady WJ, Roberts D, Morris F. The nondiagnostic ECG in the chest pain patient: Normal and nonspecific initial ECG presentations of acute MI. *Am J Emerg Med* 1999;**17**:394–7.

6 Smith SW, Zvosec DL, Henry TD, Sharkey SW. *The ECG in Acute MI: an Evidence-Based Manual of Reperfusion Therapy*. Philadelphia: Lippincott, Williams, and Wilkins, 2002:358.

7 Fesmire FM, Percy RF, Bardoner JB, *et al.* Usefulness of automated serial 12-lead ECG monitoring during the initial emergency department evaluation of patients with chest pain. *Ann Emerg Med* 1998;**31**:3–11.

8 Fesmire FM, Percy RF, Wears RL. Diagnostic and prognostic importance of comparing the initial to the previous

electrocardiogram in patients admitted for suspected acute myocardial infarction. *South Med J* 1991;**84**:841–6.

9 Braunwald E, Jones RH, Mark DB, *et al*. Diagnosing and managing unstable angina. Agency for Health Care Policy and Research. *Circulation* 1994;**90**:613–22.

10 Brush JE, Brand DA, Acampora D, *et al*. Use of the initial electrocardiogram to predict in-hospital complications of acute myocardial infarction. *N Engl J Med* 1985;**312**:1137–41.

11 Rouan GW, Lee TH, Cook EF, *et al*. Clinical characteristics and outcome of acute myocardial infarction in patients with initially normal or nonspecific electrocardiograms (a report from the Multicenter Chest Pain Study). *Am J Cardiol* 1989;**64**:1087–92.

12 Welch RD, Zalenski RJ, Frederick PD, *et al*. Prognostic value of a normal or nonspecific initial electrocardiogram in acute myocardial infarction. *JAMA* 2001;**286**:1977–84.

13 Zalenski RJ, Rydman RJ, Sloan EP, *et al*. The emergency department electrocardiogram and hospital complications in myocardial infarction patients. *Acad Emerg Med* 1996;**3**:318–25.

14 Velez J, Brady WJ, Perron AD, Garvey L. Serial electrocardiography. *Am J Emerg Med* 2002;**20**:43–9.

15 Kligfield P, Gettes LS, Bailey JJ, *et al*. Recommendations for the Standardization and Interpretation of the Electrocardiogram: Part I: The Electrocardiogram and Its Technology: A Scientific Statement From the American Heart Association Electrocardiography and Arrhythmias Committee, Council on Clinical Cardiology; the American College of Cardiology Foundation; and the Heart Rhythm Society Endorsed by the International Society for Computerized Electrocardiology. *Circulation* 2007;**115**:1306–24.

16 Drew BJ, Pelter MM, Wung SF, *et al*. Accuracy of the EASI 12-lead electrocardiogram compared to the standard 12-lead electrocardiogram for diagnosing multiple cardiac abnormalities. *J Electrocardiol* 1999;**32**(Suppl):38–47.

17 Roe MT, Ohman EM, Maas AC, *et al*. Shifting the open-artery hypothesis downstream: the quest for optimal reperfusion. *J Am Coll Cardiol* 2001;**37**:9–18.

18. Drew BJ, Adams MG. Clinical consequences of ST-segment changes caused by body position mimicking transient myocardial ischemia: hazards of ST-segment monitoring? *J Electrocardiol* 2001;**34**:261–4.

19 Fesmire FM, Wharton DR, Calhoun FB. Instability of ST segments in the early stages of acute myocardial infarction in patients undergoing continuous 12-lead ECG monitoring. *Am J Emerg Med* 1995;**13**:158–63.

20 Krucoff MW, Croll MA, Pope JE, *et al*. Continuous 12-lead ST-segment recovery analysis in the TAMI 7 study. Performance of a non-invasive method for real-time detection of failed myocardial reperfusion. *Circulation* 1993;**88**:437–46.

21 Krucoff MW, Green CE, Satler LF, *et al*. Noninvasive detection of coronary artery patency using continuous ST-segment monitoring. *Am J Cardiol* 1986;**57**:916–22.

22 Doevendans PA, Gorgels AP, van der Zee R, *et al*. Electrocardiographic diagnosis of reperfusion during thrombolytic therapy in acute myocardial infarction. *Am J Cardiol* 1995;**75**:1206–10.

Chapter 21 | What QRS complex abnormalities result in ST segment elevation that may mimic or obscure AMI?

Stephen W. Smith[1], *David M. Larson*[2]

[1]University of Minnesota, Hennepin County Medical Center, Minneapolis, MN, USA
[2]University of Minnesota Medical School, St Paul, MN, USA

Case presentations

Case 1: A 59-year-old male presents via emergency medical services (EMS) with weakness and dizziness followed by anterior chest pain, rated 4/10 in severity. He has a history of hypertension and dyslipidemia. Vital signs are: blood pressure (BP) of 184/89, heart rate (HR) of 84, and SpO_2 of 97%. His initial ECG shows non-specific intraventricular conduction delay (QRS = 126 ms) with ST segment elevation (STE) in leads III, AVF, and V1–V3, with some reciprocal ST depression in I and aVL (Figure 21.1). He is sent for emergent angiography with anticipation of percutaneous coronary intervention (PCI) for ST elevation myocardial infarction (STEMI).

Case 2: A 70-year-old male complains of chest pain radiating to his jaw while shoveling snow. He has no prior history of coronary artery disease (CAD), but he has three risk factors. He is brought to the emergency department (ED) by co-workers. His initial vital signs are as follows: BP 165/94, HR 76, respiration rate 22, and SpO_2 97% on ambient air. His exam is otherwise normal. His initial ECG demonstrates left bundle branch block (LBBB) with concordant STE in I, aVL, V5, and V6, as well as discordant STE, out of proportion to the preceding S wave (ST/S ratio ≥ 0.25 in at least one lead), in leads V1–V4 (Figure 21.2). This is diagnostic of LAD occlusion. After adjunctive medications, he is taken for angiography and anticipated PCI.

Case 3: A 56-year-old with history of hypertension, coronary stents placed 2 years prior, and aortic and mitral valve replacements, presents with 2 h of "oppressive" 9/10 constant chest pressure radiating to the back and neck, associated with diaphoresis and shortness of breath (SOB). On exam, the patient is diaphoretic and appears to be in moderate distress. Blood pressure is 140/70. The cath. lab. is activated based on the ECG (Figure 21.3).

Conditions that obscure MI because of an abnormal QRS

There are several conditions where abnormal depolarization of the ventricle results in repolarization changes that can obscure or mimic STE or T wave inversion, making it difficult to evaluate patients who present with symptoms suggestive of cardiac ischemia. Among these are: left ventricular hypertrophy (LVH), left or right bundle branch block or intraventricular conduction delays, ventricular paced rhythms, and pre-excitation syndromes such as Wolff-Parkinson-White (WPW). Brugada syndrome is discussed in Chapter 14.

Left ventricular hypertrophy: This is associated with secondary repolarization changes that include STE, ST depression, and/or T wave prominence or inversion. Left ventricular hypertrophy is a common cause of false positive STE (see Figures 21.1, 21.3, 21.4, and 21.5) [1–3], and in one study it accounted for 25% of STE in chest pain patients who did not have myocardial infarction (MI) [4]. ST depression and T inversion may mimic or obscure findings of non-ST elevation myocardial infarction (NSTEMI) [2].

In order to attribute ST-T changes to LVH, specific electrocardiographic criteria must be met. There are several published criteria for LVH that are imbedded in computerized ECG algorithms. A simply applied summary of the criteria follows [5].

1. QRS < 0.12 s, and one or more of the following:
2. R wave in lead I + S wave in lead III > 25 mm
3. R wave in aVL > 11 mm
4. R wave in aVF > 20 mm
5. S wave in aVR > 14 mm

Critical Decisions in Emergency and Acute Care Electrocardiography, 1st edition. Edited by W.J. Brady and J.D. Truwit. © 2009 Blackwell Publishing, ISBN: 9781405159067

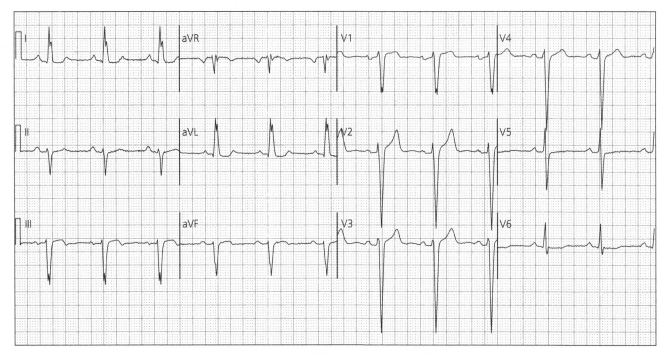

Figure 21.1 LVH and intraventricular conduction delay. See STE in inferior leads with reciprocal ST depression in lead aVL. An astute interpreter should recognize that this is not due to coronary occlusion because the STE is minimal and proportional to the QRS. See case description.

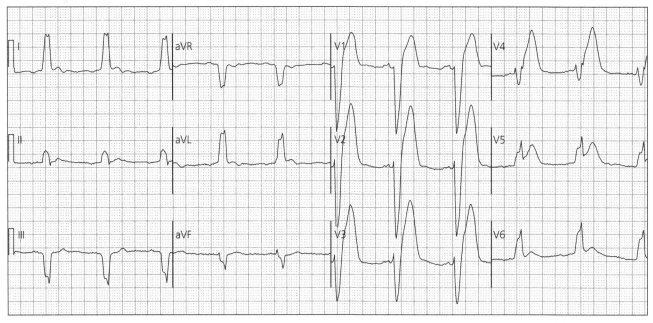

Figure 21.2 Case 2. LBBB with anterior MI due to proximal LAD occlusion. The STE is discordant, but is both > 5 mm (Sgarbossa criteria [21]) and > 25% of the previous S wave (Smith criteria [17]). There is also concordant STE in I, aVL, V5, and V6. Each of leads V1–V6, I, and aVL is diagnostic of STEMI on its own. See case description.

6 R wave in V5 or V6 > 26 mm
7 R wave in V5 or V6 + S wave in V1 > 35 mm
8 Largest R wave + largest S wave in precordial leads > 45 mm

One simple way to remember the criteria based on QRS voltage in the precordial leads is to remember the "rule of 35": the amplitude of the S wave in V1 or V2 plus the

amplitude of the R wave in V5 or V6 > 35 mm, in a patient of age > 35.

In LVH, the rightward precordial leads (V1–V3) show poor R wave progression with a large S wave, or even a QS wave, and pronounced discordant STE (see Figures 21.3–21.5). The ST segment is usually concave upward, but is frequently

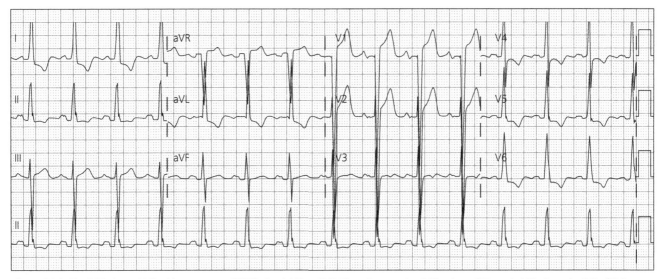

Figure 21.3 The ECG shows LVH with pronounced STE in leads V1 and V2. There is a massive QRS voltage (40 mm in V1); thus, the STE of 3.5 mm in V1 is < 10% of the depth of the S wave, and this is expected for LVH. The fact that there is no STE in V3 decreases the likelihood of STEMI. In a patient with chest pain and some risk of CAD, and this ECG, it would be prudent to do an immediate echocardiogram or to activate the cath. lab., as in this case. See case description.

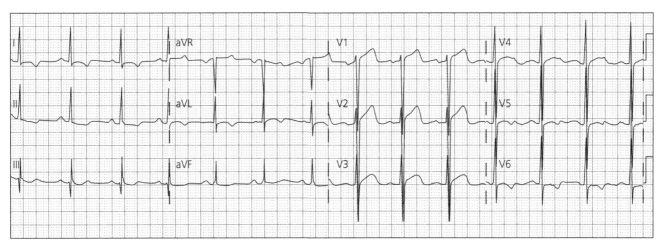

Figure 21.4 LVH with convex ST segments. There was no MI.

(confusingly) convex, mimicking STEMI (see Figure 21.4). Leftward leads (I, aVL, V5–V6) frequently show large monophasic R waves with discordant ST depression and T wave inversion, sometimes very deeply inverted. The ST segments are downsloping (formerly known as "left ventricular strain"). The STE or ST depression is *proportionate to the size of the QRS*, though no numerical definition of proportionate is yet available. When there is secondary STE in the limb leads, there may be reciprocal ST depression (Figure 21.1), mimicking AMI [6]. Other notable features include: (1) T wave asymmetry with rapid return to baseline of negative T waves, and (2) overshoot, such that the terminal T wave may be slightly positive (Figures 21.1 and 21.3, leads V5 and V6) [7].

Several features of repolarization abnormalities in LVH with superimposed ischemia may help to distinguish it from LVH alone [5]:

1 Disproportionate discordant (in relation to the QRS) STE or ST depression (disproportionate to R wave or S wave amplitude). See Figure 15.9.

2 Concordant STE or ST depression. Concordant ST depression in V1–V3 is not due to LVH and may be due to posterior infarction or subendocardial ischemia. See Figure 15.9, lead V3.

3 Flat ST depression (as opposed to downsloping).

4 Convex ST segments weakly suggest STEMI; this feature is not as specific for STEMI as it is in the presence of a normal QRS (see Figure 21.4, leads V3 and V4).

Left bundle branch block (also see Chapter 24, indications for reperfusion therapy): In LBBB the left ventricle depolarizes in reverse order, by radial spread from the point of termination of the right bundle [8]. This abnormal depolarization completely obscures Q waves that might

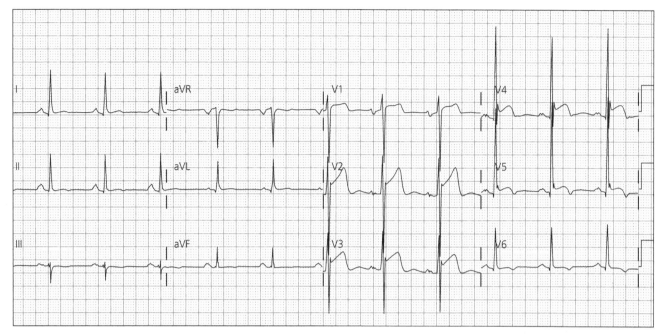

Figure 21.5 LVH with STE up to 4 mm, in leads V1–V5; the patient ruled out for MI. Concordance in V4 suggests STEMI, but pronounced J wave in the same lead suggests an element of early repolarization. QTc-B is 410 ms, relatively short for anterior MI. In the setting of ischemic symptoms, it is appropriate to initiate reperfusion therapy. In lower risk settings, echocardiography is useful.

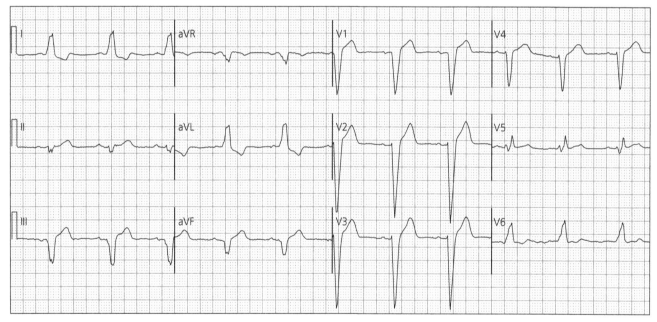

Figure 21.6 Typical LBBB without MI or ischemia. Notice that ST segments and most T waves are in the opposite direction (discordant) from the major deflection of QRS.

otherwise be present from an old MI. More importantly for critical care, it results in repolarization changes that may either mimic or obscure the typical ST segment deviation due to acute ischemia or infarction. Normally in LBBB, the ST-T wave complex will demonstrate deviation from the baseline in the opposite (discordant) direction of the QRS deflection. For example, in leads V1–V3 the QRS deflection is negative, resulting normally in STE and positive T wave. This STE might prompt the unsuspecting physician to diagnose anter-

ior STEMI. However, anterior STEMI can only be diagnosed when this discordant STE is excessive or out of proportion to the size of the S wave and upright T waves. In lateral leads (I, AVL, V5–V6), the QRS deflection is normally positive with downsloping ST depression and T wave inversion (Figure 21.6). Inferior leads may have a positive or negative QRS, but the ST-T complex should be opposite.

Criteria for LBBB are [5]: (1) QRS duration > 0.12 s, (2) lead I: wide, monophasic R wave, (3) QS or RS in V1, and

(4) delayed intrinsicoid deflection in V5–V6 (> 0.04 s to peak of R).

AMI with BBB (LBBB or RBBB): Acute myocardial infarction in the presence of bundle branch block (BBB), whether left or right, is associated with much higher in-hospital and 30-day mortality than AMI in patients with normal conduction [9,10]. Most of the excess mortality is in the cohort with persistent, as opposed to transient, BBB [10–12]. Patients who present with BBB, especially if new and persistent, are at greater risk of death, congestive heart failure, cardiogenic shock or ventricular arrhythmias (see Chapter 27 on ECG predictors of cardiovascular risk). In randomized trials of fibrinolytics, the group of patients with BBB who were randomized to fibrinolytics (versus placebo), had significantly lower mortality [13]. Unfortunately, these studies do not specify, for the most part, left versus right BBB, or which ECG subgroups of patients will benefit, and whether certain criteria specific for AMI in the presence of BBB would distinguish between those BBB patients who benefit and those who do not (see Sgarbossa criteria, below).

Left bundle branch block interferes with the orderly depolarization of the left ventricle, and is believed to distort the surface ECG such that further analysis is insufficient to exclude MI. This reputation comes mostly from old literature in which ECG Q wave analysis was used to diagnose old MI, and LBBB most certainly obscures Q waves. Whether it obscures the ST segment to such an extent that one cannot rely upon ST segment analysis to exclude large acute and persistent epicardial coronary occlusion is not entirely certain. Thus, current American College of Cardiology/American Heart Association (ACC/AHA) guidelines recommend reperfusion therapy (either fibrinolysis or PCI) for patients with ischemic symptoms and new, or presumably new, LBBB [13,14]. Right bundle branch block is not believed to sufficiently alter the analysis of the ECG, and, thus, new RBBB with ischemic symptoms is only an indication for reperfusion if there is abnormal STE (or excessive ST depression compatible with posterior MI). The American College of Emergency Physicians guidelines, but not the ACC [14], recommend reperfusion in the patient with typical chest pain and RBBB if the ST segment analysis is obscured [15].

From clinical guidelines and randomized trials, a documented new LBBB in the setting of presumably ischemic chest pain, without any specific criteria, is, in itself, believed to be sufficient to institute reperfusion therapy [14,15]. Despite guideline recommendations that patients with new, or presumably new, LBBB and ischemic symptoms receive reperfusion therapy, only about one-third prove to have a MI based on positive CK-MB [3,5,16]. Not all of these CK-MB-diagnosed MIs have acute persistent epicardial coronary occlusion, with TIMI-0 or -1 flow, without collateral circulation (true STEMI, with ongoing irreversibly infarcting myocardium, in need of emergent reperfusion). In 1042 consecutive cases of primary PCI for presumed STEMI, only one

had LBBB and confirmed LAD occlusion, as defined by LAD occlusion or culprit lesion *and* troponin I > 10 (unpublished data). In a 12-year span at another busy center, there were only 13 confirmed LAD occlusions with LBBB [17]. Thus, following the guideline will probably subject most of the patients to unnecessary emergent reperfusion therapy. In practice, only a minority of patients with LBBB and symptoms suggestive of ischemia receive any reperfusion therapy according to guidelines [9,18–20]. However, until it is better established which of the new LBBB patients with ischemic symptoms can be ruled out for coronary occlusion, it is prudent to follow the guidelines. In the absence of criteria specific for STEMI (see below), mechanical reperfusion is preferred to thrombolysis because of the uncertainty of the diagnosis. Finally, some BBB is rate-dependent, only manifesting at higher heart rates [5]. See Figure 19.3.

Certain ECG criteria can be used that increase the specificity of AMI in patients that present with chest pain and presumably new LBBB, or with previously present LBBB. In 1996, Sgarbossa and colleagues published a clinical prediction rule based on a set of ECG criteria for the diagnosis of AMI in patients with chest pain and LBBB [21]. In their analysis of GUSTO-1 data and ECGs, the criterion standard for MI was elevated CK-MB; they did not use an angiographic outcome. These criteria have high specificity for AMI by CK-MB, but have been criticized for lack of sufficient sensitivity (30–42%) to rule out AMI [22–24]. However, given that even in normal conduction, STE is only 45–50% sensitive for MI as diagnosed by CK-MB [25–29], but 80–90% sensitive for diagnosis of complete, persistent occlusion [30], then the Sgarbossa criteria may be much more sensitive for STEMI than has been acknowledged [31]. In studies with angiographic outcomes, rather than CK-MB, the ECG had sensitivity for occlusion in the presence of LBBB as high as that in normal conduction [17,32].

Sgarbossa criteria are: (1) concordant (in same direction as QRS) ST elevation of ≥ 1 mm in one lead (five points), (2) concordant ST depression ≥ 1 mm in one of leads V1–V3 (three points), and (3) discordant ST elevation ≥ 5 mm (two points).

In Sgarbossa's study, discordant STE ≥ 5 mm was less specific than concordant STE or ST depression. However, a score ≥ 2 was > 85% specific for AMI [21,24]. Smith and colleagues found in the only study using strict angiographic outcomes (n = 13 LAD occlusions, 225 controls) that the degree of discordant STE was proportional to the size of the preceding S wave, and that an STE to S wave ratio > 0.25 in any one of leads V1–V4 was highly sensitive (92%) and specific (> 97%) for LAD occlusion, significantly more accurate than the absolute value of ≥ 5 mm suggested by Sgarbossa [17]. Specificity is also very important, as LBBB without MI but with high QRS voltage is frequently associated with ≥ 5 mm STE (Figure 21.7) [33].

Comparison with a previous ECG, if available, is invaluable in patients with LBBB (see Figure 19.4). As mentioned, new LBBB, or LBBB with a concordant ST segment, are each alone

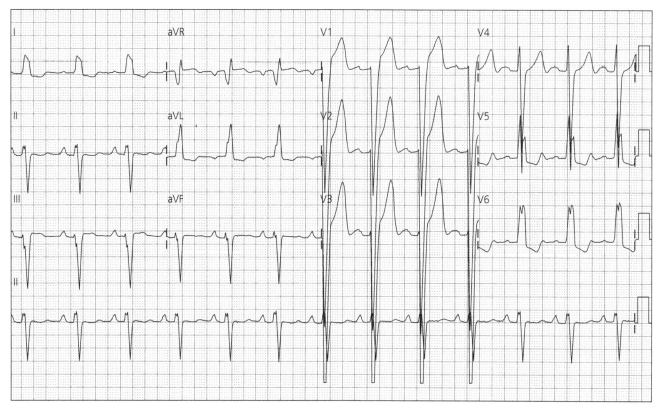

Figure 21.7 LBBB with high voltage has proportionately high ST elevation: in lead V2, there is 6 mm of STE and 69 mm of S wave, the ST/S ratio is a rather low 0.087. This patient with chest pain ruled out for acute MI.

sufficient to initiate reperfusion. However, LBBB with ST segments that have changed since a previous tracing are even more specific [31,32,34]. New concordant STE or ST depression, or even a *relative* ST shift, even pseudo-normalization (see Figure 21.8a, lead V2, compared with previous V2 in Figure 21.8b), may be diagnostic (see Figures 21.8a and b).

Right bundle branch block: Criteria for RBBB are (see Figure 21.9): (1) QRS duration ≥ 0.12 s, (2) late intrinsicoid deflection in V1 with M- or "rabbit ears-" shape of QRS (RSR′); the R′ is larger and wider than the R, (3) often the R is replaced by a Q, resulting in qR wave with large, wide R, and (4) wide S wave in lateral leads, especially lead I.

In contrast to LBBB, RBBB does not interfere with the order of left ventricular depolarization and does not, for the most part, obscure the ST segment deviation of STEMI. However, the widened end of the QRS is frequently mistaken for the ST segment and confuses the interpreter. The key to evaluating the ECG in the presence of RBBB is to find the true end of the QRS and the true beginning of the ST segment, so that the ST segment itself can be measured. The technique described by Smith is helpful in this regard [5]:

(1) Find the lead in which it is easiest to measure the QRS duration (the computer algorithm will measure this very accurately).

(2) Using the QRS duration, you can then determine the end of the QRS in any lead.

(3) This is where the ST segment begins (J point).

(4) Measure the ST segment deviation at the J point and relative to the TP segment.

RBBB without AMI does not have secondary discordant STE, as does LBBB. Therefore, any STE, even if discordant to the QRS, is abnormal (see Figures 21.10–21.12). However, often in leads V1–V3 there is up to 1 mm (0.1 mV) of ST *depression*, discordant to the R′ wave (see Figure 21.9, lead V3). As a result, anterior MI may have only minimal STE. The presence of RBBB in the setting of AMI is associated with a higher risk of complications (see Chapter 27 on ECG predictors of cardiovascular risk).

Anterior and posterior hemiblock: These do not typically result in confusing ST-T repolarization patterns.

Ventricular paced rhythms: In patients with right ventricular (RV)-paced rhythms, similar to LBBB, activation of the ventricles is altered because of abnormal right to left depolarization, which also results in abnormal repolarization. Right ventricular pacing usually produces a LBBB pattern in the right precordial leads with a negative QRS in V1–V4, but, unlike LBBB, also usually has a negative QRS in V5–V6 (Figure 21.13). The inferior leads are typically negative

(a)

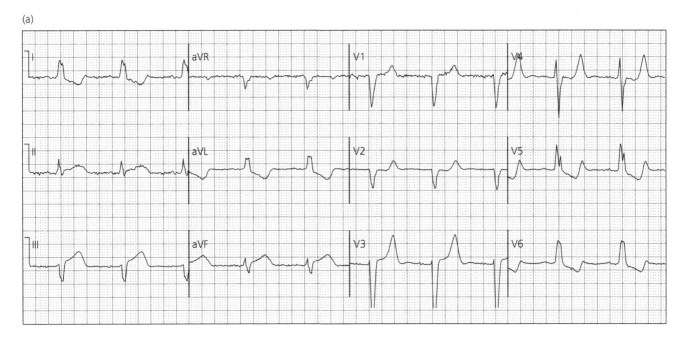

(b)

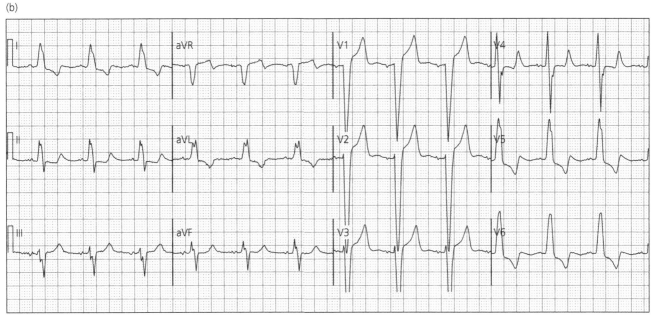

Figure 21.8 Chest pain with LBBB and ECG diagnostic for STEMI. (a) There is concordant STE in lead II, sufficient for a diagnosis of STEMI. Lead V2 does not have normal discordant STE; this is suspicious for relative ST depression. Suspicions are confirmed with comparison with the previous tracing (b), after which it is obvious that there is new STE in III and aVF and *relative* ST depression in V1 and V2, diagnostic of inferior-posterior MI. Angiography found a total thrombotic occlusion of the RCA.

as the pacer lead is usually in the RV apex and the depolarization begins in the inferior part of the heart and travels superiorly away from the inferior leads. Occasionally, if the lead is displaced to the RV outflow tract the inferior leads may be positive. A biventricular pacemaker with the RV lead in the apex and the LV lead in the coronary sinus will produce a positive QRS in V1 and/or V2 (see Figure 21.14).

The abnormal repolarization in paced rhythms results in discordant (opposite of the QRS complex) STE in most leads.

Similar to LBBB, there are ECG criteria for AMI that are highly specific but with low sensitivity. A small study found that the most sensitive criteria for MI as diagnosed by CK-MB (58% sensitivity, 88% specificity) were discordant STE ≥ 5 mm in leads with a negative QRS (see Figure 21.14) [35]. Other less sensitive but specific criteria include concordant STE of ≥ 1 mm in one lead or concordant ST depression of ≥ 1 mm in one of leads V1–V3 (see Figures 21.15 and 21.16). As with LBBB, it is helpful to compare ST segments with a

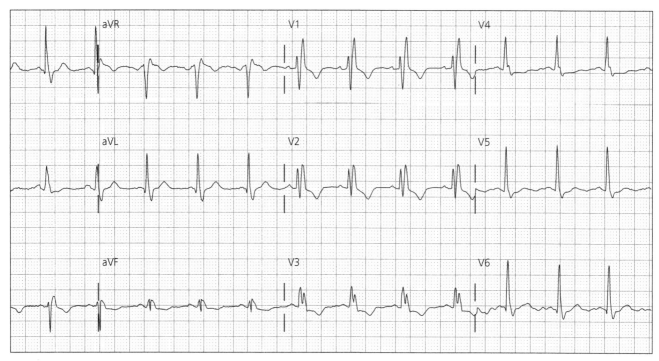

Figure 21.9 Normal RBBB. Note some normal ST depression, discordant to the positive R', in lead V3; up to 1 mm may be present in RBBB without MI. STE is never normal.

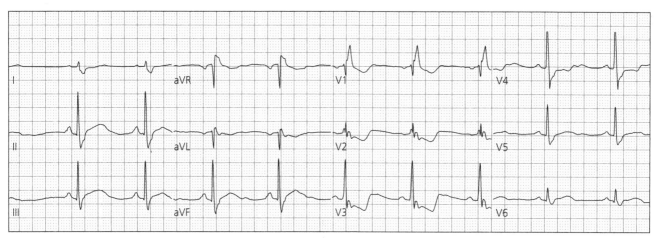

Figure 21.10 RBBB and inferior STEMI. There is STE in leads II, III, and AVF. More impressive is 2 mm of ST depression V2–V3, diagnostic of an inferior-posterior STEMI. Angiography revealed total occlusion of the RCA.

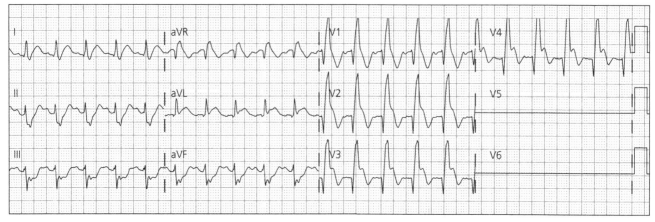

Figure 21.11 RBBB with anterior STEMI. Leads V5 and V6 are artifactual. The QRS is 154 ms, as read by the computer. Thus, in all of leads V1–V4, the ST segment begins at 154 ms after the start of the QRS and is 1–3 mm elevated, diagnostic of STEMI.

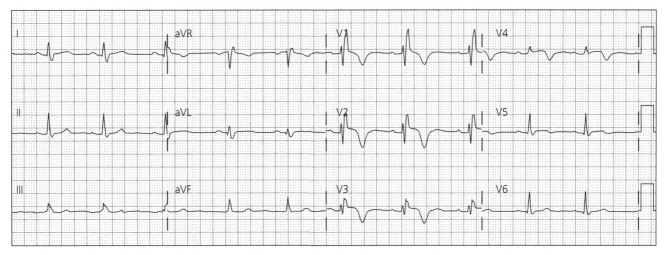

Figure 21.12 RBBB with acute anterior STEMI. There is STE where there should never be STE normally: V2 and V3. The T wave inversion does not necessarily imply reperfusion or open artery, as it would in normal conduction. In RBBB, the T wave often remains inverted with occlusion. See Figure 21.9 for RBBB with normal V1–V3.

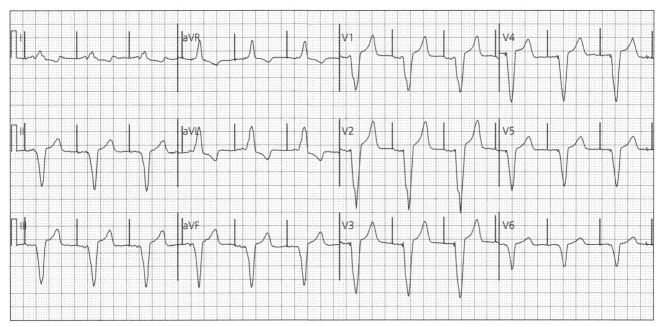

Figure 21.13 Biventricular pacemaker, without ischemia; note discordant ST segments.

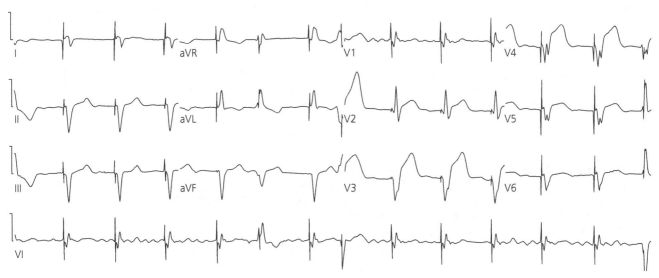

Figure 21.14 Paced with disproportionate discordant STE in V3 and V4, both ≥ 5 mm and with ST/S ratio ≥ 0.25; this is diagnostic of LAD occlusion.

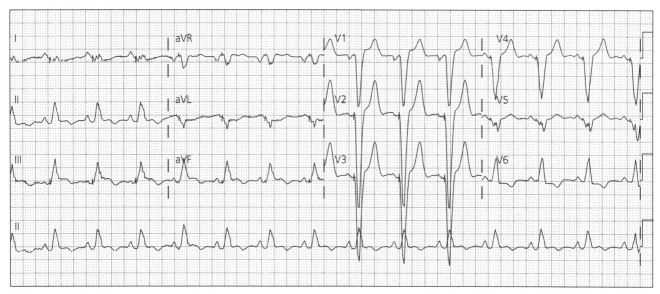

Figure 21.15 Concordant inferior STE from RCA occlusion in a patient with a pacemaker.

(a)   (b)

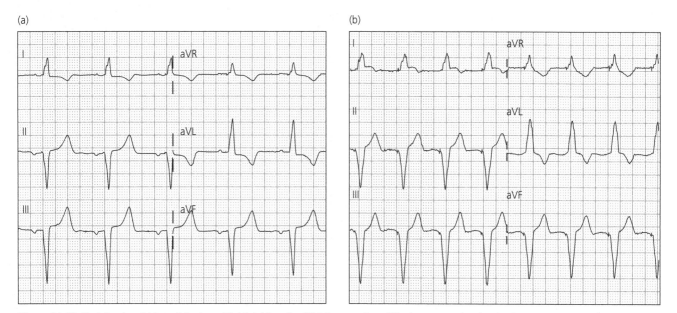

Figure 21.16 (limb leads only) Paced rhythm with MI. (a) Baseline ECG (pacer spikes difficult to appreciate here). There is normal discordant ST depression in leads I and aVL. (b) There is 1 mm of concordant STE in lead I; the ST segment is isoelectric in lead aVL, but, *relatively*, it is 1 mm elevated from baseline. There was an acute occlusion of the first obtuse marginal (lateral MI).

previous ECG. New STE, or *relative* STE (change in depth of depression, see Figure 21.16) in the setting of ischemic symptoms is significant. Though not proven, proportionality is probably as important in paced rhythms as in LBBB (see Figure 21.14).

Wolff-Parkinson-White syndrome (WPW): This may also present as a pseudo-infarction, and is caused by ventricular pre-excitation due to an accessory pathway manifested with a short PR interval, a prolonged upstroke of the QRS complex (delta wave), and QRS prolongations (Figures 21.17 and 21.18). Q waves in II, III, and AVF, and/or tall R waves

in V1–V3 may mimic inferior and/or posterior MI, and even manifest reciprocal ST depression (Figure 21.17). Patients with WPW and pseudo-infarction patterns may present with supraventricular tachycardia or with non-cardiac chest pain, but have a pseudo-infarction pattern on the 12-lead when in sinus rhythm.

Case conclusions

In Case 1, cardiac catheterization demonstrated normal coronary arteries. The patient had non-cardiac chest pain and STE

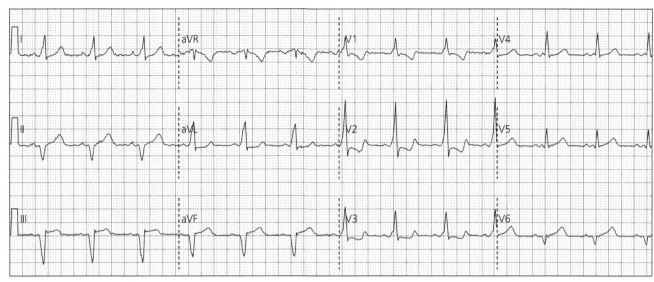

Figure 21.17 WPW syndrome. Notice the short PR interval and slurring of the upstroke of the QRS (delta wave, most prominent in V2 and V3). This abnormal QRS results in repolarization abnormalities that may mimic AMI; in this case, it results in STE in inferior leads, with reciprocal depression in aVL, and pseudo-posterior MI in V2 and V3, with tall R waves and ST depression.

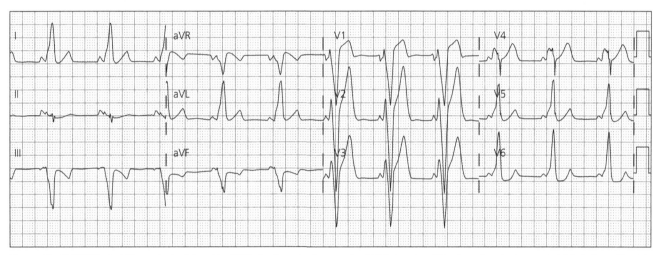

Figure 21.18 WPW mimicking anterior MI and/or LBBB. Again, note the very short PR interval and the slurred upstroke, most visible in lateral leads I, aVL, V5, and V6.

with reciprocal ST depression, which was due to LVH with secondary repolarization abnormalities. The patient in Case 2 was found to have a thrombotic occlusion of the left anterior descending coronary artery. He underwent a thrombectomy and deployment of a bare metal stent with a good outcome. The patient in Case 3 had relief of the discomfort and resolution of the hypertension with administration of nitroglycerine in the ED. The electrocardiographic diagnosis of AMI was questioned, thus an urgent ED bedside echocardiogram confirmed good anterior wall motion and concentric LVH. The patient was admitted to the coronary care unit and ruled out for MI with serial negative troponins. Serial ECGs showed no change. Repeat echocardiogram confirmed profound LVH and no wall motion abnormality.

References

1 Khoury NE, Borzak S, Gokli A, *et al.* "Inadvertent" thrombolytic administration in patients without myocardial infarction: clinical features and outcome. *Ann Emerg Med* 1996;**28**(3):289–93.

2 Larsen GC, Griffith JL, Beshansky JR, *et al.* Electrocardiographic left ventricular hypertrophy in patients with suspected acute cardiac ischemia: Its influence on diagnosis, triage, and short-term prognosis. *J Gen Intern Med* 1994;**9**:666–76.

3 Larson DM, Menssen KM, Sharkey SW, *et al.* "False-positive" cardiac catheterization laboratory activation among patients with suspected ST-segment elevation myocardial infarction. *JAMA* 2007;**298**(23):2754–60.

4 Brady WJ, Perron AD, Martin ML, *et al.* Cause of ST segment abnormality in ED chest pain patients. *Am J Emerg Med* 2001; **19**(1):25–8.

5 Smith SW, Zvosec DL, Henry TD, *et al.* eds. *The ECG in Acute MI: an Evidence-Based Manual of Reperfusion Therapy.* First ed. Lippincott, Williams, and Wilkins: Philadelphia, 2002:358.

6 Brady WJ, Perron AD, Syverud SA, *et al.* Reciprocal ST segment depression: Impact on the electrocardiographic diagnosis of ST segment elevation acute myocardial infarction. *Am J Emerg Med* 2002;**20**(1):35–8.

7 Brady WJ. ST segment and T wave abnormalities not caused by acute coronary syndromes. *Emerg Med Clin North Am* 2006; **24**(1):91–111, vi.

8 Wellens HJ. Acute myocardial infarction and left bundle-branch block – can we lift the veil? (editorial;comment). *N Engl J Med* 1996;**334**(8): 528–9.

9 Go AS, Barron HV, Rundle AC, *et al.* Bundle-branch block and in-hospital mortality in acute myocardial infarction. National Registry of Myocardial Infarction. *Ann Int Med* 1998;**129**(9):690–7.

10 Newby KH, Pisano O, Krucoff MW, *et al.* Incidence and clinical relevance of the occurrence of bundle-branch block in patients treated with thrombolytic therapy. *Circulation* 1996;**94**(10):2424–8.

11 Melgarejo-Moreno A, Galcera-Tomas J, Garcia-Alberola, *et al.* Incidence, clinical characteristics, and prognostic significance of right bundle-branch block in acute myocardial infarction: a study in the thrombolytic era. *Circulation* 1997;**96**(4):1139–44.

12 Moreno AM, Alberola AG, Tomas JG, *et al.* Incidence and prognostic significance of right bundle branch block in patients with acute myocardial infarction receiving thrombolytic therapy. *Int J Cardiol* 1997;**61**(2):135–41.

13 Fibrinolytic Therapy Trialists' (FTT) Collaborative Group. Indications for fibrinolytic therapy in suspected acute myocardial infarction: collaborative overview of early mortality and major morbidity results from all randomised trials of more than 1000 patients. *Lancet* 1994;**343**:311–22.

14 Antman EM, Anbe DT, Armstrong PW, *et al.* ACC/AHA guidelines for the management of patients with ST-elevation myocardial infarction – executive summary. A report of the American College of Cardiology/American Heart Association Task Force on Practice Guidelines (Writing Committee to revise the 1999 guidelines for the management of patients with acute myocardial infarction). *J Am Coll Cardiol* 2004;**44**(3):671–719.

15 Fesmire FM, Brady WJ, Hahn S, *et al.* Clinical policy: indications for reperfusion therapy in emergency department patients with suspected acute myocardial infarction. American College of Emergency Physicians Clinical Policies Subcommittee (Writing Committee) on Reperfusion Therapy in Emergency Department Patients with Suspected Acute Myocardial Infarction. *Ann Emerg Med* 2006;**48**(4):358–83.

16 Cannon CP, McCabe CH, Stone PH, *et al.* The electrocardiogram predicts one-year outcome of patients with unstable angina and non-Q wave myocardial infarction: results of the TIMI III Registry ECG Ancillary Study. Thrombolysis in Myocardial Ischemia. *J Am Coll Cardiol* 1997;**30**(1):133–40.

17 Smith SW, Bertog SC, Lathrop LM, *et al.* ST/S ratio distinguishes left bundle branch block from left bundle branch block with simultaneous anterior myocardial infarction (abstract). *Acad Emerg Med* 2006;**13**(5 Suppl):S160–1.

18 Shlipak MG, Go AS, Frederick PD. Treatment and outcomes of left bundle-branch block patients with myocardial infarction who present without chest pain. *J Am Coll Cardiol* 2000;**36**(3): 706–12.

19 Barron HV, Bowlby LJ, Breen T, *et al.* Use of reperfusion therapy for acute myocardial infarction in the United States: data from the National Registry of Myocardial Infarction 2. *Circulation* 1997;**97**(12):1150–6.

20 Krumholz HM, Murillo JE, Chen J, *et al.* Thrombolytic therapy for eligible elderly patients with acute myocardial infarction. *JAMA* 1997;**277**(21):1683–8.

21 Sgarbossa EB, Pinski SL, Barbagelata A, *et al.* Electrocardiographic diagnosis of evolving acute myocardial infarction in the presence of left bundle-branch block. *N Engl J Med* 1996; **334**(8):481–7.

22 Li SF, Walden PL, Marcilla O, *et al.* Electrocardiographic diagnosis of myocardial infarction in patients with left bundle branch block. *Ann Emerg Med* 1999;**36**(6):561–6.

23 Kontos MC, McQueen RH, Jesse RL, *et al.* Can myocardial infarction be rapidly identified in emergency department patients who have left bundle branch block? *Ann Emerg Med* 2001;**37**(5): 431–8.

24 Rodriguez RM, Tabas J. A meta-analysis of the Sgarbossa criteria for acute myocardial infarction in the presence of left bundle branch block. *Acad Emerg Med* 2006;**13** (5 Suppl 1):S33–4.

25 Fesmire FM, Percy RF, Bardoner JB, *et al.* Usefulness of automated serial 12-lead ECG monitoring during the initial emergency department evaluation of patients with chest pain. *Ann Emerg Med* 1998;**31**(1):3–11.

26 Fesmire FM, Percy RF, Wears RL, *et al.* Initial ECG in Q wave and non-Q wave myocardial infarction. *Ann Emerg Med* 1989;**18**(7): 741–6.

27 Rouan GW, Lee TH, Cook EF, *et al.* Clinical characteristics and outcome of acute myocardial infarction in patients with initially normal or nonspecific electrocardiograms (a report from the Multicenter Chest Pain Study). *Am J Cardiol* 1989 **64**(18): 1087–92.

28 Rude RE, Poole WK, Muller J, *et al.* Electrocardiographic and clinical criteria for recognition of acute myocardial infarction based on analysis of 3,697 patients. *Am J Cardiol* 1983;**52**(8): 936–42.

29 Menown IB, Mackenzie G, Adgey AA. Optimizing the initial 12-lead electrocardiographic diagnosis of acute myocardial infarction. *Eur Heart J* 2000;**21**(4):275–83.

30 Schmitt C, Lehmann G, Schmieder S, *et al.* Diagnosis of acute myocardial infarction in angiographically documented occluded infarct vessel: limitations of ST-segment elevation in standard and extended ECG leads. *Chest* 2001;**120**(5):1540–6.

31 Wackers FJT. The diagnosis of myocardial infarction in the presence of left bundle branch block. *Cardiol Clin* 1987;**5**(3):393–401.

32 Stark KS, Krucoff MW, Schryver B, *et al.* Quantification of ST-segment changes during coronary angioplasty in patients with left bundle branch block. *Am J Cardiol* 1991;**67**(15):1219–22.

33 Madias JE, Sinha A, Agarwal H, *et al.* ST-Segment elevation in leads V1–V3 in patients with left bundle branch block (LBBB). *J Electrocardiol* 2001;**34**(1):87–8.

34 Fesmire FM. ECG diagnosis of acute myocardial infarction in the presence of left bundle-branch block in patients undergoing continuous ECG monitoring. *Ann Emerg Med* 1995;**26**(1):69–82.

35 Sgarbossa EB, Pinski SL, Gates KB, *et al.* Early electrocardiographic diagnosis of acute myocardial infarction in the presence of ventricular paced rhythm. GUSTO-I investigators. *Am J Cardiol* 1996;**77**(5):423–4.

Chapter 22 | What are the electrocardiographically silent areas of the heart?

Samuel J. Stellpflug[1], Joel S. Holger[2], Stephen W. Smith[3]
[1]Regions Hospital, St Paul, MN, USA
[2]Senior Staff Physician, Regions Hospital, St Paul, MN, USA
[3]University of Minnesota, Hennegin County Medical Center, Minneapolis, MN, USA

Case presentations

Case 1: A 75-year-old female is brought to the emergency department (ED) from the bronchoscopy suite with chest pain, dyspnea, and systolic blood pressure (BP) in the 70s–80s. The initial electrocardiogram (ECG) is shown in Figure 22.1. The ECG computer algorithm and the physician diagnose non-specific findings. Blood pressure improves with fluids. With a normal initial troponin, the patient undergoes chest computed tomography (CT) to rule out pulmonary embolism (PE), aortic dissection, and obvious bronchus injury; this result is normal and she is admitted to the intensive care unit (ICU), where intermittent chest pain continues.

Case 2: A 51-year-old female presents to the ED with 1 h of chest pain. The initial ECG is shown in Figure 22.2a. This ECG shows only 0.5–1.0 mm ST depression in leads V2 and V3, highly suspicious for ischemia. The previous ECG is obtained (Figure 22.2b, V1–V3 only), confirming a delta ST (relative ST depression) of 2 mm in V2 and V3.

Case 3: A 60-year-old male presents with 2 h of 4/10 chest pain. His exam, including vital signs, is normal. The ECG in Figure 22.3a was recorded 40 min later, the pain was rated 6–8/10, and a second ECG was recorded (Figure 22.3b).

The electrocardiographically silent areas of the heart

These patients experienced acute coronary events that were evident only to the prepared ECG interpreter. The high left lateral wall and posterior wall of the left ventricle, and the right ventricle, may harbor large areas of ischemic myocardium at risk of infarction, but manifest minimal or subtle ECG findings, or none at all. These regions may be "electrocar-

diographically silent." Other regions may also manifest minimal ECG changes, partly because ischemia is a dynamic process and the ECG must be recorded at the appropriate time.

Normal and non-specific ECGs in ACS

A non-specific initial ECG, and even a normal ECG, does not rule out myocardial infarction (MI). Many patients with MI by biomarkers have normal or non-specific initial ECGs; in two similar studies of ED patients with chest pain and a normal ECG, 3.5% were later diagnosed with acute MI by serum cardiac markers. Of those with a "non-specific" ECG, 9% were shown to have MI [1,2]. Conversely, 6–8% of a group of patients with chest pain later shown to have MI based on a rise in CK-MB had an initially normal ECG, and 22–35% had an initial non-specific ECG [1–5].

Patients with normal or non-specific ECGs have better short-term clinical outcomes and fewer complications, if their ECGs do not become positive [2,5–7]. Zalenski and colleagues saw no significant differences in the rate of in-hospital complications between MI patients with negative and positive ECGs, but all complications in ECG-negative patients occurred only after development of serial ECG positivity [8].

Serial ECGs can improve the sensitivity of the ECG for acute MI and acute coronary syndrome (ACS). In a series of 1000 patients with chest pain, the sensitivities of the initial ECG for diagnosing acute MI and ACS were 55.4 and 27.5%, respectively. When ECGs were recorded every 20 min and evaluated by an automated ST segment analyzer, these numbers improved to 68.1 and 34.2%, respectively [9]. See Chapter 20 for more discussion of serial ECGs.

In patients with potential myocardial ischemia there is a difference between "normal" and "non-specific." A normal ECG has normal sinus rhythm, a normal QRS with normal R wave progression, no left ventricular hypertrophy (LVH), no abnormal Q waves, no ST elevation (STE) or depression ≥ 0.5 mm (relative to the corresponding PR segments), no upsloping or downsloping ST segment, and T waves with size proportional to the QRS and an axis close to that of the QRS.

Critical Decisions in Emergency and Acute Care Electrocardiography,
1st edition. Edited by W.J. Brady and J.D. Truwit. © 2009 Blackwell Publishing. ISBN: 9781405159067

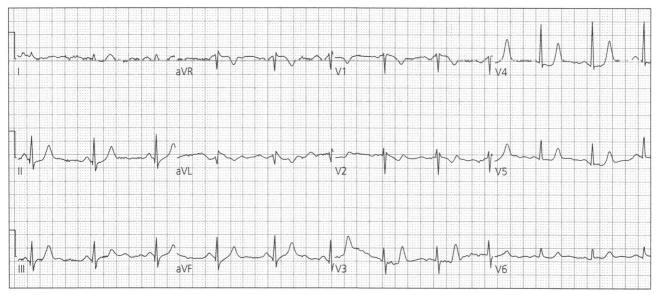

Figure 22.1 Subtle ST depression in V3–V5, with non-specific T wave changes in I and aVL, later proven to be due to a large inferolateral MI from occlusion of a dominant circumflex.

The non-specific ("non-diagnostic") ECG is abnormal but non-diagnostic of ACS: no diagnostic ST elevation or depression, T wave inversion, or inverted U wave (see Chapter 15). The abnormalities may consist of previously formed Q waves, LVH, or very minor ST or T wave abnormalities. The T waves may be "flattened" in multiple leads [10]. Patients with non-specific ECGs are more likely to have acute MI than those with normal ECGs [1,2]. Before thrombolytic therapy and percutaneous coronary intervention, patients with acute myocardial infarction with normal or non-specific ECGs clearly had a better prognosis than those with a diagnostic ECG [7]. In the era of reperfusion therapy, acute MI patients with non-specific ECGs and MI may actually have a worse prognosis than the patient with a diagnostic ECG, due to the latter group meeting qualification for reperfusion therapy [11].

Lateral myocardial infarction

The vascular supply of the lateral wall of the heart is comprised of the circumflex artery and its obtuse marginal branches, the first diagonal artery branching off the left anterior descending (LAD) artery, and occasionally branches off a large and dominant right coronary artery (RCA).

As previously stated, infarction in any area of the heart can be missed due to the imperfect sensitivity of the ECG, and the dynamic nature of the process. The lateral wall is particularly silent. The lateral leads are typically defined as precordial leads V5 and V6, and limb leads I and aVL. With left circumflex occlusion there is: (1) STE in either inferior and/or lateral leads, with or without ST depression, in approximately 1/3 of cases (and lateral ST elevation is rarely ≥ 2 mm) (2) ST depression alone in 1/3 and (3) neither ST depression nor elevation in approximately 1/3 [10]. The low sensitivity for lateral wall infarctions is highlighted by comparison with LAD or RCA

occlusions (anterior or inferior wall infarctions), which demonstrate ST segment elevation in 70–95% of cases [12–14].

Electrocardiogram changes in lateral wall MI, when seen, are STE in aVL, I, V5, and/or V6. In high lateral wall injury, there may be STE limited to aVL only. Inferior lead reciprocal ST depression, typically in leads III and aVF, may be more prominent than STE in aVL (see Figure 22.4 and Figure 13.1b) [15]. Furthermore, because the axis of aVL is often perpendicular to the QRS axis, QRS voltage may be very small in aVL. Because STE amplitude cannot be greater than QRS amplitude, STE in the presence of transmural ischemia may be < 1 mm. Thus, STE must be evaluated relative to the QRS voltage, with proportionality in mind. This also applies to T wave enlargement (hyperacute T waves, see Figure 13.1b).

In posterolateral MI, STE is often apparent in leads I, aVL, V5, and V6. Additionally, there may be anterior lead ST depression in V1–V3 due to posterior wall infarction, with STE in posterior leads V7, V8, and V9. Figure 22.5a is the initial ECG of a 93-year-old female presenting with severe nausea, which shows evidence of a high posterolateral MI. Notice the anterior precordial lead and inferior lead depression, and the STE in lead aVL that is also minimally present in lead I. Figure 22.5b is the improved ECG after initial ED treatment with medical therapy.

With inferolateral MI, there may be the same lateral lead STE, but also STE in II, III, and aVF. In Figure 22.6, an inferior posterolateral MI is shown, and there is evidence of inferior STE, anterior STE, and lateral STE.

Posterior myocardial infarction

Posterior MI is usually associated with inferior or lateral MI. However, when it is isolated to just the posterior wall, it is relatively electrocardiographically silent. Complete occlusion of

(a)

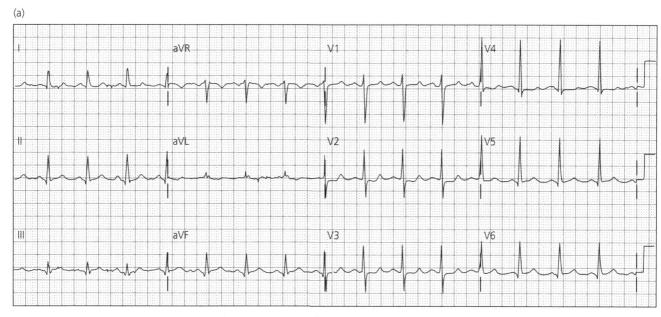

(b)

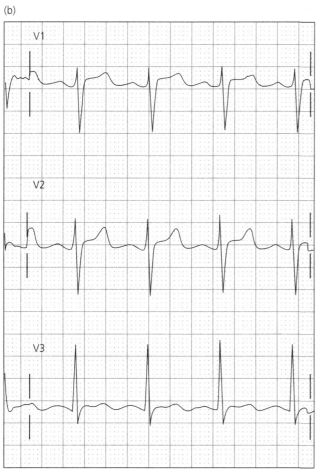

Figure 22.2 (a) Anterior ST depression, minimal, reflecting significant posterior wall STEMI from obtuse marginal occlusion. (b) Previous ECG, showing baseline J-point elevation, and demonstrating that the small amount of ST depression seen in (a) is a large relative ST deviation (large delta-ST). Reprinted with permission from Smith SW, Zvosec DL, Sharkey SW, Henry TD. *The ECG in Acute MI: an Evidence-Based Manual of Reperfusion Therapy.* 2002:140 (figure 16-1) [10].

the blood supply to the posterior wall, which is from the circumflex and its obtuse marginal branches or the RCA and its posterior descending branch, may manifest no STE even with large amounts of myocardium at risk [16]. From 3.3 to 8.5% of all acute MI, as diagnosed by serum cardiac markers, are isolated posterior MIs that present without STE on the standard ECG, and thus the diagnosis is often missed (Figures 22.6 and 22.7) [16–20].

If isolated posterior ST elevation myocardial infarction (STEMI) does manifest findings on the standard 12-lead

(a)

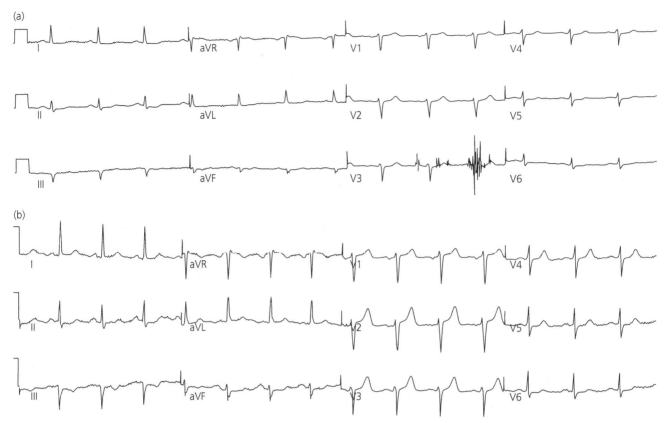

(b)

Figure 22.3 (a) Normal ECG. (b) Minimal STE of lead V2, and somewhat prominent T waves. It is tempting to diagnose early repolarization, but the R wave amplitude is insufficient to do so. When compared with the previous V1–V3 (a), it is definitely changed. Several interpreters missed this change, but it is clearly present.

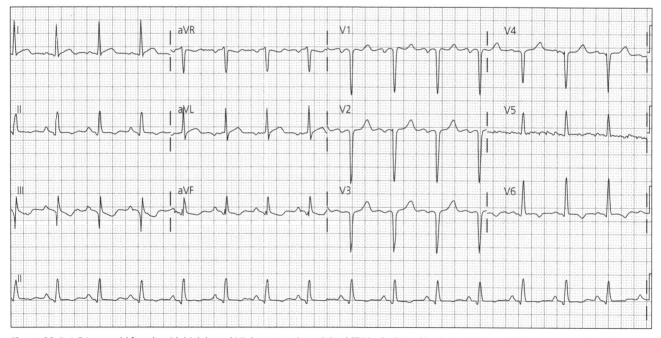

Figure 22.4 A 54-year-old female with high lateral MI demonstrating minimal STE in the lateral leads I and aVL, and ST depression in the inferior leads. There are anterior QS waves of old MI. Her troponin peaked at 100 ng/mL. An occluded first diagonal artery was stented.

(a)

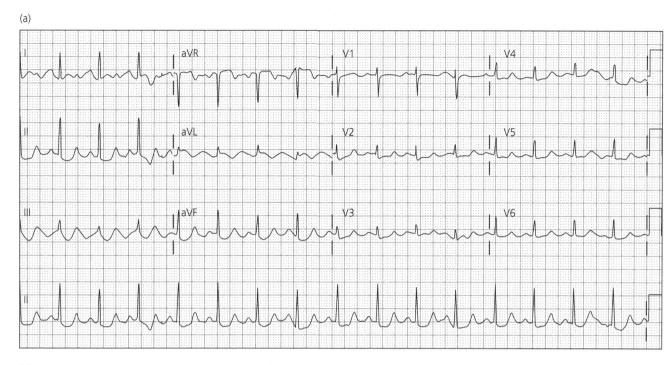

(b)

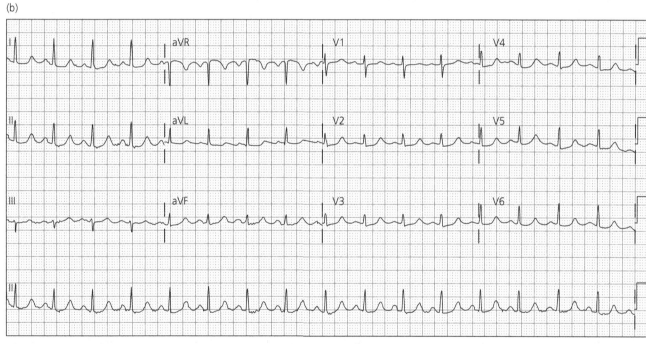

Figure 22.5 (a) Initial ECG of high posterolateral infarction pattern. Note 1 mm STE in aVL, with reciprocal inferior ST depression, as well as anterior ST depression with large R/S ratio in V2, both indicative of posterior MI. (b) ST findings resolved after immediate reperfusion.

ECG, it manifests ST depression in V1–V4, occasionally extending into V5 and V6 (see Figure 22.6). Unfortunately, ST depression may also be due to subendocardial ischemia of a different coronary distribution, for which fibrinolytics are not indicated. Transient ST depression may represent transient posterior wall transmural ischemia or anterior wall subendocardial ischemia [21–23]. Persistent ST depression in V1–V4 is most likely posterior MI. ST depression > 2 mm

in V1–V3 is 90% specific for posterior STEMI, whereas ST depression in V4–V6 is more likely to be subendocardial ischemia [24]. Most people have some STE in right precordial leads, and any ST depression may be a significant ST shift, or delta ST, from baseline (see Figure 22.2). In posterior STEMI, the T waves may be inverted or upright, and increased R wave amplitude (representing the anterior view of a posterior evolving Q wave, as would be seen in the posterior leads

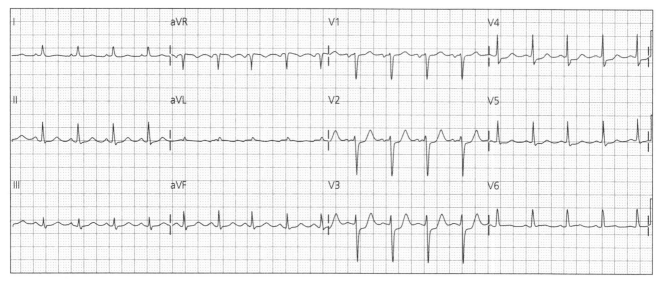

Figure 22.6 Isolated posterior MI presenting with ST depression only, in V2 and V3. The ECG is of a 64-year-old woman with chest pain, which resolved with aspirin and nitroglycerine. ST depression resolved also, and the patient was treated medically. Maximum troponin was 12.68 ng/mL, and angiogram revealed TIMI 2 flow and thrombus in a large obtuse marginal branch, removed with thrombectomy. Echo showed a large posterolateral wall motion abnormality that later resolved.

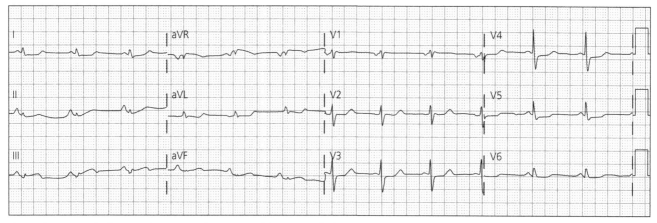

Figure 22.7 Missed inferoposterior MI. Another 64-year-old woman with chest pain. There is ST depression from V2 to V6 and aVL (1 mm in V3 and V4), with minimal STE in lead III. This was missed in the ED. Troponin later peaked at 30 ng/mL. Non-urgent angiogram showed occlusion of the circumflex distal to second obtuse marginal, but proximal to two posterolateral branches. Echo showed an inferoposterior wall motion abnormality.

V7–V9) may not be present initially. With infarction, the R wave eventually becomes greater than the S wave (R > S, or R/S ratio > 1). Additionally, ST depression is absent in many patients with posterior MI.

If there is high suspicion for MI, and there is isolated ST depression in precordial leads, placement of posterior leads V7–V9 is indicated to differentiate posterior MI from subendocardial ischemia. In the presence of posterior MI, there should be ≥ 0.5 mm STE in two leads (see Chapter 18). At 1 mm of STE, the sensitivities (80%) of the standard leads and the posterior leads are approximately equal, but posterior leads are more specific (84% versus 57%) [25]. At an STE

cutoff of ≥ 0.5 mm, the sensitivity of posterior leads improves to 94%, without significant loss of specificity [20]. Suspicious ST segments in the precordial leads (see Figures 22.2, 22.6 and 22.7) should prompt the use of posterior leads.

Routine use of posterior leads may be unwarranted. Zalenski and colleagues found that recording posterior leads on all patients with suspected MI, at a 1 mm cutoff, increased the sensitivity of the ECG for MI from 57.7 to 59.7%, with a decrease in specificity from 91 to 89.4% [26]. Brady and colleagues applied posterior leads to 595 patients in a chest pain unit and detected no additional MIs [27]. Posterior leads may help to determine whether the culprit blood vessel is the

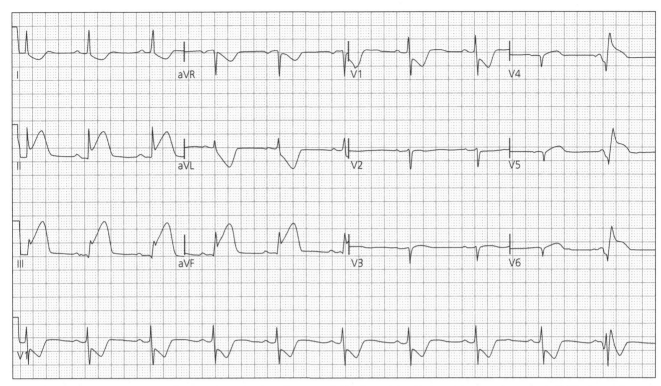

Figure 22.8 Right-sided ECG with inferior and RV infarction. The precordial leads are right-sided, and the second complex in RV4 is aberrantly conducted.

circumflex or the RCA [28,29]. Posterior leads are essential to confirm posterior STEMI, as opposed to subendocardial ischemia, as the etiology of right precordial ST depression, prior to administering fibrinolytics (see Case 1, Chapter 18).

Right ventricular myocardial infarction

Most right ventricular MI (RVMI) is seen in the context of inferior STEMI, and thus the ACS is obvious, though the RV involvement may not be. In the setting of inferior MI, especially with ST depression in lead I (indicates RCA, not circumflex, as the involved artery) or STE in lead V1, RVMI should be high on the differential and right-sided ECG should be recorded. See Figure 22.8.

Isolated RVMI is much more electrocardiographically silent and much more rare, and happens in three circumstances: first, with occlusion of the proximal RCA when the left coronary artery is dominant (left circumflex artery supplying the posterior descending artery and RCA only supplying the RV); second, if the RCA is dominant, with branch occlusion of the RV marginal artery; third, in the setting of previous completed inferior QS wave MI due to a distal lesion is now followed by occlusion of a proximal lesion. In this latter case, the inferior wall may show no ST changes although the RV is injured. Isolated RVMI should be suspected if there is STE in lead V1 on the standard 12-lead ECG.

Subtle inferior or anterior MI

The inferior and anterior walls are the most easily recorded by the ECG. Nevertheless, sometimes large MI shows little ST deviation (Case 3, Figure 22.3). Some reasons for this are clear, others speculative. The artery may supply a relatively small amount of myocardium, there may be good collateral circulation, or there may be subtotal occlusion with barely adequate flow and perfusion. There may be a large ischemic penumbra, still viable, but injured and slowly infarcting. Furthermore, it may be early after occlusion; in one study of a series of LAD occlusions, 41% had < 2 mm of ST elevation [30]. There was correlation with a short time since onset of pain.

Conclusion

Acute coronary syndrome cannot be ruled out with a normal or non-specific ECG. Up to 5% of patients with chest pain from MI have a normal ECG, and > 20% have a non-specific ECG. Large MIs of the lateral and posterior walls of the left ventricle, and of the right ventricle, are not always detected by the standard 12-lead. Even the entire inferior or anterior walls can be at risk, but manifest minimal STE.

Expertise in detecting subtle abnormalities is crucial. In a patient who has a high likelihood for ischemia, close inspection should be given for enlarged T waves, terminal QRS distortion, R wave diminution, Q waves, straightening of the ST segment, subtle ST depression, reciprocal ST depression in inferior leads as reciprocal to aVL, abnormal T inversion, U wave inversion, and abnormal proportionality. Combining the patient's clinical presentation, the practitioners' clinical suspicion, the detection of subtle abnormalities, and adjunctive studies, gives the best chance of recognizing ACS, and particularly coronary occlusion, in a timely fashion.

Case conclusions

In Case 1, the troponin levels climbed from negative to 85 ng/mL in the 12 h following her initial evaluation, with no ECG changes. Cardiac cath. showed complete proximal occlusion of a dominant circumflex artery at the site of a previous stent, with marked inferolateral hypokinesis. Follow-up ECG showed some minimal resolution of ST depression. In Case 2, these interval changes are highly suggestive of posterior infarction. This progression, however, was not recognized and the patient was treated conservatively until the troponin returned very elevated. Subsequent echocardiogram (echo) showed akinetic posterior wall, and angiography revealed 95% stenosis of the second obtuse marginal, which was then dilated and stented. In Case 3, the change from the first ECG was not appreciated. Complete anterior MI ensued. The patient did not receive reperfusion therapy. Subsequent angiogram confirmed LAD occlusion; there was significant loss of myocardium with subsequent low ejection fraction and congestive heart failure.

References

1 Karlson BW, Herlitz J, Wiklund O, *et al.* Early prediction of acute myocardial infarction from clinical history, examination and electrocardiogram in the emergency room. *Am J Cardiol* 1991; **68**:171–5.

2 Rouan GW, Lee TH, Cook EF, *et al.* Clinical characteristics and outcome of acute myocardial infarction in patients with initially normal or non-specific electrocardiograms (a report from the Multicenter Chest Pain Study). *Am J Cardiol* 1989;**64**:1087–92.

3 Karlson BW, Herlitz J. Hospitalisations, infarct development, and mortality in patients with chest pain and a normal admission electrocardiogram in relation to gender. *Coron Artery Dis* 1996; **7**:231–7.

4 McCarthy BD, Wong JB, Selker HP. Detecting acute cardiac ischemia in the emergency department: a review of the literature. *J Gen Intern Med* 1990;**5**:365–73.

5 Welch RD, Zalenski RJ, Frederick PD, *et al.* Prognostic value of a normal or non-specific initial electrocardiogram in acute myocardial infarction. *JAMA* 2001;**286**:1977–84.

6 Braunwald E, Jones RH, Mark DB, *et al.* Diagnosing and managing unstable angina. Agency for Health Care Policy and Research. *Circulation* 1994;**90**:613–22.

7 Brush JE, Brand DA, Acampora D, *et al.* Use of the initial electrocardiogram to predict in-hospital complications of acute myocardial infarction. *New Engl J Med* 1985;**312**:1137–41.

8 Zalenski RJ, Rydman RJ, Sloan EP, *et al.* The emergency department electrocardiogram and hospital complications in myocardial infarction patients. *Acad Emerg Med* 1996;**3**:318–25.

9 Fesmire FM, Percy RF, Bardoner JB, *et al.* Usefulness of automated serial 12-lead ECG monitoring during the initial emergency department evaluation of patients with chest pain. *Ann Emerg Med* 1998;**31**:3–11.

10 Smith SW, Zvosec DL, Henry TD, Sharkey SW. *The ECG in Acute MI: an Evidence-Based Manual of Reperfusion Therapy.* Philadelphia: Lippincott, Williams, and Wilkins, 2002:358.

11 Cragg DR, Friedman HZ, Bonema JD, *et al.* Outcome of patients with acute myocardial infarction who are ineligible for thrombolytic therapy. *Ann Int Med* 1991;**115**:173–7.

12 Berry C, Zalewsky A, Kovach R, *et al.* Surface electrocardiogram in the detection of transmural myocardial ischemia during coronary artery occlusion. *Am J Cardiol* 1989;**63**:21–6.

13 Huey BL, Beller GA, Kaiser D, Gibson RS. A comprehensive analysis of myocardial infarction due to left circumflex artery occlusion: comparison with infarction due to right coronary artery and left anterior descending artery occlusion. *J Am Coll Cardiol* 1988;**12**:1156–66.

14 Schmitt C, Lehmann G, Schmieder S, *et al.* Diagnosis of acute myocardial infarction in angiographically documented occluded infarct vessel: limitations of ST-segment elevation in standard and extended ECG leads. *Chest* 2001;**120**:1540–6.

15 Kosuge M, Kimura K, Toshiyuki I, *et al.* Electrocardiographic criteria for predicting total occlusion of the proximal left anterior descending coronary artery in anterior wall acute myocardial infarction. *Clin Cardiol* 2001;**24**:33–8.

16 O'Keefe JHJ, Sayed-Taha K, Gibson W, *et al.* Do patients with left circumflex coronary artery-related acute myocardial infarction without ST-segment elevation benefit from reperfusion therapy? (see comments). *Am J Cardiol* 1995;**75**:718–20.

17 Melendez LJ, Jones DT, Salcedo JR. Usefulness of three additional electrocardiographic chest leads (V7, V8, V9) in the diagnosis of acute myocardial infarction. *Can Med Assoc J* 1978;**119**: 745–8.

18 Oraii S, Maleki I, Tavakolian AA, *et al.* Prevalence and outcome of ST-segment elevation in posterior electrocardiographic leads during acute myocardial infarction. *J Electrocardiol* 1999;**32**:275– 8.

19 Smith SW, Whitwam W. Acute Coronary Syndromes. *Emerg Med Clin North Am* 2006;**24**:53–89.

20 Wung SF, Drew BJ. New electrocardiographic criteria for posterior wall acute myocardial ischemia validated by a percutaneous transluminal coronary angioplasty model of acute myocardial infarction. *Am J Cardiol* 2001;**87**:970–4; A4.

21 Boden WE, Kleiger RE, Gibson RS, *et al.* Electrocardiographic evolution of posterior acute myocardial infarction: importance of early precordial ST-segment depression. *Am J Cardiol* 1987;**59**: 782–7.

22 Matetzky S, Friemark D, Feinberg MS, *et al.* Acute myocardial infarction with isolated ST-segment elevation in posterior chest leads V7–V9: "hidden" ST-segment elevations revealing acute posterior infarction. *J Am Coll Card* 1999;**34**:748–53.

23 Bairey CN, Shah PK, Lew AS, Hulse S. Electrocardiographic differentiation of occlusion of the left circumflex versus the right coronary artery as a cause of inferior acute myocardial infarction. *Am J Cardiol* 1987;**60**:456–9.

24 Shah A, Wagner GS, Green CL, *et al.* Electrocardiographic differentiation of the ST-segment depression of acute myocardial injury due to the left circumflex artery occlusion from that of myocardial ischemia of nonocclusive etiologies. *Am J Cardiol* 1997;**80**:512–3.

25 Matetzky S, Freimark D, Chouraqui P, *et al.* Significance of ST segment elevations in posterior chest leads (V7–V9) in patients with acute inferior myocardial infarction: application for thrombolytic therapy. *J Am Coll Card* 1998;**31**:506–11.

26 Zalenski RJ, Rydman RJ, Sloan EP, *et al.* Value of posterior and right ventricular leads in comparison to the standard 12-lead electrocardiogram in evaluation of ST-segment elevation in suspected acute myocardial infarction. *Am J Cardiol* 1997;**79**: 1579–85.

27 Brady WJ, Hwang V, Sullivan R. A comparison of 12- and 15-lead ECGS in ED chest pain patients: impact on diagnosis, therapy, and disposition. *Am J Emerg Med* 2000;**18**:239–43.

28 Agarwal JB, Khaw K, Aurignac F, LoCurto A. Importance of posterior chest leads in patients with suspected myocardial infarction, but non-diagnostic, routine 12-lead electrogram. *Am J Cardiol* 1999;**83**:323–6.

29 Kulkarni AU, Brown R, Ayoubi M, Banks VS. Clinical use of posterior electrocardiographic leads: a prospective electrocardiographic analysis during coronary occlusion. *Am Heart J* 1996;**131**: 736–41.

30 Smith SW. Upwardly concave ST segment morphology is common in acute left anterior descending coronary occlusion. *J Emerg Med* 2006;**31**:69–77.

Chapter 23 | What is the value of the prehospital acquired 12-lead ECG?

Michael Christopher Kurz
Virginal Commonwealth University Medical Center, Richmond, VA, USA

Case presentations

In each case the arriving ambulance is advanced life support (ALS) and 12-lead electrocardiogram (ECG) capable.

Case 1: An ambulance arrives at a shopping center to meet a 53-year-old female with "crushing" chest pain and dyspnea for 1 h. The patient is in clear distress, pale, diaphoretic, and feels "weak all over." Her blood pressure (BP) is 85/50, pulse 125, RR 22, and O_2 saturation 97% on room air. The paramedics suspect ST segment elevation myocardial infarction (STEMI) and acquire a 12-lead ECG that reveals STE in leads II, III, aVF, and V3–V6 (Figure 23.1).

Case 2: Emergency medical services (EMS) arrive at a farm to meet a 40-year-old female clutching her chest because of "pressure" for 45 min. The patient denies any medical history. She is diaphoretic. her BP is 200/103, pulse 90, RR 26, and O_2 saturation 100% on oxygen. Emergency medical services suspect STEMI and acquires a 12-lead ECG that reveals STE in leads V1–V3 with reciprocal ST segment depression in II, III, and aVF (Figure 23.2a). Recognizing a STEMI, EMS prepare the patient for transport to the percutaneous coronary intervention (PCI) center, and administer aspirin and nitroglycerin. En route, the patient's symptoms largely resolve, and upon arrival to the PCI center, the hospital ECG demonstrates T wave inversion in V2 and V3 (Figure 23.2b).

Case 3: Emergency medical services arrive at a residence to find a 57-year-old male with 30 min of "squeezing" chest pain that radiates to his left jaw and is accompanied with nausea and diaphoresis. He has a history of diabetes and hypercholestemia. His BP is 134/90, pulse 64, RR 24, and O_2 saturation 98% on 2 L via nasal cannula, and the exam is otherwise normal. Emergency medical services acquire a 12-lead ECG that demonstrates an acute inferior myocardial

infarction (MI) not shown. Travel times to the closest hospital and the closest tertiary care center with PCI are 60 min and 2 h, respectively. Weather precludes summoning aeromedical resources.

Case 4: Emergency medical services arrive at the home of a 48-year-old male who has had 30 min of chest pain. They record the first ECG (Figure 23.3a). It is non-diagnostic of STEMI, but diagnostic of acute coronary syndrome (ACS). After aspirin and nitroglycerine, the chest pain resolved. Upon arrival at the emergency department (ED), the second ECG was obtained (Figure 23.3b). The providers did not see the prehospital ECG; they interpreted the ED ECG as non-diagnostic and admitted the patient to a chest pain unit for "rule out MI."

The value of the prehospital 12-lead electrocardiogram

In 2004, the American College of Cardiology/American Heart Association (ACC/AHA) published guidelines recommending that every STEMI patient receive reperfusion therapy in a timely manner: within 30 min of presentation to the hospital for fibrinolysis, and within 90 min for PCI [1]. While a distinct relationship between delay to fibrinolysis and increasing mortality is well established [2], it was recently demonstrated that for each 30 min of PCI delay there is an associated 7.5% relative increase in 12-month mortality [3]. Percutaneous coronary intervention performed in a timely manner by experienced operators is now the preferred method of reperfusion, with reduction in short-term mortality and long-term morbidity over fibrinolysis [4]. Unfortunately, only one in four hospitals have PCI capability [5], only 79% of the United States population lives within 60 min of a PCI center [6], and of those receiving PCI only 4.2% receive reperfusion within the 90 min ACC/AHA guideline [7]. These facts are even more concerning for those STEMI patients in cardiogenic shock at time of presentation and at high risk of death without PCI [8]. Regardless of the method of reperfusion undertaken, the overriding emphasis of the ACC/AHA guidelines is on reducing the total ischemic

Critical Decisions in Emergency and Acute Care Electrocardiography, 1st edition. Edited by W.J. Brady and J.D. Truwit. © 2009 Blackwell Publishing, ISBN: 9781405159067

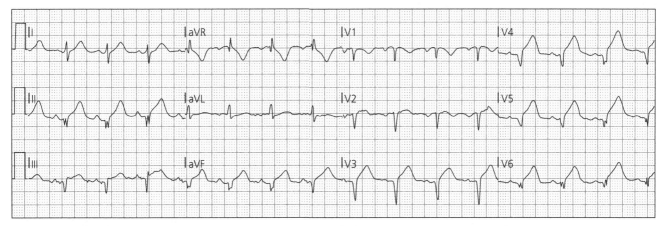

Figure 23.1 There is ST elevation with hyperacute T waves in leads II, III, aVF, and V3–V6, diagnostic of inferolateral STEMI.

(a)

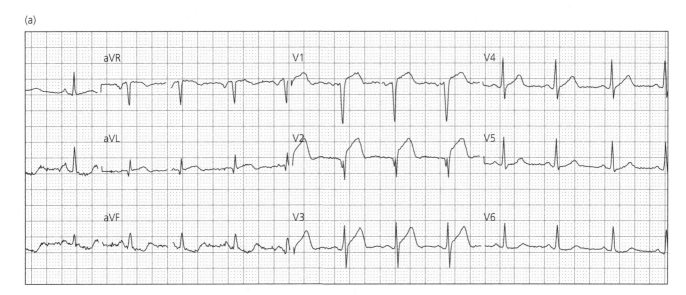

(b)

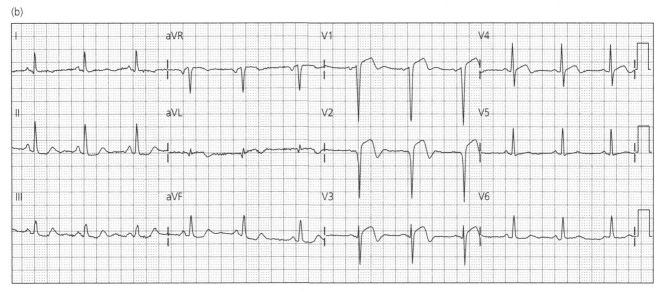

Figure 23.2 (a) There is STE in leads V1–V3 and aVL, with a hyperacute T wave in V2, and also reciprocal inferior ST depression, all diagnostic of anterior STEMI. (b) STE remains, but there is now terminal T wave inversion in V1–V3, typical of spontaneous reperfusion, and identical to Wellens' pattern A T waves.

(a)

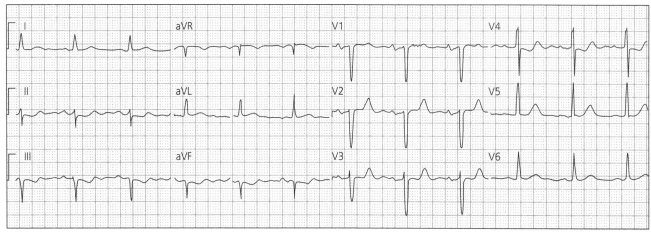

(b)

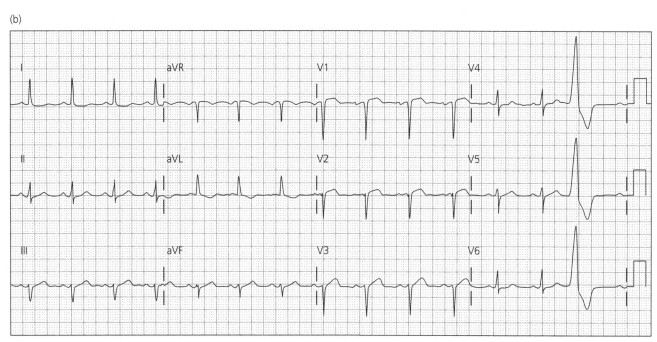

Figure 23.3 Compare (a) (earlier prehospital ECG) with (b) (ECG in the ED). In leads I and aVL, the T waves were upright in the prehospital ECG; in the ED, they were down. In V5 and V6, the T waves were large, in the ED, they were normal. In II, III, and aVF, the T waves were inverted; in the ED, they were upright. The patient had a subtotal LAD occlusion. The ST depression in the inferior leads is suggestive of high lateral STEMI (reciprocal depression); the anterior T waves are somewhat large, and the ST segment in V4 is depressed.

time. Minimizing the interval from symptom onset to restoration of coronary blood flow results in a direct reduction in morbidity and mortality [7].

As the diagnosis of STEMI is based fundamentally on the 12-lead ECG, the largest opportunity for shortening total ischemic time relies on shrinking the interval between onset of symptoms and obtaining an ECG. The ideal beginning of the reperfusion timeline should start with "first medical contact," shifting the burden of STEMI recognition from the door of the hospital to the door of the ambulance. This change in paradigm acknowledges the potential reduction in ischemic time that a system-wide response can provide when prehospital providers have 12-lead ECG capability.

Despite the ACC/AHA Class IIa recommendation for prehospital ALS providers to perform a 12-lead ECG [1], current performance rates are less than 10% nationally [9]. Furthermore, the current National Highway Traffic Safety Administration Emergency Medicine Technician–Paramedic (EMT-P) Standard Curriculum considers 12-lead ECG training as an "enhanced" rather than a core skill [10]. Those paramedics undergo up to 12 hours of classroom instruction to achieve competency and, once trained, must undergo periodic assessment. In addition to these personnel expenses, the $9000–25,000 cost of modern monitor/defibrillator devices with integrated 12-lead ECG capability represents a significant capital investment. Equipping and training prehospital providers to acquire and interpret 12-lead ECGs presents significant financial and operational challenges, but these considerations must be weighed against the potential benefits, namely the reduction of ischemic time, of such prehospital capability [9].

Impact of prehospital 12-lead electrocardiogram on hospital-based reperfusion

Once acquired, the main benefit of prehospital 12-lead ECG acquisition comes from prompt recognition of patients with STEMI and a reduction in their total ischemic time. While many sources have shown that paramedics can be trained to interpret a 12-lead ECG for STEMI as well as a board-certified emergency physician or cardiologist [11], many EMS systems are too large or diverse for all prehospital providers to retain proficiency. Therefore, in Los Angeles County, California [12], an EMS system with 27 separate agencies and > 2500 paramedics, relies upon the electronic interpretation of the ECG using the Marquette 12SL algorithm, i.e. "* * * ACUTE MI * * *", for its high rate of specificity [13]. One EMS system instituted prehospital activation for those who have a Marquette 12SL-diagnosed acute MI, with the additional requirement of chest pain. Chest pain and algorithm-positive ECG was present in 70% of all STEMIs transported by EMS, and in a before and after analysis of such patients, the mean door-to-balloon time (DBT) was decreased by 30 min, from 86 to 56 min; all patients had a DBT < 90 min [14]. By having chest pain as a requirement, there were very few false-positives, and for those, the cath. lab. was deactivated by the emergency physician upon arrival of the patient. An alternative is transmission of the prehospital 12-lead ECG via cellular, landline, wireless broadband, or Wi-Fi technology to a facsimile machine, a direct digital writer, or an internet site accessible by any number of hand-held devices, allowing an emergency physician or cardiologist to confirm the diagnosis. However, this requires expensive technology that can readily fail, and the time used for transmission and interpretation by the hospital-based physician could be used to prepare the cath. team [10,15,16].

A number of large EMS systems have demonstrated that prehospital 12-lead ECGs can be performed safely, accurately, and with minimal impact upon scene time [17,18]. The diagnostic quality of a correctly performed prehospital ECG is equal to those acquired within the hospital [17,19]. A short delay of 5 min for acquiring the tracing is inconsequential when one considers the 15–80 min reduction in door to treatment times for those patients who had a prehospital 12-lead ECG performed and advanced notification received [20,21].

These benefits of prehospital ECGs can be maximized with implementation of a regional STEMI care system modeled after the current trauma system as in Case 1 [22]. In each system, those patients most critically ill or injured are preferentially transported to predesignated receiving centers best able to deliver specialized care [12]. However, an important distinction exists: the trauma system encourages over-triage as it focuses upon sensitivity, while a STEMI system of care should focus upon specificity to avoid a significant reallocation of non-STEMI patients to designated PCI centers.

The first example of such STEMI systems emerged in January, 2003 in Boston, Massachusetts. In Boston, STEMI patients are identified by paramedics interpreting prehospital 12-lead ECGs and transported to one of eleven designated centers that agree to use PCI as their primary reperfusion strategy [23]. Since its inception, median DBTs for patients transported by Boston EMS have dropped from 91 to 67.5 min with 92% of patients going immediately to PCI [24].

The prehospital 12-lead ECG has the most impact on total ischemic time when the STEMI patient is recognized, diverted to an appropriate PCI center, and the receiving hospital is notified while the patient is still en route. In the United States and abroad, STEMI systems with advance notification may bypass the ED completely during daylight hours, traveling directly to the Cardiac Catheterization Lab on the EMS stretcher resulting in some sub-30 min DBTs [21,25]. The quantitative reduction in these times is just as dramatic when EMS prenotification occurs "after hours," allowing the cardiac catherization team and the patient to travel to the destination hospital in parallel [26]. While complex, a prehospital acquired 12-lead ECG allows such STEMI systems to significantly reduce both total ischemic time and in-hospital mortality without sacrificing patient safety [21], even in patients most at risk who present in cardiogenic shock [27].

Finally, just as serial ECGs are of use for ED patients, they may improve prehospital sensitivity for ACS or STEMI. Leads may be kept in place, with serial recordings during transport (see Figures 20.2 and 20.4).

Utility of prehospital ECG on the diagnosis of unstable angina and non ST elevation MI

In addition to reducing total ischemic time in STEMI, prehospital 12-lead ECG may also help to identify symptomatic cardiac ischemia that resolves prior to ED arrival. The prehospital ECG is often acquired by EMS while the patient is symptomatic and before any therapy has begun. As in Cases 2 and 4, this prehospital ECG, when used in combination with serially obtained hospital ECGs, may identify evolving [28] or resolving ischemic changes that would have been otherwise missed [16]. Thus, the prehospital ECG may aid in the diagnosis of chest pain because abnormalities on the prehospital ECG may no longer be present by the time of

ED arrival, and the changes can be diagnostic, as in Case 4 [29,30].

The impact of the prehospital 12-lead electrocardiogram on prehospital care

The initial introduction of the prehospital 12-lead ECG came at the behest of the investigation and then introduction of prehospital fibrinolysis. As early as 1985, Gotsman reported the successful use of prehospital streptokinase in Jerusalem, Israel [31]. Where PCI may not be available, as in Case 3, this strategy has proven to be feasible, safe, and effective, and confers up to a 15% mortality benefit as the time savings approach 60 min [32,33].

As part of their 2004 guidelines, the ACC/AHA has suggested that prehospital fibrinolysis may be reasonable only if: (1) a physician is present in the ambulance, or (2) in well-organized EMS systems with career paramedics equipped with 12-lead ECG with electronic interpretation or direct medical oversight and a medical director with experience in STEMI management and an ongoing program of quality improvement [1]. Aside from fibrinolytic therapy, the prehospital diagnosis of STEMI may also allow for early administration of adjunctive therapies beyond aspirin including low molecular weight heparin [34], clopidogrel [35], and even a glycoprotein IIb/IIIa antagonist [36].

Case conclusions

In Case 1, EMS recognized that their patient was in shock and suffering a STEMI, and transported her to a PCI center. During the 14-min transport to the PCI hospital, EMS passed two closer non-PCI capable hospitals. Upon arrival, the ECG was reviewed by the emergency physician and EMS were directed to the catheterization laboratory where an interventional team was waiting. The patient underwent PCI with placement of a stent in the proximal LAD. Her prehospital recognition to reperfusion time was 46 min.

In Case 2, based upon the serial ECG changes demonstrated on prehospital ECG, the patient went directly to the catheterization laboratory where angiography demonstrated a proximal LAD lesion, but with TIMI-3 flow. There was extension of the lesion into the left main coronary artery. No PCI was attempted and the patient went emergently to the operating room for coronary artery bypass grafting.

Paramedics prepared the patient in Case 3 for transport and completed a fibrinolytic administration checklist. En route to the local hospital, the paramedics contacted online medical direction in the destination ED to authorize prehospital fibrinolysis. Twenty minutes after administration of fibrinolytic therapy, the patient had a 14-beat run of ventricular tachycardia, relief of systems, and resolution of ST segment changes on ECG.

In the chest pain unit, the patient in Case 4 had recurrence of pain. Repeat ECG showed diffuse anterolateral ST elevation and the patient went emergently to the catheterization laboratory for PCI of an occluded LAD. Later, the prehospital ECG was found and it was noted that the T waves in I and aVL had been upright in the prehospital ECG (in the ED, they were negative). The T waves had been large in V5 and V6, (in the ED, they were normal). The T waves had been inverted in II, III, and aVF (in the ED, they were upright). This change is unequivocally diagnostic of ACS and would have prompted anti-thrombotic therapy and administration of GPIIb-IIIa inhibitors, admission to a higher intensity unit, or possibly immediate angiography.

References

1 Antman EM, Anbe DT, Armstrong PW, *et al.* ACC/AHA guidelines for the management of patients with ST-elevation myocardial infarction – executive summary. A report of the American College of Cardiology/American Heart Association Task Force on Practice Guidelines (Writing Committee to revise the 1999 guidelines for the management of patients with acute myocardial infarction). *J Am Coll Cardiol* 2004;**44**(3):671–719.

2 Cannon CP, Gibson CM, Lambrew CT, *et al.* Relationship of symptom-onset-to-balloon time and door-to-balloon time with mortality in patients undergoing angioplasty for acute myocardial infarction. *JAMA* 2000;**283**(22):2941–7.

3 De Luca G, Suryapranata H, Ottervanger JP, *et al.* Time delay to treatment and mortality in primary angioplasty for acute myocardial infarction: every minute of delay counts. *Circulation* 2004;**109**(10):1223–5.

4 Keeley EC. Primary angioplasty versus intravenous thrombolytic therapy for acute myocardial infarction: A quantitative review of 23 randomized trials. *Lancet* 2003;**361**:13–20.

5 Wennberg DE, Lucas FL, Siewers AE, *et al.* Outcomes of percutaneous coronary interventions performed at centers without and with onsite coronary artery bypass graft surgery. *JAMA* 2004;**292**(16):1961–8.

6 Nallamothu BK, Bates ER, Wang Y, *et al.* Driving times and distances to hospitals with percutaneous coronary intervention in the United States: implications for prehospital triage of patients with ST-elevation myocardial infarction. *Circulation* 2006;**113**(9): 1189–95.

7 Nallamothu BK, Bradley EH, Krumholz HM. Time to treatment in primary percutaneous coronary intervention. *N Engl J Med* 2007;**357**(16):1631–8.

8 Hochman JS, Sleeper LA, Webb JG, *et al.* Early revascularization in acute myocardial infarction complicated by cardiogenic shock. *N Engl J Med* 1999;**341**(9):625–34.

9 Curtis JP, Portnay EL, Wang Y, *et al.* The prehospital electrocardiogram and time to reperfusion in patients with acute myocardial infarction, 2000–2002: findings from the National Registry of Myocardial Infarction-4. *J Am Coll Cardiol* 2006;**47**(8): 1544–52.

10 Garvey JL, MacLeod BA, Sopko G, *et al.* Prehospital 12-lead electrocardiography programs: a call for implementation by emergency medical services systems providing advanced life

support – National Heart Attack Alert Program (NHAAP) Coordinating Committee; National Heart, Lung, and Blood Institute (NHLBI); National Institutes of Health. *J Am Coll Cardiol* 2006;**47**(3): 485–91.

11 Feldman JA, Brinsfield K, Bernard S, *et al.* Real-time paramedic compared with blinded physician identification of ST-segment elevation myocardial infarction: results of an observational study. *Am J Emerg Med* 2005;**23**(4):443–8.

12 Rokos IC, Larson DM, Henry TD, *et al.* Rationale for establishing regional ST-elevation myocardial infarction receiving center (SRC) networks. *Am Heart J* 2006;**152**(4):661–7.

13 Kudenchuk PJ, Ho MT, Weaver WD, *et al.* Accuracy of computer-interpreted electrocardiography in selecting patients for thrombolytic therapy. *J Am Coll Card* 1991;**17**(7):1486–91.

14 Bachour FA, Smith SW, Hildebrandt DA, *et al.* Paramedic prehospital cath lab activation for STEMI, without ECG transmission, dramatically reduces door to balloon time. *Am Heart Assoc* 2007.

15 Dhruva VN, Abdelhadi SI, Anis A, *et al.* ST-Segment Analysis Using Wireless Technology in Acute Myocardial Infarction (STAT-MI) trial. *J Am Coll Cardiol* 2007;**50**(6):509–13.

16 Drew BJ, Dempsey ED, Joo TH, *et al.* Prehospital synthesized 12-lead ECG ischemia monitoring with trans-telephonic transmission in acute coronary syndromes: pilot study results of the ST SMART trial. *J Electrocardiol* 2004;**37**(Suppl):214–21.

17 Aufderheide TP, Keelan MH, Hendley GE, *et al.* Milwaukee Prehospital Chest Pain Project – phase I: feasibility and accuracy of prehospital thrombolytic candidate selection. *Am J Cardiol* 1992;**69**(12):991–6.

18 Millar-Craig MW, Joy AV, Adamowicz M, *et al.* Reduction in treatment delay by paramedic ECG diagnosis of myocardial infarction with direct CCU admission. *Heart* 1997;**78**(5):456–61.

19 Grim P, Feldman T, Martin M, *et al.* Cellular telephone transmission of 12-lead electrocardiograms from ambulance to hospital. *Am J Cardiol* 1987;**60**(8):715–20.

20 Bradley EH, Herrin J, Wang Y, *et al.* Strategies for reducing the door-to-balloon time in acute myocardial infarction. *N Engl J Med* 2006;**355**(22):2308–20.

21 Carstensen S, Nelson GC, Hansen PS, *et al.* Field triage to primary angioplasty combined with emergency department bypass reduces treatment delays and is associated with improved outcome. *Eur Heart J* 2007;**28**(19):2313–9.

22 Henry TD, Atkins JM, Cunningham MS, *et al.* ST-segment elevation myocardial infarction: recommendations on triage of patients to heart attack centers: is it time for a national policy for the treatment of ST-segment elevation myocardial infarction? *J Am Coll Cardiol* 2006;**47**(7):1339–45.

23 Moyer P, Feldman J, Levine J, *et al.* Thrombolytic controversy for ST Segment Elevation Myocardial Infarction on the Organization of Emergency Medical Services. *Crit Pathways Cardiol* 2004;**3**(2): 53–61.

24 Moyer P. *Emergency Cardiovascular Care 2007: Strategies for Building Regional Integrated STEMI Systems for Reperfusion in Management of STEMI in Boston.* Washington, DC: American College of Cardiology Emergency Cardiovascular Care, 2007.

25 Blackwell TH, Garvey JL, Wilson BH, *et al.* Improved time to percutaneous coronary intervention following the implementation of a prehospital "Code STEMI" protocol (abstract). *Prehosp Emerg Care* 2007;**11**:110–1.

26 Bachour FA, Smith SW, Hildebrandt DA, *et al.* Effect Of Prehospital Cath Lab Activation On Door To Balloon Time Of STEMI Patients Presenting During Normal Workday Hours vs. After Hours. Abstract 2403. *Am Heart Assoc* 2007.

27 Ortolani P, Marzocchi A, Marrozzini C, *et al.* Usefulness of prehospital triage in patients with cardiogenic shock complicating ST-elevation myocardial infarction treated with primary percutaneous coronary intervention. *Am J Cardiol* 2007;**100**(5):787–92.

28 Kudenchuk PJ, Maynard C, Cobb LA, *et al.* Utility of the prehospital electrocardiogram in diagnosing acute coronary syndromes. *J Am Coll Cardiol* 1998;**32**(1):17–27.

29 Aufderheide TP, Hendley GE, Woo J, *et al.* A prospective evaluation of prehospital 12-lead ECG application in chest pain patients. *J Electrocardiol* 1992;**24**(Suppl):8–13.

30 Purvis GM, Weiss SJ, Gaffney FA. Prehospital ECG monitoring of chest pain patients. *Am J Emerg Med* 1999;**17**(6):604–7.

31 Koren G, Weiss AT, Hasin Y, *et al.* Prevention of myocardial damage in acute myocardial ischemia by early treatment with intravenous streptokinase. *N Engl J Med* 1985;**313**(22):1384–9.

32 European Myocardial Infarction Project Group. Prehospital thrombolytic therapy in patients with suspected acute myocardial infarction. *N Engl J Med* 1993;**329**(6):383–9.

33 GREAT Group. Feasibility, safety, efficacy of domiciliary thrombolysis by general practitioners: Grampian region early anistreplase trial. *BMJ* 1992;**305**:548–53.

34 Wallentin L, Goldstein P, Armstrong PW, *et al.* Efficacy and safety of tenecteplase in combination with the low-molecular-weight heparin enoxaparin or unfractionated heparin in the prehospital setting: the Assessment of the Safety and Efficacy of a New Thrombolytic Regimen (ASSENT)-3 PLUS randomized trial in acute myocardial infarction. *Circulation* 2003;**108**(2): 135–42.

35 Verheugt FW, Montalescot G, Sabatine MS, *et al.* Prehospital fibrinolysis with dual antiplatelet therapy in ST-elevation acute myocardial infarction: a substudy of the randomized double blind CLARITY-TIMI 28 trial. *J Thromb Thrombolysis* 2007;**23**(3): 173–9.

36 Montalescot G, Borentain M, Payot L, *et al.* Early vs late administration of glycoprotein IIb/IIIa inhibitors in primary percutaneous coronary intervention of acute ST-segment elevation myocardial infarction: a meta-analysis. *JAMA* 2004;**292**(3): 362–6.

Chapter 24 | What are the electrocardiographic indications for reperfusion therapy?

William Brady[1], David Burt[2], Chris Ghaemmaghami[2], Robert O'Connor[2], Stephen W. Smith[3]

[1]University of Virginia Health System, Life Support Learning Center, Charlottesville, VA, USA
[2]University of Virgina, Charlottesville, VA, USA
[3]University of Minnesota, Hennepin County Medical Center, Minneapolis, MN, USA

Case presentations

The setting is a mid-sized community hospital without invasive cardiac capabilities. Weather precludes timely transfer of the patient to a tertiary center approximately 3 h distant.

Case 1: A 46-year-old previously healthy male presents to the emergency department (ED) with 2 h of pressure-like chest pain. He appears ill, with marked diaphoresis; blood pressure (BP) is 100/60 mmHg, pulse 110 beats per minute (bpm), RR 26, and O_2 saturation 96% on 2 L via nasal cannula. His examination is otherwise normal. The electrocardiogram (ECG) is shown in Figure 24.1.

Case 2: A 61-year-old male with history of previous myocardial infarction (MI) presents to the ED with 4 h of dyspnea and chest pain similar to previous MI. He is anxious, pale, and diaphoretic; BP is 95/70 mmHg, pulse 110 bpm, RR 26, and O_2 saturation 93% on 2 L via nasal cannula. His examination is otherwise significant for rales in the lung bases bilaterally. The ECG is shown in Figure 24.2. A rapid review of his medical record reveals a past ECG with normal sinus rhythm and normal intraventricular conduction. A bedside qualitative test is positive for elevated troponin.

Case 3: A 63-year-old female, with past history of hypertension, diabetes mellitus, and congestive heart failure, presents to the ED with intermittent chest discomfort, associated with diaphoresis, nausea, and vomiting. The pain has become constant over the past 3 h. She is in no apparent distress;

BP 150/90 mmHg, pulse 90 bpm, RR 20, with O_2 saturation of 94% on 2 L via nasal cannula. Her primary examination is unremarkable for acute issues. The 12-lead ECG (Figure 24.3) demonstrates ST segment depression in leads V1 to V3. A bedside qualitative test is positive for elevated troponin.

These three patients are likely experiencing acute coronary syndrome (ACS). Each patient has a different ECG presentation, including ST segment elevation (STE), ST depression, and, presumably, new left bundle branch block (LBBB). Assuming each patient continues with worrisome chest pain and lacks contraindication for fibrinolysis, in which case, if any, would you initiate fibrinolysis and/or percutaneous coronary intervention (PCI)?

The electrocardiographic indications for reperfusion (fibrinolysis or percutaneous coronary intervention) in presumed acute myocardial infarction

The 12-lead ECG provides extremely important clinical information in the adult patient presenting with potential acute myocardial infarction (AMI). In fact, data from the ECG represent the major criteria for reperfusion therapy in the patient with presumed ST elevation myocardial infarction (STEMI). The ECG must, of course, be interpreted in the context of clinical symptoms, the duration of symptoms, and the presence of any contraindications to reperfusion therapy.

The ECG indications [1,2] for emergent reperfusion therapy in the patient with presumed STEMI include the following (STE is measured at the J point). They are summarized in Table 24.1.

Critical Decisions in Emergency and Acute Care Electrocardiography,
1st edition. Edited by W.J. Brady and J.D. Truwit. © 2009 Blackwell Publishing, ISBN: 9781405159067

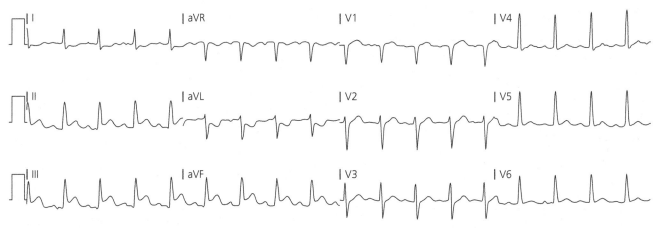

Figure 24.1 Patient #1 with inferior wall STEMI, with significant STE in leads II, III, and aVF. Note the reciprocal ST depression in the lateral leads I and aVL, and also the minimal STE in lead V1, potentially consistent with a right ventricular AMI.

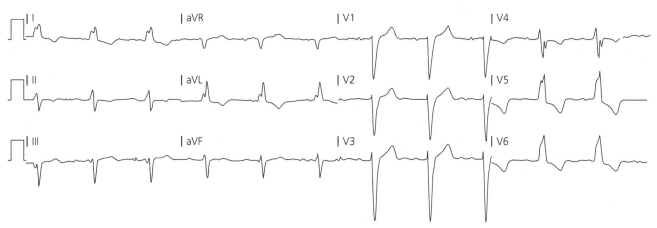

Figure 24.2 Patient #2 with new-onset LBBB. The ST segment changes seen here are appropriate for LBBB.

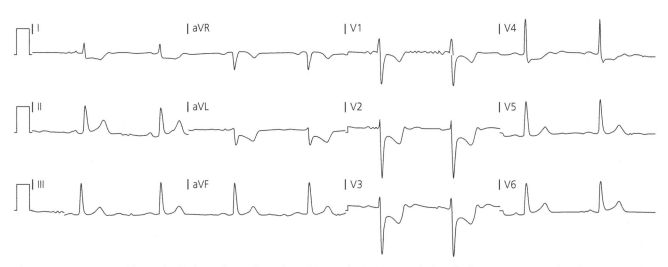

Figure 24.3 Patient #3 with anterior ST depression and prominent T wave. The QRS is normal. These findings represent an isolated posterior wall STEMI.

Table 24.1 Electrocardiographic indications for fibrinolysis in presumed acute myocardial infarction

ST segment elevation: ST segment elevation ≥ 1 mm in at least two anatomically oriented leads (note that the ST segment elevation lacks features of non-infarction syndromes). Note that there is greater specificity if 2 mm STE (in women, 1.5 mm) is required in leads V2 and V3.

Left bundle branch block: (1) New, or presumably new LBBB, with a strong clinical suspicion for AMI, and (2) pre-existing LBBB with abnormal ST segments in the setting of a strong clinical suspicion for AMI; abnormal ST segments such as:

a Concordant ST segment elevation ≥ 1 mm in one lead
b Concordant ST segment depression ≥ 1 mm in one of leads V1–V3
c Discordant ST segment deviation ≥ 5 mm in one lead.

Right bundle branch block (criteria identical to normal conduction): ST segment elevation.

ST segment depression: "Marked" ST segment depression in V2 and V3, associated prominent R wave and upright T waves in patients with a strong clinical suspicion for AMI (of the posterior wall of the left ventricular wall). Diagnosis is much more certain with 0.5 mm of STE in posterior leads V7–V9 or with echocardiograhic posterior wall motion abnormality. Alternatively, STE of 1 mm in two consecutive posterior leads V7–V9.

---

(1) ST segment elevation ≥ 1 mm in at least two anatomically oriented leads [1]. Additionally, STE must not be the result of a pseudo-infarction syndrome (see Chapters 14 and 21). See comments below under "Magnitude of ST elevation" regarding low specificity of this criterion.

(2) New or presumably new LBBB, with a strong clinical suspicion for AMI (Figure 24.2) [1]. It is possible that the benefit of immediate reperfusion is limited to a subgroup of LBBB patients who have either concordant ST segments or discordant ST segments that are out of proportion to the preceding S wave (see Chapter 21). However, randomized trials did not do subgroup analyses on these patients. Therefore, new LBBB remains an indication for reperfusion in the setting of typical symptoms (persistent typical chest discomfort).

(3) LBBB, if not new, should have *one* of the following unanticipated or abnormal ST segments, with a strong clinical suspicion for AMI (see Chapter 21):

a Concordant STE ≥ 1 mm in a *single* lead (Figure 24.4)
b Concordant ST segment depression ≥ 1 mm in *one* of leads V1–V3 (Figure 24.5)
c Discordant ST segment deviation ≥ 5 mm in a *single* lead, especially if > 25% of the preceding S wave (Figure 24.6).

(4) Isolated posterior STEMI

a "Marked" ST depression in two consecutive leads (V1–V4), with either associated prominent R wave and upright T waves, or with associated STE of ≥ 0.5 mm in two posterior leads V7–V9, or associated posterior wall motion abnormality on echocardiogram (Figure 24.3) [1,3].

b manifesting ≥ 1 mm of STE in two consecutive posterior leads V7–V9.

(5) For PCI only, *not fibrinolytics*: angina with persistent ischemic ST depression refractory to medical therapy.

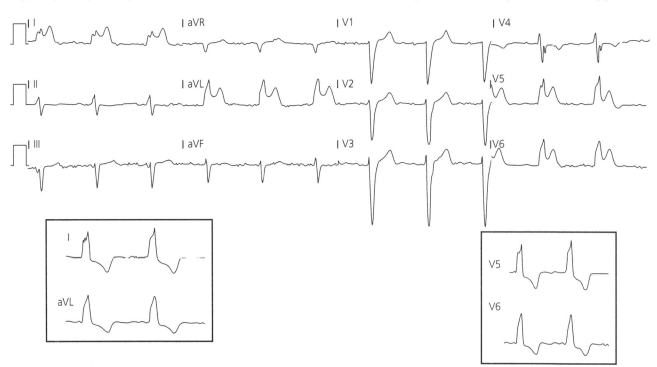

Figure 24.4 Note the concordant STE in the lateral leads I, aVL, V5, and V6 as seen in this LBBB pattern. This finding is diagnostic of STEMI. Leads I, aVL, V5, and V6 in the insert describe the appropriate, or normal, ST configurations in this region of the LBBB pattern.

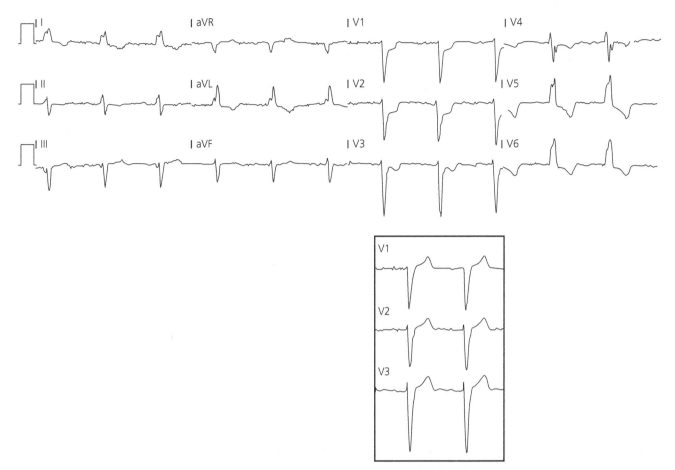

Figure 24.5 Note the concordant ST depression in the right precordial leads V1 to V3 in this LBBB. This finding is consistent with posterior injury. Leads V1 to V3 in the insert describe the appropriate, or normal, ST segment configurations in this region of the LBBB pattern.

Criteria 1 and 2 represent the most frequently encountered clinical presentations in the patient with presumed AMI; these presentations also are supported by the most robust literature base. Criterion 3, the so-called Sgarbossa criteria [4], represents reasonable ECG indications for fibrinolysis; it must be stressed, however, that large clinical trials supporting this approach are lacking. Criteria 4 is an ECG presentation that is associated with posterior STEMI, but there are no randomized trials of reperfusion establishing benefit. There are also no randomized trials of emergent PCI for refractory angina.

Right bundle branch block: To the experienced interpreter, STE is not obscured by RBBB (Figure 24.7). Therefore, new RBBB alone is not an ECG indication for fibrinolytics; there must be STE, or ST depression consistent with posterior STEMI.

ST segment elevation

The most commonly encountered and widely accepted ECG criterion for fibrinolysis is STE. Magnitude, distribution, and morphology of STE are important.

Magnitude of ST segment elevation

There is no established method to measure STE, making it difficult to interpret the many studies using various cutoffs [5]. Nevertheless, measurement at the J point, relative to the PR segment, has become standard. Contiguity is defined in the precordial leads by the lead sequence V1–V6, and in the frontal plane (limb leads) by aVL, I, inverted aVR, II, aVF, and III.

No STE cutoff is both an adequately sensitive or specific indicator of coronary occlusion (the anatomic correlate of "STEMI"). For anterior STEMI, a 2 mm cutoff in right precordial leads V1 to V3 or V4 is relatively specific but not sensitive, and a cutoff of 1 mm is relatively sensitive but not specific. Using only the minimal 1 mm cutoff in precordial leads, especially V2 and V3, will optimize the detection of STEMI yet place a significant burden on physician interpretation because many patients have this degree of STE on their baseline non-pathologic ECG [6,7].

Many fibrinolytic investigations have largely focused on 1 mm of STE in the limb leads and 2 mm in the precordial

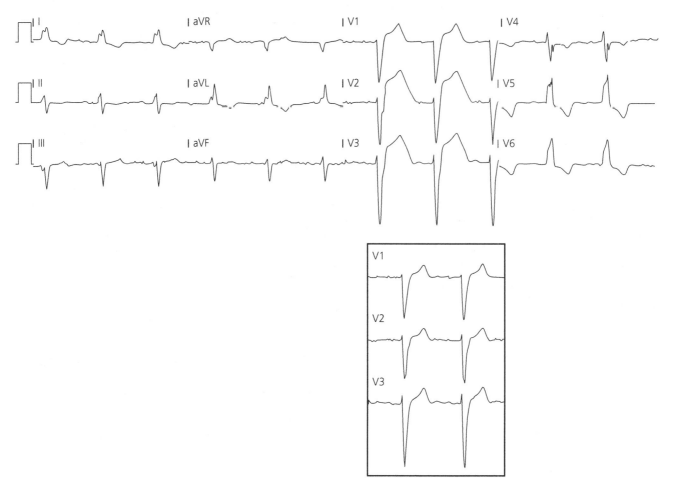

Figure 24.6 Excessive, discordant STE in LBBB. This finding is suggestive of electrocardiographic AMI. V2 had ≥ 5 mm of STE, but both V2 and V3 have an ST/S ratio > 0.25. Leads V1 to V3 in the insert describe the appropriate, or normal, ST configurations in this region of the LBBB pattern.

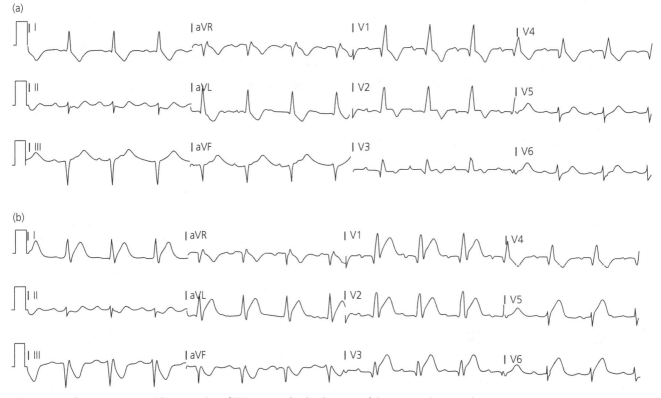

Figure 24.7 The RBBB pattern with progression of STEMI; note the development of the abnormal ST waveforms. (a) The ST segment in V2 is slightly elevated, when it should be isoelectric or depressed in V2. (b) Now there is obvious ST elevation in leads I, aVl, V1, V2, V3, V5, and V6. ST elevation is never present in normal RBBB, even if concordant to a negative QRS. These ECGs are consistent with an anterolateral STEMI in the setting of RBBB.

leads, without specifying the method of measurement [8–13]. Unfortunately, 2 mm of STE is very insensitive for lateral injury. The 2004 American College of Cardiology (ACC)/American Heart Association (AHA) guidelines, although commenting on the poor specificity, recommended 1 mm STE in any two consecutive leads, including precordial leads, as the diagnostic criterion for "fibrinolysis" [1]. This ACC/AHA recommendation enables the clinician to include numerous "electrocardiographically borderline" situations in the consideration of fibrinolysis for STEMI; a single mm of STE in two consecutive leads is a not uncommon STEMI presentation, particularly early in the progression of inferior and lateral acute MI. ST elevation must not be a result of non-MI syndromes, such as benign early repolarization, bundle branch block, left ventricular hypertrophy, etc. (see Chapters 14 and 21).

The ACC and European Society published guidelines for "ECG changes indicative of myocardial ischemia that may progress to MI" (but do not specifically recommend fibrinolysis) [14]. This cutoff requires 2 mm in V1–V3, while retaining the 1 mm criteria in V4–V6 and in limb leads, and is more sensitive and accurate than the universal 1 mm cutoff [15,16] The 2007 ACC/AHA STEMI guidelines update did not change the STE fibrinolysis criteria [17]. However, the AHA published new guidelines for diagnosis of MI (but not specifically for fibrinolysis) in late 2007, which offer better sensitivity with minimal loss of specificity [18]. These criteria require 2 mm STE only in leads V2 and V3, and, for women, require only 1.5 mm STE in these two leads [18].

In a study of 1190 patients with symptoms of ACS and 335 with acute MI, the optimal sensitivity and specificity were criteria of ≥ 1 mm in ≥ *one* limb lead or V5 or V6, and ≥ 2 mm in *one* of anteroseptal leads V1–V4. ST elevation was 45–55% sensitive for MI by CK-MB, depending on the criteria used [16]. In another study, however, 40% of consecutive left anterior descending (LAD) occlusion had no lead with 2 mm of STE [19]. In yet another, STE was encountered in approximately one-fifth of all ED chest pain patients, though the majority were ultimately diagnosed with a non-ACS cause of the STE, including normal variant, left ventricular hypertrophy, and LBBB; STEMI accounted for only 20% of these patients with STE [20]. In fact, the majority of males under age 50 have baseline STE ≥ 1 mm [1,2,6,7]. In the major study described above, "significant" STE was found in 18% of non-AMI patients [16]. The ECG differential diagnosis of STE in the adult chest pain patient is extensive, and includes STEMI, left ventricular aneurysm, myocarditis, cardiomyopathy, benign early repolarization, ventricular-paced rhythm, and pericarditis, as well as BBB and left ventricular hypertrophy, the latter two being the most common cause of STE, whether the population considered is prehospital, ED, or coronary care unit (CCU) [2,20–22]. Fortunately, the majority of the time the clinicians can discern the etiology of STE, such that most initiation of reperfusion therapy is appropriate [23,24]. In fact, a well

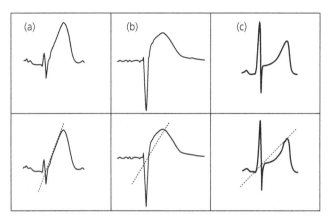

Figure 24.8 Morphologic considerations in the elevated ST segment. Three basic contours of ST elevation are seen in clinical medicine. The obliquely straight and convex forms – considered together as the non-concave morphologies – are often seen in STEMI, while the concave contour is almost always seen in non-STEMI syndromes; exceptions to both of these statements are seen, with STEMI presenting with concave morphologies and non-STEMI presenting with non-concave shapes (especially left ventricular hypertrophy). A line is drawn between the J point and apex of the T wave. (a) Obliquely straight. (b) Convex. (c) Concave.

informed subjective interpretation performs better than any measured criteria [25]. Pseudo-infarction patterns, and the differentiation from STEMI, are discussed in much greater detail in Chapters 14 and 21.

Because a single mm of STE is very often seen in chest pain patients without an ultimate ACS diagnosis, as well as in patients with coronary occlusion requiring immediate therapy, the clinician must employ other ECG analysis methods, including QRS and ST segment waveform analysis, proportionality, and reciprocal ST depression, as well as adjuncts such as serial ECGs, echocardiography, biomarkers, and angiography.

Morphology of ST segment elevation: The majority of patients with STEMI will manifest a "typical" ST morphology with the ST segment upwardly straight or convex (bulging upward, see Figure 24.8a and b) in at least one lead. An upwardly concave ST morphology (Figure 24.8c) is concave in all leads of a coronary distribution and is the normal configuration, and is present in most ECGs of patients with non-AMI causes of STE [26,27]. The use of this waveform analysis in ED chest pain patients demonstrates very high specificity (97%) and positive predictive value (94%) for correct ECG diagnosis of STEMI [26]. Non-concave morphologies are unusual in non-AMI syndromes, with the exception of convex ST segments in left ventricular hypertrophy. See Figure 21.4. Unfortunately, the sensitivity of non-concave ST morphology for anterior MI due to LAD occlusion is low, especially early in the process [19,28], yet its specificity is quite high and, therefore, of value in the "rule-in" strategy for STEMI. Non-concave morphology in just one of leads V2–V6 was encountered in only 56% of STEMI patients with

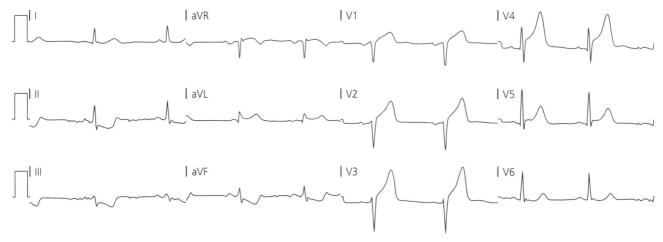

Figure 24.9 Reciprocal ST depression in early anterior wall STEMI. The reciprocal ST segment depression is seen here in leads II, III, and aVF. In this example, the STE is concave in morphology, less suggestive of STEMI. The presence of reciprocal ST depression strongly supports the diagnosis of STEMI of the anterior wall, as does the low R-wave amplitude in V2–V4.

LAD occlusion; importantly, concave morphology was seen in 43% and was associated with a shorter duration of symptoms.

Reciprocal ST segment depression: Reciprocal ST depression, also referred to as reciprocal change (Figure 24.9), is a common finding in STEMI; Its presence on the ECG not only strongly supports the ECG diagnosis of STEMI but also identifies a patient with a greater risk of cardiovascular complication, poor left ventricular function, and death [22,29]. Reciprocal ST depression is defined as ST depression of at least 0.5 mm in a single lead that is electrically opposite the lead(s) with STE. In the presence of abnormal conduction (e.g. left ventricular hypertrophy [LVH], bundle branch block [BBB], or intraventricular conduction delay [IVCD]), "reciprocal" ST depression only signifies ischemia if out of proportion to the repolarization abnormalities that are to be expected after this abnormal QRS complex [29]. Absence of reciprocal ST depression does not rule out STEMI. In both prehospital and ED chest pain populations suspected of STEMI, reciprocal change supported the ECG diagnosis of STEMI with both high specificity and high positive predictive values [29].

Inferior STEMI almost universally presents with true reciprocal ST depression in lead aVL (electrically opposite), so much so that the diagnosis must be in doubt if there is no reciprocal depression. Absence only occurs in simultaneous inferior and lateral injury (see Figure 10.1), or commonly in the pseudo-infarction patterns of peri- or myocarditis. On the contrary, anterior MI presents with inferior ST depression in only approximately half of cases. When present, it is strongly correlated with proximal LAD occlusion [30].

QRS analysis: The presence of terminal QRS distortion (loss of S wave in V2 or V3) is highly suggestive of MI and is not seen in normal variants, unless replaced by a J wave. Furthermore, mean R wave amplitude of < 5 mm in V2–V4 is very unusual in normal variants.

Summary: With precordial STE in V2–V4, if any one of the following is present, normal ECG is very unlikely, and a provisional diagnosis of anterior STEMI should be made (see Figures 24.10a and 24.10b):

(1) single lead with > 5 mm of STE
(2) anterior or inferior reciprocal ST depression
(3) terminal QRS distortion
(4) one lead with a straight or convex ST segment
(5) mean STE (V2–V4) of ≥ 2 mm
(6) mean R wave (V2–V4) of ≤ 5 mm.

Bundle branch block

See indications for fibrinolysis above, and see Chapter 21. Patients with BBB and AMI are at an increased risk of adverse outcome, and, thus, should be rapidly and aggressively managed in the ED with appropriate revascularization therapies, including fibrinolysis. Left bundle branch block obscures ST segment analysis such that most consider a new, or presumably new LBBB, an indication for fibrinolysis. Because the ST segment is not obscured by RBBB, and because RBBB should not have STE unless associated with MI, most would not give fibrinolysis to new RBBB without STE [1].

The presence of a new or presumably new LBBB in the setting of suspected AMI is considered an indication for fibrinolysis, based on randomized trials of fibrinolytics that did not attempt to further interpret the ECG [31–33]. The development of LBBB in the setting of AMI suggests occlusion of the proximal LAD and is associated with high mortality, lower ejection fraction, and increased incidence of complications [31–33]. Despite this increased risk, patients with LBBB less often receive fibrinolytic agents; however, when managed aggressively, these individuals, as a group, show significant benefit [32].

(a)

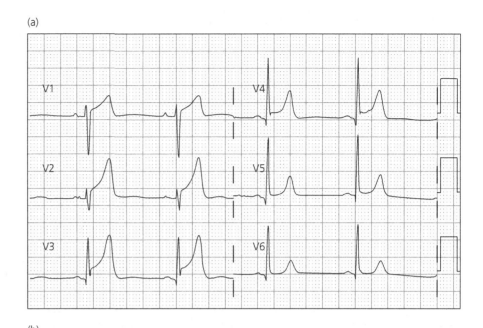

(b)

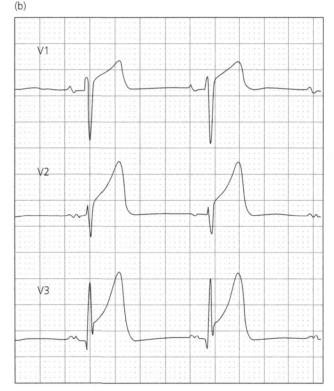

Figure 24.10 (a) Acute MI mistaken for early repolarization (only V1–V6 shown, limb leads were normal). There is upward concavity in all leads. The mean R wave amplitude in V2–V4 is > 5 mm. However, there is loss of the S wave (terminal QRS distortion) in lead V3. There is also a mean STE at the J point (V2–V4) of > 2 mm (= 2.33 mm). Both these are quite specific for AMI. This was missed and another ECG is recorded later (b). Note the straightening of the ST segment in V2, compared with the initial ECG. This straightening is diagnostic of STEMI. The patient had a complete LAD occlusion.

While a pre-existing (i.e. previously noted) LBBB is also associated with an increased chance of poor outcome, its presence alone is not a readily accepted indication for fibrinolysis. With pre-existing LBBB, fibrinolysis is only indicated with abnormal ST segment morphologies [1,2]. It must be noted, however, that the incidence of AMI in chest pain patients with LBBB is low, with one study demonstrating that only approximately 10% of these individuals actually experienced any acute MI (diagnosis by CK-MB, with or without complete persistent coronary occlusion) [34].

These abnormal ST segment morphologies, best known as the Sgarbossa criteria (Figures 24.4–24.6), are best described as alterations in the appropriate discordant pattern of the major, terminal portion of the QRS complex and the ST segment (Figure 24.2) [4]. Recall that in a "normal" relationship, the ST-T complex is located in the opposite direction ("discordant") of the major, terminal portion of the QRS complex. Thus, in the lateral leads, the QRS complex is usually a large R wave (i.e. predominantly or entirely positive) and is appropriately associated with a depressed ST segment;

conversely, leads V1 to V3 possess a predominantly negative QRS complex (QS, QR, or QRS complexes) and therefore demonstrate an elevated ST segment (Figure 24.2). These findings represent the "normal," or expected, ST segment morphologies in the LBBB pattern. Variations from the normal discordant QRS complex-ST segment relationship represent alterations in the concept of appropriate discordance and can be the sole ECG manifestation of an ACS [2].

The findings as described by Sgarbossa and colleagues [4] include "concordant" (in the same direction as the majority of the QRS) STE ≥ 1 mm in at least one lead (Figure 24.4), concordant ST depression ≥ 1 mm in one of leads V1 to V3 (Figure 24.5), and one lead with excessive discordant STE ≥ 5 mm (Figure 24.6). A more recent study, comparing patients with LAD occlusion with control subjects with no LAD occlusion (in contrast to CK-MB positive versus negative), found that discordant STE out of proportion to the preceding S wave (ratio of STE at the J point to the depth of the S wave ≥ 0.25) was a very sensitive and specific indicator of LAD occlusion, significantly more accurate than an absolute criterion of ≥ 5 mm discordant STE [35]. The Sgarbossa criteria were found to be independently predictive of AMI, as diagnosed by CK-MB, with impressive specificity. The sensitivity, in the range of 40%, has been (inappropriately) criticized; one must remember that even in normal conduction, the initial ECG is only about 45% sensitive for MI as diagnosed by CK-MB [36]. In normal conduction, the ECG is only sensitive for complete persistent coronary occlusion, not for any MI [37]. The degree to which LBBB obscures ST segment analysis during complete occlusion (requiring reperfusion therapy) may be greatly exaggerated. Indeed, Stark and colleagues found that a change in the ST segments of 1 mm was 80% sensitive for angiographic balloon occlusion in 10 cases of LBBB (mean delta ST was 2.7 mm) versus 75% sensitivity in 20 patients with normal conduction [38]. Smith found that an ST/S ratio in any of leads V1–V4 was > 90% sensitive and specific for LAD occlusion [35]. Both of these studies support the notion that the ECG may be just as sensitive for STEMI in the presence of LBBB as in normal conduction. Left bundle branch block does indeed greatly obscure the Q wave diagnosis of completed MI, and that is the primary source of its reputation.

Without randomized trials, or subgroup analyses of previous fibrinolytic trials, the sensitivity of the criteria is uncertain. Thus, in a patient with new LBBB, one should not exclude urgent reperfusion based on this uncertainty. However, they should prompt fibrinolysis if present in a patient with high suspicion for acute MI and a previous history of LBBB.

Right bundle branch block: There is some controversy over RBBB. Right bundle branch block with acute MI is associated with very high mortality, unless it is transient [39–43]. Patients with MI and RBBB are undertreated with reperfusion therapy [40]. However, RBBB only minimally obscures ST segment analysis of the ECG. One must find the end of the QRS; this is where the ST segment begins. Then STE or ST depression can be identified as with normal conduction. The one difficulty is in leads V1–V3, in which there is frequently up to 1 mm of ST depression, with a negative T wave, and both are discordant to the positive R' wave. Anterior MI in RBBB may present with normalization of a previously depressed ST segment, or minimal STE (Figure 24.7a), and posterior MI may present with exaggeration of the ST depression. ST elevation, even discordant STE, is not seen in RBBB in the absence of pathology (e.g. ischemia). Finally, if the interpreter finds that the RBBB obscures the ST segment analysis because of either a particularly bizarre QRS, or due to inexperience, it may be reasonable, when there is high suspicion of ongoing MI, to administer fibrinolysis.

ST segment depression

Fibrinolytics are not indicated for ACS with ST depression, unless that ST depression represents posterior wall injury (STEMI) [1,44]. However, PCI is not contraindicated and is recommended if there are symptoms with persistent ST depression.

The only subset of patients with ST depression (without STE) for whom fibrinolysis is recommended is the patient with acute isolated posterior wall MI (Figure 24.3). See also Chapters 15, 18, and 22. The posterior wall is a segment of the left ventricle, and isolated posterior wall AMI is associated with a significant amount of myocardium in jeopardy [45]. Isolated posterior MI (Figure 24.3) presents with ST depression in at least two anatomically oriented right precordial leads (leads V1 to V4) as well as a prominent R wave and inverted or upright T wave in these same leads; the ST depression is most often horizontal in contour [1,2].

Unfortunately, anterior subendocardial ischemia, for which fibrinolysis is ineffective, also has anterior ST depression. Determining the etiology of anterior ST depression is, therefore, quite difficult, and the literature does not provide an easy, direct answer to this clinical dilemma. The AHA/ACC notes an exception to ST segment depression fibrinolysis exclusion when "marked ST-segment depression is confined to leads V1 through V4" [1]. The support for this statement is less than substantial. The LATE trial and related commentary reported that a subset of patients managed with fibrinolysis and significant ST depression demonstrated a reduction in mortality; it is theorized that this subset of patients were actually experiencing an isolated, acute posterior wall myocardial infarction [46,47]. Boden and colleagues investigated patients with isolated precordial ST segment depression, noting that posterior wall myocardial infarction is a not uncommon cause of this ECG finding. They recommended that this subtype of ACS patient be considered for fibrinolytic therapy if AMI is suspected based on clinical grounds [48]. The only two reliable means of establishing that anterior ST depression is posterior MI are: (1) recording

STE on posterior leads, or (2) finding a posterior wall motion abnormality on echocardiogram.

Acuteness – when is it too late for reperfusion?

In deciding on reperfusion, particularly on fibrinolytic therapy, it is important to assess the amount of viable injured myocardium at risk of infarction. This is traditionally done by assessing time since pain onset, and randomized trials of fibrinolytics found no significant advantage if pain duration was > 12 h [12,32,49]. However, time since pain onset is a crude way of assessing amount of infarcted (irreversible) versus ischemic (viable, salvageable) myocardium. Often, occlusion is incomplete, or collateral circulation maintains the viability of ischemic myocardium, or there is ischemic preconditioning, and myocardium that is fully salvageable may have pain duration of days. Fortunately, the ECG is probably a better indicator of salvageable myocardium than pain duration.

High ECG "acuteness" is associated with significant salvageable myocardium. An ECG has a high acuteness score if it has tall T waves, and lower acuteness if there are Q waves or T wave inversion is present [50]. In 395 patients, this score was shown to add the most value in situations of data disagreement: (1) in acute anterior MI when the history indicates symptom onset of > 2 h but the acuteness score is high, or (2) in acute inferior MI, if history indicates a time since symptom onset of < 2 h but the acuteness score is low [51]. More recently, a high acuteness score was found on single photon emission computed tomography (SPECT) scanning to be associated with a large amount of salvageable myocardium, and to be superior to time since pain onset for determining myocardium at risk (but not yet infarcted) [52]. This corresponds to other data showing that tall T waves are an independent marker of benefit from fibrinolytics [53], and that, among those with positive T waves, mortality after thrombolytics is the same for those who have < 2 h versus > 2 h of symptoms [54]. It is also important to know that QR waves are present in 50% of anterior MI within the first hour, and represent ischemia of the conducting system, not infarction [55]. Figure 24.11 helps to demonstrate acuteness.

There are no randomized fibrinolytic trials based on ECG characteristics of acuteness. However, PCI has proven beneficial in a randomized trial of patients with persistent pain and ST elevation at > 12 h [56].

Finally, ischemic discomfort is far less predictive of ongoing ischemia than persistent STE and tall T waves. Electrocardiogram acuteness should not be ignored because of resolution of symptoms [57].

In summary, tall T waves indicate a large amount of viable, salvagable, myocardium. Q waves indicate lower acuteness, but may be present early in anterior MI; thus, in anterior MI, T waves are more important. Inverted T waves signify either low acuteness or an open artery (see Chapter 25 on reperfusion). Figures 24.11a and b demonstrate high and low acuteness in V1–V3 in the same patient at different times.

Case conclusions

Cases 1 and 2 represent ACS presentations with unequivocal ECG indications for fibrinolysis, assuming no absolute contraindications. Both patients received fibrinolysis with resolution of the chest discomfort and normalization of the ECG – resolution of the ST segment elevation in Case 1 and a disappearance of the LBBB pattern in Case 2. Case 3 represents a more difficult set of clinical circumstances – an ACS presentation with electrocardiographic ST segment depression. This presentation is more problematic with the clinical electrocardiographic differential diagnosis including anterior wall ischemia and acute posterior wall myocardial infarction. The presence of the prominent R wave in these same leads suggests AMI as the cause of this ST segment depression. This presentation is a somewhat controversial indication for fibrinolysis. Yet, based upon an analysis of the clinical presentation and the electrocardiogram, a fibrinolytic agent was administered with good outcome.

References

1 Antman EM, *et al.* ACC/AHA guidelines for the management of patients with ST-elevation myocardial infarction – executive summary. A report of the American College of Cardiology/American Heart Association Task Force on Practice Guidelines (Writing Committee to revise the 1999 guidelines for the management of patients with acute myocardial infarction). *J Am Coll Cardiol* 2004;**44**(3):671–719.

2 Fesmire FM, *et al.* Clinical policy: indications for reperfusion therapy in emergency department patients with suspected acute myocardial infarction. American College of Emergency Physicians Clinical Policies Subcommittee (Writing Committee) on Reperfusion Therapy in Emergency Department Patients with Suspected Acute Myocardial Infarction. *Ann Emerg Med* 2006;**48**(4): 358–83.

3 Wung SF, Drew BJ. New electrocardiographic criteria for posterior wall acute myocardial ischemia validated by a percutaneous transluminal coronary angioplasty model of acute myocardial infarction. *Am J Cardiol* 2001;**87**(8):970–4; A4.

4 Sgarbossa EB, *et al.* Electrocardiographic diagnosis of evolving acute myocardial infarction in the presence of left bundle-branch block. *N Engl J Med* 1996;**334**(8):481–7.

5 Smith SW. ST Elevation in anterior acute myocardial infarction differs with different methods of measurement. *Acad Emerg Med* 2006;**13**(4):406–12.

6 Wang K, Asinger RW, Marriott HJ. ST-segment elevation in conditions other than acute myocardial infarction. *N Engl J Med* 2003;**349**(22):2128–35.

7 Surawicz B, Parikh SR. Prevalence of male and female patterns of early ventricular repolarization in the normal ECG of males and females from childhood to old age. *J Am Coll Cardiol* 2002; **40**(10):1870–6.

(a)

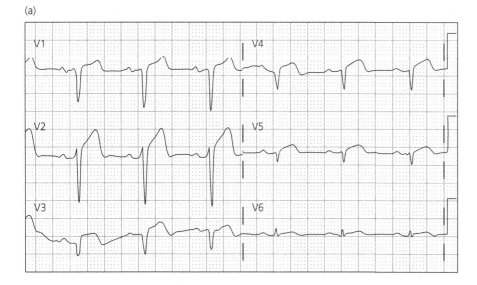

(b)

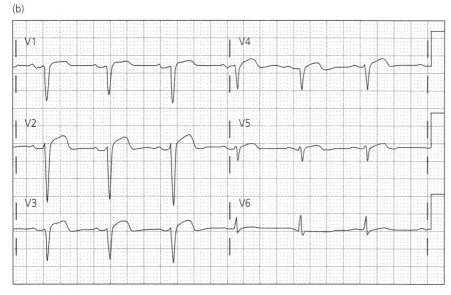

Figure 24.11 (a) LAD occlusion at < 12 h. The tall T wave (8 mm) in V2 shows reasonably high acuteness, in spite of 12 h of chest pain and QS-waves in V3 and V4, indicating significant completed infarction. Care must be taken if denying reperfusion to this patient with AMI. (b) The same patient 24 h later. This shows the height of a typical T wave when there is low acuteness. There is persistent STE but the T wave is only 4 mm in height.

8 AIMS (APSAC Intervention Mortality Study) Trial Study Group. Effect of intravenous APSAC on mortality after acute myocardial infarction: preliminary report of a placebo-controlled clinical trial. AIMS Trial Study Group. *Lancet* 1988;**1**(8585):545–9.

9 ISAM (Intravenous Streptokinase in Acute Myocardial Infarction) Study Group, A prospective trial of intravenous streptokinase in acute myocardial infarction (I.S.A.M.). Mortality, morbidity, and infarct size at 21 days. The I.S.A.M. Study Group. *N Engl J Med* 1986;**314**(23):1465–71.

10 ISIS-2 (Second International Study of Infarct Survival) Collaborative Group, Randomised trial of intravenous streptokinase, oral aspirin, both, or neither among 17,187 cases of suspected acute myocardial infarction: ISIS-2. *Lancet* 1988; **2**(8607):349–60.

11 ISIS-3 (Third International Study of Infarct Survival) Collaborative Study Group. ISIS-3: a randomised comparison of streptokinase vs. tissue plasminogen activator vs anistreplase and of aspirin plus heparin vs aspirin alone among 41,299 cases of suspected acute myocardial infarction. *Lancet* 1992;**339**(8796): 753–70.

12 LATE Study Group. Late assessment of thrombolytic efficacy (LATE) study with alteplase 6–24 hours after onset of acute myocardial infarction. *Lancet* 1993;**342**:759–66.

13 Rossi P, Bolognese L. Comparison of intravenous urokinase plus heparin versus heparin alone in acute myocardial infarction. Urochinasi per via Sistemica nell'Infarto Miocardico (USIM) Collaborative Group. *Am J Cardiol* 1991;**68**(6):585–92.

14 Joint European Society of Cardiology/American College of Cardiology Committee. Myocardial infarction redefined: A consensus document of the Joint European Society of Cardiology/ American College of Cardiology committee for the redefinition of myocardial infarction. *J Am Coll Cardiol* 2000;**36**:959–69.

15 Martin TN, *et al.* ST-segment deviation analysis of the admission 12-lead electrocardiogram as an aid to early diagnosis of acute myocardial infarction with a cardiac magnetic resonance imaging gold standard. *J Am Coll Cardiol* 2007;**50**:1021–8.

16 Menown IB, Mackenzie G, Adgey A. Optimizing the initial 12-lead electrocardiographic diagnosis of acute myocardial infarction. *Eur Heart J* 2000;**21**(4):275–83.

17 Anderson JL, *et al.* ACC/AHA 2007 Guidelines for the Management of Patients With Unstable Angina/Non ST-Elevation Myocardial Infarction. A Report of the American College of Cardiology/American Heart Association Task Force on Practice Guidelines. *J Am Coll Cardiol* 2007;**50**:1–157.

18 Thygesen K, *et al.* Universal definition of myocardial infarction. *Circulation* 2007;**116**:2634–53.

19 Smith SW. Upwardly concave ST segment morphology is common in acute left anterior descending coronary occlusion. *J Emerg Med* 2006;**31**(1):69–77.

20 Brady WJ, *et al.* Cause of ST segment abnormality in ED chest pain patients. *Am J Emerg Med* 2001;**19**(1):25–8.

21 Larsen GC, *et al.* Electrocardiographic left ventricular hypertrophy in patients with suspected acute cardiac ischemia: Its influence on diagnosis, triage, and short-term prognosis. *J Gen Intern Med* 1994;**9**:666–76.

22 Otto LA, Aufderheide TP. Evaluation of ST segment elevation criteria for the prehospital electrocardiographic diagnosis of acute myocardial infarction. *Ann Emerg Med* 1994;**23**(1):17–24.

23 Khoury NE, *et al.* "Inadvertent" thrombolytic administration in patients without myocardial infarction: clinical features and outcome. *Ann Emerg Med* 1996;**28**(3):289–93.

24 Larson DM, *et al.* "False-positive" cardiac catheterization laboratory activation among patients with suspected ST-segment elevation myocardial infarction. *JAMA* 2007;**298**(23):2754–60.

25 Massel D, Dawdy JA, Melendez LJ. Strict reliance on a computer algorithm or measurable ST segment criteria may lead to errors in thrombolytic therapy eligibility. *Am Heart J* 2000;**140**(2):221–6.

26 Brady WJ, *et al.* Electrocardiographic ST segment elevation: the diagnosis of acute myocardial infarction by morphologic analysis of the ST segment. *Acad Emerg Med* 2001;**8**(10):961–7.

27 Kosuge M, *et al.* Value of ST-segment elevation pattern in predicting infarct size and left ventricular function at discharge in patients with reperfused acute anterior myocardial infarction. *Am Heart J* 1999;**137**(3):522–7.

28 Kosuge M, *et al.* Electrocardiographic criteria for predicting total occlusion of the proximal left anterior descending coronary artery in anterior wall acute myocardial infarction. *Clin Cardiol* 2001;**24**:33–38.

29 Brady WJ, *et al.* Reciprocal ST segment depression: Impact on the electrocardiographic diagnosis of ST segment elevation acute myocardial infarction. *Am J Emerg Med* 2002;**20**(1):35–8.

30 Smith SW, Whitwam W. Acute coronary syndromes. *Emerg Med Clin North Am* 2006;**24**(1):53–89.

31 Col JJ, Weinberg SL. The incidence and mortality of intraventricular conduction defects in acute myocardial infarction. *Am J Cardiol* 1972;**29**(3):344–50.

32 Fibrinolytic Therapy Trialists' (FTT) Collaborative Group. Indications for fibrinolytic therapy in suspected acute myocardial infarction: collaborative overview of early mortality and major morbidity results from all randomised trials of more than 1000 patients. *Lancet* 1994;**343**:311–22.

33 Hindman MC, *et al.* The clinical significance of bundle branch block complicating acute myocardial infarction. 2. Indications for temporary and permanent pacemaker insertion. *Circulation* 1978;**58**(4):689–99.

34 Fesmire FM, *et al.* Initial ECG in Q wave and non-Q wave myocardial infarction. *Ann Emerg Med* 1989;**18**(7):741–6.

35 Smith SW, *et al.* ST/S ratio distinguishes left bundle branch block from left bundle branch block with simultaneous anterior myocardial infarction (abstract). *Acad Emerg Med* 2006;**13**(5 Suppl): S160–1.

36 Smith SW. Beyond left bundle-branch block: looking for the acute transmural myocardial infarction (letter). *Ann Emerg Med* 2002;**39**(1):95.

37 Schmitt C, *et al.* Diagnosis of acute myocardial infarction in angiographically documented occluded infarct vessel: limitations of ST-segment elevation in standard and extended ECG leads. *Chest* 2001;**120**(5):1540–6.

38 Stark KS, *et al.* Quantification of ST-segment changes during coronary angioplasty in patients with left bundle branch block. *Am J Cardiol* 1991;**67**(15):1219–22.

39 Dubois C, *et al.* Short- and long-term prognostic importance of complete bundle-branch block complicating acute myocardial infarction. *Clin Cardiol* 1988;**11**(5):292–6.

40 Go AS, *et al.* Bundle-branch block and in-hospital mortality in acute myocardial infarction. National Registry of Myocardial Infarction. *Ann Int Med* 1998;**129**(9):690–7.

41 Melgarejo-Moreno A, *et al.* Incidence, clinical characteristics, and prognostic significance of right bundle-branch block in acute myocardial infarction: a study in the thrombolytic era. *Circulation* 1997;**96**(4):1139–44.

42 Moreno AM, *et al.* Incidence and prognostic significance of right bundle branch block in patients with acute myocardial infarction receiving thrombolytic therapy. *Int J Cardiol* 1997; **61**(2):135–41.

43 Newby KH, *et al.* Incidence and clinical relevance of the occurrence of bundle-branch block in patients treated with thrombolytic therapy. *Circulation* 1996;**94**(10):2424–8.

44 TIMI IIIB Investigators. Effects of tissue plasminogen activator and a comparison of early invasive and conservative strategies in unstable angina and non-Q-wave myocardial infarction. Results of the TIMI IIIB Trial. Thrombolysis in Myocardial Ischemia. *Circulation* 1994;**89**(4):1545–56.

45 Smith SW, *et al.* eds. *The ECG in Acute MI: an Evidence-Based Manual of Reperfusion Therapy.* First ed. Lippincott, Williams, and Wilkins: Philadelphia, 2002: 358.

46 Braunwald E, Cannon CP. Non-Q-wave and ST segment depression myocardial infarction: Is there a role for thrombolytic therapy? *J Am Coll Cardiol* 1996;**27**(6):1333–4.

47 Langer A, *et al.* Late assessment of thrombolytic efficacy (LATE) study: prognosis in patients with non-Q wave myocardial infarction. *J Am Coll Cardiol* 1996;**27**(6):1327–32.

48 Boden WE, *et al.* Electrocardiographic evolution of posterior acute myocardial infarction: importance of early precordial ST-segment depression. *Am J Cardiol* 1987;**59**(8):782–7.

49 EMERAS (Estudio Multicentro Estreptoquinsa Republicas de America del Sur). Randomised trial of late thrombolysis in patients with suspected acute myocardial infarction. *Lancet* 1993; **342**(8874):767–72.

50 Wilkins ML, *et al.* An electrocardiographic acuteness score for quantifying the timing of a myocardial infarction to guide decisions regarding reperfusion therapy. *Am J Cardiol* 1995;**75**(8): 617–20.

51 Corey KE, *et al.* Combined historical and electrocardiographic timing of acute anterior and inferior myocardial infarcts for

prediction of reperfusion achievable size limitation. *Am J Cardiol* 1999;**83**(6):826–31.

52 Engblom H, *et al.* ECG estimate of ischemic acuteness and time from pain onset for predicting myocardial salvage in patients undergoing primary percutaneous coronary intervention. AHA Abstract 2404. *Circulation* 2007;**116**(Suppl II):II_528.

53 Hochrein J, *et al.* Higher T-wave amplitude associated with better prognosis in patients receiving thrombolytic therapy for acute myocardial infarction (a GUSTO-1 substudy). Global Utilization of Streptokinase and Tissue plasminogen activator for Occluded Coronary Arteries. *Am J Cardiol* 1998;**81**(9):1078–84.

54 Herz I, *et al.* The prognostic implications of negative T-waves in the leads with ST segment elevation on admission in acute myocardial infarction. *Cardiology* 1999;**92**(2):121–7.

55 Raitt MH, *et al.* Appearance of abnormal Q waves early in the course of acute myocardial infarction: implications for efficacy of thrombolytic therapy. *J Am Coll Cardiol* 1995;**25**(5):1084–8.

56 Schomig A, *et al.* Mechanical reperfusion in patients with acute myocardial infarction presenting more than 12 hours from symptom onset: a randomized controlled trial. *JAMA* 2005;**293**(23):2865–72.

57 2007 Writing Group to Review New Evidence and Update the ACC/AHA 2004 Guidelines for the Management of Patients With ST-Elevation Myocardial Infarction. 2007 Focused Update of the ACC/AHA 2004 Guidelines for the Management of Patients with ST-Elevation Myocardial Infarction. *J Am Coll Cardiol* 2008;**51**(2).

Chapter 25 | What are the ECG manifestations of reperfusion and reocclusion?

Daniel T. O'Laughlin

University of Minnesota School of Medicine, Minneapolis, MN, USA

Case presentations

Case 1: A 47-year-old man presents with chest pain at 4:30 pm. A 12-lead electrocardiogram (ECG) shows an inferior ST elevation myocardial infarction (STEMI). He receives a fibrinolytic agent at 5:40 pm and is transferred to the cardiac care unit on a two-lead continuous ST segment monitor. Figure 25.1 shows the course of the ST segments.

Case 2: A 56-year-old female presents to the emergency department (ED) of a community hospital without percutaneous coronary intervention (PCI) facilities; they are available at a tertiary cardiac hospital 90 min away. She has chest pain, weakness, diaphoresis, and dyspnea, which began approximately 25 min prior to her arrival and has steadily worsened since onset. She appears ill. The first ECG is in Figure 25.2a and b. Compared with a previous tracing, the physician identifies new ST elevation (STE) in leads V1–V3 and aVR; and new ST depression in leads I, II, aVF, and V5–V6, and diagnoses her with an acute anterior STEMI. He initiates the hospital's facilitated PCI protocol partial dose fibrinolytic agent in combination with aspirin, heparin, and a glycoprotein IIb/IIIa inhibitor, then transports her to the PCI-capable facility.

Case 3: A 56-year-old male presents by emergency medical services (EMS) to an urban PCI-capable hospital with chest pain of 2 h duration, associated with dyspnea and diaphoresis. The paramedics diagnosed STEMI and activated the hospital's catheterization laboratory via a prehospital STEMI alert. Figure 25.3a is the ED ECG.

The electrocardiographic manifestations of reperfusion and reocclusion

In acute STEMI, the goal is successful reperfusion of the infarct-related epicardial vessel and of the downstream micro-

vasculature. Percutaneous coronary intervention is superior to thrombolytics when performed by experienced operators in a timely manner, especially if symptoms have been present for at least 3 h [1,2]. However, the use of thrombolytic agents remains a major therapeutic intervention for STEMI and is the most common reperfusion method for STEMI in the United States and worldwide [3]. Failure to achieve TIMI 3 flow (Table 25.1) through the infarct-related artery (IRA) at 90 minutes occurs in 40–50% of cases treated with thrombolytic agents [3–5]. Early reocclusion of those with reperfusion occurs in 4.3% of GUSTO-1 and GUSTO-3 cases [6], although newer adjunctive treatments such as enoxaparin

Table 25.1 The TIMI Grade Flow. A grading system developed by the TIMI Study Group to describe the coronary artery flow following reperfusion therapy

TIMI Grade Flow	Definition
0	**No perfusion** – No antegrade flow beyond the point of occlusion.
1	**Penetration without perfusion** – The contrast material passes beyond the area of obstruction, but "hangs up" and fails to opacify the entire coronary bed distal to the obstruction for the duration of the cine run.
2	**Partial reperfusion** – The contrast material passes across the obstruction and opacifies the coronary bed distal to the obstruction. However, the rate of entry of contrast into the vessel distal to the obstruction and/or its rate of clearance from the distal bed are perceptibly slower than its entry into and/or clearance from comparable areas not perfused by the culprit vessel (e.g. the opposite coronary artery or coronary bed proximal to the obstruction).
3	**Complete reperfusion** – Antegrade flow into the bed distal to the obstruction occurs as promptly as into the bed proximal to the obstruction *and* clearance of contrast material from the involved bed is as rapid as from an uninvolved bed in the same vessel or the opposite artery.

Critical Decisions in Emergency and Acute Care Electrocardiography, 1st edition. Edited by W.J. Brady and J.D. Truwit. © 2009 Blackwell Publishing, ISBN: 9781405159067

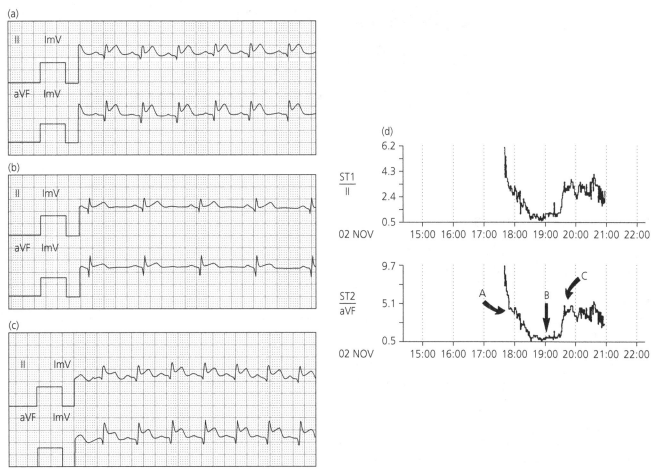

Figure 25.1 Continuous ST monitoring. (a) Continuous leads II and aVF show STE at 17:49, also reflected in the graph in (d). (b) At 19:02, with no CP, the ST segments are normalized (ST resolution), confirming reperfusion. The graph in (d) also illustrates this. (c) ST segments are re-elevated, and an alarm sounded (reocclusion, with recurrent chest pain). (d) Graphs of ST segments versus time in leads II and aVF. Times A, B, and C correspond to tracings a, b, c.

(versus unfractionated heparin) appears to reduce the rate from 4.7 to 2.7% [7].

The phenomenon of inadequate myocardial perfusion through a given segment of the coronary circulation without angiographic evidence of mechanical vessel obstruction has been termed "no-reflow," and is a result of the downstream occlusion of the microvasculature by small platelet-rich thrombi [8]. No-reflow occurs in 19–30% of patients after thrombolysis or mechanical intervention, despite optimal recanalization of the epicardial vessel [5,8,9], and can be visualized on an angiogram as absence of "myocardial blush," which may be graded by the TIMI myocardial perfusion (TMP) grades of 0–3, with 3 as the best flow. TIMI myocardial perfusion and TIMI flow are independent predictors of outcome from MI; a patient with an open vessel may have TMP flow of 0 or 1 [10–12].

Rapid evaluation of the success or failure of reperfusion therapies in a non-invasive manner allows the clinician to quickly determine if rescue therapies, which are proven successful [13], may be required, and to initiate those inter-

ventions as emergently as possible. Non-invasive markers for epicardial IRA reperfusion, such as resolution of chest pain, changes in the ST segments, accelerated idioventricular rhythms (AIVR) and changes in T wave morphology have been re-examined in the context of not only IRA patency, but also restoration of the downstream myocardial tissue [14,15].

ECG manifestations of reperfusion

Since the introduction of reperfusion therapies, ECG characteristics including ST segment changes, T wave morphology changes and reperfusion arrhythmias have been evaluated for their ability to accurately assess the perfusion status of an IRA following therapeutic interventions. Electrocardiogram evaluation currently provides the best continuous, non-invasive method of assessing IRA and myocardial perfusion. Subjective clinical changes in a patient's chest pain following

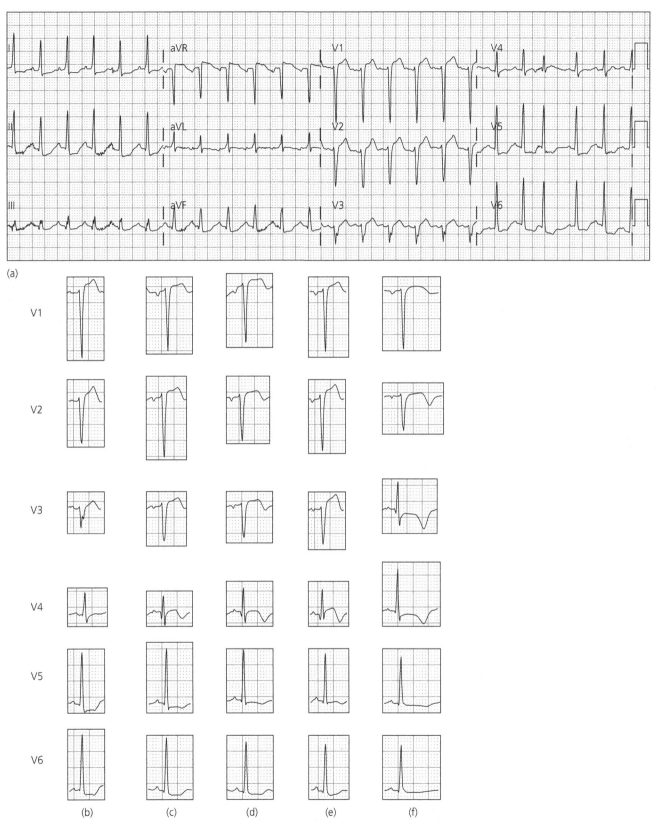

Figure 25.2 Reperfusion and reocclusion. (a) ECG #1 obtained at presentation, t = 0. There is STE in leads V1–V3 and aVR, with ST depression in leads I, II, aVF, and V5–V6. Findings are consistent with an anterior wall STEMI involving the proximal LAD. TNK-tPA was given at t = 22 min. (b) The same precordial leads as in (a), for comparison. (c) ECG #2 obtained at t = 42 min. Note the initial improvement in the ST segments in V1 and V5, and early T wave inversion now present in V4, all suggesting the beginning of early reperfusion. (d) ECG #3, t = 65 min. Terminal T wave inversion is noted in V1–V3; reperfusion is more advanced, but not complete. (e) ECG #4 at t = 100 min. ST segments have re-elevated, with upright T-waves (reocclusion with pseudo-normalization of T waves). (f) ECG #5 at t = 123 min and after PCI. There is > 70% resolution of the maximal ST segment deviation. T waves are again inverted, all indicative of successful reperfusion.

(a)

(b)

(c)

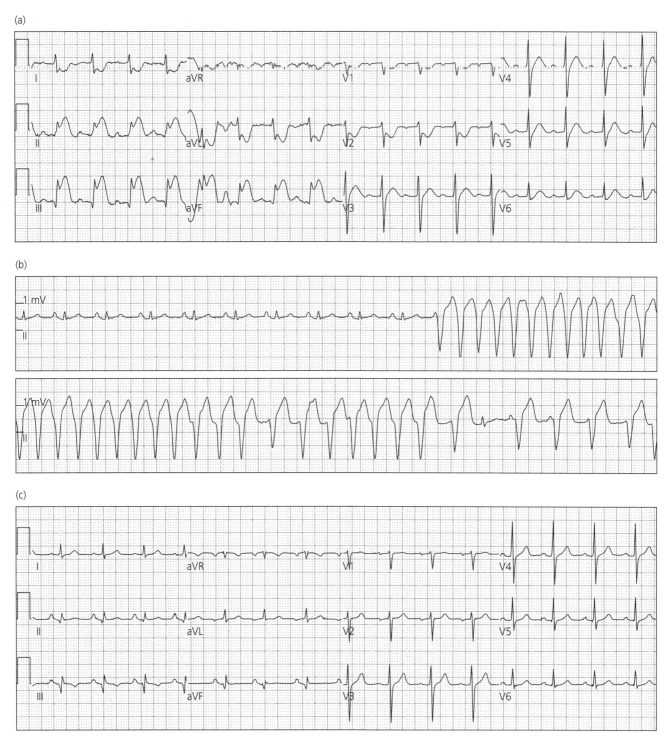

Figure 25.3 (a) ECG #1 obtained on arrival at the ED shows inferior and posterior (inferobasal) STEMI. (b) Reperfusion arrhythmia generated after PCI. Lead II strip demonstrates a sinus rhythm that converts to a brief run of ventricular tachycardia and then into an accelerated idioventricular rhythm. (c) ECG #2 obtained after the events noted in (b). Sinus rhythm with complete resolution of STE. The ECG shows minimal residual infarct: lead III has minimal T inversion and a Q wave. The prognosis is good.

Table 25.2 The TIMI Myocardial Perfusion Grade. A grading system developed by the TIMI Study Group to define myocardial perfusion of the microvasculature following reperfusion therapy

TIMI Myocardial Perfusion Grade (TMPG)	Definition
0	Failure of dye to enter the microvasculature.
1	Dye slowly enters but fails to exit the microvasculature.
2	Delayed entry and exit of dye from the microvasculature.
3	Normal entry and exit of dye from the microvasculature.

reperfusion therapy have poor reliability as a single indicator of reperfusion and/or reocclusion [14,16,17]. Chest pain may increase due to cyclical changes to IRA patency that frequently occur during the early stages of coronary reperfusion, but these may also be asymptomatic. Chest pain is also impacted through the use of analgesic and anti-ischemic medications [5,14,16,18,19].

ST segments

The ST segment is a physiologic reflection of the perfusion of the myocardium and the transmembrane ion gradients of the myocytes, rather than epicardial vessel blood flow [15,20,21]. ST segment elevation correlates with the loss of the ion gradient of the myocytes that occurs during the disruption of oxygen delivery to the cells [19,22]. Thus, the best non-invasive predictor of myocardial perfusion, as measured by TMP flow, is the ST segment on the ECG [23,24]. Reperfusion following thrombolytic administration is a dynamic process. Intermittent IRA recanalization and reocclusion will frequently occur, with 35–50% of patients demonstrating wide fluctuations in the ST segment amplitude, with multiple episodes of both ST segment resolution and re-elevation [5,25].

Evaluation of the ST segment is the most frequently used assessment of reperfusion and reocclusion following reperfusion therapy. Continuous monitoring is superior to serial studies because it has more frequent sampling. Unlike serial ECGs, there are no missed intervals (see Case 1, Figure 25.1) [5,19,26]. The optimal interval between serial ECG studies is not well established, but should balance the issues of the labor involved versus the likelihood of missing critical information with more prolonged study intervals. Further discussion on serial ECGs and continuous ST segment monitoring can be found in Chapter 20.

The rapid resolution of STE ("ST resolution," or "ST recovery") together with angiographic evidence for microvascular reperfusion are the best predictors of outcome from STEMI [10,27]. However, the ability to obtain rapid angiographic evidence for myocardial reperfusion is not universally available. Multiple studies have evaluated the prognostic value of ST segment recovery [28–35]. Whether ST segment resolution should be evaluated at 30, 60, or 90 min or beyond, and whether ST resolution should be defined as ≥ 50% or ≥ 70%, is not absolutely determined. Patients who received thrombolytics for STEMI within 6 h of onset of chest pain were studied with continuous vector cardiography and 12-lead monitoring for 24 h. Time intervals to achieve 20%, 30%, 50%, and 70% ST resolution (STR) from the maximal STE were measured. Patients were also assessed for percentage of STR at each time interval of 60, 90, and 180 min. The group with 50% STR at each time point had significantly lower mortality than the group without this degree of STR; the group with 50% STR at ≤ 60 minutes of treatment had the lowest 30-day mortality [36]. The taskforce that developed the American College of Cardiology/American Heart Association (ACC/AHA) 2007 update to the guidelines for management of patients with STEMI believes that a 50% reduction in STE at 90 min after the initiation of thrombolysis was the best criterion for evaluating the need for rescue PCI [37].

Patients without ST resolution are at higher risk for complications, especially if the T wave remains upright in the first 24–48 h after therapy (see Figure 25.4, and T wave section below). Those who develop early Q waves that do not resolve with reperfusion are also at higher risk [38–40]. Patients with diminished total R wave voltage that does not recover have significantly reduced LV dysfunction and a worse prognosis [41].

T waves

The significance and prognosis of T wave changes that occur during and following an AMI may vary based on the duration of the ischemia, the area of myocardium involved, and the speed at which reperfusion occurs. Development of terminal T wave inversion within the first hour after initiation of reperfusion therapy is a less sensitive indicator of reperfusion than ST resolution, but is very specific (94%) [27]. T wave inversion that develops within 24 h following a STEMI is associated with greater IRA patency and perfusion grade. Very early T inversion is a sign of a patent infarct artery and is independently associated with improved survival [42,43]. Absence of early T inversion is associated with poor outcome (see Figure 25.4). This is in contrast to the gradual development of T wave inversion to a depth of < 3 mm over 48–72 h, which is associated with failed reperfusion, especially when associated with development of QS waves [27].

Wellens' syndrome is a pattern of ECG T wave changes that are associated with a critical stenosis of the proximal left anterior descending (LAD) coronary artery, with probable

(a)

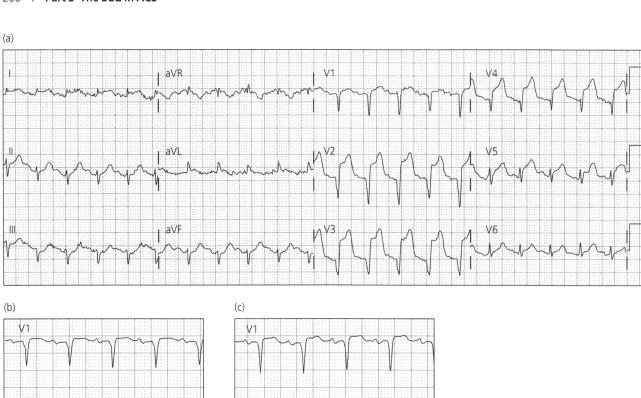

(b)

(c)

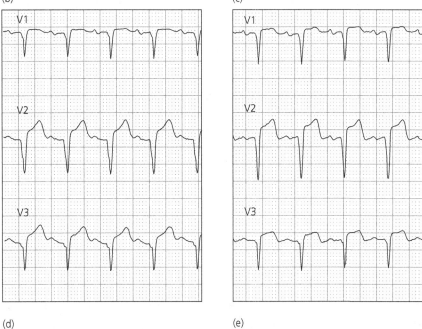

(d)

(e)

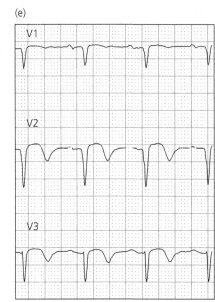

Figure 25.4 Early and complete infarct artery reperfusion, but poor microvascular perfusion and poor outcome. (a) A 72-year-old woman with 30 min of acute onset chest pain while on a treadmill. There are already deep Q waves at < 1 h, 6 mm of STE in V2; there is also STE V2–V5, I, and aVL, with reciprocal ST depression in inferior leads. She went for immediate PCI, with a symptom onset to balloon time of 70 min, and a 100% occluded proximal LAD was opened, with subsequent TIMI-3 flow. (b) (V1–V3 only) Postreperfusion ECG, with 2.5 mm STE in V2 (40% resolution). However, there is no T inversion, and no recovery of the R wave; both are negative prognostic signs. (c) and (d) (V1–V3 only) V1–V3 over the next 2 days, with persistent STE, Q waves, and upright T waves. Maximum CK-MB was very high, at 216.3 ng/mL. (e) After 2 weeks, T waves finally invert, with some residual STE. Echocardiography at this time shows left ventricular aneurysm, and the patient has clinical congestive heart failure.

transient STEMI that has spontaneously opened or received collateral flow. This ECG pattern is demonstrated in (see Figure 19.1, Figure 23.2, and Figures 15.1 and 15.2). The T wave morphology present in Wellens' syndrome is identical to the T wave changes that occur during reperfusion.

T wave inversion is associated with myocardial stunning effect. By 3–4 weeks, normalization of negative T waves is associated with myocardial viability and predicts recovery of regional dysfunction compared with patients with persistent T wave inversion at 4 weeks [44]. Although early normalization of T wave inversion portends clinical improvement, a benefit is still present if T waves normalize within the first 12 months following a STEMI; after 12 months, patients that have normalization of their T waves demonstrate similar LV function to patients with persistently inverted T waves [45].

Reperfusion arrhythmias

Reperfusion-related ventricular arrhythmias (RA) include premature ventricular complexes, AIVR, and ventricular fibrillation [46]. Reperfusion-related ventricular arrhythmia occurs in approximately 50% of successful reperfusions and is considered a marker for the recanalization of the infarct-related epicardial coronary artery [26,46–49]. However, RA is also more frequently seen in patients with no-reflow of the myocardium than in those with reflow [46,50]. There has been some debate over the prognostic implications for not only the presence, but also the timing of RAs following reperfusion therapy.

Very early onset of AIVR, in contrast to later onset, seems to be associated with favorable prognosis. Engelen and colleagues studied 62 patients with acute anterior wall MI treated with either thrombolytics or PCI; 82% had ≥ one episode of AIVR when monitored over the first 24 h following reperfusion therapy [46]. Patients with repetitive, frequent, and early AIVR episodes, especially patients with > 100 AIVRs during the first 6 h after treatment, demonstrated significant deterioration in left ventricular function at 1 to 2-month follow-up [46]. In contrast, Ilia and colleagues found a decrease in short-term mortality of patients undergoing PCI for STEMI if the patient had TIMI grade 3 flow established, and developed RA within 1 min of balloon deflation [51].

ECG manifestations of reocclusion

From discussion above, reperfusion results in resolution or normalization of the ST segment and/or inversion of the T wave. Accordingly, re-elevation of the ST segment and/or normalization ("pseudo-normalization") of inverted T wave to the upright or normal position, are the salient ECG indicators of reocclusion of the IRA. During the early stages of STEMI reperfusion with thrombolytics, there is often sig-

nificant variability and instability in the ST segments, which may occur during or following the resolution of STE [25,52,53]. One-third of these transient ST segment deviations that occur in the initial 24 h after STEMI are a result of persistence of IRA thrombus or TIMI 0 or 1 flow [53]. Of the approximately 2.7–6.4% of successful thrombolytics cases that will have reocclusion, one-third will be asymptomatic [25]. In contrast, IRA reocclusion occurs in up to 15% of patients treated with PCI, and up to 5% of patients treated with stenting [54]. Many authors believe that continuous ST segment monitoring provides the best method for early identification of IRA reocclusions. As discussed previously, frequent serial static 12-lead ECGs may provide adequate information, but may suffer from undersampling.

Each STEMI generates a 12-lead ECG "fingerprint," and, if reocclusion of the original IRA location occurs, will produce the same ECG pattern, including re-elevation of the ST segments [27]. T waves that have become inverted from the initial infarction will rapidly "pseudo-normalize," becoming upright. This "pseudo-normalization" of T waves is seen in Figure 25.2e from Case 2. Postinfarction regional pericarditis may mimic the ECG findings of reocclusion. However, these changes tend to develop in a gradual fashion over 24–72 h following a STEMI [27].

Conclusion

Ideal reperfusion following AMI involves sustained patency of the infarct-related epicardial vessel as well as successful reperfusion at the microvascular and cellular level of the myocardium. Patients that are at higher risk for ventricular dysfunction may be more readily identified through the use of non-invasive monitoring for reperfusion arrhythmias and ST segment recovery, as well as the more invasive angiographic evaluation of TIMI myocardial perfusion grading.

Case conclusions

In Case 1, the ST segment abnormalities and chest pain resolved after administration of the fibrinolytic agent (see Figure 25.1b). Unfortunately, after approximately 45 min, the patient's pain returned, with development of ST segment elevation (Figure 25.1c). He was taken for rescue PCI with demonstration of a 100% occluded right coronary artery (RCA). The artery was opened via stent placement with good flow and an uneventful hospital course thereafter. In Case 2, serial ECGs were obtained during transport and following angiogram (Figure 25.3c–f). The patient experienced partial reperfusion following facilitated PCI and was found to have TIMI grade 2 flow in the LAD on subsequent angiogram. She had stents placed. She experienced cardiogenic shock during the initial hours of her STEMI, but did recover. At her 6-month follow-up she was found to have an ejection fraction of 45%. In Case 3, the patient underwent successful PCI of the RCA There were reperfusion arrhythmias and resolution of STE, as seen in Figure 25.3b and c.

References

1 Keeley EC. Primary angioplasty versus intravenous thrombolytic therapy for acute myocardial infarction: A quantitative review of 23 randomized trials. *Lancet* 2003;**361**:13–20.

2 Boden WE, Eagle K, Granger CB. Reperfusion strategies in acute ST-segment elevation myocardial infarction: a comprehensive review of contemporary management options. *J Am Coll Cardiol* 2007;**50**:917–29.

3 Wijeysundera HC, Vijayaraghavan R, Nallamothu BK, *et al.* Rescue angioplasty or repeat fibrinolysis after failed fibrinolytic therapy for ST-segment myocardial infarction. A meta-analysis of randomized trials. *J Am Coll Cardiol* 2007;**49**:422–30.

4 GUSTO-I Angiographic Investigators. The effects of tissue plasminogen activator, streptokinase or both on coronary artery patency, ventricular function, and survival after acute myocardial infarction. *N Engl J Med* 1993;**329**:673–82.

5 Krucoff MW, Croll MA, Pope JE *et al.* Continuous 12-lead ST-segment recovery analysis in the TAMI 7 study. Performance of a non-invasive method for real-time detection of failed myocardial reperfusion. *Circulation* 1993;**88**:437–46.

6 Hudson MP, Granger CB, Topol EJ, *et al.* Early reinfarction after fibrinolysis: experience from the global utilization of streptokinase and tissue plasminogen activator (alteplase) for occluded coronary arteries (GUSTO I) and global use of strategies to open occluded coronary arteries (GUSTO III) trials. *Circulation* 2001; **104**:1229–35.

7 Armstrong PW, Chang WC, Wallentin L, *et al.* Efficacy and safety of unfractionated heparin versus enoxaparin: a pooled analysis of ASSENT-3 and -3 PLUS data. *Can Med Assoc J* 2006;**174**:1421–6.

8 Eeckhout E, Kern MJ. The coronary no-reflow phenomenon: a review of mechanisms and therapies [see comment]. *Eur Heart J* 2001;**22**:729–39.

9 Carrabba N, Parodi G, Valenti R, *et al.* Significance of additional ST segment elevation in patients with no reflow after angioplasty for acute myocardial infarction. *J Am Soc Echocardio* 2007;**20**: 262–9.

10 van't Hof AW, Liem A, Suryapranata H, *et al.* Angiographic assessment of myocardial reperfusion in patients treated with primary angioplasty for acute myocardial infarction: myocardial blush grade. Zwolle Myocardial Infarction Study Group. *Circulation* 1998;**97**:2303–6.

11 Gibson CM, Cannon CP, Murphy SA, *et al.* Relationship of TIMI myocardial perfusion grade to mortality after administration of thrombolytic drugs. *Circulation* 2000;**101**:125–30.

12 Gibson CM, Cannon CP, Murphy SA, *et al.* Relationship of the TIMI myocardial perfusion grades, flow grades, frame count, and percutaneous coronary intervention to long-term outcomes after thrombolytic administration in acute myocardial infarction. *Circulation* 2002;**105**:1909–13.

13 Gershlick AH, Stephens-Lloyd A, Hughes S, *et al.* Rescue angioplasty after failed thrombolytic therapy for acute myocardial infarction. *N Engl J Med* 2005;**353**:2758–68.

14 Oude Ophuis AJ, Bar FW, Vermeer F, *et al.* Angiographic assessment of prospectively determined non-invasive reperfusion indices in acute myocardial infarction [see comment]. *Heart* 2000;**84**:164–70.

15 de Lemos JA. ST-Segment resolution as a marker of epicardial and myocardial reperfusion after thrombolysis: insights from the TIMI 14 and in TIME-II trials. *J Electrocardiol* 2000;**33**(Suppl):67–72.

16 Caldwell MA, Pelter MM, Drew BJ. Chest pain is an unreliable measure of ischemia in men and women during PTCA. *Heart Lung* 1996;**25**:423–9.

17 de Lemos JA, Morrow DA, Gibson CM, *et al.* Early noninvasive detection of failed epicardial reperfusion after fibrinolytic therapy. *Am J Cardiol* 2001;**88**:353–8.

18 Califf RM, O'Neill WW, Stack RS, *et al.* Failure of simple clinical measurements to predict perfusion status after intravenous thrombolysis. *Ann Int Med* 1988;**108**:658–62.

19 Krucoff MW, Johanson P, Baeza R, *et al.* Clinical utility of serial and continuous ST-segment recovery assessment in patients with acute ST-elevation myocardial infarction: assessing the dynamics of epicardial and myocardial reperfusion. *Circulation* 2004;**110**:e533–9.

20 Drew BJ, Dempsey ED, Joo TH, *et al.* Pre-hospital synthesized 12-lead ECG ischemia monitoring with trans-telephonic transmission in acute coronary syndromes: pilot study results of the ST SMART trial. *J Electrocardiol* 2004;**37**(Suppl):214–21.

21 Zeymer U, Schroder K, Wegscheider K, *et al.* ST resolution in a single electrocardiographic lead: a simple and accurate predictor of cardiac mortality in patients with fibrinolytic therapy for acute ST-elevation myocardial infarction. *Am Heart J* 2005;**149**:91–7.

22 Kleber AG. ST-segment elevation in the electrocardiogram: a sign of myocardial ischemia. *Cardiovasc Res* 2000;**45**:111–8.

23 Angeja BG, Gunda M, Murphy SA, *et al.* TIMI myocardial perfusion grade and ST segment resolution: association with infarct size as assessed by single photon emission computed tomography imaging. *Circulation* 2002;**105**:282–5.

24 Aasa M, Kirtane AJ, Dellborg M, *et al.* Temporal changes in TIMI myocardial perfusion grade in relation to epicardial flow, ST-resolution and left ventricular function after primary percutaneous coronary intervention. *Coron Artery Dis* 2007;**18**:513–8.

25 Kwon K, Freedman SB, Wilcox I, *et al.* The unstable ST segment early after thrombolysis for acute infarction and its usefulness as a marker of recurrent coronary occlusion. *Am J Cardiol* 1991; **67**:109–15.

26 Doevendans PA, Gorgels AP, van der Zee R, *et al.* Electrocardiographic diagnosis of reperfusion during thrombolytic therapy in acute myocardial infarction. *Am J Cardiol* 1995;**75**:1206–10.

27 Smith SW, Zvosec DL, Henry TD, Sharkey SW. *The ECG in Acute MI: an Evidence-Based Manual of Reperfusion Therapy.* Philadelphia: Lippincott, Williams, and Wilkins, 2002:358.

28 Shah A, Wagner GS, O'Connor CM, *et al.* Prognostic implications of TIMI flow grade in the infarct related artery compared with continuous 12-lead ST-segment resolution analysis. Reexamining the "gold standard" for myocardial reperfusion treatment. *J Am Coll Cardiol* 2000;**35**:666–72.

29 Schroder R, Wegscheider K, Schroder K, *et al.* Extent of early ST segment elevation resolution: a strong predictor of outcome in patients with acute myocardial infarction and a sensitive measure to compare thrombolytic regimens. A substudy of the International Joint Efficacy Comparison of Thrombolytics (INJECT) trial. *J Am Coll Cardiol* 1995;**26**:1657–64.

30 van't Hof AW, Liem A, de Boer MJ, *et al.* Clinical value of 12-lead electrocardiogram after successful reperfusion therapy for acute myocardial infarction. Zwolle Myocardial Infarction Study Group. *Lancet* 1997;**350**:615–9.

31 Santoro GM, Antoniucci D, Valenti R, *et al.* Rapid reduction of ST-segment elevation after successful direct angioplasty in acute myocardial infarction. *Am J Cardiol* 1997;**80**:685–9.

32 Syed MA, Borzak S, Asfour A, *et al.* Single lead ST-segment recovery: a simple, reliable measure of successful fibrinolysis after acute myocardial infarction. *Am Heart J* 2004;**147**:275–80.

33 Watanabe J, Nakamura S, Sugiura T, *et al.* Early identification of impaired myocardial reperfusion with serial assessment of ST segments after percutaneous transluminal coronary angioplasty during acute myocardial infarction. *Am J Cardiol* 2001;**88**:956–9.

34 Santoro GM, Valenti R, Buonamici P, *et al.* Relation between ST-segment changes and myocardial perfusion evaluated by myocardial contrast echocardiography in patients with acute myocardial infarction treated with direct angioplasty. *Am J Cardiol* 1998;**82**:932–7.

35 Anderson RD, White HD, Ohman EM, *et al.* Predicting outcome after thrombolysis in acute myocardial infarction according to ST-segment resolution at 90 minutes: a substudy of the GUSTO-III trial. Global Use of Strategies To Open occluded coronary arteries. *Am Heart J* 2002;**144**:81–8.

36 Johanson P, Jernberg T, Gunnarsson G, *et al.* Prognostic value of ST-segment resolution – when and what to measure. *Eur Heart J* 2003;**24**:337–45.

37 2007 Writing Group to Review New Evidence and Update the ACC/AHA 2004 Guidelines for the Management of Patients With ST-Elevation Myocardial Infarction. 2007 Focused Update of the ACC/AHA 2004 Guidelines for the Management of Patients with ST-Elevation Myocardial Infarction. *J Am Coll Cardiol* 2008;**51**.

38 Bar FW, Volders PG, Hoppener B, *et al.* Development of ST-segment elevation and Q- and R-wave changes in acute myocardial infarction and the influence of thrombolytic therapy. *Am J Cardiol* 1996;**77**:337–43.

39 Blanke H, Scherff F, Karsch KR, *et al.* Electrocardiographic changes after streptokinase-induced recanalization in patients with acute left anterior descending artery obstruction. *Circulation* 1983;**68**:406–12.

40 Barbagelata A, Califf RM, Sgarbossa EB, *et al.* Thrombolysis and Q wave versus non-Q wave first acute myocardial infarction: a GUSTO-I substudy. Global Utilization of Streptokinase and Tissue Plasminogen Activator for Occluded Arteries Investigators. *J Am Coll Cardiol* 1997;**29**:770–7.

41 Askenazi J, Parisi AF, Cohn PF, *et al.* Value of the QRS complex in assessing left ventricular ejection fraction. *Am J Cardiol* 1978;**41**:494–9.

42 Sgarbossa EB, Meyer PM, Pinski SL, *et al.* Negative T waves shortly after ST-elevation acute myocardial infarction are a powerful marker for improved survival rate. *Am Heart J* 2000;**140**:385–94.

43 Herz I, Birnbaum Y, Zlotikamien B, *et al.* The prognostic implications of negative T-waves in the leads with ST segment elevation on admission in acute myocardial infarction. *Cardiology* 1999;**92**:121–7.

44 Pierard LA, Lancellotti P. Determinants of persistent negative T waves and early versus late T wave normalisation after acute myocardial infarction. *Heart* 2005;**91**:1008–12.

45 Sakata K, Yoshino H, Houshaku H, *et al.* Myocardial damage and left ventricular dysfunction in patients with and without persistent negative t waves after q-wave anterior myocardial infarction. *Am J Cardiol* 2001;**87**:510–5.

46 Engelen DJ, Gressin V, Krucoff MW, *et al.* Usefulness of frequent arrhythmias after epicardial recanalization in anterior wall acute myocardial infarction as a marker of cellular injury leading to poor recovery of left ventricular function [see comment]. *Am J Cardiol* 2003;**92**:1143–9.

47 Goldberg S, Greenspon AJ, Urban PL, *et al.* Reperfusion arrhythmia: a marker of restoration of antegrade flow during intra-coronary thrombolysis for acute myocardial infarction. *Am Heart J* 1983;**105**:26–32.

48 Gorgels AP, Vos MA, Letsh IS, *et al.* Usefulness of the accelerated idioventricular rhythm as a marker for myocardial necrosis and reperfusion during thrombolytic therapy in acute myocardial infarction. *Am J Cardiol* 1988;**61**:231–5.

49 Hohnloser SH, Zabel M, Kasper W, *et al.* Assessment of coronary artery patency after thrombolytic therapy: accurate prediction using the combined analysis of three noninvasive markers. *J Am Coll Cardiol* 1991;**18**:44–9.

50 Ito H, Iwakura K. Assessing the relation between coronary reflow and myocardial reflow. *Am J Cardiol* 1998;**81**:8G–12G.

51 Ilia R, Zahger D, Cafri C, *et al.* Predicting survival with reperfusion arrhythmias during primary percutaneous coronary intervention for acute myocardial infarction. *Isr Med Assoc J* 2007;**9**:21–3.

52 Hackett D, Davies G, Chierchia S, Maseri A. Intermittent coronary occlusion in acute myocardial infarction. Value of combined thrombolytic and vasodilator therapy. *N Engl J Med* 1987;**317**:1055–9.

53 Johanson P, Wallentin L, Nilsson T, *et al.* ST-segment analyses and residual thrombi in the infarct-related artery: A report from the ASSENT PLUS ST-monitoring substudy. *Am Heart J* 2004;**147**:853–8.

54 Antman EM, Anbe DT, Armstrong PW, *et al.* ACC/AHA guidelines for the management of patients with ST-elevation myocardial infarction – executive summary. A report of the American College of Cardiology/American Heart Association Task Force on Practice Guidelines (Writing Committee to revise the 1999 guidelines for the management of patients with acute myocardial infarction). *J Am Coll Cardiol* 2004;**44**:671–719.

Chapter 26 | Does localization of the anatomic segment/ identification of the infarct-related artery affect early care?

Wayne Whitwam[1], Stephen W. Smith[2]
[1]University of California, San Diego, CA, USA
[2]University of Minnesota, Hennepin County Medical Center, Minneapolis, MN, USA

Case presentations

Case 1: A 62-year-old male with no past history presents at 9:00 pm with 2 days of increasing and intermittent chest discomfort; at presentation, his pain is minimal. The examination is largely unremarkable. He is managed with aspirin and other appropriate medical therapies while chest radiographs and serum laboratory studies are performed. His ECG at presentation is shown in Figure 26.1a. At 9:40 pm, his pain increases significantly, at which time the ECG in Figure 26.1b is recorded.

Case 2: A 63-year-old male with a history of hypertension and known left bundle branch block (LBBB) presents at 3:30 am with chest pressure. The examination demonstrates no acute concerns. Anti-anginal and anti-platelet therapies are administered while diagnostic studies are performed. His initial ECG is shown in Figure 26.2a. It is interpreted as LBBB without evidence of ischemia. The discomfort resolves. The initial troponin is negative. He is admitted to the coronary care unit (CCU). At 6:00 pm, he complains of recurrent discomfort and the ECG in Figure 26.2b is recorded.

Case 3: A 58-year-old female presents with altered mental status, weakness, dizziness, and syncope, but denies chest pain. Her blood pressure is 50/38 with a pulse of 38. She is pale, diaphoretic, and anxious in appearance. The cardiopulmonary examination is remarkable only for a slow heart rate. The presenting ECG is shown in Figure 26.3. Appropriate anti-ischemic therapy is started while the patient is resuscitated.

Critical Decisions in Emergency and Acute Care Electrocardiography,
1st edition. Edited by W.J. Brady and J.D. Truwit. © 2009 Blackwell Publishing, ISBN: 9781405159067

Localization of the anatomic segment/identification of the infarct-related artery and early management issues

ST segment elevation (STE) is the cardinal ECG sign of epicardial injury, such that the vector of the deviated ST segment is directed toward the site of ischemia. Thus, STE in anterior leads is indicative of acute anterior myocardial infarction (MI); whereas STE in inferior leads corresponds with inferior STEMI. The specificity of the ECG to localize the site of acute myocardial injury is precluded by variations of coronary anatomy as well as by the presence of coronary artery disease (CAD), including prior MI, collateral blood flow, and prior coronary artery bypass operation (CABG). Nonetheless, the use of an ECG to assess anatomic correlates of acute injury is helpful in understanding the pathologic process, as well as assessing the amount of myocardium at risk and directing treatment toward its resolution.

Anterior myocardial infarction

Anatomy: The left main coronary artery (LMCA) supplies the left anterior descending artery (LAD) and the (left) circumflex artery (LCX). The LMCA is the principle blood supply of the left ventricle. A persistent complete occlusion of the LMCA usually leads to cardiogenic shock and death (see Case 4, Chapter 27). The LAD may extend distally around the apex to the inferior wall, where it is termed a "wraparound LAD." The LAD supplies the anterior wall, with branches supplying the anterolateral wall (diagonal arteries) and most of the septum (septal arteries). The first septal branch (S1) usually originates from the LAD proximal to the first diagonal

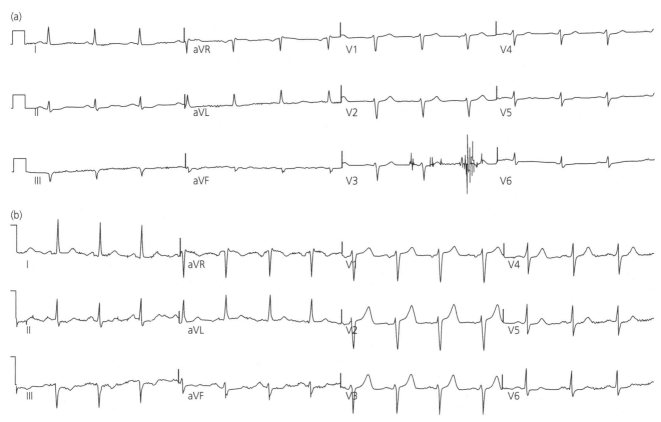

Figure 26.1 (a) This ECG shows no acute ischemia, though it does manifest a wide QS wave in lead III, suggestive of old inferior MI. (b) There is now borderline STE in leads V1–V3 and minimal STE in leads I and aVL, with minimal reciprocal depression in inferior leads. The T-waves are greatly enlarged. Electrocardiographically, this LAD occlusion could be either proximal or distal to the first diagonal. In this case, it was distal.

(D1); but in some it originates distal to D1. There is a wide variability in the number and size of the diagonal branches. More than 90% have one to three such branches [1]. A ramus intermedius (RM), arising at the division of the LMCA and producing a trifurcation of this vessel, instead of the usual bifurcation, was present in over one-third of 418 subjects studied. Only two patients were found to be lacking either diagonal branches or the RM; both had large obtuse marginal branches (OM) of the LCX, which appeared to serve areas of the anterolateral LV wall [1].

Left main coronary artery occlusion: A significant but incomplete occlusion of the LMCA produces STE in lead aVR and less STE in lead V1, while STE in both aVR and aVL predicts occlusion of the LMCA with higher specificity than that in only aVR. Occlusion of the LMCA may also manifest ST segment depression in leads II, III, or aVF, and left anterior fasicular block (see Figure 27.4). While this occlusion is rare, it is life-threatening, requiring immediate therapeutic intervention, often aortocoronary bypass surgery rather than angioplasty [2,3].

Proximal left anterior descending occlusion: A complete occlusion of the LAD proximal to D1 affects anterior, and lateral left ventricular walls, manifesting STE in leads V2–V4 (also often V4–V6), maximally in V2–V3. The differentiation of occlusion proximal versus distal to D1 rests primarily on the presence or absence of inferior reciprocal ST depression in leads II, III, and aVF (see Figure 26.4). There is also frequently STE in leads I and aVL, and occasionally lead V1. ST elevation in aVL > 0.5 mm is very sensitive, and > 1.0 mm is very specific for, occlusion of the LAD proximal to D1 (see Figure 17.1) [4]. However, in the absence of marked precordial STE, STE in aVL may reflect occlusion of D1 alone, or of the first obtuse marginal (OM1) of the circumflex artery (see remarks below). With proximal LAD occlusion, reciprocal ST depression is nearly always present in the inferior leads [5,6], and is usually > 1 mm [7]. This ST depression often co-exists with STE in leads I and aVL. Another predictor of LAD occlusion proximal to D1 is ST depression in lead III > STE in aVL (85% sensitivity, 95% specificity) [8].

If the occlusion is proximal to S1 (see Figures 26.5a and b), the septum may be affected, but it is commonly protected by a conal branch off the RCA (see below). S1 is most often proximal to D1, though not always [7,9]. Occlusion proximal to S1 is predicted on the ECG by STE in aVR (43% sensitivity, 95% specificity); ST depression in V5 (17% sensitivity, 98% specificity); new right bundle branch block (RBBB) (14% sensitivity, 100% specificity); or STE > 2.5 mm in lead V1 (see Figure 26.5a, 12% sensitivity, 100% specificity) [7,9,10].

(a)

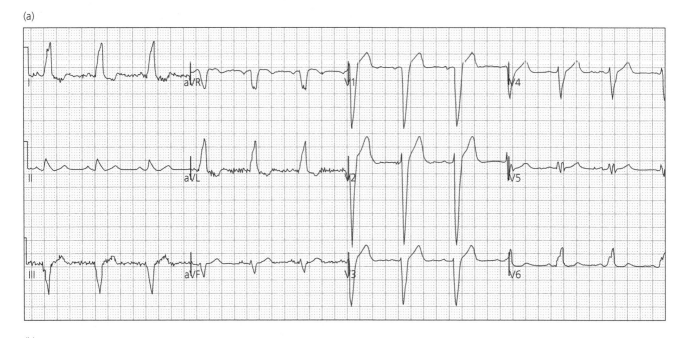

(b)

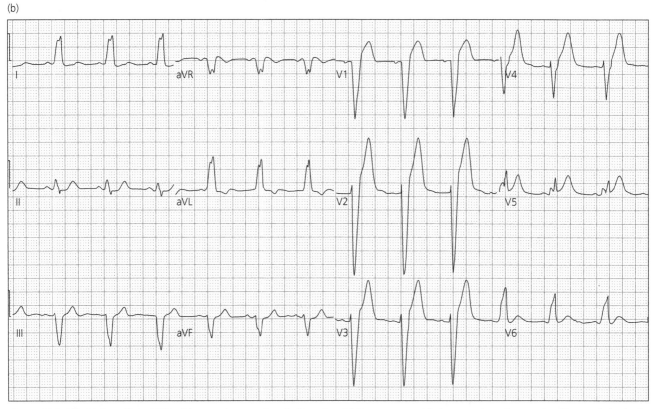

Figure 26.2 This ECG manifests LBBB with normal, proportionally discordant ST-T complexes, with the exception of concordant T waves in leads V5 and V6 (which should make one suspicious of ischemia). (b) LBBB persists, but the T waves in all precordial leads are now much more pronounced (hyperacute T waves). The discordant STE is also more pronounced, and out of proportion, with the ST/S ratio in lead V2 at 7.5 mm/30 mm = 0.25. A ratio ≥ 0.25 is consistent with acute LAD occlusion. As there is no change in I or aVL, and no concordant ST depression in inferior leads, this is consistent with an occlusion distal to the first diagonal; angiography done too late to salvage myocardium proved this correct.

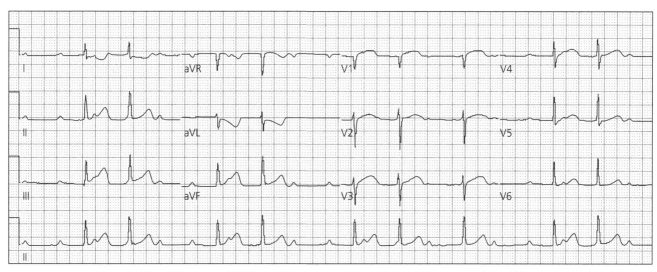

Figure 26.3 The P waves are not associated with a QRS; thus this is complete (third-degree) heart block. There is STE in leads II, III, and aVF, with reciprocal ST depression in I and aVL, diagnostic of inferior STEMI. The presence of significant ST depression in lead I, as well as greater STE in lead III than lead II, is consistent with an RCA (as opposed to LCX) occlusion. Additionally, there is ST elevation in leads V1–V4. This is consistent with additional RVMI, though it could also be seen with a "wraparound" LAD that supplies the inferior wall. The predominance of STE in lead V1 over the other precordial leads argues strongly against this. A right-sided ECG (not available) showed greater STE in right-sided leads than left-sided, confirming RCA occlusion, which was confirmed at angiography.

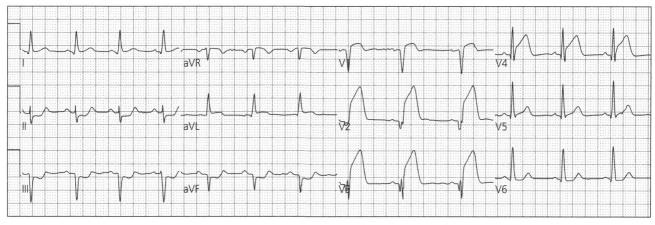

Figure 26.4 LAD occlusion proximal to D1, but distal to S1. There is STE in V1–V4. There can be up to 2.5 mm of STE in V1 without septal involvement, as in this case. The occlusion is proximal to D1; this is manifested as STE (though minimal) in aVL with reciprocal ST depression in inferior leads; the ST depression in lead III > STE in aVL.

Distal or mid-left anterior descending occlusion: When the LAD is occluded distal to S1 and D1, it is called a distal or mid-LAD occlusion; these manifest STE in V2–V4 (± STE in V1, V5, I, and aVL) (see Figure 26.6). However, there is less reciprocal ST depression (≤ 1 mm) in the inferior leads II, III, and aVF. STE in lead aVL, if present, is usually greater than the reciprocal ST depression in lead III [8]. In wraparound LAD (see Figure 20.1), there is STE in II, III and aVF; in such cases LAD, the inferior STE of inferior injury is not offset by the vector of reciprocal ST depression [7]. In echocardiographic studies comparing proximal and distal LAD occlusions, there is no difference in apical wall motion [5].

Mid-anterolateral AMI: Occlusion of the D1 may produce a mid-anterior or mid-anterolateral infarction sparing the apex and septum (see Figure 26.7). Occlusion of D1 may also produce a high lateral MI (see below). A similar pattern may be suggested by occlusion of a RM or high OM branch of the circumflex. These lesions are not to be confused with occlusion of the LAD proximal to D1. If, in addition to the STE in aVL, there is STE in leads V2–V5, the occlusion is most likely at the proximal LAD. Occlusion of D1 produces STE in aVL, and also often the additional non-contiguous V2, and sometimes V1. There may be isoelectric or depressed ST segments in leads V3–V5 [11].

(a)

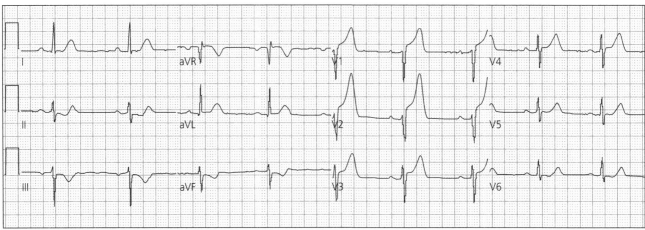

(b)

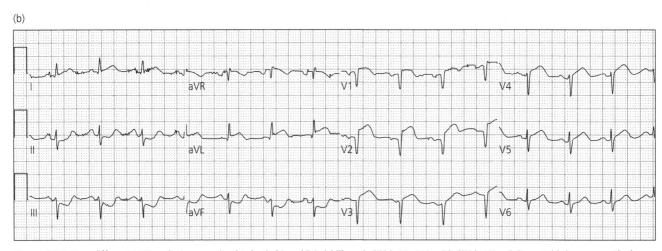

Figure 26.5 Two different LAD occlusions proximal to both S1 and D1. (a) There is STE in V1–V4, with STE in V1 = 2.5 mm; this is very specific for septal involvement and indicates septal injury. The septum did not have collateral circulation off of the conal branch of the RCA, as it does in many cases. (b) There is STE in V1–V4, but this does not mean that the septum is injured; STE in V1 is frequently seen in anteroapical injury. There are no specific indicators of septal involvement. Findings specific for occlusion proximal to D1 are STE in I and aVL, with reciprocal depression in III > STE in aVL.

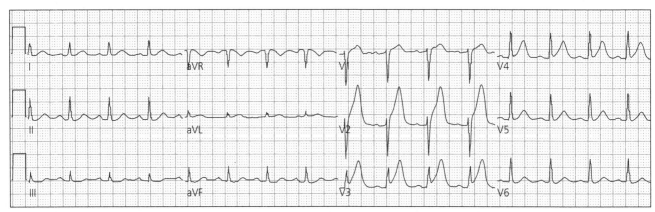

Figure 26.6 Mid- or distal LAD occlusion. There is STE in leads V2–V4, with only minimal, if any, inferior ST depression.

(a)

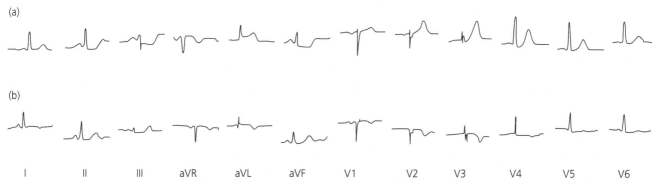

(b)

| I | II | III | aVR | aVL | aVF | V1 | V2 | V3 | V4 | V5 | V6 |

Figure 26.7 Mid-anterolateral MI due to occlusion of the first diagonal artery (no LAD occlusion). (a) Acute STE in leads aVL and V2, with hyperacute T waves in V2–V4 and ST depression in leads III, and aVF (with negative T waves), and also V4–V5 (with positive T waves) (b) ECG on the third day shows a fully evolved T wave inversion in leads V2 and aVL with resolution of the ST depression in the inferior leads. Reprinted with permission from Sclarovsky S, et al. *Int J Cardiol* 1994;**46**:37–47 [11].

Septal AMI: Traditionally, Q waves in V1 and V2 have represented a septal infarction. This assessment was based upon ECG comparisons to autopsy findings of MI in the subacute and chronic phases. It was naturally assumed that STEs in V1 and V2 also correspond with septal injury, but non-invasive imaging techniques in the more acute phases of MI have revised this assumption. Two-thirds of patients receive dual blood supply to the septum from a conal branch of the right coronary artery (RCA), resulting in absence of STE in lead V1 during acute LAD-AMI [12]. However, even in those patients with moderate (< 1.5 mm) STE in V1 (to V3), echocardiographic assessment has demonstrated anteroapical dysfunction but *normal* septal motion [13]. Thus, what appears to be anteroseptal STEMI, with STE in V1–V3, is actually anteroapical. In those patients with V1 STE, the occlusion was the mid-LAD in 80%, the distal LAD in 5%, and the proximal LAD in only 15% of patients [13]. Similarly, another study demonstrated that STE in V1–V3 was associated with LAD occlusion distal to the septal branches in 80% of subjects; however, a STE > 2.5 mm in V1 does predict LAD occlusion proximal to the first septal branch [7].

Other commonly held beliefs correlating location of STE to myocardial location may be called into question with preliminary research. Residual STE in the subacute phase of MI was studied in 55 patients and, when present in lead V3, it was associated more with the apical portion of the inferior wall rather than the anterior wall [14].

Lateral and posterior acute myocardial infarction

Anatomy: The LMCA bifurcates into the LAD and LCX. The lateral wall of the left ventricle (LV) is supplied by the LCX and its OM branches and by D1. When the circumflex is the dominant vessel, the LCX wraps around the obtuse margin of the heart, supplying the posterobasal wall of the left ventricle. Occlusions of vessels that supply the posteroapical wall

manifest as inferior MI; although there is not a clear demarcation anatomically. Branches of a large dominant RCA may also supply the posterolateral wall [15]. Occlusion of a LCX or one of its OM branches accounts for a majority of isolated posterior AMIs (lateral AMI may be present, but rarely pronounced); whereas an RCA occlusion causes concurrent posterior and inferior AMI.

Lateral AMI: Lateral AMI manifests as STE in leads aVL, I, and/or V5–V6, often with STE < 1 mm (0.1 mV) or no STE at all (see Figure 2.1b). The STE may be in lead aVL only, with or without lead I (see Figure 26.8; also see Figure 22.5a). When occlusion of a dominant LCX is present, STE is also seen in leads II, III, and aVF (see Figure 26.9) [16]. The sensitivity of STE for detection of lateral AMI is low because the LCX artery supplies a relatively electrocardiographically silent area of the myocardium. With left circumflex occlusion there is: (1) STE in either inferior and/or lateral leads, with or without ST depression, in approximately 1/3 of cases (and lateral ST elevation is rarely ≥ 2 mm) (2) ST depression alone in 1/3 and (3) neither ST depression nor elevation in approximately 1/3. (4) either or both STE or ST depression (two-thirds), and (5) neither STE nor ST depression in one-third of cases [5,17]. This contrasts markedly with complete LAD occlusion (anterior AMI) or RCA occlusion (inferior AMI), which manifests STE in at least 85–95% of cases [17]. ST segment deviation in the lateral leads (V5, V6, and aVL), but not inferior leads, typically corresponds with acute occlusion of either the LAD proximal to D1, occlusion of D1, or occlusion of OM1, as discussed above.

Posterior AMI (the "inferobasal" segment): From 3.3 to 8.5% of all AMIs, as diagnosed by CK-MB, are posterior AMIs that present without STE on the standard 12-lead ECG. The diagnosis is often missed as the standard 12-lead ECG does not include posterior leads [5]. The ST segment changes are seen indirectly in the anterior precordial leads. Anterior leads face the endocardial surface of the "posterior" wall of

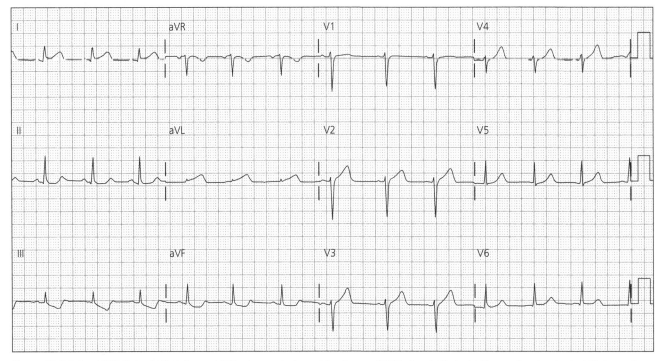

Figure 26.8 Lateral STEMI due to first diagonal (D1) artery occlusion, with < 1 mm of STE in I and aVL, but with prominent reciprocal ST depression in III and aVF.

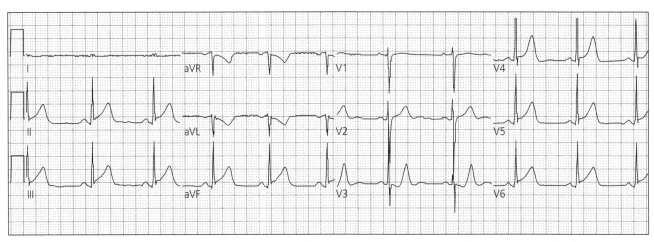

Figure 26.9 Inferolateral STEMI due to occlusion of a large second obtuse marginal off of the (dominant) circumflex. There is inferior STE, as well as STE in V4–V6. The reciprocal ST depression in aVL is attenuated by the lateral STE (it would have been more pronounced without the involvement of the lateral wall).

the LV, recording from the opposite side of the heart instead of directly over the infarct; thus, the changes of posterior injury are reversed in these leads (see Figure 15.10 and Figure 18.1). The development of more prominent R waves in leads V1–V2 are usually associated with the lateral component of a posterior (inferobasal) MI, typically seen following a dominant LCX occlusion [18]. ST depression in V1–V4 may be due to subendocardial ischemia, but persistent ST depression suggests posterior occlusion of an artery supplying the posterior ("inferobasal") wall (either the RCA or LCX). See Chapter 18 for use of additional posterior leads in diagnosis of posterior MI.

Inferior and right ventricular acute myocardial infarction

Anatomy: The RCA is the *dominant* vessel in approximately 80–90% of individuals, meaning it supplies blood to the inferior myocardium. The LCX artery is the dominant vessel in the remaining population; leaving the RCA to supply the right margin of the heart, but not the inferior wall.

Hence, an RCA occlusion is the most common cause of inferior AMI. Proximal occlusion of the RCA results in inferior AMI and concurrent right ventricular (RV) AMI

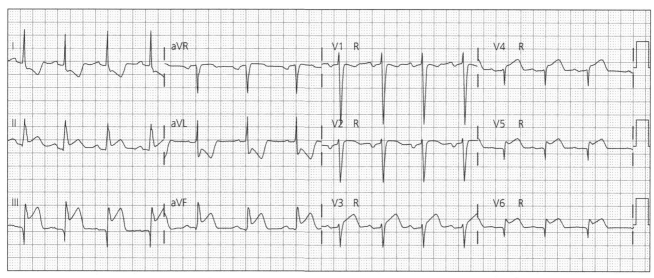

Figure 26.10 Inferior and RVMI (right-sided leads only): limb leads are identical to the limb leads on a standard 12-lead ECG, and show STE in II, III, aVF with reciprocal ST depression in I and aVL. Reciprocal ST depression in I, and STE in lead III > lead II, are found in inferior MI due to RCA, as opposed to LCX, occlusion. The RCA (but never the LCX) supplies the RV; thus, such an inferior pattern may involve the RV as well. The precordial leads are of the RV, proving RVMI by STE in V2R–V6R. This was an occlusion of the RCA proximal to the RV marginal branch. (Courtesy of K. Wang. *Atlas of Electrocardiograph*).

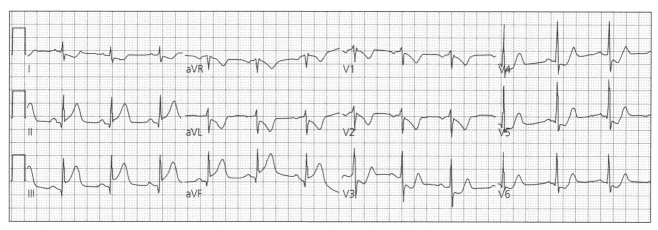

Figure 26.11 Inferoposterior MI due to RCA occlusion. Again, reciprocal ST depression in lead I strongly suggests the RCA, not LCX, as the culprit for this inferior MI. ST depression in V1–V4 is reciprocal to posterior injury (occlusion of the RCA proximal to posterior ["inferobasal"] branches).

(see Figures 26.3 and 26.10). Right coronary artery occlusion distal to the acute marginal branch spares the right ventricle. Occlusion of the RCA with a large posterolateral branch (also known as posterolateral vessel) leads to inferolateral, inferoposterior (see Figure 26.11), and/or inferoposterolateral AMI. Occlusion of the LCX in a left-dominant heart will manifest as an inferolateral or inferoposterolateral AMI. Although RCA and LCX are treated in much the same manner, routine use of nitrates or diuretics in a patient with RCA occlusion, and concurrent RV infarction, may significantly compound hypotension. See Figure 26.12 for a case of inferoposterolateral MI from simultaneous RCA and LCX occlusion. See Figure 26.13 for an inferoposterior MI from circumflex occlusion. See Figures 26.14 and 26.15 for two cases of occlusion of the circumflex or its obtuse marginal branches; both have subtle STE.

Inferior AMI: An RCA (versus LCX) occlusion is suggested with STE in lead III > lead II and with reciprocal ST depression ≥ 1 mm in leads I and AVL (see Figures 26.3 and 26.10) [5]. There may also be STE in leads V1–V4 and/or V4R, a sign of concomitant RV involvement (see Figure 26.3 and 26.10) (see also Figure 24.1) [5].

ST elevation in II ≥ III predicts a dominant LCX as the culprit vessel with 97% sensitivity and 90% specificity [5]. There may also be an isoelectric or elevated ST segment in lead I and/or aVL [5]; an abnormal R wave in lead V1 [16]; or STE in lateral precordial leads (V5, V6) [5].

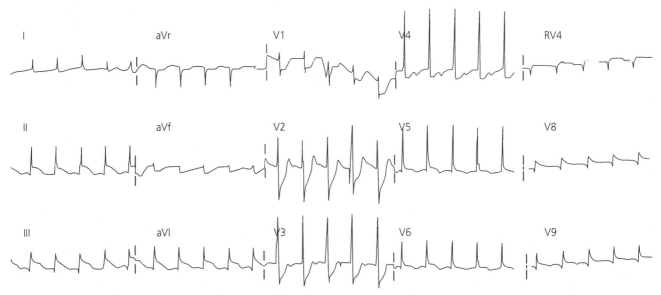

Figure 26.12 Inferoposterolateral AMI due to simultaneous RCA and circumflex occlusion. On this 15-lead ECG, there is STE in II, III, and aVF with reciprocal ST depression in aVL and minimal ST depression in lead I, strongly suggesting LCX as the culprit. There is also posterior injury (ST depression anterior is reciprocal to posterior STE, as proven by STE in posterior leads V7–V9) and lateral injury (V5, V6). Angiography revealed thrombus in both the RCA and LCX, with additional LAD disease.

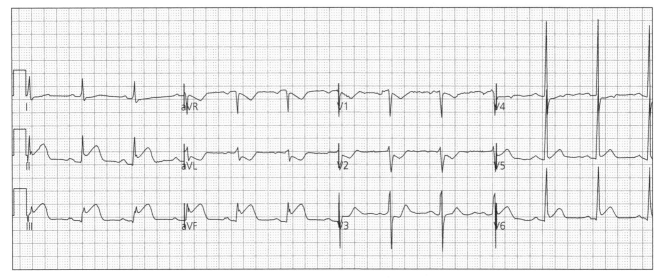

Figure 26.13 Inferoposterolateral AMI due to 100% proximal dominant circumflex occlusion. The lateral STE is minimal.

ST depression in the precordial leads V1–V4 concurrent with inferior lead STE reflects concurrent posterior wall injury. These additional changes reflect a larger amount of myocardium at risk, higher mortality, and greater benefit from reperfusion, but their presence does not discriminate between LCX or RCA occlusions. See Figures 26.11 and 26.12, and Figure 13.2a and Figure 24.3.

Right ventricular AMI: Ischemic involvement of the RV is almost exclusively seen with RCA occlusion. Its presence with inferior AMI is useful in differentiating the anatomic location of the lesion. Right coronary artery occlusion prox-

imal to the RV marginal branch (or acute marginal branch) causes concurrent RV and inferior AMI. With RV AMI, there is RV distention within a fixed pericardial space. The distended RV compromises filling of the LV during diastole, and hypotension follows. There is also an acute risk of complete atrioventricular (AV) block that responds well to atropine, but may require temporary pacing to restore AV synchrony and hemodynamic function [19,20]. As a result, there is a higher short-term morbidity and mortality rate of RV AMI, especially without reperfusion [5,20].

Right ventricle AMI manifests as STE in the precordial leads, especially lead V1 (see Figure 26.3) [21], but also in

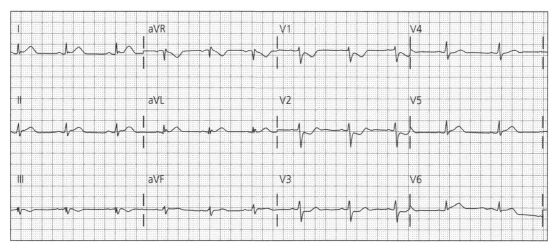

Figure 26.14 Inferoposterolateral AMI due to 100% proximal dominant circumflex occlusion. The STE is minimal in all regions (I, V5, and V6); however, this was a very large MI with CK measured at 6000 IU/L that resulted in a reduction of the ejection fraction from normal to 45%.

(a)

(b)

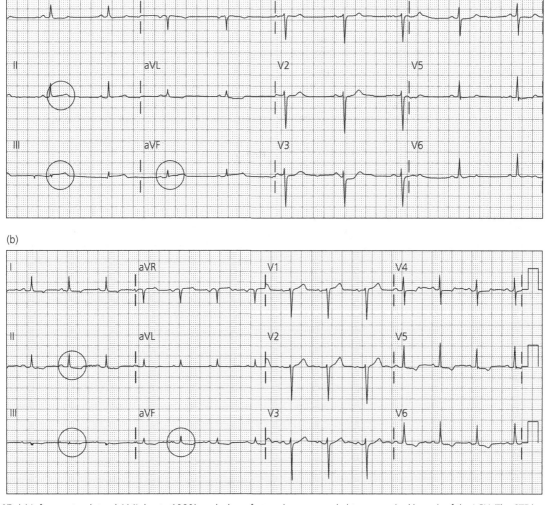

Figure 26.15 (a) Inferoposterolateral AMI due to 100% occlusion of a very large second obtuse marginal branch of the LCX. The STE is minimal, < 1 mm in all leads; however, this also was a large MI with CK measured at 2500 IU/L and a resulting ejection fraction of 55%. (b) ECG of the same patient after reperfusion, as demonstrated by the encircled T waves.

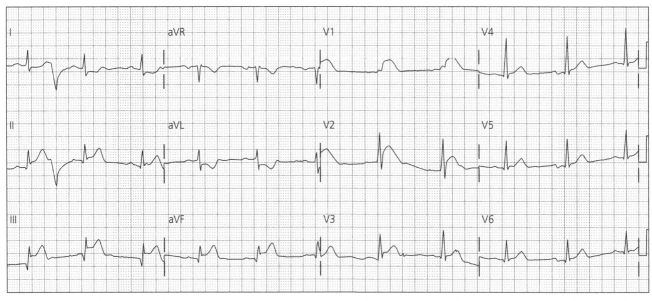

Figure 26.16 "Pseudo-anteroseptal MI" appears to be a simultaneous left ventricular inferior and anterior MI, with STE in II, III, and aVF, as well as V1–V3, but this anterior STE is due to injury of the RV, not LV.

leads V2–V5. These changes occur in addition to the concomitant STE in leads II, III, and aVF of inferior AMI, but may present in the rare event of isolated RV infarction in patients with right ventricular hypertrophy [5,22]. This STE mimics the pattern of anteroseptal AMI (see Figure 26.16, "pseudo-anteroseptal MI"), except that the STE declines progressively toward V5, whereas the anterior LV injury pattern is more elevated in lead V2 to V3, and less in V1 [5,22]. The use of right-sided precordial leads V2R–V7R improves sensitivity for RV AMI (see Figure 26.10). Lead V4R alone has a sensitivity and predictive accuracy for RV infarction of 93% [20]. ST elevation as high as 0.6 mm in V4R can be found in normal individuals, but in the context of inferior AMI, should be interpreted as RV involvement [23,24].

Case conclusions

Case 1: The ECG in Figure 26.1b was interpreted as normal. However, there is a definite change in ST elevation from Figure 26.1a to 26.1b that was not discerned. The patient was not sent for immediate angiography; rather, he was admitted for observation. Subsequently, he suffered significant myocardial loss; delayed angiogram showed a mid-LAD occlusion.

Case 2: The change in ST elevation in leads V1–V5 was not appreciated from Figure 26.2a to 26.2b; the anterior STEMI was missed. Eventual angiography showed a mid-LAD occlusion. There was significant loss of myocardium.

Case 3: The ECG (Figure 26.3) shows third-degree heart block and inferior MI with evidence of RVMI. She was given intravenous fluids, atropine, and dopamine, but required temporary transcutaneous pacing for her heart block; heart rate and blood pressure responded. On right heart catheterization, the patient had elevated right heart pressures (right atrium mean 32 mmHg; RV systolic 40 mmHg); there was a proximal RCA occlusion that was opened.

References

1 Levin DC, Harrington DP, Bettmann MA, *et al.* Anatomic variation of the coronary arteries supplying the anterolateral aspect of the left ventricle: possible explanation of the unexplained anterior aneurysm. *Invest Radiol* 1982;**17**:458–62.

2 Yamaji H, Iwasaki K, Kusachi S, *et al.* Prediction of acute left main coronary artery obstruction by 12-lead electrocardiography. ST segment elevation in lead aVR with less ST segment elevation in lead V(1). *J Am Coll Cardiol* 2001;**38**:1348–54.

3 Gorgels AP, Engelen DJ, Wellens HJ. Lead aVR, a mostly ignored but very valuable lead in clinical electrocardiography. *J Am Coll Cardiol* 2001;**38**:1355–6.

4 Birnbaum Y, Sclarovsky S, Solodky A, *et al.* Prediction of the level of left anterior descending coronary artery obstruction during anterior wall acute myocardial infarction by the admission electrocardiogram. *Am J Cardiol* 1993;**72**:823–6.

5 Smith SW, Whitwam W. Acute Coronary Syndromes. *Emerg Med Clin North Am* 2006;**24**:53–89.

6 Tamura A, Kataoka H, Mikuriya Y, Nasu M. Inferior ST segment depression as a useful marker for identifying proximal left anterior descending artery occlusion during acute anterior myocardial infarction. *Eur Heart J* 1995b;**16**:1795–9.

7 Engelen DJ, Gorgens AP, Cheriex EC, *et al.* Value of the electrocardiogram in localizing the occlusion site in the left anterior descending coronary artery in acute myocardial infarction. *J Am Coll Cardiol* 1999;**34**:389–95.

8 Kosuge M, Kimura K, Toshiyuki I, *et al.* Electrocardiographic criteria for predicting total occlusion of the proximal left anterior descending coronary artery in anterior wall acute myocardial infarction. *Clin Cardiol* 2001;**24**:33–8.

9 Martinez-Dolz L, Arnau MA, Almenar L, *et al.* [Usefulness of the electrocardiogram in predicting the occlusion site in acute anterior myocardial infarction with isolated disease of the left anterior descending coronary artery.] *Rev Esp Cardiol* 2002; **55**:1036–41.

10 Vasudevan K, Manjunath CN, Srinivas KH, *et al.* Electrocardiographic localization of the occlusion site in left anterior descending coronary artery in acute anterior myocardial infarction. *Indian Heart J* 2004;**56**:315–9.

11 Sclarovsky S, Birnbaum Y, Solodky A, *et al.* Isolated mid-anterior myocardial infarction: a special electrocardiographic sub-type of acute myocardial infarction consisting of ST-elevation in non-consecutive leads and two different morphologic types of ST-depression. *Int J Cardiol* 1994;**46**:37–47.

12 Ben-Gal T, Sclarovsky S, Herz J, *et al.* Importance of the conal branch of the right coronary artery in patients with acute anterior wall myocardial infarction: electrocardiographic and angiographic correlation. *J Am Coll Cardiol* 1997;**29**:506–11.

13 Shalev Y, Fogelman R, Oettinger M, Caspi A. Does the electrocardiographic pattern of "anteroseptal" myocardial infarction correlate with the anatomic location of myocardial injury? *Am J Cardiol* 1995;**75**:763–6.

14 Zafrir B, Zafrir N, Ben-Gal T, *et al.* Correlation between ST elevation and Q waves on the predischarge electrocardiogram and the extent and location of MIBI perfusion defects in anterior myocardial infarction. *Ann Noninvasive Electrocardiol* 2004;**9**:101–12.

15 Assali AR, Sclarovsky S, Herz I, *et al.* Comparison of patients with inferior wall acute myocardial infarction with versus without ST-segment elevation in leads V5 and V6. *Am J Cardiol* 1998;**81**:81–3.

16 Huey BL, Beller GA, Kaiser D, Gibson RS. A comprehensive analysis of myocardial infarction due to left circumflex artery occlusion: comparison with infarction due to right coronary artery and left anterior descending artery occlusion. *J Am Coll Cardiol* 1988;**12**:1156–66.

17 Schmitt C, Lehmann G, Schmieder S, *et al.* Diagnosis of acute myocardial infarction in angiographically documented occluded infarct vessel: limitations of ST-segment elevation in standard and extended ECG leads. *Chest* 2001;**120**:1540–6.

18 Bayes de Luna A, Wagner G, Birnbaum Y, *et al.* A new terminology for left ventricular walls and location of myocardial infarcts that present Q wave based on the standard of cardiac magnetic resonance imaging: a statement for healthcare professionals from a committee appointed by the International Society for Holter and Noninvasive Electrocardiography. *Circulation* 2006;**114**:1755–60.

19 Braat SH, de Zwaan C, Brugada P, *et al.* Right ventricular involvement with acute inferior wall myocardial infarction indentfies high risk of developing atrioventricular nodal conduction disturbances. *Am Heart J* 1984;**107**:1183–7.

20 Zehender M, Kasper W, Schonthaler M, *et al.* Right ventricular infarction as an independent predictor of prognosis after acute inferior myocardial infarction. *N Engl J Med* 1993;**328**:981–8.

21 Zimetbaum PJ, Krishnan S, Gold A, *et al.* Usefulness of ST-segment elevation in lead III exceeding that of lead II for identifying the location of the totally occluded coronary artery in inferior wall myocardial infarction. *Am J Cardiol* 1998;**81**:918–9.

22 Smith SW, Zvosec DL, Henry TD, Sharkey SW. *The ECG in Acute MI: an Evidence-Based Manual of Reperfusion Therapy.* Philadelphia: Lippincott, Williams, and Wilkins, 2002:358.

23 Andersen HR, Nielsen D, Hanse LG. The normal right chest electrocardiogram. J Electrocardiol 1987;**20**:27–32.

24 Simon R, Angehrn W. Right ventricular involvement in infero-posterior myocardial infarct: clinical significance of ECG diagnosis. *Schweiz Med Wochenschr* 1993;**123**:1499–507.

Chapter 27 | Can the ECG be used to predict cardiovascular risk and acute complications in ACS?

Wayne Whitwam[1], Nima Taha[2], Khaled Bachour[3]
[1]University of California, San Diego, CA, USA
[2]Los Angeles County / University of California Medical Center, Los Angeles, CA, USA
[3]Wayne State University School of Medicine, Detroit, MI, USA

Case presentations

Case 1: A 77-year-old female presents to the emergency department (ED) with dyspnea on exertion associated with brief episodes of chest tightness with low levels of activity. Physical examination reveals mild respiratory distress with RR 24 and O_2 saturation of 94% on room air. There are bilateral wheezes. The electrocardiogram (ECG, Figure 27.1) demonstrates subendocardial ischemia manifesting as ST depression in leads V1–V6, I, and aVL. Initial troponin I is 15.9 ng/mL.

Case 2: A 58-year-old female is brought to the ED after syncope, with continued weakness and lightheadedness. Blood pressure (BP) is 50/38 mmHg, with a pulse of 38. She is somnolent and confused. Her ECG reveals complete heart block and subtle ST segment changes (Figure 27.2a). Her initial troponin is normal. Shortly after, a second ECG shows ST elevation (STE) in II, III, and aVF, and STE in V1, indicative of proximal right coronary artery (RCA) occlusion with inferior and right ventricular (RV) infarct (Figure 27.2a and b).

Case 3: A 57-year-old female presents to the ED complaining of progressive dyspnea. She is hypoxic, but remaining vital signs are stable. She has jugular venous distention, bilateral lung crackles, a faint S3 cardiac sound, and mild dependent pitting edema. There is subtle STE in V5 and V6, with ST depression in V1–V4 and aVR, and inferior Q waves, as well as loss of R waves in the precordial leads (Figure 27.3).

Critical Decisions in Emergency and Acute Care Electrocardiography,
1st edition. Edited by W.J. Brady and J.D. Truwit. © 2009 Blackwell Publishing, ISBN: 9781405159067

The electrocardiogram in the assessment of cardiovascular risk at presentation of acute coronary syndrome

Early aggressive medical and interventional treatment of acute coronary syndrome (ACS) has been shown to substantially reduce complications, particularly in high-risk patients. Current practice guidelines emphasize risk-stratification upon hospital admission, based on clinical history, physical examination, biochemical markers of myocardial demand, and 12-lead ECG [1]. There are prognostic factors that can be accessed using the ECG during ACS. The presenting ECG allows immediate risk-stratification across the spectrum of ACS. While the introduction of troponin assays have aided in the process of risk-stratification [2,3], the time required for efflux of this biomarker from cardiac myocytes delays treatment, and thus the negative predictive value of troponin at the time of arrival is poor (Case 2, Figure 27.2). Three general categories of probability that signs and symptoms represent ACS are commonly used [4,5]:

(1) High likelihood: new, or presumably new, transient ST segment deviation (1 mm or greater) or T wave inversion in multiple precordial leads.

(2) Intermediate likelihood: fixed Q waves, ST depression 0.5–1 mm, or T wave inversion greater than 1 mm.

(3) Low likelihood: T wave flattening or inversion less than 1 mm in leads with dominant R waves (such as I, aVL, and V1–V6), or normal ECG.

ST elevation myocardial infarction (STEMI) is often defined by the presence of STE ≥ 1 mm (0.1 mV) in at least two contiguous leads. It is associated with a current of injury during transmural myocardial ischemia, and is usually caused by a sudden acute complete atherosclerotic or thrombotic occlusion of a large coronary artery. With STEMI, the myocardial injury is often severe and progressive. Unless

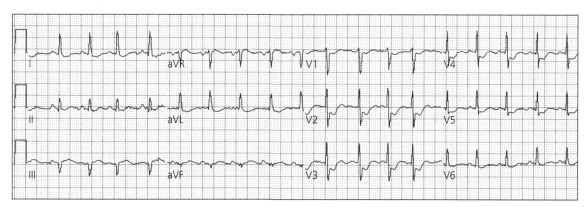

Figure 27.1 Case 1 developed subendocardial ischemia that manifested as 3-mm downsloping ST segment depressions in the anterior precordial leads V1–V6, I, and aVL. Troponin I was moderately elevated at 15.9 ng/mL. The presence of ≥ 2 mm ST segment depression in three or more leads is associated with a high incidence of left main or three-vessel disease and significant increase in the risk of death at 1 year. This patient had three-vessel coronary artery disease requiring surgical bypass.

(a)

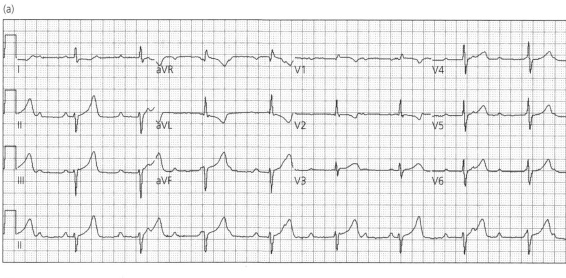

(b)

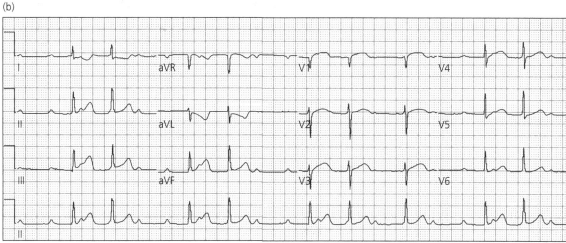

Figure 27.2 Case 2. Complete AV block, with later development of inferior STE. (a) Sinus rhythm (rate 125 bpm) with complete AV block and junctional escape at 51 bpm; there is a suggestion of inferior STE and reciprocal ST depression in aVL. (b) Repeat ECG one-half hour later with obvious inferior STEMI; there is STE in V1 (right ventricular MI) and continued AV block. There is evidence of proximal occlusion of the RCA that manifested as ST segment elevation in the inferior leads (II, III, and aVF), in addition to lead V1. Conduction disturbances like sinus bradycardia, Mobitz type I (Wenckebach) and second- and third-degree AV block are commonly seen with inferior MI, and occasionally anterior MI, and are associated with higher in-hospital and 30-day mortalities.

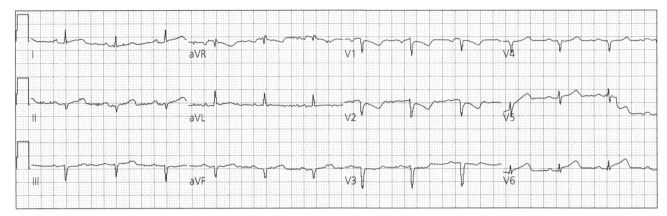

Figure 27.3 Case 3. Posterior acute MI in the presence of old inferior and anterior MI. There is ST depression in V1–V3 and STE in V5 and V6, as well as Q waves in inferior and anterior leads. Angiogram showed acutely occluded LCX and tight LAD stenosis. Although, at first glance, this is not a visually stunning ECG (and the findings were not appreciated), high risk is indicated by Q waves (old infarct both anterior and inferior) and by new ST deviation in the territory of the LCX.

intervention or spontaneous reperfusion (by lysis of thrombus or by collateral circulation) occurs, myocardial necrosis develops in areas where STE was present, with subsequent elevation of serial cardiac troponins. Thus, patients with STEMI should be treated acutely with thrombolysis or primary percutaneous coronary intervention (PCI), if admitted within 12 h of symptom onset.

Patients with large ST deviations (sum of both STE and ST depression) have a more elevated troponin, more reduced left ventricular (LV) function, and higher hospital mortality than those without large ST deviations [6–9]. In the GUSTO-1 database, the sum of the absolute ST deviation, of 19 mm (versus 8 mm) was independently associated with an increased risk [10]. Anterior MI, especially a proximal left anterior descending (LAD) occlusion, has much ST deviation and has the highest 1-year rate of recurrent myocardial infarction (MI) or death [11]. See Figure 25.4 for a case with a large ST sum.

Some investigators showed no relationship between the sum of ST segment deviations and infarct size [12–15]. There are several possible explanations: the magnitude of ST deviation is influenced by the shape and size of the chest wall or infarction site [16]. Also, the ECG in anterior MI can change dramatically within a period of hours; thus, classifying the sum of ST segment deviation may be different depending on the time of recording the acute event. Furthermore, in spite of a large amount of myocardium at risk [17,18], circumflex or first diagonal occlusion may present with minimal or no ST deviation on a standard 12-lead ECG (Case 3, Figure 27.3a; see also Chapter 22) [19–21].

Anterior MI with large STE, though associated with more myocardium at risk and worse outcomes, is also more likely to be detected and receive prompt reperfusion therapy on admission, and this limits its poor prognosis [22].

Independent of ST deviation, distortion of the terminal portion of the QRS (loss of S wave in leads with RS configuration, or J point ≥ 50% the height of the R wave) is associated with a higher hospital mortality [23–25].

Resolution of ST and T wave changes (see also Chapter 25)

Persistent STE following STEMI is associated with both poor short- and long-term outcome in patients, despite complete restoration of TIMI grade 3 flow in the infarct-related artery. Prompt resolution of these changes is a marker of coronary artery patency and microvascular reperfusion, and is associated with smaller infarct size and improved cardiac function [26–29]. In one study, patients with complete (> 70%), partial (30–70%), and < 30% ST resolution at 60 min had 30-day mortalities of 2.1%, 5.2%, and 5.5%, while those with worsening STE had a mortality of 8.1% [30].

Presence of Q waves or loss of R amplitude (see also Chapter 17)

Pathologic Q waves form in the leads overlying the infarcted myocardium. The presence of Q waves at the time of presentation of acute MI may be due to prior MI or due to early formation during the acute MI. In acute anterior MI, Q waves are frequently due to ischemia and injury of the conducting system, as opposed to (irreversible) infarction, and appear within 1 hour of onset of symptoms in 50% of cases, and rapidly resolve with reperfusion [31,32]. Patients who develop Q waves have, on average, larger MI, and thus have less myocardial reserve and are at higher risk if they suffer another MI. The prognostic power of Q waves is mirrored in patients who undergo non-emergent PCI, in whom the development of Q wave MI is the single most powerful negative prognostic indicator [33].

Q waves at presentation in the same leads that demonstrate acute STEMI predict a higher 30-day mortality. Patients who do not ultimately develop Q waves have a greater patency of the infarct-related artery and a smaller MI as demonstrated by a lower CK-MB and a higher LV ejection fraction (EF) before discharge [34]. Absence of Q waves after thrombolytic therapy predicts less severe MI and better outcomes [35]. With anterior MI, there is similar loss of R wave voltage in the precordial leads, seen as a Q wave equivalent. Patients with diminished total R wave voltage have significantly reduced LV dysfunction and a worse prognosis [36].

Similarly, Q waves in leads distant from the acute STEMI, demonstrating evidence of previous MI, carry a higher mortality risk. In a GUSTO-1 analysis, patients with acute inferior MI had better survival than other locations, unless there was ECG evidence of previous MI in another location (either anterior or lateral). In contrast, a previous MI in those with new acute anterior MI carried no increased risk for 30-day mortality compared with patients with no previous MI [10,37].

ST segment depression (see also Chapter 15)

ST depression – if not due to posterior STEMI, or reciprocal changes to STE – is an ECG sign of subendocardial ischemia, and, in the context of ACS, indicates unstable angina/non-ST elevation myocardial infarction (UA/NSTEMI). Whether the ST depression is due to subendocardial ischemia or reciprocal to STEMI, its presence is associated with higher morbidity and mortality. Furthermore, the more leads with ST depression, and the greater the ST depression, the higher the mortality (Case 1, Figure 27.1). ST depression of even 0.5 mm from baseline is associated with increased mortality, but it is particularly significant when ≥ 1 mm (0.10 mV) in two or more contiguous leads [38,39].

ST depression > 2 mm and present in more than three leads is associated with a high probability of elevated CK-MB and almost always with elevated troponin, as well as a high incidence of left main or three-vessel disease [40,41]. Lesser degrees of ST depression (in the absence of PCI) are associated with 30-day mortality rates from 10 to 26% [7,42]. The greater the sum of ST depression in all ECG leads, the greater the risk of mortality at 1 month [40,43].

Persistent ST depression with angina, in spite of maximal medical therapy, is an indication for urgent angiography with possible percutaneous coronary intervention, but not for fibrinolytic therapy [44–46]. In the pre-interventional era, patients with ST depression and acute MI (by CK-MB) (who did not receive fibrinolytics because they are not indicated for ST depression) had a higher mortality than those cohorts with STEMI who did receive fibrinolytic therapy [42,47]. Recent clinical studies continue to support an early routine invasive strategy, particularly with unstable, very high-risk UA/NSTEMI patients [41,48–52]. In stable patients, results from the ICTUS trial suggests that one may achieve similar outcomes with a carefully managed, selective invasive approach, with optimal medical therapy. However, 54% of the selective group had invasive therapy by 1 year [4,53].

Reciprocal ST depression in STEMI

True "reciprocal" ST depression (r-ST depression) is an electrical mirroring phenomenon observed on the ventricular wall opposite transmural injury. In common usage, r-ST depression refers to any ST depression concomitant with STEMI; it improves the specificity for the ECG diagnosis of STEMI (in the anatomic territory of the STE), but does not reflect ischemia in the territory of the ST depression. ST depression seen in posterior STEMI (i.e. ST depression in leads V1–V4) is truly reciprocal only to posterior leads (if present), not to any concomitant inferior or lateral STE. Anterior acute MI manifests r-ST depression in at least one of leads II, III, and aVF in 40–70% of cases; this ST depression correlates strongly with a proximal LAD occlusion [54–57]. With inferior acute MI, reciprocal ST depression is usually present in leads I and aVL; the r-ST depression in precordial leads in most inferior MI is due to concomitant posterior MI and is not true reciprocity.

R-ST depression is associated with a higher mortality [7,10], but also with greater benefit from fibrinolytics [6], especially in inferior AMI, because the r-ST depression is reciprocal to posterior STEMI in approximately 90% of cases and thus represents a second area of transmural MI [58–62]. When STEMI has r-ST depression that remains after resolution of STE, in-hospital mortality is higher [63]. In a minority of inferior STEMI, r-ST depression is a result of subendocardial ischemia in the territory of a second coronary vessel, rather than a mirroring phenomenon. Inferior MI with reciprocal ST depression in leads V4–V6 (versus V1–V3 or those without ST depression), is more likely to have subendocardial ischemia and to have associated three-vessel disease (36% versus 16% and 14%) [64], and derive greater absolute benefit from reperfusion therapy with thrombolytic agents or angioplasty [65]. Acute inferior MI with persistent (≥ 12 h) r-ST depression is associated with multivessel coronary disease, more complications (heart failure, cardiogenic shock, or intraventricular conduction delays) and increased 30-day and 1-year mortality when compared to the absence of these changes [66–69].

T wave inversion (see Chapter 15)

In the undifferentiated patient with chest pain, T wave inversion is associated with increased risk because of its association with ACS. However, for a patient who has known ACS, there is generally less associated mortality risk with T wave inversion than with STE or ST depression.

In the presence of symptoms suggesting ACS, abnormally inverted T waves should be assumed to be a manifestation of ischemia. In patients with ACS, isolated or minimally inverted non-dynamic T waves (< 1 mm), compared to a normal ECG, have not been shown to be associated with adverse outcomes [41]. In contrast, markedly inverted T waves (≥ 2 mm or in ≥ two leads) in patients with angina are predictive of significant coronary artery stenosis, and associated with higher risk when treated medically [70–72]. Such T waves are associated with resolution of symptoms and are a sign of reperfusion of a previously unrecorded coronary occlusive event. These patients require prompt revascularization in order to resolve a critical stenosis of the LAD (see Figure 19.1, Figure 23.2, and Figures 15.1 and 15.2).

T wave inversion due to ACS may be transient (reversible), and may be without significant ST segment shift, indicating transient ischemia (without an elevated troponin), whereas sustained and evolving regional T wave inversion suggests either: (1) spontaneous reperfusion (of the infarct artery, or through collaterals), or (2) in the presence of QS waves, prolonged occlusion both are associated with elevated troponin. After prolonged non-reperfused coronary occlusion (12–72 h), as regional ST segments resolve toward the isoelectric level, T waves have shallow (< 3 mm) inversion in the same region [73].

Very early T inversion is a sign of a patent infarct artery and is independently associated with improved survival [74,75]. Over a time period of weeks to months, the T waves in the infarcted region usually normalize. Absence of T wave resolution, or late appearance of new negative T waves, predicts more pronounced left ventricular enlargement and progressive deterioration of ventricular function. In contrast, normalization of T waves is related to functional recovery of viable myocardium and may be more predictive than QRS changes [76,77].

Lead aVR

In practice, most interpreters neglect lead aVR [78] because it is exactly opposite lateral leads aVL, I, and II, and STE in aVR is often reflected by ST depression in these leads. However, STE in lead aVR independently predicts higher rates of in-hospital death, recurrent ischemic events, and heart failure [79,80]. ST elevation in aVR ≥ STE in V1 is associated with acute left main coronary artery obstruction (Figure 27.4) [81,82]. Similarly, inferior or lateral acute STEMI with ST depression in aVR confers higher risk and larger infarct size [83].

Conduction abnormalities

Bradyarrhythmias and conduction disturbances are well recognized complications of acute MI. They are induced by either autonomic imbalance or ischemia and necrosis of the conduction system, and may either be transient or progress to irreversible and symptomatic high-degree atrioventricular (AV) block. While the incidence of conduction abnormalities associated with acute MI has diminished with prompt revascularization, the mortality and morbidity associated with these abnormalities remains unchanged.

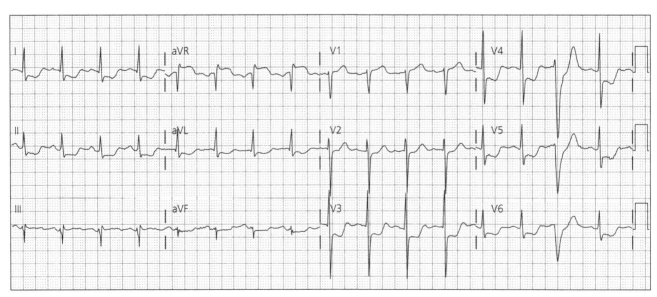

Figure 27.4 Left main occlusion. This 38-year-old male presented with severe dyspnea, chest pain, and agitation. He quickly arrested and was not resuscitated. ST elevation (2 mm) in aVR, along with diffuse ST depression, most pronounced in lead V4, is strongly associated with left main insufficiency and poor outcome.

Bundle branch block

In the presence of acute MI, patients with new right (R) or left (L) bundle branch block (BBB) have a worse prognosis, with a greater incidence of congestive heart failure, cardiogenic shock, and ventricular arrhythmias [84], and a higher 1-year mortality (up to 55%) than either STEMI (21%) or NSTEMI (31%) with normal conduction [85]. Higher mortality is associated with persistent (22% of BBB, 19% mortality), as opposed to transient, BBB (78% of BBB, 6% mortality) [86]. Patients with BBB are typically older, more frequently have diabetes mellitus, peripheral vascular disease, and previous coronary artery bypass grafting. They have lower EF and more multivessel disease [87]. The true incidence of new-onset BBB at acute MI is unknown because it is often transient, under-recognized, and under-reported. Even RBBB is greatly undertreated with reperfusion therapy [88], despite its very high associated mortality [88–90]. Pre-existing BBB in the presence of an acute MI also has a poor prognosis.

Bundle branch block with acute MI varies between 8 and 18%, with a higher incidence of RBBB, although LBBB is more prevalent in patients with chronic ischemic disease. Some studies suggest that RBBB with acute MI portends a higher risk than LBBB; these studies do not differentiate between new or pre-existing BBB [88,91,92]. This is counter-intuitive because more widespread ischemia is necessary for the destruction of the two fascicles of the left bundle versus the one right bundle.

This higher mortality in the presence of RBBB [89,92] is most likely due to selection bias: clinical trial criterion for receiving thrombolytics for LBBB was "LBBB not known to be old." Thus, many patients with LBBB and NSTEMI, who are at lower immediate risk, would have received thrombolytics and been included in this study. In contrast, STE in the setting of RBBB is more easily recognized, and thus nearly all the patients who received thrombolytics would have had STEMI. In RBBB, assessment of ST segment amplitude is only slightly more difficult than in normal conduction, whereas LBBB significantly distorts STE patterns. Although there is reason to believe that coronary occlusion may be nearly as detectable for LBBB as for normal conduction, current recommendations are to treat patients with chest pain and new, or presumably new, LBBB with prompt aggressive reperfusion or interventional therapy [93].

Despite the higher clinical risk profile, clinicians often remain reluctant to provide prompt therapy in patients with acute MI and new BBB. In the NRMI database, patients who had LBBB were less likely to receive aspirin, beta-blockers, heparin, and intravenous nitroglycerin. They were also 4.2 times less likely to receive reperfusion therapy than patients who did not have LBBB [88].

ST elevation myocardial infarction, when associated with non-specific intraventricular conduction delay, or incomplete BBB (QRS interval 100–120 ms), is also associated with a higher risk of short- and long-term mortality, even after accounting for age, gender, and clinical factors [94,95]. Left ventricular hypertrophy (LVH) [96] or paced rhythm also confer a higher short-term mortality.

Second- and third-degree heart block

Conduction disturbances associated with acute MI can occur acutely or after hours or days. They are usually transient, but are nevertheless associated with increased risk, and this is especially true of high-grade AV block. Sinus bradycardia, Mobitz Type I (Wenckebach) and second- and third-degree AV block are commonly seen with inferior MI, as the sinoatrial (SA) node, AV node, and His bundle are primarily supplied by the RCA (Case 2, Figure 27.2). Heart block in anterior MI may occur (2.5%, versus 9.4% of inferior MI) and is usually complete, with widened QRS complexes and associated Stokes-Adams attacks; it is associated with higher mortality [97,99]. Patients with heart block during MI are also more likely to be elderly, female, have diabetes mellitus and hypertension, use tobacco, and have a worse Killip class upon presentation [99]. The incidence of heart block and mortality rates have been generally unchanged in the reperfusion era: recently reported short-term mortality rates have ranged from 8.4 [100] to 29.6% [101].

Sinus bradycardia is the most common arrhythmia associated with inferior MI, present in up to 40% of patients in the first 2 h. It is usually attributable to increased vagal tone in the first 24 h after MI onset and is responsive to atropine. Transient sinus node dysfunction occurring later may be due to sinus node or atrial ischemia. First-degree AV block due to occlusion of the RCA with involvement of the AV node is usually transient, generally resolving in 5–7 days; it requires no therapy.

Sustained ventricular arrhythmias

Ventricular fibrillation (VF) or ventricular tachycardia (VT) during acute MI is associated with complete vessel occlusion and with early mortality, even in the absence of congestive heart failure and hypotension. Most VF and VT occurs in the first 48 h (Case 3, Figure 27.3). Mortality risk is pronounced in the first 30 days, but not thereafter [102]. When compared with patients with VF and polymorphic VT, patients with monomorphic VT during the early phase of acute MI have been found to have more extensive infarctions, more hemodynamic complications, a wider QRS (> 130 ms), higher in-hospital recurrence rate of arrhythmia, and higher in-hospital mortality [103,104]. By 1992, the incidence of primary VF during the first hours in the cardiac care unit had declined to 0.35% [105]. Thus, routine use of anti-arrhythmics has since been discouraged. Only a small fraction of those with "warning arrhythmias" such as ventricular premature beats (VPB or premature ventricular contraction, PVC) subsequently suffer VF [106].

In spite of reperfusion therapy, VT and VF still occur. Some investigations have suggested that these ventricular arrhythmias are associated with coronary reperfusion, others have related them to suboptimal reperfusion [107–112]. For those patients who make it to the catheterization laboratory for primary percutaneous intervention, VF and VT occur in 4.3% of presentations, and are associated with shorter time to treatment, TIMI-0 flow, RCA infarct, smoking, and lack of preprocedural beta-blockers. When these arrhythmias do occur, if they are treated promptly with beta-blockers and anti-arrhythmics, they do not affect PCI success or in-hospital or 1-year outcomes [113]. Late occurrence of these arrhythmias, especially monomorphic VT, is associated with scar formation.

The most frequent reperfusion arrhythmias are VPB, accelerated idioventricular rhythm (AIVR), and non-sustained VT, rather than VF or sustained VT. Accelerated idioventricular rhythm is a marker of restoration of antegrade flow and myocardial reperfusion; its presence supports an improved 30-day prognosis [114]. Early occurrence (< 6 h) of AIVR can be a specific (76%) sign of a patent coronary artery after thrombolytic therapy [109].

Atrial fibrillation

Atrial fibrillation (AF) may be present in as many as 22% of patients with AMI, NSTEMI, or STEMI. In one study, 10.8% of patients had AF on arrival, and 11.3% developed AF during hospitalization [115]. Patients presenting with AF and AMI are more likely to be elderly, female, have a history of hypertension, have more advanced heart failure, and to have had a prior MI and undergone coronary revascularization [115,116]. Atrial fibrillation is usually a premorbid condition, not related to the acute MI.

Several studies have shown increased hospital and long-term death rates associated with AF in the setting of MI [115,117–120], but others have shown no independent effect of this rhythm disturbance on in-hospital or long-term mortality [121–123]. In one registry, patients with AF and ACS are 2.5–4 times more likely to suffer death, reinfarction, cardiogenic shock, pulmonary edema, cardiac arrest, major bleeding, and stroke than those patients without AF [116]. Only new-onset AF was found to be an independent predictor of worse in-hospital outcomes in patients with ACS [116].

Heart rate

During acute MI, sinus tachycardia (heart rate, HR ≥ 100 beats per minute, bpm) may be a manifestation of heightened adrenergic tone (a source of further stress) or lower stroke volume and impending hemodynamic failure [124]. It is a negative prognostic sign, and an independent risk predictor of mortality [125–127]. With an elevated HR there is an increase in cardiac work and myocardial oxygen consumption, producing myocardial ischemia that facilitates arrhythmias. A HR ≥ 90 bpm is associated with increased in-hospital and 1-year mortalities [128]. Similar results were observed in the GUSTO-1 database of 41,021 subjects with a HR of 84 bpm (versus 60 bpm) [10].

In early studies of MI, beta-blockers demonstrated beneficial clinical effects in acute MI when started in the first 24 h. However, their use in the largest randomized trial was associated with cardiogenic shock [129]; the American College of Cardiology/American Heart Association (ACC/AHA) now advise against the use of beta-blockers in MI patients at risk of shock; this would include those with tachycardia [130].

The normal or non-specific ECG

Fewer than half of the patients who are admitted with chest pain have a final diagnosis of ACS [131]. However, up to 6% of those discharged from the ED have a missed MI, with associated higher mortality [132,133]. Many of these patients, in fact, have ischemic changes on an ECG that were missed by the interpreting physician (Case 3, Figure 27.3) see also Cases 1 and 2 in Chapter 26 [134]. Others present with normal or non-specific ECGs. Patients with normal or non-specific ECGs (NoNsECG), as compared with diagnostic ECGs, have lower in-hospital mortality and event rates. However, 20% of patients who presented with NoNsECGs eventually developed ECG changes consistent with ischemia, in which case the mortality rates exceeded that for patients with initially diagnostic ECGs [135]. In most cases, a single ECG recording provides only a single snapshot view of dynamic process (Case 2, Figure 27.2) [136]. Both serial and continuous ECG recordings can provide improved sensitivity for ischemic changes not observed in a single recording [137,138]. Although risk may be low if the initial ECG has no high-risk features, risk is greatly increased if subsequent ECGs develop high-risk features [139]. Serial troponins will have a higher diagnostic yield, but their presence does not provide therapeutic criteria for thrombolytics [93,140]. Outcome is not different if the NoNsECG is recorded during the presence or absence of symptoms; the rate of 30-day cardiovascular events is the same [141].

Multivariable risk algorithms

Clinical triage decisions based on ECG and troponin elevation alone have been developed from large randomized trials of patients with known ACS, but are often applied to all patients with chest pain. Risk assessment may be based on the ECG alone, or also on additional testing such as troponin, with or without additional independent clinical predictors. Application of models may be limited to either STEMI or UA/NSTEMI, or to the whole spectrum of ACS. Some of the earlier models predicted only mortality, while more recent ones provide information on recurrent MI and ischemia, taking advantage of new or emerging prognostic variables.

Brush and colleagues proposed a simple risk assessment criteria based solely on the ECG criteria and found that life-threatening complications were 23 times more likely in patients with ECGs suggestive of ischemia or infarction [142]. Patients classified in the negative group had a low incidence of life-threatening complications (0.6%), but had a higher number of infarctions than expected (15%), and up to 48% were diagnosed with unstable angina.

Clinical signs and history were added to the ECG-only model to create a better predictive instrument that would improve sensitivity without jeopardizing specificity. Two

widely used models added clinical signs and history to the ECG-only model, improving sensitivity without harming specificity. The Goldman Chest Pain Protocol [143] and the Acute Cardiac Ischemia Time Insensitive Predictive Instrument (ACI-TIPI) [144] were developed prior to the routine use of reperfusion therapy. Both may improve decision-making, improving safety and utilization of the coronary care unit (CCU) [145–147].

A multivariate analysis of 41,021 patients demonstrated ECG variables in predicting 30-day mortality in patients with STEMI [10]. These included sum of ST segment deviation in all leads (STE plus ST depression) ≥ 19 mm, new inferior MI with prior ECG evidence of MI in either lateral or anterior territory, HR ≥ 84 bpm, or QRS duration ≥ 100 ms for anterior MI. Variables such as LVH, first- or second-degree AV block, and, surprisingly, complete heart block were not significant predictors of 30-day mortality [10].

The Thrombolysis in Myocardial Infarction (TIMI) study group developed a ten-point risk score for STEMI [148],

Table 27.1 Risk calculator for 6-month postdischarge mortality after hospitalization for acute coronary syndrome [126]

Medical history		Findings at initial hospital presentation		Findings during hospitalization	
1. Age in years	Points	**4.** Resting heart rate, bpm	Points	**7.** Initial serum creatinine, mg/dL	Points
≤ 29	0		0		1
30–39	0	≤ 49.9	3	0–0.39	3
40–49	18	50–69.9	9	0.4–0.79	5
50–59	36	70–89.9	14	0.8–1.19	7
60–69	55	90–109.9	23	1.2–1.59	9
70–79	73	110–149.9	35	1.6–1.99	15
80–89	91	150–199.9	43	2–3.99	20
≥ 90	100	≥ 200		≥ 4	
2. History of congestive heart failure	24	**5.** Systolic blood pressure, mmHg	24	**8.** Elevated cardiac enzymes	15
			22		
		≤ 79.9	18		
		80–99.9	14		
		100–119.9	10		
		120–139.9	4		
		140–159.9	0		
		160–199.9			
		≥ 200			
3. History of myocardial infarction	12	**6.** ST segment depression	11	**9.** No in-hospital percutaneous coronary intervention	14
Points					
1. _____		5. _____		9. _____	
2. _____		6. _____		**Total risk score** _____ (sum of points)	
3. _____		7. _____			
4. _____		8. _____		**Mortality risk** _____ (from plot)	

Record the points for each variable at the bottom left and add the points to calculate the total risk score. Find the score on the x-axis of the nomogram plot (Figure 27.5). The corresponding probability on the y-axis is the estimated probability of all-cause mortality from hospital discharge to 6 months.

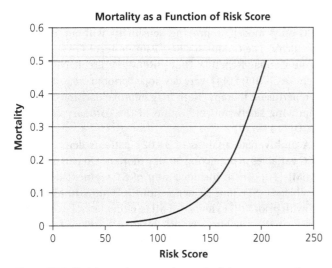

Figure 27.5 Find the total score on the x-axis of the nomogram plot. The corresponding probability on the y-axis is the estimated probability of all-cause mortality from hospital discharge to 6 months.

and a seven-point score for UA/NSTEMI [125]. The risk algorithm for UA/NSTEMI (TIMI risk score) has since been validated as a model for unselected patients in the ED presenting with chest pain [149–151]. This clinical tool is available at www.timi.org

The Global Registry of Acute Coronary Events (GRACE) is an international database designed to track outcomes of patients presenting with ACS. A risk score calculator compiled from their database of patients with ACS predicts in-hospital mortality as well as recurrent MI [126,152]. The calculator (see Table 27.1 and Figure 27.5) was validated in subsequent GRACE and GUSTO IIb cohorts, and found to have superior predictive accuracy in ACS populations, compared with the TIMI or PURSUIT scores [153]. This clinical tool is available at www.outcomes-umassmed.org/grace for download to computers and handhelds.

Case conclusions

In Case 1, after aspirin, heparin, eptifibatide, and nitroglycerin, the ECG changes resolved. The next day, a coronary angiogram revealed severe three-vessel disease including a 100% chronic RCA occlusion with left-to-right collaterals. An echocardiogram (echo) revealed EF of 45%, with anteroseptal hypokinesis. After four-vessel bypass, she was discharged home.

The patient in Case 2 received intravenous fluids, atropine, and dopamine, with good response and resolution of heart block. Initial troponin I was normal. A coronary angiogram revealed a proximally occluded dominant RCA, and right heart cath. revealed elevated pressures (right atrium: mean 32 mmHg). After stenting of the proximal RCA, troponin increased sharply. Predischarge echo demonstrated pre-

served bi-ventricular function with no regional wall motion abnormalities (WMA) and EF of 60%. She was discharged 3 days later in a stable condition.

In Case 3, the ECG findings were not appreciated and the patient was admitted to the CCU without going to the cath. lab. She developed multiple episodes of monomorphic ventricular tachycardia. Troponin I was 43 ng/mL (normal < 2.1). Echo revealed severe systolic dysfunction with an EF of 30%, and new inferoposterior and distal lateral wall severe hypokinesis, and severe mitral regurgitation. Cardiogenic shock ensued, requiring pressors and endotracheal intubation with mechanical ventilation. A balloon pump was placed and immediate cardiac cath. demonstrated a diffusely narrowed LAD and discrete 100% occlusion of the proximal circumflex (LCX), which was opened with balloon angioplasty.

References

1 Braunwald E, Antman EM, Beasley JW, *et al.* ACC/AHA guideline update for the management of patients with unstable angina and non-ST-segment elevation myocardial infarction – 2002: summary article: a report of the American College of Cardiology/American Heart Association Task Force on Practice Guidelines (Committee on the Management of Patients With Unstable Angina). *Circulation* 2002;**106**:1893–900.

2 Scirica BM, Morrow DA. Troponins in acute coronary syndromes. *Prog Cardiovasc Dis* 2004;**47**:177–88.

3 Antman EM, Tanasijevic MJ, Thompson B, *et al.* Cardiac-specific troponin I levels to predict the risk of mortality in patients with acute coronary syndromes. *N Engl J Med* 1996;**335**:1342–9.

4 Anderson JL, Adams CD, Antman EM, *et al.* ACC/AHA 2007 Guidelines for the Management of Patients With Unstable Angina/Non ST-Elevation Myocardial Infarction. A Report of the American College of Cardiology/American Heart Association Task Force on Practice Guidelines. *J Am Coll Cardiol* 2007;**50**:1–157.

5 Braunwald E, Jones RH, Mark DB, *et al.* Diagnosing and managing unstable angina. Agency for Health Care Policy and Research. *Circulation* 1994;**90**:613–22.

6 Willems JL, Willems RJ, Willems GM, *et al.* Significance of initial ST segment elevation and depression for the management of thrombolytic therapy in acute myocardial infarction. *Circulation* 1990;**82**:1147–58.

7 Savonitto S, Ardissino D, Granger CB, *et al.* Prognostic value of the admission electrocardiogram in acute coronary syndromes. *JAMA* 1999;**281**:707–13.

8 Bar FW, Vermeer F, de Zwaan C, *et al.* Value of admission electrocardiogram in predicting outcome of thrombolytic therapy in acute myocardial infarction. *Am J Cardiol* 1987;**59**:6–13.

9 Clements IP, Kaufmann UP, Bailey KR, *et al.* Electrocardiographic prediction of myocardial area at risk. *Mayo Clin Proc* 1991;**66**:985–90.

10 Hathaway WR, Peterson ED, Wagner GS, *et al.* Prognostic significance of the initial electrocardiogram in patients with acute myocardial infarction. GUSTO-I Investigators. Global Utilization of Streptokinase and t-PA for Occluded Coronary Arteries. *JAMA* 1998;**279**:387–1.

11 Haim M, Hod H, Reisin L, *et al.* Comparison of short- and long-term prognosis in patients with anterior wall versus inferior or lateral wall non-Q-wave acute myocardial infarction. Secondary Prevention Reinfarction Israeli Nifedipine Trial (SPRINT) Study Group. *Am J Cardiol* 1997;**79**:717–21.

12 Madias JE, Venkataraman K, Hodd WB, Jr. Precordial ST-segment mapping 1. Clinical studies in the coronary care unit. *Circulation* 1975;**52**:799–809.

13 Murray RG, Peshock RM, Parkey RW, *et al.* ST isopotential precordial surface maps in patients with acute myocardial infarction. *J Electrocardiol* 1979;**12**:55–64.

14 Thompson PL, Katavatis V. Acute myocardial infarction. Evaluation of precordial ST segment mapping. *Br Heart J* 1976;**38**: 1020–4.

15 Norris RM, Barratt-Boyes C, Heng MK, Singh BN. Failure of ST segment elevation to predict severity of acute myocardial infarction. *Br Heart J* 1976;**38**:85–92.

16 Yusuf S, Lopez R, Maddison A, *et al.* Value of electrocardiogram in predicting and estimating infarct size in man. *Br Heart J* 1979;**42**:286–93.

17 Christian TF, Clements IP, Gibbons RJ. Noninvasive identification of myocardium at risk in patients with acute myocardial infarction and nondiagnostic electrocardiograms with technetium-99m-sestamibi. *Circulation* 1991;**83**:1615–20.

18 O'Keefe JHJ, Sayed-Taha K, Gibson W, *et al.* Do patients with left circumflex coronary artery-related acute myocardial infarction without ST-segment elevation benefit from reperfusion therapy? (see comments). *Am J Cardiol* 1995;**75**:718–20.

19 Huey BL, Beller GA, Kaiser D, Gibson RS. A comprehensive analysis of myocardial infarction due to left circumflex artery occlusion: comparison with infarction due to right coronary artery and left anterior descending artery occlusion. *J Am Coll Cardiol* 1988;**12**:1156–66.

20 Berry C, Zalewsky A, Kovach R, *et al.* Surface electrocardiogram in the detection of transmural myocardial ischemia during coronary artery occlusion. *Am J Cardiol* 1989;**63**:21–6.

21 Veldkamp RF, Sawchak S, Pope JE, *et al.* Performance of an automated real-time ST segment analysis program to detect coronary occlusion and reperfusion. *J Electrocardiol* 1996;**29**: 257–63.

22 Sharkey SW, Berger CR, Brunette DD, Henry TD. Impact of the electrocardiogram on the delivery of thrombolytic therapy for acute myocardial infarction. *Am J Cardiol* 1994;**73**:550–3.

23 Smith SW, Zvosec DL, Henry TD, Sharkey SW. *The ECG in Acute MI: an Evidence-Based Manual of Reperfusion Therapy.* Philadelphia: Lippincott, Williams, and Wilkins, 2002: 358.

24 Birnbaum Y, Maynard C, Wolfe S, *et al.* Terminal QRS distortion on admission is better than ST-segment measurements in predicting final infarct size and assessing the Potential effect of thrombolytic therapy in anterior wall acute myocardial infarction. *Am J Cardiol* 1999;**84**:530–4.

25 Birnbaum Y, Criger DA, Wagner GS, *et al.* Prediction of the extent and severity of left ventricular dysfunction in anterior acute myocardial infarction by the admission electrocardiogram. *Am Heart J* 2001;**141**:915–24.

26 Schroder K, Wegscheider K, Zeymer U, *et al.* Extent of ST-segment deviation in a single electrocardiogram lead 90 min after thrombolysis as a predictor of medium-term mortality in acute myocardial infarction. *Lancet* 2001;**358**:1479–86.

27 van't Hof AW, Liem A, de Boer MJ, *et al.* Clinical value of 12-lead electrocardiogram after successful reperfusion therapy for acute myocardial infarction. Zwolle Myocardial Infarction Study Group. *Lancet* 1997;**350**:615–9.

28 Angeja BG, Gunda M, Murphy SA, *et al.* TIMI myocardial perfusion grade and ST segment resolution: association with infarct size as assessed by single photon emission computed tomography imaging. *Circulation* 2002;**105**:282–5.

29 Lepper W, Sieswerda GT, Vanoverschelde JL, *et al.* Predictive value of markers of myocardial reperfusion in acute myocardial infarction for follow-up left ventricular function. *Am J Cardiol* 2001;**88**:1358–63.

30 Cura FA, Roffi M, Pasca N, *et al.* ST-segment resolution 60 minutes after combination treatment of abciximab with reteplase or reteplase alone for acute myocardial infarction (30-day mortality results from the resolution of ST-segment after reperfusion therapy substudy). *Am J Cardiol* 2004;**94**: 859–63.

31 Barold SS, Falkoff MD, Ong LS, Heinle RA. Significance of transient electrocardiographic Q waves in coronary artery disease. *Cardiol Clin* 1987;**5**:367–80.

32 Raitt MH, Maynard C, Wagner GS, *et al.* Appearance of abnormal Q waves early in the course of acute myocardial infarction: implications for efficacy of thrombolytic therapy. *J Am Coll Cardiol* 1995;**25**:1084–8.

33 Stone GW, Mehran R, Dangas G, *et al.* Differential impact on survival of electrocardiographic Q-wave versus enzymatic myocardial infarction after percutaneous intervention: a device-specific analysis of 7147 patients. *Circulation* 2001;**104**:642–7.

34 Huey BL, Gheorghiade M, Crampton RS, *et al.* Acute non-Q wave myocardial infarction associated with early ST-segment elevation: evidence for spontaneous coronary reperfusion and implications for thrombolytic trials. *J Am Coll Cardiol* 1987; **9**:18–25.

35 Barbagelata A, Califf RM, Sgarbossa EB, *et al.* Thrombolysis and Q wave versus non-Q wave first acute myocardial infarction: a GUSTO-I substudy. Global Utilization of Streptokinase and Tissue Plasminogen Activator for Occluded Arteries Investigators. *J Am Coll Cardiol* 1997;**29**:770–7.

36 Askenazi J, Parisi AF, Cohn PF, *et al.* Value of the QRS complex in assessing left ventricular ejection fraction. *Am J Cardiol* 1978; **41**:494–9.

37 Mauri F, Franzosi MG, Maggioni AP, *et al.* Clinical value of 12-lead electrocardiography to predict the long-term prognosis of GISSI-1 patients. *J Am Coll Cardiol* 2002;**39**:1594–600.

38 Hyde TA, French JK, Wong CK, *et al.* Four-year survival of patients with acute coronary syndromes without ST-segment elevation and prognostic significance of 0.5-mm ST-segment depression. *Am J Cardiol* 1999;**84**:379–85.

39 Cannon CP, McCabe CH, Stone PH, *et al.* The electrocardiogram predicts one-year outcome of patients with unstable angina and non-Q wave myocardial infarction: results of the TIMI III Registry ECG Ancillary Study. Thrombolysis in Myocardial Ischemia. *J Am Coll Cardiol* 1997;**30**:133–40.

40 Kaul P, Fu Y, Chang WC, *et al.* Prognostic value of ST segment depression in acute coronary syndromes: insights from PARAGON-A applied to GUSTO-IIb. PARAGON-A and GUSTO IIb Investigators. Platelet IIb/IIIa Antagonism for the Reduction of Acute Global Organization Network. *J Am Coll Cardiol* 2001; **38**:64–71.

41 Diderholm E, Andren B, Frostfeldt G, *et al.* ST depression in ECG at entry indicates severe coronary lesions and large benefits of an early invasive treatment strategy in unstable coronary artery disease; the FRISC II ECG substudy. The Fast Revascularisation during InStability in Coronary artery disease. *Eur Heart J* 2002; **23**:41–9.

42 Wong PS, el Gaylani N, Griffith K, *et al.* The clinical course of patients with acute myocardial infarction who are unsuitable for thrombolytic therapy because of the presenting electrocardiogram. UK Heart Attack Study Investigators. *Coron Artery Dis* 1998;**9**:747–52.

43 Savonitto S, Cohen MG, Politi A, *et al.* Extent of ST-segment depression and cardiac events in non-ST-segment elevation acute coronary syndromes. *Eur Heart J* 2005;**26**:2106–13.

44 Fibrinolytic Therapy Trialists' (FTT) Collaborative Group. Indications for fibrinolytic therapy in suspected acute myocardial infarction: collaborative overview of early mortality and major morbidity results from all randomised trials of more than 1000 patients. *Lancet* 1994;**343**:311–22.

45 Anderson HV, Cannon CP, Stone PH, *et al.* One-year results of the Thrombolysis in Myocardial Infarction (TIMI) IIIB clinical trial. A randomised comparison of tissue-type plasminogen activator versus placebo and early invasive versus early conservative strategies in unstable angina and non-Q wave myocardial infarction. *J Am Coll Cardiol* 1995;**26**:1643–50.

46 Ryan TJ, Anderson JL, Antman EM, *et al.* ACC/AHA Guidelines for the management of patients with acute myocardial infarction: a report of the American College of Cardiology/American Heart Association Task Force on Practice Guidelines (Committee on Management of Acute Myocardial Infarction). *J Am Coll Cardiol* 1996;**28**:1328–428.

47 Cragg DR, Friedman HZ, Bonema JD, *et al.* Outcome of patients with acute myocardial infarction who are ineligible for thrombolytic therapy. *Ann Int Med* 1991;**115**:173–7.

48 Bavry AA, Kumbhani DJ, Quiroz R, *et al.* Invasive therapy along with glycoprotein IIb/IIIa inhibitors and intracoronary stents improves survival in non-ST-segment elevation acute coronary syndromes: a meta-analysis and review of the literature. *Am J Cardiol* 2004;**93**:830–5.

49 Mehta SR, Cannon CP, Fox KA, *et al.* Routine vs selective invasive strategies in patients with acute coronary syndromes: a collaborative meta-analysis of randomized trials. JAMA 2005; **293**:2908–17.

50 Biondi-Zoccai GG, Abbate A, Agostoni P, *et al.* Long-term benefits of an early invasive management in acute coronary syndromes depend on intracoronary stenting and aggressive antiplatelet treatment: a metaregression. *Am Heart J* 2005;**149**: 504–11.

51 Holmvang L, Clemmensen P, Lindahl B, *et al.* Quantitative analysis of the admission electrocardiogram identifies patients with unstable coronary artery disease who benefit the most from early invasive treatment. *J Am Coll Cardiol* 2003;**41**:905–15.

52 Cannon CP, Weintraub WS, Demopoulos LA, *et al.* Comparison of early invasive and conservative strategies in patients with unstable coronary syndromes treated with the glycoprotein IIb/IIIa inhibitor tirofiban. (TACTICS)-TIMI 18. *N Engl J Med* 2001;**344**:1879–87.

53 de Winter RJ, Windhausen F, Cornel JH, *et al.* Early invasive versus selectively invasive management for acute coronary syndromes. *N Engl J Med* 2005;**353**:1095–104.

54 Birnbaum Y, Sclarovsky S, Solodky A, *et al.* Prediction of the level of left anterior descending coronary artery obstruction during anterior wall acute myocardial infarction by the admission electrocardiogram. *Am J Cardiol* 1993;**72**:823–6.

55 Tamura A, Kataoka H, Nagase K, *et al.* Clinical significance of inferior ST elevation during acute anterior myocardial infarction. *Br Heart J* 1995;**74**:611–4.

56 Engelen DJ, Gorgens AP, Cheriex EC, *et al.* Value of the electrocardiogram in localizing the occlusion site in the left anterior descending coronary artery in acute myocardial infarction. *J Am Coll Cardiol* 1999;**34**:389–95.

57 Kosuge M, Kimura K, Toshiyuki I, *et al.* Electrocardiographic criteria for predicting total occlusion of the proximal left anterior descending coronary artery in anterior wall acute myocardial infarction. *Clin Cardiol* 2001;**24**:33–8.

58 Peterson ED, Hathaway WR, Zabel KM, *et al.* Prognostic significance of precordial ST segment depression during inferior myocardial infarction in the thrombolytic era: results in 16,521 patients. *J Am Coll Cardiol* 1996;**28**:305–12.

59 Edmunds JJ, Gibbons RJ, Bresnahan JF, Clements IP. Significance of anterior ST depression in inferior wall acute myocardial infarction. *Am J Cardiol* 1994;**73**:143–8.

60 Matetzky S, Freimark D, Chouraqui P, *et al.* Significance of ST segment elevations in posterior chest leads (V7–V9) in patients with acute inferior myocardial infarction: application for thrombolytic therapy. *J Am Coll Cardiol* 1998;**31**:506–11.

61 Ruddy TD, Yasuda T, Gold HK, *et al.* Anterior ST segment depression in acute myocardial infarction as a marker of greater inferior, apical, and posterolateral damage. *Am Heart J* 1986; **112**:1210–6.

62 Wong CK, Freedman SB. Usefulness of continuous ST monitoring in inferior wall acute myocardial infarction for describing the relation between precordial ST depression and inferior ST elevation. *Am J Cardiol* 1993;**72**:532–7.

63 Shah A, Wagner GS, Califf RM, *et al.* Comparative prognostic significance of simultaneous versus independent resolution of ST segment depression relative to ST segment elevation during acute myocardial infarction. *J Am Coll Cardiol* 1997;**30**: 1478–83.

64 Birnbaum Y, Wagner GS, Barbash GI, *et al.* Correlation of angiographic findings and right (V1 to V3) versus left (V4 to V6) precordial ST-segment depression in inferior wall acute myocardial infarction. *Am J Cardiol* 1999;**83**:143–8.

65 Evans MA, Clements IP, Christian TF, Gibbons RJ. Association between anterior ST depression and increased myocardial salvage following reperfusion therapy in patients with inferior myocardial infarction. *Am J Med* 1998;**104**:5–11.

66 Chaitman BR, Waters DD, Corbara F, Bourassa MG. Prediction of multivessel disease after inferior myocardial infarction. *Circulation* 1978;**57**:1085–90.

67 Tzivoni D, Chenzbraun A, Keren A, *et al.* Reciprocal electrocardiographic changes in acute myocardial infarction. *Am J Cardiol* 1985;**56**:23–6.

68 Tendera M, Campbell WB. Significance of early and late anterior precordial ST-segment depression in inferior myocardial infarction. *Am J Cardiol* 1984;**54**:994–6.

69 Salcedo JR, Baird MG, Chambers RJ, Beanlands DS. Significance of reciprocal S-T segment depression in anterior precordial leads in acute inferior myocardial infarction: concomitant left anterior descending coronary artery disease? *Am J Cardiol* 1981;**48**:1003–8.

70 de Zwaan C, Bar FW, Janssen JHA, *et al.* Angiographic and clinical characteristics of patients with unstable angina showing an ECG pattern indicating critical narrowing of the proximal LAD coronary artery. *Am Heart J* 1989;**117**:657–65.

71 de Zwaan C, Bar FW, Wellens HJJ. Characteristic electrocardiographic pattern indicating a critical stenosis high in left anterior descending coronary artery in patients admitted because of impending myocardial infarction. *Am Heart J* 1982;**103**:730–6.

72 Haines DE, Raabe DS, Gundel WD, Wackers FJ. Anatomic and prognostic significance of new T-wave inversion in unstable angina. *Am J Cardiol* 1983;**52**:14–8.

73 Oliva PB, Hammill SC, Edwards WD. Electrocardiographic diagnosis of postinfarction regional pericarditis: ancillary observations regarding the effect of reperfusion on the rapidity and amplitude of T wave inversion after acute myocardial infarction. *Circulation* 1993;**88**:896–904.

74 Sgarbossa EB, Meyer PM, Pinski SL, *et al.* Negative T waves shortly after ST-elevation acute myocardial infarction are a powerful marker for improved survival rate. *Am Heart J* 2000; **140**:385–94.

75 Herz I, Birnbaum Y, Zlotikamien B, *et al.* The prognostic implications of negative T-waves in the leads with ST segment elevation on admission in acute myocardial infarction. *Cardiology* 1999;**92**:121–7.

76 Bosimini E, Giannuzzi P, Temporelli PL, *et al.* Electrocardiographic evolutionary changes and left ventricular remodeling after acute myocardial infarction: results of the GISSI–3 Echo substudy. *J Am Coll Cardiol* 2000;**35**:127–35.

77 Nagase K, Tamura A, Mikuriya Y, Nasu M. Spontaneous normalization of negative T waves in infarct-related leads reflects improvement in left ventricular wall motion even in patients with persistent abnormal Q waves after anterior wall acute myocardial infarction. *Cardiology* 2001;**96**:94–9.

78 Pahlm US, Pahlm O, Wagner GS. The standard 11-lead ECG. Neglect of lead aVR in the classical limb lead display. *J Electrocardiol* 1996;**29** (Suppl):270–4.

79 Barrabes JA, Figueras J, Moure C, *et al.* Prognostic value of lead aVR in patients with a first non-ST-segment elevation acute myocardial infarction. *Circulation* 2003;**108**:814–9.

80 Barrabes JA, Figueras J, Moure C, *et al.* Prognostic significance of ST segment depression in lateral leads I, aVL, V5 and V6 on the admission electrocardiogram in patients with a first acute myocardial infarction without ST segment elevation. *J Am Coll Cardiol* 2000;**35**:1813–9.

81 Gorgels AP, Vos MA, Mulleneers R, *et al.* Value of the electrocardiogram in diagnosing the number of severely narrowed coronary arteries in rest angina pectoris. *Am J Cardiol* 1993; **72**:999–1003.

82 Yamaji H, Iwasaki K, Kusachi S, *et al.* Prediction of acute left main coronary artery obstruction by 12-lead electrocardiography. ST segment elevation in lead aVR with less ST segment elevation in lead V(1). *J Am Coll Cardiol* 2001;**38**:1348–54.

83 Menown IB, Adgey AA. Improving the ECG classification of inferior and lateral myocardial infarction by inversion of lead aVR. *Heart* 2000;**83**:657–60.

84 Stephenson K, Skali H, McMurray JJ, *et al.* Long-term outcomes of left bundle branch block in high-risk survivors of acute myocardial infarction: The VALIANT experience. *Heart Rhythm* 2007;**4**:308–13.

85 Terkelsen CJ, Lassen JF, Norgaard BL, *et al.* Mortality rates in patients with ST-elevation vs. non-ST-elevation acute myocardial infarction: observations from an unselected cohort. *Eur Heart J* 2005;**26**:18–26.

86 Newby KH, Pisano O, Krucoff MW, Green C, Natale A. Incidence and clinical relevance of the occurrence of bundle-branch block in patients treated with thrombolytic therapy. *Circulation* 1996;**94**:2424–8.

87 Guerrero M, Harjai K, Stone GW, *et al.* Comparison of the prognostic effect of left versus right versus no bundle branch block on presenting electrocardiogram in acute myocardial infarction patients treated with primary angioplasty in the primary angioplasty in myocardial infarction trials. *Am J Cardiol* 2005;**96**: 482–8.

88 Go AS, Barron HV, Rundle AC, *et al.* Bundle-branch block and in-hospital mortality in acute myocardial infarction. National Registry of Myocardial Infarction. *Ann Int Med* 1998;**129**:690–7.

89 Sgarbossa EB, Pinski SL, Topol EJ, *et al.* Acute myocardial infarction and complete bundle branch block at hospital admission: clinical characteristics and outcome in the thrombolytic era. *J Am Coll Cardiol* 1998;**31**:105–10.

90 Hod H, Goldbourt U, Behar S. Bundle branch block in acute Q-wave inferior wall myocardial infarction. A high risk subgroup of interior myocardial infarction patients. The SPRINT Study Group. Secondary Prevention Reinfarction Israeli Nifedipine Trial. *Eur Heart J* 1995;**16**:471–7.

91 Barron HV, Bowlby LJ, Breen T, *et al.* Use of reperfusion therapy for acute myocardial infarction in the United States: data from the National Registry of Myocardial Infarction 2. *Circulation* 1997;**97**:1150–6.

92 Wong CK, Stewart RA, Gao W, *et al.* Prognostic differences between different types of bundle branch block during the early phase of acute myocardial infarction: insights from the Hirulog and Early Reperfusion or Occlusion (HERO)-2 trial. *Eur Heart J* 2006;**27**:21–8.

93 Antman EM, Anbe DT, Armstrong PW, *et al.* ACC/AHA guidelines for the management of patients with ST-elevation myocardial infarction – executive summary. A report of the American College of Cardiology/American Heart Association Task Force on Practice Guidelines (Writing Committee to revise the 1999 guidelines for the management of patients with acute myocardial infarction). *J Am Coll Cardiol* 2004;**44**:671–719.

94 Pudil R, Feinberg MS, Hod H, *et al.* The prognostic significance of intermediate QRS prolongation in acute myocardial infarction. *Int J Cardiol* 2001;**78**:233–9.

95 Brilakis ES, Mavrogiorgos NC, Kopecky SL, *et al.* Usefulness of QRS duration in the absence of bundle branch block as an early predictor of survival in non-ST elevation acute myocardial infarction. *Am J Cardiol* 2002;**89**:1013–8.

96 Larsen GC, Griffith JL, Beshansky JR, *et al.* Electrocardiographic left ventricular hypertrophy in patients with suspected acute cardiac ischemia: Its influence on diagnosis, triage, and short-term prognosis. *J Gen Intern Med* 1994;**9**:666–76.

97 Norris RM. Heart block in posterior and anterior myocardial infarction. *Br Heart J* 1969;**31**:352–6.

98 Aplin M, Engstrom T, Vejlstrup NG, *et al.* Prognostic importance of complete atrioventricular block complicating acute myocardial infarction. *Am J Cardiol* 2003;**92**:853–6.

99 Meine TJ, Al-Khatib SM, Alexander JH, *et al.* Incidence, predictors, and outcomes of high-degree atrioventricular block

complicating acute myocardial infarction treated with thrombolytic therapy. *Am Heart J* 2005;**149**:670–4.

100 Berger PB, Ruocco NA, Jr., Ryan TJ, *et al*. Incidence and prognostic implications of heart block complicating inferior myocardial infarction treated with thrombolytic therapy: results from TIMI II. *J Am Coll Cardiol* 1992;**20**:533–40.

101 Rathore SS, Gersh BJ, Berger PB, *et al*. Acute myocardial infarction complicated by heart block in the elderly: prevalence and outcomes. *Am Heart J* 2001;**141**:47–54.

102 Henkel DM, Witt BJ, Gersh BJ, *et al*. Ventricular arrhythmias after acute myocardial infarction: a 20-year community study. *Am Heart J* 2006;**151**:806–12.

103 Mont L, Cinca J, Blanch P, *et al*. Predisposing factors and prognostic value of sustained monomorphic ventricular tachycardia in the early phase of acute myocardial infarction. *J Am Coll Cardiol* 1996;**28**:1670–6.

104 Hatzinikolaou-Kotsakou E, Tziakas D, Hotidis A, *et al*. Could sustained monomorphic ventricular tachycardia in the early phase of a prime acute myocardial infarction affect patient outcome? *J Electrocardiol* 2007;**40**:72–7.

105 Antman EM, Berlin JA. Declining incidence of ventricular fibrillation in myocardial infarction. Implications for the prophylactic use of lidocaine. *Circulation* 1992;**86**:764–73.

106 El-Sherif N, Myerburg RJ, Scherlag BJ, *et al*. Electrocardiographic antecedents of primary ventricular fibrillation. Value of the R-on-T phenomenon in myocardial infarction. *Br Heart J* 1976;**38**:415–22.

107 Zehender M, Utzolino S, Furtwangler A, *et al*. Time course and interrelation of reperfusion-induced ST changes and ventricular arrhythmias in acute myocardial infarction. *Am J Cardiol* 1991;**68**:1138–42.

108 Six AJ, Louwerenburg JH, Kingma JH, *et al*. Predictive value of ventricular arrhythmias for patency of the infarct-related coronary artery after thrombolytic therapy. *Br Heart J* 1991;**66**:143–6.

109 Gressin V, Louvard Y, Pezzano M, Lardoux H. Holter recording of ventricular arrhythmias during intravenous thrombolysis for acute myocardial infarction. *Am J Cardiol* 1992;**69**:152–9.

110 Buckingham TA, Devine JE, Redd RM, Kennedy HL. Reperfusion arrhythmias during coronary reperfusion therapy in man. Clinical and angiographic correlations. *Chest* 1986;**90**:346–51.

111 Berger PB, Ruocco NA, Ryan TJ, *et al*. Incidence and significance of ventricular tachycardia and fibrillation in the absence of hypotension or heart failure in acute myocardial infarction treated with recombinant tissue-type plasminogen activator: results from the Thrombolysi in Myocardial Infarction (TIMI) Phase II trial. *J Am Coll Cardiol* 1993;**22**:1773–9.

112 Newby KH, Thompson T, Stebbins A, *et al*. Sustained ventricular arrhythmias in patients receiving thrombolytic therapy: incidence and outcomes. The GUSTO Investigators. *Circulation* 1998;**98**:2567–73.

113 Mehta RH, Harjai KJ, Grines L, *et al*. Sustained ventricular tachycardia or fibrillation in the cardiac catheterization laboratory among patients receiving primary percutaneous coronary intervention: incidence, predictors, and outcomes. *J Am Coll Cardiol* 2004;**43**:1765–72.

114 Ilia R, Zahger D, Cafri C, *et al*. Predicting survival with reperfusion arrhythmias during primary percutaneous coronary intervention for acute myocardial infarction. *Isr Med Assoc J* 2007;**9**:21–3.

115 Rathore SS, Berger AK, Weinfurt KP, *et al*. Acute myocardial infarction complicated by atrial fibrillation in the elderly: prevalence and outcomes. *Circulation* 2000;**101**:969–74.

116 Mehta RH, Dabbous OH, Granger CB, *et al*. Comparison of outcomes of patients with acute coronary syndromes with and without atrial fibrillation. *Am J Cardiol* 2003;**92**:1031–6.

117 Behar S, Zahavi Z, Goldbourt U, Reicher-Reiss H. Long-term prognosis of patients with paroxysmal atrial fibrillation complicating acute myocardial infarction. SPRINT Study Group. *Eur Heart J* 1992;**13**:45–50.

118 Eldar M, Canetti M, Rotstein Z, *et al*. Significance of paroxysmal atrial fibrillation complicating acute myocardial infarction in the thrombolytic era. SPRINT and Thrombolytic Survey Groups. *Circulation* 1998;**97**:965–70.

119 Crenshaw BS, Ward SR, Granger CB, *et al*. Atrial fibrillation in the setting of acute myocardial infarction: the GUSTO-I experience. Global Utilization of Streptokinase and TPA for Occluded Coronary Arteries. *J Am Coll Cardiol* 1997;**30**:406–13.

120 Sakata K, Kurihara H, Iwamori K, *et al*. Clinical and prognostic significance of atrial fibrillation in acute myocardial infarction. *Am J Cardiol* 1997;**80**:1522–7.

121 Goldberg RJ, Seeley D, Becker RC, *et al*. Impact of atrial fibrillation on the in-hospital and long-term survival of patients with acute myocardial infarction: a community-wide perspective. *Am Heart J* 1990;**119**:996–1001.

122 Madias JE, Patel DC, Singh D. Atrial fibrillation in acute myocardial infarction: a prospective study based on data from a consecutive series of patients admitted to the coronary care unit. *Clin Cardiol* 1996;**19**:180–6.

123 Vaage-Nilsen M, Hansen JF, Mellemgaard K, *et al*. Short- and long-term prognostic implications of in-hospital postinfarction arrhythmias. DAVIT II Study Group. *Cardiology* 1995;**86**:49–55.

124 Crimm A, Severance HW, Jr., Coffey K, *et al*. Prognostic significance of isolated sinus tachycardia during first three days of acute myocardial infarction. *Am J Med* 1984;**76**:983–8.

125 Antman EM, Cohen M, Bernink PJLM, *et al*. The TIMI risk score for unstable angina/non–ST elevation MI: a method for prognostication and therapeutic decision making. *JAMA* 2000;**284**:835–42.

126 Eagle KA, Lim MJ, Dabbous OH, *et al*. A validated prediction model for all forms of acute coronary syndrome: estimating the risk of 6-month postdischarge death in an international registry. *JAMA* 2004;**291**:2727–33.

127 Boersma E, Pieper KS, Steyerberg EW, *et al*. Predictors of outcome in patients with acute coronary syndromes without persistent ST-segment elevation. Results from an international trial of 9461 patients. The PURSUIT Investigators. *Circulation* 2000;**101**:2557–67.

128 Hjalmarson A, Gilpin EA, Kjekshus J, *et al*. Influence of heart rate on mortality after acute myocardial infarction. *Am J Cardiol* 1990;**65**:547–53.

129 Chen ZM, Pan HC, Chen YP, *et al*. COMMIT: Early intravenous then oral metoprolol in 45,852 patients with acute myocardial infarction: randomised placebo-controlled trial. *Lancet* 2005;**366**:1622–32.

130 2007 Writing Group to Review New Evidence and Update the ACC/AHA 2004 Guidelines for the Management of Patients With ST-Elevation Myocardial Infarction. 2007 Focused Update of the ACC/AHA 2004 Guidelines for the Management of

Patients with ST-Elevation Myocardial Infarction. *J Am Coll Cardiol* 2008;**51**.

131 Blatchford O, Capewell S, Murray S, Blatchford M. Emergency medical admissions in Glasgow: general practices vary despite adjustment for age, sex, and deprivation. *Br J Gen Pract* 1999; **49**:551–4.

132 Pope JH, Aufderheide TP, Ruthazer R, *et al.* Missed diagnosis of acute cardiac ischemia in the emergency department. *N Engl J Med* 2000;**342**:1163–70.

133 Collinson PO, Premachandram S, Hashemi K. Prospective audit of incidence of prognostically important myocardial damage in patients discharged from emergency department. *BMJ* 2000; **320**:1702–5.

134 McCarthy BD, Beshansky JR, D'agostino RB, Selker HP. Missed diagnosis of acute myocardial infarction in the emergency department: results from a multicenter study. *Ann Emerg Med* 1993;**22**:579–82.

135 Welch RD, Zalenski RJ, Frederick PD, *et al.* Prognostic value of a normal or nonspecific initial electrocardiogram in acute myocardial infarction. *JAMA* 2001;**286**:1977–84.

136 Fesmire FM, Wharton DR, Calhoun FB. Instability of ST segments in the early stages of acute myocardial infarction in patients undergoing continuous 12-lead ECG monitoring. *Am J Emerg Med* 1995;**13**:158–63.

137 Fesmire FM, Percy RF, Bardoner JB, *et al.* Usefulness of automated serial 12-lead ECG monitoring during the initial emergency department evaluation of patients with chest pain. *Ann Emerg Med* 1998;**31**:3–11.

138 Patel DJ, Knight CJ, Holdright DR, *et al.* Long-term prognosis in unstable angina. The importance of early risk stratification using continuous ST segment monitoring. *Eur Heart J* 1998; **19**:240–9.

139 Goldman L, Cook EF, Johnson PA, *et al.* Prediction of the need for intensive care in patients who come to the emergency departments with acute chest pain. *N Engl J Med* 1996;**334**: 1498–504.

140 Hedges JR, Young GP, Henkel GF, *et al.* Serial ECGs are less accurate than serial CK-MB results for emergency department diagnosis of myocardial infarction. *Ann Emerg Med* 1992; **21**:1445–50.

141 Chase M, Brown AM, Robey JL, *et al.* Prognostic value of symptoms during a normal or nonspecific electrocardiogram in emergency department patients with potential acute coronary syndrome. *Acad Emerg Med* 2006;**13**:1034–9.

142 Brush JE, Brand DA, Acampora D, *et al.* Use of the initial electrocardiogram to predict in-hospital complications of acute myocardial infarction. *N Engl J Med* 1985;**312**:1137–41.

143 Goldman L, Cook EF, Brand DA, *et al.* A computer protocol to predict myocardial infarction in emergency department patients with chest pain. *N Engl J Med* 1988;**318**:797–803.

144 Pozen MW, D'agostino RB, Selker HP, *et al.* A predictive instrument to improve Coronary-Care-Unit admission practices in acute ischemic heart disease. *N Engl J Med* 1984;**310**:1273–8.

145 Selker HP, Beshansky J, Griffith JL, *et al.* Use of the Acute Cardiac Time-Insensitive Predictor Instrument (ACI-TIPI) to assist with triage of patients with chest pain or other symptoms suggestive of acute cardiac ischemia. A multicenter, controlled clinical trial. *Ann Int Med* 1998;**129**:845–55.

146 Selker HP, Griffith JL, D'Agostino RB. A time-insensitive predictive instrument for acute myocardial infarction mortality: a multicenter study. *Med Care* 1991;**29**:1196–211.

147 Lee TH, Pearson SD, Johnson PA, *et al.* Failure of information as an intervention to modify clinical management. A time-series trial in patients with acute chest pain. *Ann Intern Med* 1995; **122**:434–7.

148 Morrow DA, Antman EM, Charlesworth A, *et al.* TIMI risk score for ST-elevation myocardial infarction: A convenient, bedside, clinical score for risk assessment at presentation: An intravenous nPA for treatment of infarcting myocardium early II trial substudy. *Circulation* 2000;**102**:2031–7.

149 Pollack CV, Jr., Sites FD, Shofer FS, *et al.* Application of the TIMI risk score for unstable angina and non-ST elevation acute coronary syndrome to an unselected emergency department chest pain population. *Acad Emerg Med* 2006;**13**:13–8.

150 Soiza RL, Leslie SJ, Williamson P, *et al.* Risk stratification in acute coronary syndromes – does the TIMI risk score work in unselected cases? *QJM* 2006;**99**:81–7.

151 Scirica BM, Cannon CP, Antman EM, *et al.* Validation of the thrombolysis in myocardial infarction (TIMI) risk score for unstable angina pectoris and non-ST-elevation myocardial infarction in the TIMI III registry. *Am J Cardiol* 2002;**90**:303–5.

152 Granger CB, Goldberg RJ, Dabbous O, *et al.* Predictors of hospital mortality in the global registry of acute coronary events. *Arch Intern Med* 2003;**163**:2345–53.

153 de Araujo Goncalves P, Ferreira J, Aguiar C, Seabra-Gomes R. TIMI, PURSUIT, and GRACE risk scores: sustained prognostic value and interaction with revascularization in NSTE-ACS. *Eur Heart J* 2005;**26**:865–72.

Part 4 | **The Dysrhythmic ECG**

Chapter 28 | **Can the electrocardiogram determine the rhythm diagnosis in narrow complex tachycardia?**

Lisa M. Filippone, Claire C. Caldwell
UMDNJ-Robert Wood Johnson Medical School, Camden, NJ, USA

Case presentations

Case 1: A 24-year-old female is brought to the emergency department (ED) via emergency medical services (EMS) for the evaluation of palpitations and lightheadedness. She states that these symptoms started suddenly while resting just prior to her calling EMS. She has never had these symptoms before and is otherwise healthy. She is afebrile with a heart rate of 200 beats per minute (bpm). Her blood pressure is 120/72 mmHg and respiratory rate is normal with an oxygen saturation of 100% on oxygen. Her examination is normal other than a rapid, regular tachycardia. On the cardiac monitor, a narrow QRS complex tachycardia is seen – regular without identifiable P waves. The 12-lead electrocardiogram (ECG) demonstrates similar findings along with ST segment depression in the lateral and inferior leads (Figure 28.1).

Case 2: A 74-year-old woman is brought to the ED via emergency EMS for shortness of breath. She has a long history of chronic obstructive pulmonary disease (COPD) for which she is currently receiving albuterol. Other than the shortness of breath, she is without complaint. Emergency medical services personnel report that her heart rate is 140 bpm with a blood pressure of 130/80 mmHg, a respiratory rate of 40 breaths per minute and oxygen saturation 92%. An oral temperature is not feasible due to the respiratory distress. Her physical examination is significant for her use of accessory muscles for respiration, decreased breath sounds with expiratory wheezing and a rapid irregular heart beat. She is placed on a cardiac monitor, which demonstrates an irregular narrow complex tachycardia with a rate of 140 bpm. P waves are difficult to discern. An ECG (Figure 28.2) is performed which confirms the irregular narrow complex tachycardia. P waves do appear, but are irregular in appearance and have varying morphologies.

Case 3: A 68-year-old male is sent to the ED from a long-term care facility for the evaluation of fever and change in his mental status. He has a long history of dementia, hypertension and recurrent urinary tract infections. As per the nursing home, he was in his usual state of health until this morning when it was noticed that he was febrile and less alert than normal. On arrival to the ED, he is awake and alert but cannot answer questions. His vital signs are significant for a rectal temperature of 102.5 °F, heart rate of 150 bpm, blood pressure of 100/60 mmHg and respiratory rate of 22 breaths per minute. His oxygen saturation is normal on room air. He is placed on the cardiac monitor, which demonstrates a regular narrow complex tachycardia. An ECG (Figure 28.3) is performed. The ECG confirms that this is a regular narrow complex tachycardia. P waves appear to be present preceding each QRS and there are diffuse non-specific ST segment/T wave changes. After anti-pyretics and intravenous crystalloid, the patient's blood pressure and temperature have improved but his heart rate remains at 150 bpm.

The electrocardiogram and the diagnosis of narrow complex tachycardia

These three patients all present with rapid narrow complex rhythms that collectively are referred to as supraventricular tachycardias (SVTs); however, their etiologies and treatments are quite different. Initial identification from a cardiac monitor may be difficult or impossible, particularly when the rates are very rapid, but close inspection of a 12-lead ECG can help determine the rhythm diagnosis.

Supraventricular tachycardia

The term supraventricular tachycardia refers to any tachycardic rhythm that originates above the ventricles, i.e. the atrioventricular (AV) node and above into the atria. The site

Critical Decisions in Emergency and Acute Care Electrocardiography, 1st edition. Edited by W.J. Brady and J.D. Truwit. © 2009 Blackwell Publishing. ISBN: 9781405159067

233

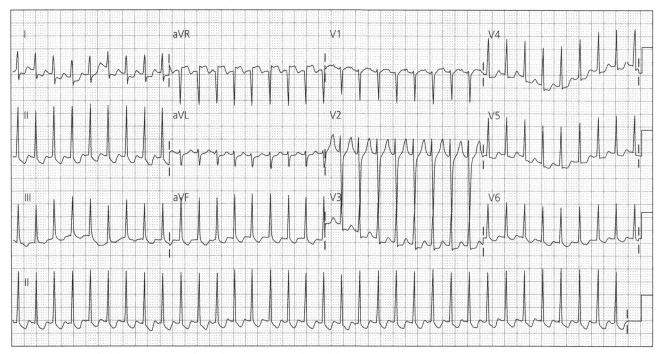

Figure 28.1 Paroxysmal supraventricular tachycardia (atrioventricular nodal re-entrant tachycardia). The rhythm is regular and narrow complex, and there are no discernable P waves. ST segment depression is noted in some leads, a common finding with some types of SVT.

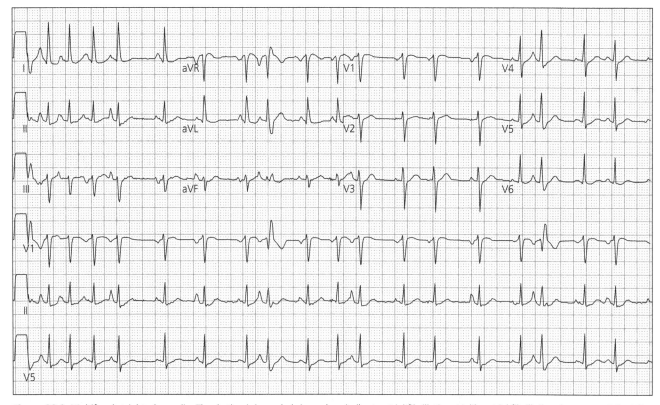

Figure 28.2 Multifocal atrial tachycardia. The rhythm is irregularly irregular, similar to atrial fibrillation. Unlike atrial fibrillation, however, distinct P waves are present and vary in morphology.

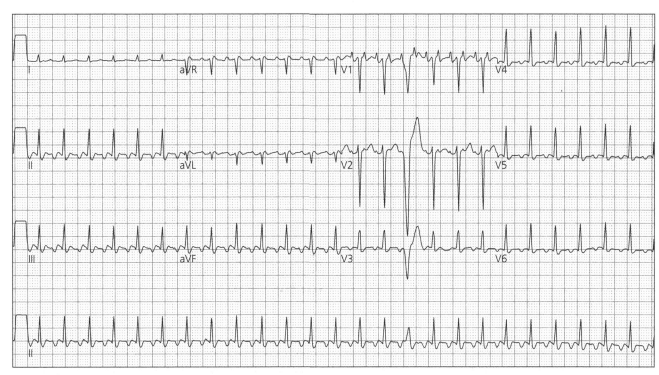

Figure 28.3 Atrial flutter. With the exception of the portion of the rhythm containing a premature ventricular complex, the rhythm is regular and narrow complex. Inverted flutter waves are noted best in the inferior leads.

of origin may be the sinus node, atrial tissue, the AV node, or the His bundle or a combination. Supraventricular tachycardias commonly encountered include sinus tachycardia (ST), atrioventricular nodal re-entrant tachycardia (AVNRT), atrioventricular re-entrant tachycardia (AVRT, tachycardia associated with Wolff-Parkinson-White syndrome), atrial tachycardia (AT), multifocal atrial tachycardia (MAT), junctional tachycardia (JT), atrial fibrillation (AF) and atrial flutter (AF1). Paroxysmal SVT (PSVT) is an inclusive term encompassing the above tachycardias; however, AF and AF1 are often segregated.

It is estimated that PSVT occurs in the general population with an incidence of 36/100,000 persons per year and a prevalence of 2.29/1000 persons. It may or may not be associated with underlying cardiovascular disease. Those patients without underlying cardiovascular disease tend to be younger at first presentation, are more often female, and are more likely to present to the emergency department [1].

Electrocardiographic characteristics of supraventricular tachycardias

Initially an SVT may be recognized by looking at the cardiac monitor. A narrow complex tachycardia can readily be seen. When a 12-lead ECG is done, the QRS width is usually less than 120 ms. The reason for the narrow QRS complexes is

that while the site of origin for a SVT may be the sinus node, atrium, AV node or His bundle, conduction down to the ventricles occurs via the Purkinje fibers and bundle branches, thus ventricular depolarization is normal. The exception to this occurs if aberrant conduction is present. This may be because of a pre-existing bundle branch block, a rate-related bundle branch block, or a pre-existing accessory pathway (e.g. Wolff-Parkinson-White syndrome). The resulting rhythm demonstrates a wide complex tachycardia (WCT).

After recognizing that the tachycardia is a narrow complex tachycardia, the next step is determining whether the ventricular rhythm is regular or irregular and whether or not there are P waves present. P waves should be sought out on the ECG, and their morphology and relationship to the QRS determined. A P wave is considered to be "normal" if it is upright in leads I, aVL, and the inferior leads, and inverted in lead aVR. The P wave axis should be between +15 to +75. The relationship of the P wave and QRS should be defined. Is there one P wave before each QRS or are there more than one P waves per QRS? Does the P wave precede the QRS or does it appear after the QRS, referred to as a retrograde P wave? By identifying the above information, often the rhythm can be diagnosed.

There are, however, times when the rhythm is still unclear and various maneuvers or medications are needed to ultimately determine the rhythm. The Valsalva maneuver can be done in a hemodynamically stable patient who is co-operative, to help identify or possibly terminate the SVT. This will increase intrathoracic pressure, which stimulates baroreceptors in the aorta which, in turn, can temporarily slow the sinoatrial (SA) node and AV nodal conduction. A similar response may be seen with carotid sinus massage; however, one should be cautious of performing this maneuver in persons at risk for atherosclerotic disease [2].

Of the medications commonly used in the evaluation of SVT, adenosine is generally the first to be administered. Depending on the type of SVT, adenosine may terminate the rhythm or simply slow the rate such that identification is possible. There is some evidence to suggest that adenosine may precipitate atrial fibrillation in a small percentage of patients. In a study of 200 patients that received adenosine for SVT, 12% of patients had a brief episode of AF or AFl. It should be noted however, that all of the patients had intracardiac catheters in place and 99% of the patients had their SVT successfully terminated by adenosine [3].

Sinus tachycardia

Sinus tachycardia is a common rhythm that can affect any age group. It is a physiologic response and the key is to recognize and treat the underlying cause. Some common causes of sinus tachycardia include hypovolemia, fever, hypoxia, pain, and anxiety.

The rate can vary between 100 and 200 bpm, with higher rates being more commonly seen in younger patients (Figure 28.4). Typically, the rate will gradually increase and decrease, and may show beat to beat variation. One P wave should be seen preceding each QRS complex. While P waves are usually clearly seen, they can be difficult to detect with faster rates, as the P wave may become buried in the preceding T wave, or in the presence of a long PR interval [4]. The P waves themselves will have normal morphology and axis, unless there is underlying atrial disease. As the rate increases, the P wave amplitude may increase and the PR interval may shorten [5]. The ventricular response typically is regular; however, it may appear irregular in the presence of premature atrial beats.

Once the diagnosis of sinus tachycardia is made, the underlying cause must be identified and treated.

Atrioventricular nodal re-entrant tachycardia

Atrioventricular nodal re-entrant tachycardia is the most common cause of paroxysmal SVT. As the name implies, it utilizes the AV node or perinodal tissue with a re-entry mechanism. Two different functional pathways are possible in this patient group – within the AV node or the perinodal atrial tissues [6]. These pathways have different conduction and refractory times such that one conducts rapidly but has a long refractory period (fast pathway) and one conducts

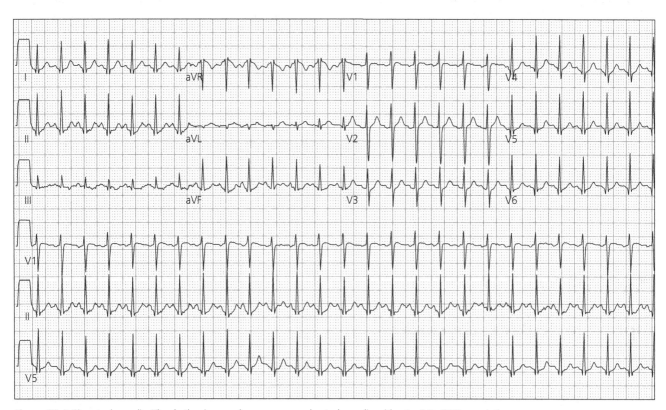

Figure 28.4 Sinus tachycardia. The rhythm is a regular narrow complex tachycardia with a 1 : 1 P : QRS association.

slowly but has a short refractory period (slow pathway). These pathways join into a final common pathway within the AV node. In the correct setting such as that precipitated by a premature atrial contraction, the fast pathway is refractory but the slow pathway is not. Conduction may occur via the slow pathway and down the His-Purkinje system to depolarize the ventricles. If the fast pathway has recovered by the time the impulse reaches the final common pathway in the AV node, conduction may also occur retrograde back to the atria. If the slow pathway has recovered its excitability, the impulse can re-enter the slow pathway and, hence, the circuitous route begins. This form of AVNRT is called the "common form," where conduction down to the ventricle uses the slow pathway and retrograde conduction uses the fast pathway. If conduction down to the ventricle is via the fast pathway and retrograde conduction is via the slow pathway, it is referred to as the "uncommon form" of AVNRT.

Typically, the ECG of a patient presenting with AVNRT is that of a regular narrow complex tachycardia with a rate between 120 and 220 bpm (Figure 28.1). In the common form of AVNRT, P waves are often unidentifiable; however, sometimes a retrograde P wave may be identified. Close inspection of the QRS complex in lead V1 may demonstrate a pseudo-R' wave. This positive, terminal deflection is actually the retrograde P wave fused with the QRS (Figure 28.5). Inspection of the QRS complex in the inferior leads may similarly display a pseudo-S wave. In the uncommon form of AVNRT, retrograde P waves may be identified appearing after the QRS. They are usually inverted in the inferior leads. The P wave may actually be closer to the subsequent QRS complex and mistaken for an ectopic atrial tachycardia. As the time from the QRS to the P wave is long, it is said to have a long RP interval. In the common form of AVNRT, if the p wave is identifiable it is close to the QRS and, thus, is said to have a short RP interval. A beat to beat alteration in QRS amplitude, termed QRS alternans is another common finding in AVNRT [7]. Unlike electrical alternans associated with pericardial effusions, the QRS amplitude is normal.

Depression of ST segments are often seen in patients with AVNRT and are not necessarily related to myocardial ischemia. In a study of patients greater than 45 years of age with paroxysmal SVT, 21 of 39 patients had at least 1 mm of ST depression. Of these 21 patients, only seven (33%)

had significant coronary artery stenosis on coronary angiography. There was no statistical difference in the rate of SVT or amount of ST segment depression between those patients with significant coronary artery disease (CAD) and those patients without significant CAD [8].

After restoration of sinus rhythm is achieved, inverted T waves may be encountered on the ECG. This may occur immediately after tachycardia termination or within the following hours and is not necessarily associated with underlying CAD. These abnormal T waves may persist for a variable length of time. In a study of 63 patients with paroxysmal re-entrant SVT, 25 (39%) had new T wave inversions within 6 h. Of these 25 patients, only two (9%) had confirmed CAD. The conclusion was that inverted T waves were a common finding that were not predicable based on clinical or ECG characteristics, and that CAD does not seem to be the cause of the inverted T wave [9].

Atrioventricular re-entrant tachycardia

Atrioventricular re-entrant tachycardia is the second-most common form of PSVT and most common in persons with pre-existing accessory pathways [10]. An accessory pathway is an anomalous connection that allows conduction between the atria and ventricles bypassing the normal cardiac conduction system. Wolff-Parkinson-White syndrome (WPW) is the classic example of a pre-excitation syndrome. In WPW, the accessory pathway known as the bundle of Kent results in earlier activation of the ventricle during sinus rhythm resulting in a shortened PR interval. Initial depolarization of the ventricle results via the accessory pathway. The slow initial upstroke of the QRS complex, referred to as the delta wave, is observed as a result of abnormal depolarization of the ventricle via the accessory pathway.

Because of the two different conduction pathways (the AV node-His-Purkinje system and the accessory pathway) in persons with pre-excitation syndromes, a properly timed premature depolarization can initiate a re-entrant tachyarrhythmia. As with AVNRT, these two different pathways have different conduction and refractory properties. If a premature atrial depolarization occurs and is able to conduct to the ventricle via the AV node but the accessory pathway is initially refractory, retrograde conduction from the ventricle to the atria via the accessory pathway may occur beginning a re-entrant loop. Similarly, if a premature ventricular depolarization occurs and is able to conduct retrograde to the atria via the accessory pathway, then the impulse follows the normal pathway back down to the ventricule via AV node, this conduction loop may continue to proceed in an automatic movement. The term orthodromic AVRT is used for this type of re-entry when the AV node is used for antegrade conduction and the accessory pathway is used for retrograde conduction. It is possible for conduction to proceed utilizing

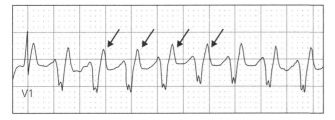

Figure 28.5 Paroxysmal supraventricular tachycardia (atrioventricular nodal re-entrant tachycardia). This lead V1 rhythm strip demonstrates a regular tachycardia with retrograde P waves that manifest as R' waves (arrows).

the accessory pathway for antegrade conduction and the AV node for retrograde conduction, termed antidromic AVRT. As antidromic AVRT results in a wide complex tachycardia, further discussion of the ECG characteristics are covered in Chapter 30. Only orthodromic AVRT will be covered here as it presents as a narrow complex tachycardia, whereas antidromic AVRT produces a wide complex tachycardia.

Patients presenting with orthodromic AVRT present with a regular narrow complex tachycardia. The ventricular rate is often 150 to 250 bpm. Interestingly, in patients with WPW, the QRS complex during orthodromic AVRT is narrower with loss of the delta wave compared with the QRS complex morphology during normal sinus rhythm. The reason for this is that during normal sinus rhythm, conduction to the ventricle is occurring both through the AV node and via the accessory pathway. During orthodromic AVRT, ventricular activation is only via the AV node and thus a narrow-appearing QRS complex is present. As conduction to the atria is retrograde via the accessory pathway, a P wave may be seen within the ST segment-T wave and is usually close to the QRS complex. It has a short RP interval. As with AVNRT, ST segment depression and T wave inversion are not uncommon and do not necessarily imply myocardial ischemia [7,11]. A beat to beat variation in QRS complex amplitude may also be noted on the ECG [7].

Atrioventricular re-entrant tachycardia may precipitate atrial fibrillation, which, in the setting of an accessory pathway, can result in very rapid ventricular rates and hemodynamic instability. Normally, however, AVRT can be terminated by prolonging conduction through the AV node and disrupting this circuit. Valsalva and carotid sinus massage may terminate the rhythm and restore sinus rhythm. If these fail, adenosine may be administered; however, caution should be used as there is some evidence that adenosine may precipitate atrial fibrillation [3,12].

Atrial tachycardia

Atrial tachycardia is the name given to the group of arrhythmias that originate in the atria but not within the sinus node. They may be paroxysmal or sustained in nature. The etiology may involve re-entry, automatic or triggered activity within the atria. Atrial flutter and MAT are specific types of atrial tachycardia but will be discussed separately below.

Despite the varied etiology and electrophysiologic properties of atrial tachycardias, they do share several characteristics on the ECG. By definition, the atrial rate should be greater than 100 bpm. There may be a gradual increase in atrial rate that can be identified on ECG during the initiation phase of the arrhythmia. Likewise during the termination phase of the rhythm, there may be a gradual decrease in rate. There are usually identifiable P waves; however, both the morphology of the P wave and P wave axis are usually abnormal (Figure 28.6) indicating an ectopic atrial origin. The

exception to this is if the site of origin of the P waves is close to the SA node. In this setting, the P wave may be very close to normal in appearance and only with comparison to an ECG in sinus rhythm may a difference in morphology be noticed. There should be an isoelectric baseline between P waves. P waves are related to the QRS complex, but depending on medications and pre-existing medical conditions, there may be an associated second-degree AV block. Patients with digoxin toxicity often present with AT with variable AV block. As with the other SVTs, the QRS complex should be of normal duration unless there is aberrant conduction due to a pre-existing bundle branch block, a rate-related bundle branch block, or an accessory pathway.

Multifocal atrial tachycardia

Multifocal atrial tachycardia is a type of AT. The term MAT was first used by Shine and colleagues in 1968 [13]. Other terminology referring to this atrial arrhythmia can be found in the literature, including chaotic atrial tachycardia and chaotic atrial rhythm. Controversy still exists as to the correct terminology for this arrhythmia but the term MAT is most commonly used.

Multifocal atrial tachycardia is one of the less commonly encountered SVTs. Its prevalence in hospitalized patients has been estimated to be 0.05–0.35% [13,14,15,16]. It is usually seen in the setting of chronic pulmonary disease, although it has also been described postoperatively and in other conditions where hypoxia exists as in pneumonia, pulmonary embolism, and congestive heart failure [13,15,17,18]. In a review of the literature by McCord and Borzak, the average age of patients with MAT was 72 years. Importantly, they also reported an overall in-hospital mortality of 45% [19]; however, this is likely related more to the serious underlying medical conditions and older age. Hypomagnesemia and hypokalemia may also play a role in development of MAT as replacement of magnesium and potassium have been shown to convert MAT to sinus rhythm [20]. The mechanism for the development of MAT has not been proven but it is likely a result of abnormal automaticity or triggered activity. Re-entry does not seem to play a role.

The ECG characteristics initially described by Shine in 1968 are still the most commonly cited criteria used [13]. As the name implies, there are multiple different P wave morphologies seen on the ECG. There is debate as to the exact number of P wave morphologies that must be seen. In general, three different P wave morphologies should be identified with an atrial rate greater than 100 bpm. They are usually best seen in leads II, III and V1 (Figure 28.2). Some authors specify that the three P waves should be distinct from the sinus P wave. Additionally, there should be an isoelectric baseline between P waves. The reason for this is to help differentiate MAT from AF and AFl. Finally, the PP interval should be irregular. Other characteristics that were not

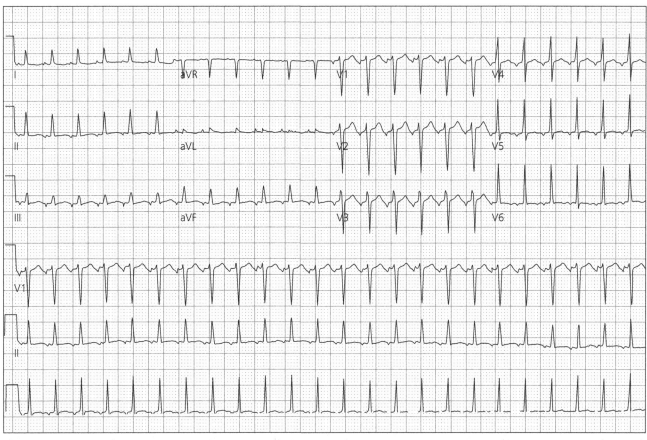

Figure 28.6 Atrial tachycardia. The rhythm is a regular narrow complex tachycardia with ventricular rate of approximately 150 bpm. Like sinus tachycardia, there is a 1 : 1 P : QRS ratio. However, the atrial beats are inverted in the inferior leads and upright in lead aVR, which rules out a sinus node origin of the atrial beats and indicates that they are originating from an ectopic atrial focus. Thus, the rhythm is referred to as ectopic atrial tachycardia, or simply "atrial tachycardia."

included in the primary criteria include a varying PR interval and varying RR interval.

The irregularity of the QRS complexes is often times the most easily recognized ECG finding and, thus, can be mistaken for AF. At faster rates, it can be quite difficult to identify the P waves required to make this distinction and this may only become more obvious with a slower ventricular rate. The distinction between MAT and atrial fibrillation is critical, as management differences between the two conditions are profound. The QRS complex itself should be normal in appearance as conduction down the His-Purkinje system is normal. As mentioned previously, the exception to this would be in the setting of a pre-existing bundle branch, rate-related aberrant conduction, or a pre-existing accessory pathway. Repolarization occurs normally; however, the superimposition of P waves on preceding T waves may result in an abnormal appearance of the ST segment-T wave complex.

The initial management of MAT involves treating the underlying cause. This involves improving oxygenation, correction of electrolyte and acid-base abnormalities, and withdrawal of medications that may be contributing factors such as theophylline. Interestingly, digitalis toxicity does not

seem to play a role in MAT [13]. Rate control may be needed on occasion. Finally, it is worth mentioning that unlike most SVTs, which should be electrically cardioverted if unstable, MAT is not responsive to electrical cardioversion [15,21].

Junctional tachycardia

Junctional tachycardia is an uncommon SVT that originates within the AV junction. Other terminology that has been used to describe this arrhythmia includes non-paroxysmal junctional tachycardia (often in adults) and junctional ectopic tachycardia (in children). In general, its mechanism for generation is thought to be enhanced automaticity of a focus within the AV junction [22,23]. It is often seen in the setting of children that have undergone surgery for congenital cardiac abnormalities. In adults it may be associated with myocardial ischemia/infarction, digoxin toxicity, cardiomyopathy, and myocarditis [23,24].

The ECG characteristics of JT can be varied because of the complexity of structure and function of the AV junction.

Normally, the main function of the AV junction is conduction of an impulse that originates from above, preferably from within the SA node down to the His-Purkinje system. This is referred to as antegrade conduction. Not uncommonly, conduction may occur in a retrograde fashion from the ventricles to atria. Additionally, cells within the AV junction possess intrinsic automaticity. Normally, this is suppressed by the faster intrinsic automaticity of the SA node; however, under certain circumstances such as that of myocardial ischemia or drug toxicity, the automaticity of the AV junction may become enhanced and become the dominant pacemaker resulting in a junctional rhythm. Terminology associated with junctional rhythms is ventricular rate-dependent: (1) junctional rhythm or junctional escape rhythm (rate 40–60 bpm) which reflects the intrinsic rate of the AV junction, (2) accelerated junctional rhythm (rate 60–100 bpm, and (3) junctional tachycardia (rate > 100 bpm).

The presence of P waves is variable in JT. If there is retrograde conduction to the atria, P waves may be identifiable either preceding the QRS complex or following the QRS complex. If the P waves precede the QRS they are often inverted in leads II, III, and aVF and the PR interval is very short (< 120 ms). Electrocardiograms with P waves following the QRS, but in close proximity, are described as having a short RP interval. However, there may be various degrees of AV block such that this 1 : 1 relationship is not constant. For example, in the presence of Wenckebach AV conduction, P waves that follow the QRS will gradually have a lengthening RP interval with a subsequent drop of the P wave.

Atrioventricular dissociation may also be present. In this situation, the ventricles are beginning depolarized by an impulse that originates in the AV junction while the atria are depolarized by another impulse such as that arising in the SA node. If this is the case, regular P waves may be seen throughout the ECG but they are unrelated to (dissociated from) the QRS complexes. The QRS rate is greater than 100 bpm, while the P waves are often at a rate slower than this. Occasionally, ventricular capture beats can be seen if an appropriately timed sinus beat is allowed antegrade conduction through the AV node

In general, the QRS complex should be narrow and regular in morphology because depolarization down the His-Purkinje system to the ventricle is normal. During the initiation of the arrhythmia there may be a gradual increase in ventricular rate. A widened QRS can be seen in the setting of pre-existing bundle branch block, rate-related aberrant conduction, or pre-existing accessory pathway. If there is intermittent block within the AV junction or AV dissociation is present, the QRS complexes may appear to be irregular and can be confused with AF. However, the irregularity of the QRS complexes is more obvious in AF and there should be no identifiable P waves.

Treatment of JT focuses on treating the underlying cause such as a decrease in digoxin level, improvement of myocardial oxygenation, or correction of electrolyte abnormalities.

Beta-blockers are usually the initial drug of choice, but ablation may be necessary in refractory cases.

Atrial flutter

Atrial flutter is a common SVT that is characterized by rapid atrial depolarizations that appear as a saw-tooth pattern on the ECG. In 1979, Wells and colleagues characterized AFl into two categories, type I AFl and type II AFl [25]. Since that time, a new classification system has been adopted based on whether the arrhythmia is dependent on the cavotricuspid isthmus [26]. The term *typical flutter* is used to refer to that type of AFl that is dependent on the cavotricuspid isthmus for part of the macrore-entrant circuit. *Atypical flutter* does not depend on the cavotricuspid isthmus and its mechanism is unclear. This distinction is of clinical significance because typical flutter is more easily amenable to catheter ablation.

The more common form of AFl is the typical variety. The atrial depolarization rate is usually around 300 bpm. In persons with a healthy AV node and not on medication that would affect conduction of the AV node, the ventricular rate is usually half of the atrial rate (2 : 1 AV conduction). Thus the ventricular rate of 150 bpm is characteristic of typical AFl (Figure 28.3). In persons with underlying heart disease or on AV-blocking medications, the ratio of atrial to ventricular depolarizations may be lower, 3 : 1, 4 : 1, etc. When looking at the ECG of a person in typical AFl, the classical saw-tooth pattern of the AFl waves can be identified in the inferior and right precordial leads. This may be difficult when 2 : 1 AV conduction exists, because some of the flutter waves may be obscured by the QRS complex or the ST-T wave. In this situation, the rhythm may be confused with sinus tachycardia; therefore, whenever the ventricular rate is approximately 150 bpm, a diagnosis of AFl should be strongly considered and the ECG should be closely scrutinized for "hidden" flutter waves (F waves). This is particularly true if the rate is relatively constant despite therapeutic measures.

When looking at the ECG of a patient in typical AFl, the F waves should display a particular pattern of polarity. The usual pattern is negatively appearing flutter waves in the inferior leads, with positive appearing flutter waves in lead V1. This is the more common ECG pattern seen and reflects a counterclockwise activation around the tricuspid annulus (Figure 28.3). If the flutter waves are positive in the inferior leads and negative in V1, this is still a typical AFl but activation around the tricuspid annulus is in a clockwise direction.

Atypical AFl refers to a tachycardia that fulfills the classical ECG definition of a continuously undulating pattern but not fitting the typical (clockwise or counterclockwise) pattern. The atrial rate may be more rapid. The underlying mechanism for this type of AFl is unclear. An example of an AFl would be a narrow complex tachycardia with an undulating baseline but with flutter waves of the same polarity in the inferior and precordial leads.

The QRS complex in AF1 should be narrow unless there is a pre-existing bundle branch block, rate-related aberrancy, or a pre-existing accessory pathway. The RR interval may be regular if the ratio of atrial to ventricular depolarization is constant, or it may be irregular if the ratio of atrial to ventricular depolarizations is variable ("atrial flutter with variable conduction").

The initial treatment in the ED for AF1 focuses on rate control. If rhythm identification is unclear because of a rapid ventricular rate and the patient is stable, adenosine or Valsalva maneuver may be employed to slow conduction through the AV node such that the AF1 waves are more readily apparent. Following rhythm identification, a longer acting agent will need to be administered to decrease the ventricular rate. As mentioned above, a hemodynamically unstable patient should be electrically cardioverted.

Atrial fibrillation

Atrial fibrillation has been called "the most common arrhythmia encountered in clinical practice" [27], and "the most common sustained dysrhythmia in adults" [28]. It is often a consequence of a pre-existing cardiovascular condition, such as hypertension, CAD, or cardiomyopathy. Other conditions including pulmonary embolism, COPD, and hyperthyroidism have been associated with the development of AF. Usually, AF is a disease of adults over 50 years of age and

is rarely seen in the pediatric population (an exception being those children who have had cardiac surgery). "Lone" AF is the term given when it occurs in a younger patient (less than 60 years old) who does not have any pre-existing cardiac disease. Atrial fibrillation can be either paroxysmal or chronic [29]. Complications include heart failure, cardiomyopathy, systemic embolization, and stroke [30].

Atrial fibrillation is triggered when a premature atrial beat, originating in an area other than the SA node, travels down an abnormal pathway to the ventricle. This leads to the development of an abnormal re-entrant circuit [28]. The atrial fibrillatory waves, which characterize AF, are conducted to the ventricles in an irregularly irregular pattern (Figure 28.7).

Typically, the ECG of a patient in AF will reveal a lack of distinct P waves, the presence of fibrillatory waves (best seen in leads V1, II, III, and aVF), a narrow QRS complex, and a ventricular rate between 90 and 170 bpm, with a variable (irregularly irregular) RR interval. However, close inspection of the ECG is necessary as not all patients present with these classic findings [31].

Although P waves are absent, fibrillatory waves may vary in amplitude (fine fibrillatory waves < 0.5 mm, coarse > 0.5 mm), morphology, and intervals. They may have sufficient amplitude to mimic P waves, thus leading the observer to conclude that the patient is in a different rhythm, such as MAT [27], AT, or AF1 with variable AV block. In patients with longstanding AF, the amplitude of the fibrillatory waves may be decreased to the point where they are no longer

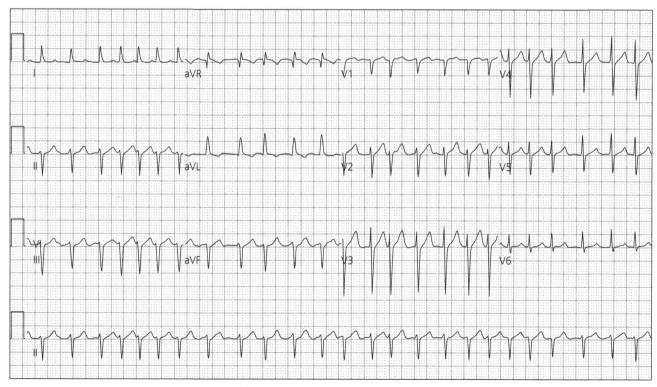

Figure 28.7 Atrial fibrillation with rapid ventricular response. The rhythm is an irregularly irregular narrow complex tachycardia. Distinct atrial activity is absent. (ECG courtesy of Amal Mattu, MD.)

apparent. Artifacts such as shivering or tremor may mimic fibrillatory waves.

As noted above, the QRS complexes in atrial fibrillation are typically narrow and appear irregularly irregular. Accordingly the RR interval varies from beat to beat. The QRS complex may be wide and abnormal in appearance in the setting of a pre-existing bundle branch block, rate-related aberrancy, or a pre-existing accessory pathway. The ventricular rate is usually between 90 and 170 bpm. The rate may be slower in the elderly and in patients taking medications that slow conduction through the AV node, such as beta-blockers and calcium channel-blockers. More rapid rates may be seen in patients with hypovolemia or other causes of tachycardia. The irregularity may be difficult to detect in patients with very rapid ventricular rates.

Case conclusions

The first case is a common example of a patient presenting with an AVNRT. Initially, vagal maneuvers were attempted to try to break the rhythm, without success. The patient had an intravenous line established and 6 mg of intravenous adenosine was rapidly administered, followed by a saline flush which within seconds terminated the arrhythmia and restored sinus rhythm. The patient was discharged home asymptomatic with outpatient follow-up with cardiology.

The second case was initially misdiagnosed as AF, but careful inspection of the ECG reveals that, while this is an irregularly irregular narrow complex tachycardia, there are P waves present preceding the QRS complexes. These P waves do have varying morphology. These ECG characteristics and patient presentation are consistent with MAT. As the patient's pulmonary status improved with oxygen, nebulized albuterol, and steroids, her heart rate decreased. She was admitted to the hospital for a COPD exacerbation.

The third case was initially misdiagnosed as sinus tachycardia. However, despite appropriate interventions for temperature reduction and intravenous fluid administration, the heart rate did not change from 150 bpm. The diagnosis of AFl with 2 : 1 AV conduction was eventually made and an intravenous bolus of diltiazem was administered, followed by a continuous infusion. The ventricular rate decreased to 70 bpm and the AFl waves were more readily apparent with a rate of 300 bpm.

References

1 Orejarena JA, Vidaillet H, DeStefano F, *et al.* Paroxysmal supraventricular tachycardia in the general population. *J Am Coll Cardiol* 1998;**31**:150–7.

2 Davies AJ, Kenny RA. Frequency of neurologic complications following carotid sinus massage. *Am J Cardiology* 1998;**81**:1256–7.

3 Strickberger SA, Man KC, Daoud EG, *et al.* Adenosine-induced atrial arrhythmia: a prospective analysis. *Ann Intern Med* 1997;**127**:417–22.

4 Pieper SJ, Stanton MS. Narrow QRS Complex Tachycardias. *Mayo Clin Proc* 1995;**70**:371–5.

5 Goodacre S, Irons R. Atrial arrhythmias. *BMJ* 2002;**324**(7337): 594–7.

6 McGuire MA, Bourke JP, Robotin MC, *et al.* High resolution mapping of Koch's triangle using sixty electrodes in humans with atrioventricular junctional (AV nodal) reentrant tachycardia. *Circulation* 1993;**88**:2315–28.

7 Erdinler I, Okmken E, Oguz E, *et al.* Differentiation of narrow QRS complex tachycardia types using the 12 lead electrocardiogram. *ANE* 2002;**7**:120–6.

8 Gulec S, Ertab F, Karaoouz R, *et al.* Value of ST-depression during paroxysmal supraventricular tachycardia in the diagnosis of coronary artery disease. *Am J Cardiol* 1999;**83**:458–60.

9 Paparella N, Ouyang F, Fuca G, *et al.* Significance of newly acquired negative T waves after interruption of paroxysmal reentrant supraventricular tachycardia with narrow QRS complex. *Am J Cardiol* 2000;**85**:261–3.

10 Munger TM, Packer DL, Hammill SC, *et al.* A population study of the natural history of Wolff-Parkinson-White Syndrome in Olmsted County, Minnesota, 1953–1989. *Circulation* 1993;**87**: 866–73.

11 Nelson SD, Kou WH, Annesley T, *et al.* Significance of ST segment depression during paroxysmal supraventricular tachycardia. *J Am Coll Cardiol* 1988;**12**:383.

12 Exner, DV, Muzyka T, Gillis AM. Proarrhythmia in patients with Wolff-Parkinson-White after standard doses of intravenous adenosine. *Ann Intern Med* 1995;**122**:351–2.

13 Shine KI, Kastor JA, Yurchak PM. Multifocal atrial tachycardia: clinical and electrocardiographic features in 32 patients. *N Engl J Med* 1968;**279**:344–9.

14 Lipson MJ, Maimi S. Multifocal atrial tachycardia: clinical associations and significance. *Circulation* 1970;**42**:397–407.

15 Kones RJ, Phillips JH, Herch J. Mechanism and management of chaotic atrial mechanism. *Cardiology* 1974;**59**:92–101.

16 Phillips J, Spano J, Burch G. Chaotic atrial mechanism. *Am Heart J* 1969;**78**:171–9.

17 Berlinerblau R, Feder W. Chaotic atrial rhythm. *J Electrocardiol* 1972;**5**:135–44.

18 Habizbadez, MA. Multifocal atrial tachycardia: a 66 month follow-up of 50 patients. *Heart Lung* 1980;**9**:328–35.

19 McCord J, Borzak S. Multifocal Atrial Tachycardia. *Chest* 1998; **113**:203–9.

20 Iseri LT, Fairshter RD, Hardemann JL *et al.* Magnesium and potassium therapy in multifocal atrial tachycardia. *Am Heart J* 1985;**110**:789–94.

21 Wang K, Goldfard BL, Gobel FL *et al.* Multifocal atrial tachycardia. *Arch Intern Med* 1977;**137**:161–4.

22 Scheinman MM, Gonzalez RP, Cooper MW *et al.* Clinical and electrophysiologic features and role of catheter ablation techniques in adult patients with automatic atrioventricular junctional tachycardia. *Am J Cardiol* 1994;**74**:565–72.

23 Rosen KM. Junctional tachycardia. *Circulation* 1973;**47**:654–64.

24 Konecke LL, Knoebel SB. Nonparoxysmal junctional tachycardia complicating acute myocardial infarction. *Circulation* 1972;**45**: 367–74.

25 Wells JL, Mclean WAH, James TN *et al.* Characterization of atrial flutter. Studies in man after open heart surgery using fixed atrial electrodes. *Circulation* 1979;**60**:665–73.

26 Saoudi N, Codia F, Waldo A, *et al.* A classification of atrial flutter and regular atrial tachycardia according to electrophysiological mechanism and anatomic bases. A statement from a Joint Expert Group from the Working Group of Arrhythmias of the European Society of Cardiology and the North American Society of Pacing and Electrophysiology. *Eur Heart J* 2001;**22**:1162–82.

27 Ganz, Leonard I. Management of atrial fibrillation. *Crit Pathways Cardiol* 2002;**1**(1):3–11.

28 Veenhuyzen GD, Simpson CS, Abdollah H. Atrial fibrillation. *Can Med Assoc J* 2004;**171**(7):755–60.

29 Fuster V, Ryden LE, Asinger RW, *et al.* ACC/AHA/ESC Guidelines for the Management of Patients With Atrial Fibrillation: Executive Summary A Report of the American College of Cardiology/ American Heart Association Task Force on Practice Guidelines and the European Society of Cardiology Committee for Practice Guidelines and Policy Conferences (Committee to Develop Guidelines for the Management of Patients With Atrial Fibrillation) Developed in Collaboration With the North American Society of Pacing and Electrophysiology. *Circulation* 2001;**104**(17):2118–50.

30 Khairy P, Nattel S. New insights into the mechanisms and management of atrial fibrillation. *Can Med Assoc J* 2002;**167**(9):1012–20.

31 Bogun F, Anh D, Kalahasty G, *et al.* Misdiagnosis of atrial fibrillation and its clinical consequences. *Am J Med* 2004;**117**:636.

Chapter 29 | Can the ECG guide treatment of narrow QRS tachycardia?

Michael A. Bohrn
York Hospital, York, PA, USA

Case presentations

Case 1: A 36-year-old female presents to the emergency department (ED) with palpitations and dizziness. She has no past medical history. She is diaphoretic and pale and her vital signs show a blood pressure of 100/60, pulse of 160, respirations of 20/minute, and oxygen saturation of 98% on room air. Her examination otherwise shows clear lung fields, and a normal mental status. The electrocardiogram (ECG) shows a narrow complex, regular tachycardia (Figure 29.1).

Case 2: A 28-year-old male presents to the ED with dizziness on a Monday morning. He has no past medical history, but does admit to drinking significant amounts of alcohol over the weekend. He has no chest pain, but notes near syncope with sudden onset of the dizziness at 8:30 am this morning. Vital signs are temperature of 37 °C (98.6 °F), blood pressure of 110/70, pulse of 140, respirations 20/minute, with oxygen saturation of 99% on room air. Physical examination shows an irregularly irregular pulse, no cardiac murmur or gallop, clear lung fields, no thyromegaly, and normal peripheral pulses. His ECG (Figure 29.2) shows atrial fibrillation with a rapid ventricular response.

Case 3: A 78-year-old female presents to the ED with dizziness and respiratory distress. The patient began feeling poorly earlier today, and her breathing worsened while she was visiting with her family. She has no chest pain, and has a long history of chronic obstructive pulmonary disease (COPD). Vital signs show a normal temperature, blood pressure of 130/70, pulse of 120, respirations 28/minute and oxygen saturation of 87% on oxygen. Examination reveals an anxious patient who is somewhat pale. Lungs show diffuse wheezes, and peripheral pulses are present but weak. The patient has a history of similar episodes, which have

required intubation in the past. Her ECG (Figure 29.3) shows an irregular narrow QRS tachycardia.

The ECG in narrow QRS tachycardia: management considerations

Approximately 50,000 ED visits per year are attributed to supraventricular tachycardia (SVT) [1]. This is a fairly common tachydysrhythmia and represents only one variation of narrow QRS tachycardias. The 12-lead ECG is an important tool in managing the adult patient presenting to the ED with tachycardia. One of the critical steps in the management of the tachycardic patient is determining whether the QRS complex is wide or narrow. Once the QRS complex has been deemed to be narrow with a regular pattern, the differential diagnosis list is limited to a manageable number of possibilities, including sinus tachycardias, atrioventricular nodal re-entrant tachycardias (AVNRT), focal and non-paroxysmal junctional tachycardias, atrioventricular re-entrant tachycardias (AVRT) with extranodal accessory pathways, focal atrial tachycardias, and atrial flutter [2]. The irregular narrow QRS tachycardias include atrial fibrillation, atrial flutter with variable conduction, and multifocal atrial tachycardia (MAT).

Patients with acute tachydysrhythmias represent typical urgent and emergent presentations. Management of these patients usually involves time-critical decisions requiring simultaneous evaluation and management to ensure the best possible patient outcome. The following chapter will discuss some of these tachycardias and how the ECG can be used to guide management decisions.

Narrow QRS tachycardias – regular

Electrocardiogram diagnosis is the key to treating narrow QRS complex tachycardias. While the focus here is on management, some discussion of the ECG diagnosis process is

Critical Decisions in Emergency and Acute Care Electrocardiography,
1st edition. Edited by W.J. Brady and J.D. Truwit. © 2009 Blackwell Publishing, ISBN: 9781405159067

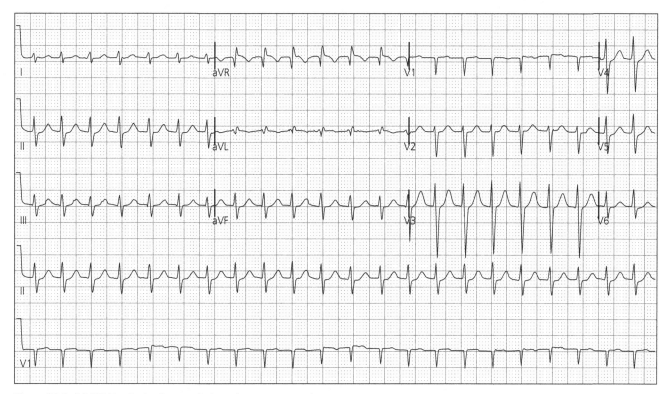

Figure 29.1 AVNRT. The rhythm has a typical regular, narrow complex pattern.

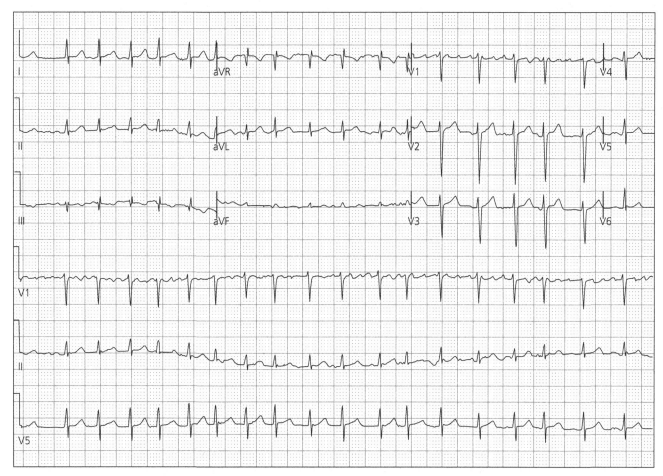

Figure 29.2 Atrial fibrillation. The rhythm is irregularly irregular with disorganized atrial activity.

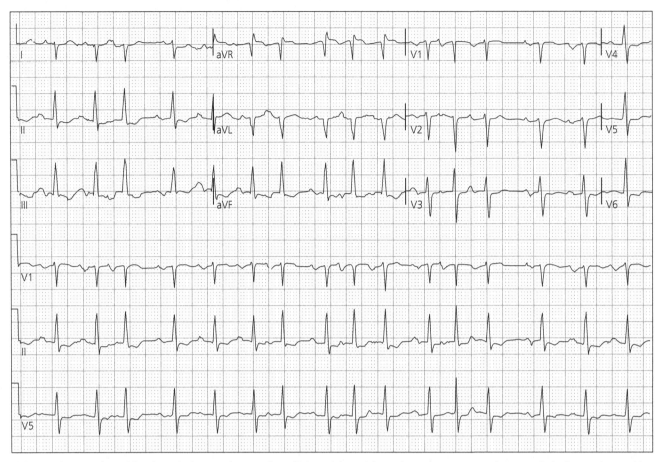

Figure 29.3 MAT. The atrial and ventricular complex occur irregularly, and the atrial complexes demonstrate ≥ three morphologies consistent with origin from various sites within the atria.

needed. Several studies have looked at the use of the surface ECG in differentiating the mechanisms of narrow QRS complex tachycardias. In one study, multiple criteria were developed for various tachycardia types. Presence of a P wave separate from the QRS complex was seen frequently with atrioventricular (AV) reciprocating tachycardia, as was QRS alternans. In lead V1, a pseudo-R′ pattern and pseudo-S wave in the inferior leads were seen commonly with AVNRT. Presence of P waves separate from the QRS, as well as RP/PR interval greater or equal to 1, were also associated with atrial tachycardias [3]. Similar findings regarding visible P waves with narrow QRS tachycardia were seen in another, more recent study, where an R′ pattern in V1 or S wave in lead II were associated with AVNRT. This study also suggests the need for consideration of AVRT in elderly and female patients with narrow QRS tachycardia and visible P waves, when pre-excitation is not noticed [4]. Several studies also focus on the more specialized, invasive diagnosis and management of narrow QRS complex tachycardia in the electrophysiology lab. [5,6]. Simultaneous diagnostic testing and management can be accomplished via use of the Valsalva maneuver or carotid sinus massage in appropriate patients [7,8]. Another technique that may aid in visualizing P waves

is to increase the speed of the ECG recording (see Figure 29.4) [9]. Despite the criteria above, the diagnosis and treatment of narrow QRS complex tachycardias remains difficult.

Initial medical management of AVNRT (Figure 29.1) usually involves vagal maneuvers, followed by intravenous (IV) adenosine if vagal maneuvers are unsuccessful. Adenosine is rapid-acting, has a very short duration of action, and a good safety profile, including use in prehospital care [10,11]. Treatment with adenosine has also been compared with verapamil and similar efficacy rates have been noted [12,13]. Additional treatment options include other calcium channel-blockers and beta-blockers, and "pill in the pocket" regimens have been proposed. Treatment involves prescribing an oral medication to be taken on an as-needed basis. The combination of oral diltiazem and propranolol seems to be effective for this purpose [14].

Atrioventricular reciprocating tachycardias involve the presence of an accessory or bypass tract around the AV node. Wolff-Parkinson-White (WPW) syndrome most commonly provides the substrate for this dysrhythmia. In sinus rhythm, widening of the QRS complex is seen along with shortened PR interval; additionally, the QRS complex is initially slurred, known as the delta wave. Wolff-Parkinson-White syndrome,

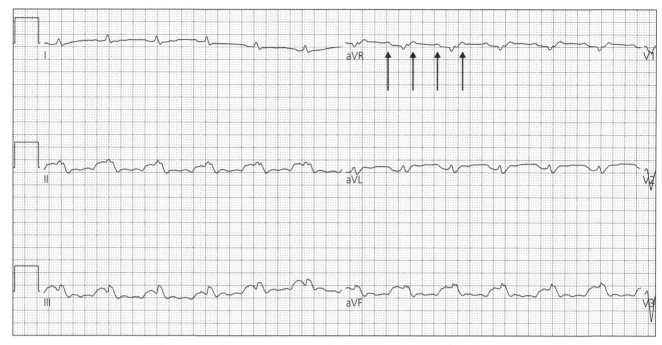

Figure 29.4 ECG recorded as 50 mm/s. Normally ECGs are recorded at 25 mm/s. In this case, the ECG computer setting was changed to "stretch out" the tracing. This allows easier distinction of the P waves (arrows). Note that because the tracing occurs at half-speed, the atrial and ventricular rates are halved as well. (ECG courtesy of Amal Mattu, MD.)

as well as other forms of AVRT, can also involve a "concealed" accessory pathway, with orthodromic conduction leading to a narrow QRS tachycardia. Because the tachycardia may manifest with a narrow QRS complex, it is important to evaluate the baseline ECG, after return to sinus rhythm for evidence of pre-excitation. ST segment elevation in lead aVR, seen with AVRT, may also help differentiate this mechanism from other types of SVT [15]. Patients with wide QRS complex AVRT due to WPW syndrome typically respond to medical treatment with procainamide or synchronized cardioversion. Long-term treatment most often involves ablation of the accessory pathway.

Electrocardiogram diagnosis of sinus tachycardia is based on verification of a sinus mechanism. P wave axis is helpful in this regard. Positive (upright) P waves in the inferior leads, with negative P waves in aVR define the ECG criteria for sinus rhythm [2]. Integrating the clinical findings is also key for sinus tachycardia. The tachycardia typically begins and ends gradually (non-paroxysmal), as opposed to the sudden onset associated with many AVRT or AVRNT. There is also some evidence that the amplitude of the QRS complex in leads V2–V5 may increase with SVT, but not with sinus tachycardia. This may be useful in differentiating these rhythms at faster rates [16]. Thus, using the ECG for patients with sinus tachycardia can guide therapy toward the underlying condition (e.g. pain, fever, hypovolemia, anxiety, etc.) [2]. Specific medications for sinus tachycardia are sometimes indicated – e.g. beta-blockers as part of the treatment regimen for thyrotoxicosis – but treatment, in general, should be focused on correcting the underlying cause.

Focal atrial tachycardias can usually be differentiated from sinus tachycardias by evaluating the P wave axis. Inverted P waves in the inferior leads (II, III, aVF) indicate an abnormal site of origin of the rhythm. A regular, narrow QRS complex tachycardia with an abnormal P wave axis should lead to consideration of an atrial tachycardia. Management of automatic atrial tachycardias is difficult as medical therapies and electrical cardioversion are often ineffective. Attempts to control ventricular rate usually involve either beta-blockers or calcium channel-blockers, often with limited success. Direct suppression of the atrial focus can be attempted by using class Ia or Ic agents, or with class III agents such as sotalol or amiodarone [2].

The ECG criteria for atrial flutter (see Figure 29.5) include organized regular atrial activity and atrial impulses at a rate of 250–350. Typically, atrial flutter is due to one of a variety of re-entry loops and manifests with 2 : 1 ventricular conduction. The organized atrial activity (saw-tooth waves) seen on ECG affects treatment planning. Class Ic agents may slow the flutter waves, but do not typically lead to conversion to sinus rhythm. Class III agents such as amiodarone tend to be more effective in terminating atrial flutter. Electrical cardioversion, often with relatively low energy levels, is very effective for atrial flutter as well [2].

Focal junctional tachycardias have ventricular rates of 100–250 and frequently show ECG evidence of AV dissociation. These rhythms are sometimes known as automatic or paroxysmal junctional tachycardias and there is a paucity of information in the medical literature regarding their management. Stress or exercise can be precipitants, and potential

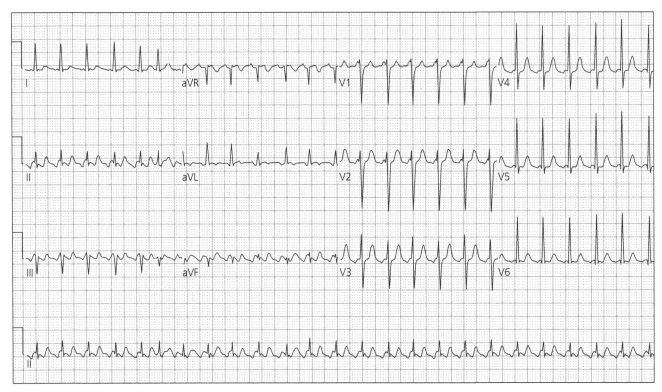

Figure 29.5 Atrial flutter with 2 : 1 AV conduction. The rhythm is regular with a ventricular rate of approximately 150 bpm, typical of this rhythm. Atrial activity manifests as the classic "saw-tooth" pattern with inverted flutter waves ("F waves") in the inferior leads with a rate of 300 bpm. (ECG courtesy of Amal Mattu, MD.)

treatments include beta-blockers and IV flecainide. Ablation via catheter can result in a cure but is associated with a risk of AV block [2].

Non-paroxysmal junctional rhythms typically manifest with a slower ventricular rate (70–120 bpm) than the focal junctional tachycardias, and usually exhibit one-to-one AV association. A "warm up" and "cool down" pattern is seen at the beginning and end of the period of dysrhythmia, and this rhythm can sometimes be a marker for serious underlying problems such as digoxin toxicity, cardiac ischemia, or hypokalemia. Treatment, similar to MAT, centers on correcting the underlying medical problems, especially digoxin toxicity. Digitalis-binding antibodies may be required in serious cases [2]. For refractory cases, calcium channel-blockers or beta-blockers may be used [17].

Narrow QRS tachycardias – irregular

The differential diagnosis of the irregular narrow QRS complex tachycardia is somewhat simpler. Atrial fibrillation comprises the vast majority of irregular tachycardias (Figure 29.2). Atrial fibrillation is usually fairly evident from the surface ECG, although rapid ventricular rates can make this diagnosis somewhat more difficult. The presence of an irregularly irregular rhythm with no evidence of organized atrial activity confirms the diagnosis of atrial fibrillation. Once this ECG diagnosis is made, treatment decisions are based on the desired end-result. Short-term management often includes ventricular rate control, accomplished by using calcium channel-blockers such as diltiazem or beta-blockers, such as esmolol or metoprolol [18,19]. Additional considerations include attempts at electrical cardioversion, pharmacologic cardioversion using amiodarone, flecainide, quinidine, ibutilide, or propafenone, as well as initiation of anticoagulation in cases of certain atrial fibrillation [18].

Multifocal atrial tachycardia is often secondary to cardiorespiratory issues, electrolyte abnormalities, or medication toxicity [2]. Electrocardiogram diagnosis hinges on identification of three or more distinct P wave morphologies, in conjunction with the appropriate clinical situation (Figure 29.3). Differentiating MAT from the more commonly seen atrial fibrillation is dependent on identification of distinct P waves and correlating this with the clinical scenario. Treatment should be aimed at the underlying condition, with specific medical management occasionally focusing on rate control with calcium channel-blockers, as cardioversion and other anti-arrhythmic medication therapy are not indicated [2]. Atrial flutter with variable conduction (see Figure 29.6) is a third, and relatively common, cause of irregular QRS tachycardia. In this rhythm, the AV conduction usually varies

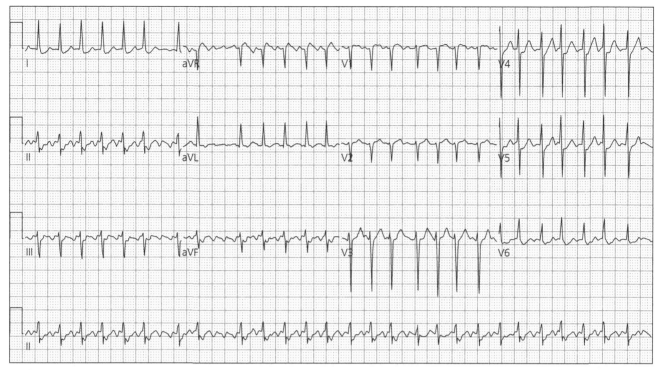

Figure 29.6 Atrial flutter with variable AV conduction. F waves are noted in the inferior leads at a rate of approximately 300 bpm, diagnostic of atrial flutter. The ventricular response is irregular because the AV conduction varies between 2 : 1, 3 : 1, and even 4 : 1. Note that in some portions of the rhythm when the conduction ratio is consecutively 2 : 1, the ventricular response is *regular*. Atrial fibrillation, on the other hand, would remain irregular throughout. (ECG courtesy of Amal Mattu, MD.)

between 2 : 1, 3 : 1, and sometimes 4 : 1 conduction producing an overall irregular rhythm. The irregularity often causes a misdiagnosis of atrial fibrillation. Treatment of this irregular atrial flutter is similar to treatment for regular atrial flutter.

Case conclusions

In Case 1, the ECG (Figure 29.1) demonstrates a regular, narrow QRS complex tachycardia; the rhythm diagnosis is AVNRT. The rhythm was compromising, yet the patient was considered hemodynamically stable. She received intravenous adenosine with prompt return to sinus rhythm. A repeat ECG was within normal limits. In Case 2, the ECG (Figure 29.2) demonstrates atrial fibrillation with an irregularly irregular rhythm and disorganized atrial activity without discernible P waves. The patient initially was managed with volume expansion with normal saline followed by rate control with intravenous diltiazem. His rate markedly slowed, yet he remained in the dysrhythmia. He was admitted to the hospital where he ultimately converted to sinus rhythm; subsequent evaluation was unremarkable. Lastly, Case 3 (Figure 29.3) illustrates MAT; the patient was experiencing an exacerbation of COPD coupled with volume depletion and hypokalemia. The underlying conditions were managed with ultimate conversion to sinus tachycardia.

References

1 Murman DH, McDonald AJ, *et al.* U.S. emergency department visits for supraventricular tachycardia, 1993–2003. *Acad Emerg Med* 2007;**14**:578–81.

2 Blomstron-Lundqvist C, Scheinman MM, *et al.* ACC/AHA/ESC guidelines for the management of patients with supraventricular arrhythmias – executive summary. *J Am Coll Cardiol* 2003;**42**: 1493–531.

3 Kalbfleisch SJ, el-Atassi R, *et al.* Differentiation of paroxysmal narrow QRS complex tachycardias using the 12-lead electrocardiogram. *J Am Coll Cardiol* 1993;**21**:85–9.

4 Maury P, Zimmerman M, Metzger J. Distinction between atrioventricular reciprocating tachycardia and atrioventricular node re-entrant tachycardia in the adult population based on P wave location. *Europace* 2003;**5**:57–64.

5 Chen SA, Chiang CE, *et al.* Accessory pathway and atrioventricular node reentrant tachycardia in elderly patients: clinical features, electrophysiologic characteristics and results of radiofrequency ablation. *J Am Coll Cardiol* 1994;**23**:702–8.

6 Knight BP, Zivin A, *et al.* A technique for the rapid diagnosis of atrial tachycardia in the electrophysiology laboratory. *J Am Coll Cardiol* 1999;**33**:775–81.

7 Lim SH, Anantharaman V, *et al.* Comparison of treatment of supraventricular tachycardia by Valsalva maneuver and carotid sinus massage. *Ann Emerg Med* 1998;**31**:30–5.

8 Delacretaz E. Supraventricular tachycardia. *N Engl J Med* 2006; **354**:1039–51.

9 Accardi AJ, Miller R, Holmes JF. Enhanced diagnosis of narrow

complex tachycardias with increased electrocardiograph speed. *J Emerg Med* 2002;**22**:123–6.

10 Glatter KA, Cheng J, *et al.* Electrophysiologic effects of adenosine in patients with supraventricular tachycardia. *Circulation* 1999; **99**:1034–40.

11 Gausche M, Persse DE, *et al.* Adenosine for the prehospital treatment of paroxysmal supraventricular tachycardia. *Ann Emerg Med* 1994;**24**:183–9.

12 Madsen CD, Pointer JE, Lynch TG. A comparison of adenosine and verapamil for the treatment of supraventricular tachycardia in the prehospital setting. *Ann Emerg Med* 1995;**25**:649–55.

13 Brady WJ, DeBehnke DJ, *et al.* Treatment of out-of-hospital supraventricular tachycardia: adenosine vs. verapamil. *Acad Emerg Med* 1996;**3**:574–85.

14 Alboni P, Tomasi C, *et al.* Efficacy and safety of out-of-hospital, self-administered single-dose oral drug treatment in the management of well-tolerated paroxysmal supraventricular tachycardia. *J Am Coll Cardiol* 2001;**37**:548–53.

15 Ho YL, Lin LY, *et al.* Usefulness of ST elevation in lead aVR during tachycardia for determining mechanism of narrow QRS complex tachycardia. *Am J Cardiol* 2003;**92**:1424–8.

16 Wakimoto H, Izumida N, *et al.* Augmentation of QRS wave amplitudes in the precordial leads during narrow QRS tachycardia. *J Cardiovasc Electrophysiol* 2000;**11**:52–60.

17 Lee KL, Chun HM, *et al.* Effect of adenosine and verapamil in catecholamine-induced accelerated atrioventricular junctional rhythm: insights into the underlying mechanism. *Pacing Clin Electrophysiol* 1999;**22**:866–70.

18 Fuster V, Ryden LE, *et al.* ACC/AHA/ESC 2006 guidelines for the management of patients with atrial fibrillation – executive summary. *J Am Coll Cardiol* 2006;**48**:854–906.

19 Wang HE, O'Connor RE, *et al.* The use of diltiazem for treating rapid atrial fibrillation in the out-of-hospital setting. *Ann Emerg Med* 2001;**37**:38–45.

Chapter 30 | How can the ECG guide the diagnosis and management of wide complex tachycardias?

Traci Thoureen, Amal Mattu
University of Maryland School of Medicine, Baltimore, MD, USA

Case presentations

The setting is a mid-sized community hospital without invasive cardiac capabilities. Bad weather conditions preclude the timely transfer of patients to a tertiary-care center approximately 3 h away.

Case 1: A 90-year-old woman is brought to the emergency department (ED), with the chief complaint of shortness of breath. Her blood pressure is 130/70 mmHg and her electrocardiogram (ECG) demonstrates a wide complex regular tachycardia with a rate of 135 beats per minute (bpm) and a right bundle branch pattern (Figure 30.1). The patient has a medical history of hypertension and hypercholesterolemia. The physician places defibrillation pads and a peripheral intravenous line. The patient is given amiodarone, 150 mg IV push, but she does not respond. She is given a second dose and converts to sinus rhythm, with a rate of 95 bpm. Another ECG is obtained and shows sinus rhythm with right bundle branch block (BBB) (Figure 30.2). A baseline ECG is retrieved from the medical record and shows an identical pattern.

Case 2: A 34-year-old man presents to the ED after an episode of syncope. On arrival, he is awake and alert. He states that he feels well and just did not eat this morning. His medical history is unremarkable. Vital signs are notable for a blood pressure of 120/70 mmHg and a heart rate of 170 bpm. The ECG demonstrates an irregular wide complex rhythm (Figure 30.3). The patient is given IV adenosine, 6 mg, without effect, but 12 mg causes the rhythm to decompensate into ventricular fibrillation. After defibrillation, the patient's rhythm returns to a sinus rhythm. A prior ECG shows evidence of Wolff-Parkinson-White (WPW) syndrome.

Critical Decisions in Emergency and Acute Care Electrocardiography,
1st edition. Edited by W.J. Brady and J.D. Truwit. © 2009 Blackwell Publishing, ISBN: 9781405159067

The ECG as a guide to the diagnosis and management of wide complex tachycardia

These cases exemplify the challenges in interpretation and management of wide complex tachycardia (WCT) in the emergent setting. Studies have shown that 70–90% of individuals with WCT have ventricular tachycardia (VT). Ventricular tachycardia is especially important to consider in patients over 35 years of age and patients with a history of heart disease [1–3]. Unfortunately, physicians have a tendency to underdiagnose VT in favor of supraventricular tachycardia (SVT) when patients have regular rhythms [4]; they also have a tendency to overlook the possibility of WPW syndrome in patients with irregular WCTs. If either of these two errors is made, the resulting incorrect treatment can result in disastrous consequences. Ultimately, the onus of preliminary diagnosis lies with emergency physicians, so they must be adept at correctly diagnosing patients who present with WCTs.

Wide complex tachycardia

Wide complex tachycardia is generally defined as an arrhythmia with a QRS complex > 0.12 s duration and a ventricular rate > 120 bpm [5]. In the emergent setting, it is important to differentiate between ventricular tachycardia versus more benign conditions. Wide complex tachycardias should initially be separated into two major categories: irregular WCTs and regular WCTs.

Irregular WCT

The differential diagnosis of an irregular WCT focuses on atrial fibrillation with aberrant conduction (e.g. BBB or non-specific intraventricular conduction delay), atrial fibrillation

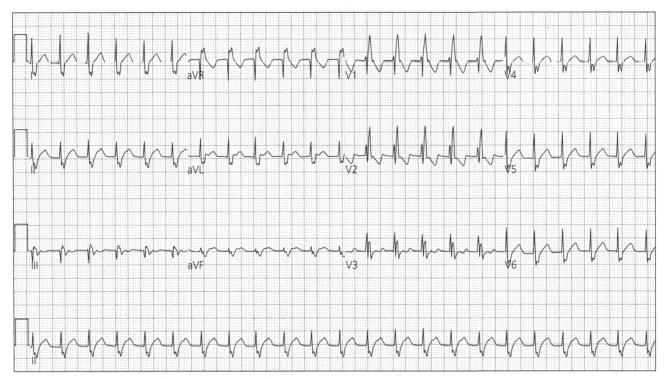

Figure 30.1 Case 1. Wide complex regular tachycardia; ventricular rate, 135 bpm. Reprinted from Mattu A, Brady W. ECGs for the Emergency Physician, Volume 1. London: BMJ Publishing, 2003.

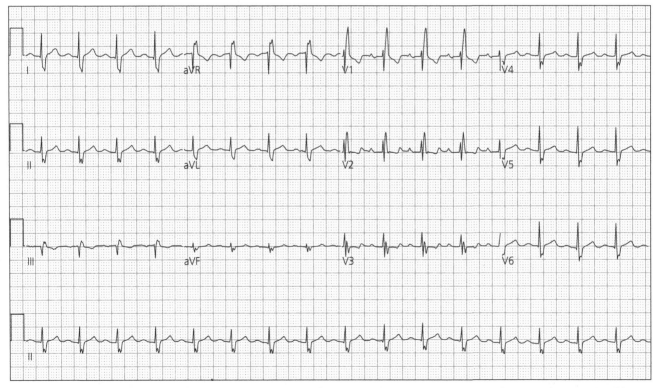

Figure 30.2 Case 1. Sinus tachycardia with right bundle branch block after conversion with amiodarone; ventricular rate, 95 bpm. Reprinted from Mattu A, Brady W. *ECGs for the Emergency Physician*, Volume 1. London: BMJ Publishing, 2003.

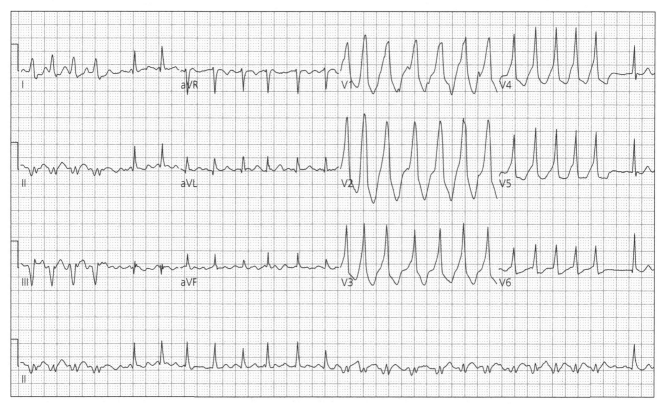

Figure 30.3 Case 2. Wide complex irregular tachycardia; ventricular rate, 170 bpm. The ECG demonstrates classic features of atrial fibrillation with Wolff-Parkinson-White syndrome: (1) irregularly irregular rhythm, (2) variations of QRS morphologies in amplitude and width, and (3) extremely rapid conduction in some areas of the rhythm, with rates approaching 250–300 bpm.

with pre-excitation (usually a WPW pattern), and polymorphic VT. A more detailed discussion of atrial fibrillation and WPW syndrome can be found in separate sections of this book. However, some simple guidelines for the distinction should be understood. All three of these entities manifest as *irregularly irregular* rhythms.

Atrial fibrillation: Atrial fibrillation with aberrant conduction (Figure 30.4), much like atrial fibrillation with normal atrioventricular conduction, usually demonstrates QRS morphologies that appear identical throughout the rhythm, and the rate rarely exceeds 180 bpm. In contrast, atrial fibrillation with pre-excitation (Figure 30.3) demonstrates QRS morphologies with significant variation in width because of the simultaneous conduction through the accessory pathway and His-Purkinje system. Wide QRS complexes are caused by conduction through the accessory pathway, narrow complexes are caused by conduction through the His-Purkinje system, and intermediate width complexes are caused by fusion of beats. Additionally, atrial fibrillation with pre-excitation often produces ventricular rates in excess of 200 bpm, including some areas on the rhythm strip that may demonstrate rates approaching 300 bpm.

Polymorphic VT (PVT): Like atrial fibrillation with pre-excitation, PVT has variable QRS morphologies within a

single electrocardiograph lead (Figure 30.5). Unlike the latter, however, PVT usually demonstrates a changing QRS axis, which can help in the distinction of PVT versus atrial fibrillation with pre-excitation. This type of VT may have a normal or long QT interval. A specific type of PVT associated with a long QT interval is torsade de pointes. Torsade de pointes has a characteristic electrocardiographic pattern, matching the translation of its name, "twisting of the pointes": the QRS amplitude increases and decreases apparently around the isoelectric line, producing the appearance that the QRS complexes are "twisting" around a central line or point (Figure 30.6). When this morphology is seen, the patient should be assessed for electrolyte abnormalities, drug toxicity (especially sodium channel-blockers), and cardiac ischemia/infarction. It is helpful to have a rhythm strip or ECG that shows the initiation of PVT, which may show an R-on-T phenomenon, in which the premature ventricular contraction falls on the T wave and initiates the arrhythmia. Polymorphic ventricular tachycardia is most frequently caused by acute ischemia or myocardial infarction. It is found in 20–25% of patients who experience cardiac arrest in the prehospital setting, and torsade de pointes is seen in a subset of 20% [6–9].

Other causes of irregular WCTs: Although atrial fibrillation with aberrant conduction, atrial fibrillation with

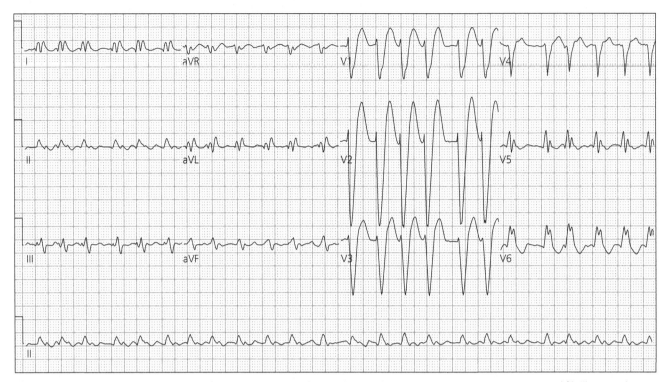

Figure 30.4 Atrial fibrillation with non-specific intraventricular conduction delay ventricular rate, 145 bpm. In contrast to atrial fibrillation with Wolff-Parkinson-White syndrome (Figure 30.3), atrial fibrillation with aberrant conduction demonstrates slower ventricular rates and minimal variation in the QRS complex morphologies.

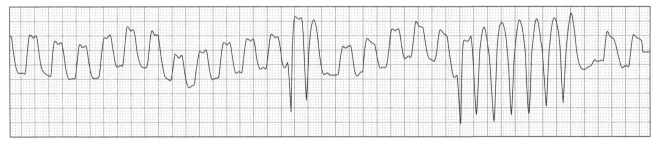

Figure 30.5 Polymorphic ventricular tachycardia. The rate is extremely rapid, with changing QRS morphologies and axis.

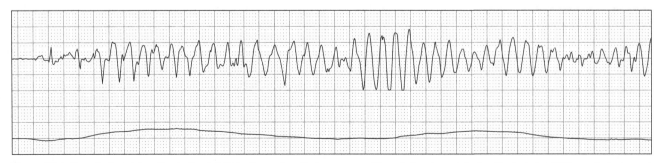

Figure 30.6 Torsade de pointes. The rhythm is initiated by an R-on-T phenomenon. The rate is extremely fast, with changing QRS morphologies and axis. The QRS complexes change smoothly in amplitude, giving the appearance they are "twisting" around a central axis.

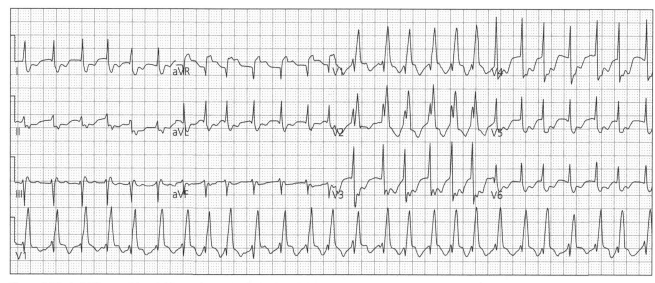

Figure 30.7 Atrial flutter with variable conduction and right bundle branch block; ventricular rate, 154 bpm. The overall rhythm is irregular, but atrial fibrillation is unlikely because the RR intervals in many areas are actually constant, i.e. the rhythm is not *irregularly* irregular. A right bundle branch block QRS morphology with rsR' complexes is present in lead V1.

pre-excitation, and PVT are the three major causes of irregular WCTs, multifocal atrial tachycardia and atrial flutter with variable AV conduction can also produce irregular WCTs if a BBB is present. In both of these conditions, however, the diagnosis is usually revealed by the presence of atrial activity. Atrial complexes (flutter waves) can be difficult to find in patients with rapid atrial flutter, but the diagnosis can be made by noting periods of regularity within the overall irregular rhythm (Figure 30.7). In contrast, as noted previously, atrial fibrillation and PVT should demonstrate irregular irregularity throughout the rhythm.

Regular WCT

Regular WCTs can be classified into three main groups: VT, SVT with aberrant conduction, and pre-excited tachycardia. Aberrant conduction is usually caused by a BBB, which may be fixed or rate-related. Other less common causes of aberrant conduction in the setting of tachycardia include hyperkalemia, drug toxicities (especially those that affect sodium channels), and non-specific intraventricular conduction delays. Pre-excitation syndromes, of which WPW syndrome is the most common, is another cause of aberrant ventricular conduction, although we and many other authors place it in its own category of WCTs to emphasize its importance in this discussion.

The physiology of ventricular conduction helps to explain the electrocardiographic appearance of the QRS complex. Normally, the ventricles are depolarized rapidly and simultaneously through the His-Purkinje system and the left and right bundle branches. Normal depolarization is accomplished within 0.12 s. When the normal routes are not used, and the conduction occurs sequentially from myocyte to myocyte, as with a BBB, VT, or an accessory pathway (WPW), or if the conduction is slowed secondary to cardiac ischemia, drugs, or electrolyte disturbances, the QRS complex is prolonged to more than 0.12 s (Figure 30.8) [10].

Ventricular tachycardia: The most common type of WCT is VT. It is defined as three or more consecutive ventricular beats at a rate of at least 120 bpm. "Non-sustained" VT lasts less than 30 s. "Sustained" VT lasts for more than 30 s, causes hemodynamic compromise, or requires a therapeutic intervention for termination (such as cardioversion) [10].

The appearance of the QRS complexes leads to further classification as monomorphic or polymorphic VT (Figure 30.9). Monomorphic VT has uniform QRS complexes. It is most commonly seen in patients with underlying coronary artery disease. It may be associated with valvular disorders or cardiomyopathies. Less frequent causes of monomorphic VT include idiopathic VT, right ventricular outflow tachycardia, VT associated with right ventricular dysplasia, and bundle branch re-entry [11,12].

Non-ischemic causes of VT are most often seen with long QT syndrome. As mentioned above, the most common causes of a prolonged QT interval are reversible (electrolyte abnormalities, drug toxicities, myocardial ischemia). If those causes are ruled out, however, the cause of the prolonged QT interval may be congenital. Patients with congenital prolonged QT syndrome are usually treated with beta-blockers, pacemaker insertion, left stellate ganglionectomy, or placement of an internal cardioverter-defibrillator. Temporary pacing, isoproterenol administration to increase heart rate, and IV magnesium are used to treat acute episodes of PVT in these patients [13].

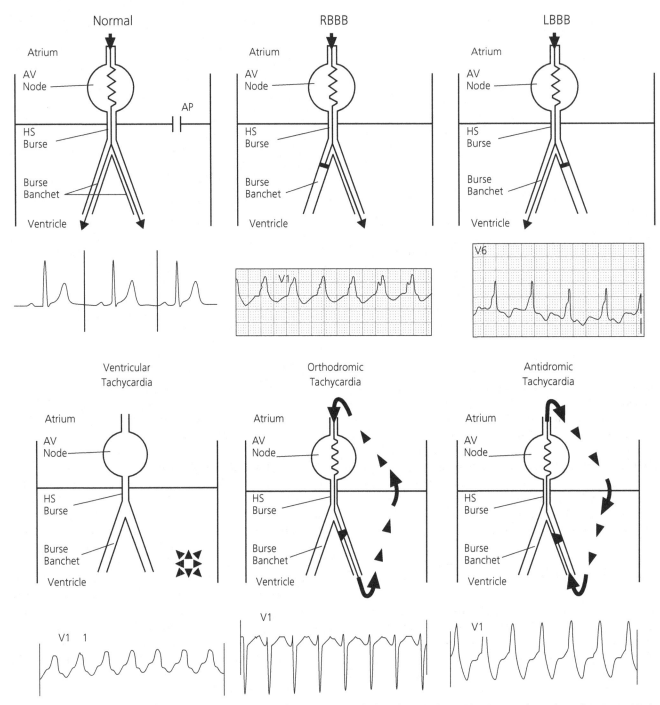

Figure 30.8 Mechanisms of wide QRS tachycardia. Reprinted from Shah CP *et al.* Clinical approach to wide QRS complex tachycardias. *Emerg Med Clin North Am* 1998;**16**:332–3. Copyright 1998, with permission from Elsevier.

SVT with aberrant conduction: SVT is defined as any tachycardia that uses the normal AV conduction system, with its origination in the atria or AV node, and that requires the AV node for its maintenance [10]. The various types and causes of SVT are discussed in further detail in the chapters on narrow complex tachycardia. Supraventricular tachycardia may also manifest as a WCT if aberrant ventricu-

lar conduction is present. Aberrancy can be caused by conduction delay or block (e.g. BBB; see Figures 30.1 and 30.2) over the normal AV conduction system. This block may be fixed or functional. A frequent cause of aberrancy is a sudden acceleration in rate at the onset of SVT; the increased rate may be continued by retrograde conduction into the blocked pathway. Right and left BBBs are the most frequent patterns,

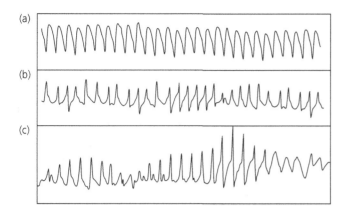

(a)

(b)

(c)

Figure 30.9 (a) Monomorphic VT. (b) Polymorphic VT. (c) Polymorphic VT with undulating pattern, suggestive of torsade de pointes. Reprinted from Hudson KB *et al.* Electrocardiographic manifestations: ventricular tachycardia. *J Emerg Med* 2003;**25**:303–14. Copyright 2003, with permission from Elsevier.

but any part of the His-Purkinje system may be involved [14].

Pre-excited tachycardia: With this type of rhythm, AV conduction occurs over two paths – the AV nodal His pathway and an accessory pathway (AP). Accessory pathways are abnormal extranodal tissues that connect the epicardial surface of the atrium and ventricle along the AV groove. Because conduction through the AP does not encounter the usual slowing of conduction that occurs in the AV node, the ventricle begins depolarization early through the AP, i.e. the ventricle becomes "pre-excited." The WPW syndrome is the most common cause of pre-excitation. Patients with this syndrome frequently develop symptomatic tachyarrhythmias [11,15]. Common forms of pre-excited tachycardia in patients with WPW syndrome are atrial fibrillation and paroxysmal SVT with ventricular activation over an AP [10]. Patients who have APs may have atrioventricular re-entrant tachycardia (AVRT). In patients with WPW, AVRT is the most common arrhythmia, occurring in 75% [15]. Atrioventricular re-entrant tachycardia may be orthodromic or antidromic. In orthodromic conduction, the anterograde (atrium to ventricle) conduction occurs over the AV node and retrograde (ventricle to atrium) conduction occurs over the AP. The QRS complex is regular and narrow, as the conduction is occurring in the normal manner, unless there is a pre-existing BBB. In contrast, in antidromic conduction, anterograde conduction occurs through the AP, and retrograde conduction is through the AV node, manifesting as regular WCT that is virtually indistinguishable from monomorphic VT. Orthodromic AVRT is more common, even in patients with WPW syndrome; antidromic tachycardia is seen in 10% of individuals with WPW syndrome [16]. Atrial fibrillation is an uncommon arrhythmia in patients with WPW syndrome, occurring in approximately 20% (Figure 30.3) [16], but it is much more deadly, as its rapid rates can

degenerate into ventricular fibrillation [15]. In the treatment of this subgroup of WCT, AV nodal blocking agents must be strictly avoided, because they can worsen the tachycardia by increasing conduction through the AP. A more detailed discussion of the tachyarrhythmias associated with WPW syndrome can be found in Chapter 34.

Other causes of regular WCT: Several other important causes of WCT should also be considered. Sinus tachycardia with pre-existing BBB (Figure 30.10) produces WCT. In this setting, close scrutiny of all leads for evidence of a regular P-QRS association confirms the diagnosis. Note that in the presence of tachycardia, P waves are not always obvious in all 12 leads, because they may become fused with or "buried within" the preceding T wave.

Wide complex tachycardias can be caused by medications that induce sodium channel-blockade (Table 30.1), such as tricyclic depressants (Figure 30.11). The cardiac effects of

Table 30.1 Sodium channel–blocking drugs that can cause wide complex tachycardia

Carbamazepine
Chloroquine
Class IA anti-arrhythmics
   Disopyramide
   Quinidine
   Procainamide
Class IC anti-arrhythmics
   Encainide
   Flecainide
   Propafenone
Citalopram
Cocaine
Cyclic anti-depressants
   Amitriptyline
   Amoxapine
   Desipramine
   Doxepine
   Imipramine
   Nortriptyline
   Maprotiline
Diphenhydramine
Hydroxychloroquine
Loxapine
Orphenadrine
Phenothiazines
   Mesoridazine
   Thioridazine
Propoxyphene
Quinine
Venlafaxine

Reprinted with permission from Hollowell H *et al.* Wide-complex tachycardia: beyond the traditional differential diagnosis of ventricular tachycardia vs supraventricular tachycardia with aberrant conduction. *Am J Emerg Med* 2005;**23**:876–89. Copyright 2005, with permission from Elsevier.

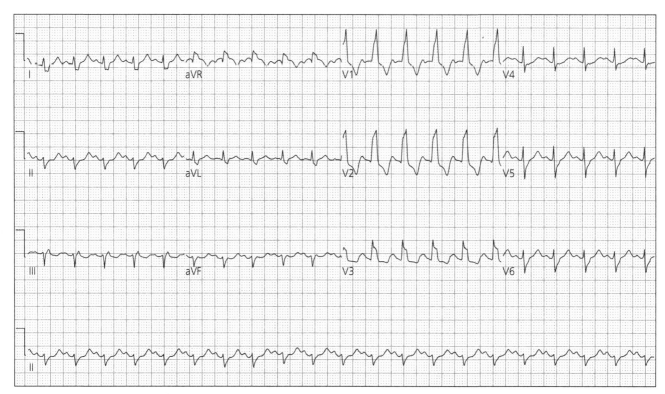

Figure 30.10 Sinus tachycardia with right bundle branch block; ventricular rate, 125 bpm.

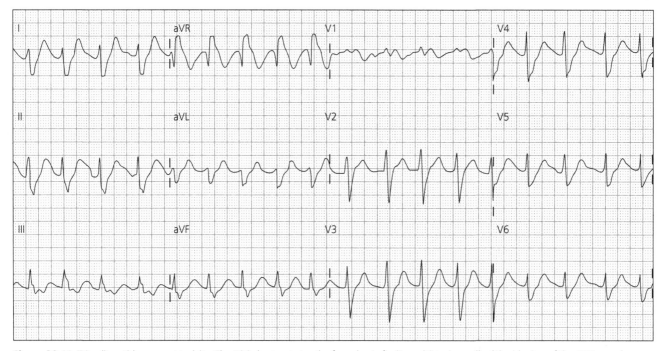

Figure 30.11 Tricyclic antidepressant toxicity. The ECG demonstrates the four classic findings: (1) tachycardia, (2) widening of the QRS complexes, (3) rightward axis, and (4) tall R wave in lead aVR. Reprinted from Hollowell H *et al.* Wide-complex tachycardia: beyond the traditional differential diagnosis of ventricular tachycardia vs supraventricular tachycardia with aberrant conduction. *Am J Emerg Med* 2005;**23**:876–89. Copyright 2005, with permission from Elsevier.

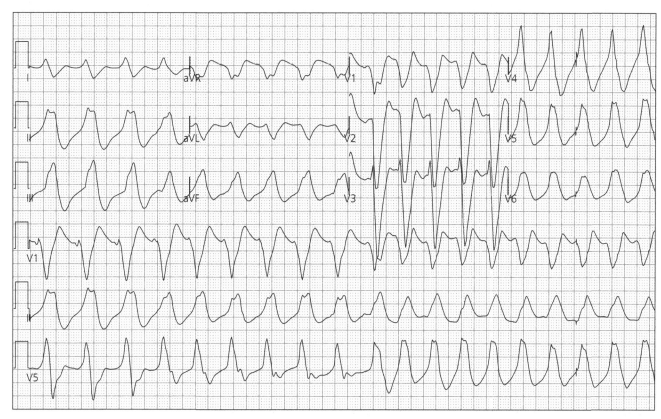

Figure 30.12 Hyperkalemia; ventricular rate, 120 bpm. Hyperkalemia often mimics VT by producing a WCT without obvious P waves. Note that the QRS duration is increased to > 200 ms, a finding that is uncommon in VT and strongly favors a metabolic abnormality or drug toxicity. This patient's serum potassium level was 9.2 mEq/L.

severe tricyclic antidepressant overdose have a characteristic electrocardiographic appearance: sinus tachycardia with QRS complex > 100 ms, right axis deviation, and tall R or R′ complexes in lead aVR (Figure 30.11) [17].

Severe hyperkalemia can also produce WCT. The electrocardiographic changes associated with hyperkalemia (serum potassium > 5.5 mEq/L) vary according to the serum potassium level. Initially, peaked T waves appear, followed by PR segment prolongation, loss of P waves, widening of the QRS complex, sine-wave formation, and then ventricular fibrillation and asystole [18]. With loss of P waves and widening of the QRS complex, a wide complex rhythm develops that, if tachycardic, can be easily mistaken for VT (Figure 30.12).

Patients who have been resuscitated from cardiac arrest often demonstrate arrhythmias, including WCTs, narrow complex tachycardias, and bradycardias. Wide complex tachycardia may occur secondary to acute bundle branch dysfunction resulting from the cardiac arrest and the administration of electrical shocks. The administration of epinephrine during the resuscitation can also induce ischemia, which can produce any of these arrhythmias. Arrhythmias that are truly caused by the resuscitation process itself, rather than ongoing ischemia and electrolyte abnormalities, usually resolve within 15–30 min after the return of spontaneous circulation [19,20].

Accelerated idioventricular rhythm (AIVR) is another cause of WCT that may be mistaken for VT (Figure 30.13). Accelerated idioventricular rhythm typically occurs in the setting of an acute myocardial infarction (MI) and is considered a marker of reperfusion; thus, it is often referred to as a "reperfusion arrhythmia." The rhythm resembles VT but has a rate < 100 bpm – note that some authors extend the rate range to < 120 bpm. The rhythm needs no acute treatment, as it is transient, usually lasting only minutes, and is not a hemodynamically destabilizing rhythm. Treatment with ventricular anti-arrhythmics (e.g. lidocaine, amiodarone, procainamide) will likely produce asystole. The patient's history plays a critical role in the correct diagnosis of these types of WCT.

One final mimicker of WCT is acute MI with massive ST segment elevation. In this setting, the QRS complexes are actually narrow, but if the ST segments are markedly elevated, they can fuse with the R wave and produce an appearance of QRS widening.

Electrocardiographic diagnosis

Numerous strategies and electrocardiographic criteria have been delineated for the identification of WCT in the

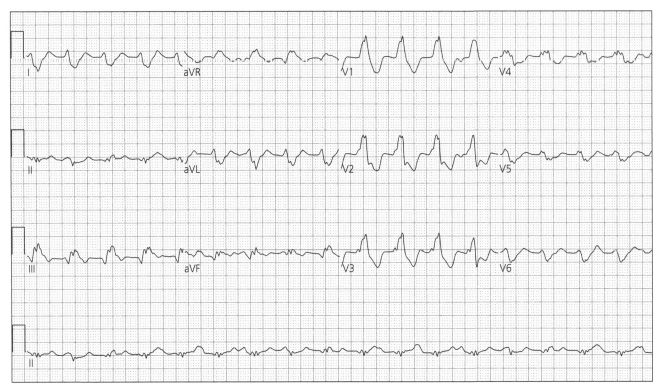

Figure 30.13 Accelerated idioventricular rhythm; ventricular rate, 105 bpm. This rhythm could easily be mistaken for VT, but the rate is too slow. The diagnosis of VT should generally be withheld when the ventricular rate is < 120 bpm.

emergent setting. They have focused on distinguishing between VT and SVT with BBB. The American Heart Association (AHA), in its Guidelines for Emergency Cardiovascular Care, recommends that the first step in the evaluation of a patient with WCT is to decide if the patient is stable or unstable. If the patient has signs of hemodynamic instability (hypotension, ischemic chest pain, acute heart failure, decreased mental status), immediate synchronized cardioversion is recommended. If the patient is hemodynamically stable, 12-lead ECG is used to distinguish between VT and SVT with BBB [21].

Attempts to establish electrocardiographic criteria that allow a definitive distinction between VT and SVT with BBB have been unsuccessful. In 1978, for example, Wellens proposed a set of criteria focused on the QRS complex morphology, but the positive predictive value for diagnosing VT was only 80% at best [22,23]. Perhaps the most well-known set of criteria was proposed in 1991 by Brugada and colleagues, who proposed a four-step algorithm for the diagnosis of VT [24]. This approach was intended as a simplified approach to ECG interpretation. The algorithm required physicians to evaluate the ECG for: (1) absence of an RS complex in all precordial leads, (2) an RS interval > 100 ms in any one precordial lead, (3) AV dissociation, and (4) various QRS morphologies in leads V1–V2 and V6. The presence of any one of the four criteria was considered diagnostic of VT,

whereas the absence of all four criteria ruled out VT in more than 98% of cases. Attempts to validate the Brugada algorithm have been disappointing. In 1996, Herbert and colleagues [25] studied interobserver agreement between emergency physicians in the use of the Brugada criteria. Twenty-seven regular WCT ECGs were given to three emergency physicians trained in the use of the criteria, and they were asked to decide whether the ECGs represented VT or SVT with aberrant conduction. The physicians disagreed on 22% of the ECGs. More recently, Isenhour and colleagues [1] studied interobserver agreement as well as accuracy in evaluating 157 regular WCT ECGs. The final diagnosis of the ECGs was confirmed electrophysiologically. Two emergency physicians and two cardiologists were asked to use the Brugada algorithm to analyze the ECGs. The sensitivities of the two emergency physicians in detecting VT were 83% and 79%, respectively, with an interobserver agreement of 82%. The cardiologists fared only slightly better, achieving sensitivities of 85% and 91%, respectively, with interobserver agreement of 81%. In other words, these four physicians using the Brugada algorithm misdiagnosed VT as SVT with aberrant conduction in 9–21% of cases.

The important takeaway point is that, although there are many criteria that help to rule in VT, there are no reliable criteria that definitively rule out VT (and rule in SVT with BBB), with the possible exception of the demonstration of

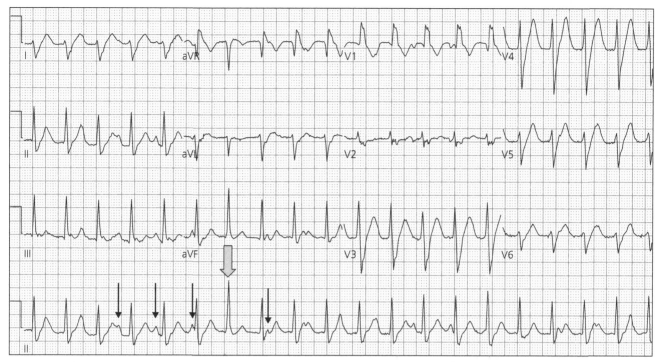

Figure 30.14 Ventricular tachycardia; rate, 125 bpm. Thin arrows demonstrate atrial activity, indicating the presence of AV dissociation. Wide arrow points out a premature narrow QRS complex, a capture beat. The patient is using amiodarone chronically, which will markedly slow the ventricular rate in VT.

identical QRS morphology on a baseline ECG (when one can be obtained) as when the patient has sinus rhythm (see Case 1). Misdiagnosis of VT as SVT with aberrant conduction and corresponding treatment for SVT with calcium channel-blockers or beta-blockers can be deadly; therefore, the safest approach is to assume and treat the WCT as VT. Nevertheless, readers should be aware of some of the electrocardiographic clues that *suggest* specific types of WCT. These are discussed below.

Rate: It was previously thought that a rate > 170 bpm favored SVT [26]. However, it is now accepted that there is too much overlap in the rates associated with SVT and VT to use this parameter to differentiate them.

Regularity: The regularity of the rhythm must be noted. A regular or only *slightly* irregular rhythm suggests VT or SVT with aberration. On the other hand, an obviously irregular WCT likely represents atrial fibrillation with aberrancy (e.g. BBB), atrial fibrillation with pre-excitation, or polymorphic VT [10]. An irregular tachycardia with wide QRS complexes and a rate > 220 bpm is most likely atrial fibrillation with pre-excitation or polymorphic VT [26].

AV dissociation: AV dissociation is virtually pathognomonic of VT (Figure 30.14) [22,23,26]. Unfortunately, it is often difficult to see this on a single-lead rhythm strip and even on a 12-lead ECG, it is present in only 25% of cases

[23]. Atrioventricular dissociation is best seen on lead V1 or II, but it may be seen in any lead. It is very rare for AV dissociation to be found in the presence of SVT [27]. Ventricular tachycardia may demonstrate retrograde P waves with 1 : 1 conduction (Figure 30.15) in up to 50% of cases. These retrograde P waves may be mistaken for AV dissociation [28]. Of greater concern, they may be mistaken for sinus P waves, resulting in a misdiagnosis of sinus tachycardia with BBB.

Capture and fusion beats: Capture and fusion beats may be seen in the presence of AV dissociation and may suggest VT (Figure 30.14). Capture beats arise when the P wave activates the entire ventricle before the VT cycle, resulting in a narrow premature beat. A fusion beat is a QRS complex that has two sources of activation – from a P wave that has activated part of the ventricle over the recovered AV node and from the next VT complex – resulting in a complex of intermediate width. Fusion complexes may occur during SVT with aberrancy, but they are very rare [29]. The occurrence of these complexes requires that there is not a 1 : 1 AV relationship during VT and that there is a relatively slow VT rate, giving the atrial complexes the chance to conduct [29]. Although these complexes help with diagnosis, they are rare, occurring in fewer than 10% of patients with VT [30].

Characteristics of the QRS complex: Various features of the QRS complex can suggest a diagnosis of VT though none of these findings is pathognomonic for the diagnosis.

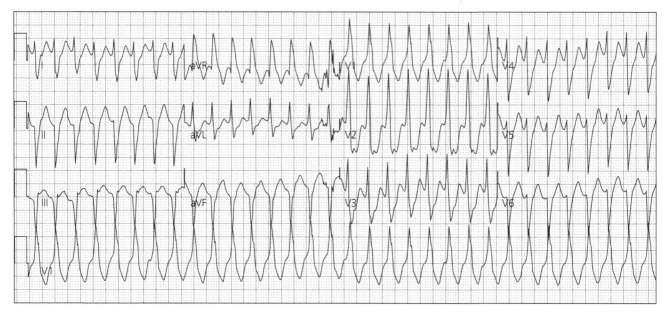

Figure 30.15 Ventricular tachycardia; rate, 190 bpm. Retrograde P waves are found following the QRS complexes, especially in leads V2 and III. A right bundle branch pattern is noted, with the typical features of VT: monophasic R wave in lead V1 and rS (R : S < 1) pattern in lead V6. Extreme right axis deviation is also noted, a finding that almost always proves the WCT is VT.

Width of QRS complex: It had been held that SVT has QRS complexes < 0.14 s, whereas VT produced complexes of much greater duration [26]. In reality, 20% of patients with VT have an interval < 0.14 s [31]. Ventricular tachycardia with relatively shorter QRS width has also been described in association with digitalis toxicity and in young children [23,24,32]. On the other hand, a QRS complex > 0.16 s may be seen in SVT or sinus tachycardia with aberrancy in association with hyperkalemia (Figure 30.12), tricyclic antidepressant overdose (Figure 30.11), anti-dysrhythmic agents, and WPW syndrome [29,31]. Some authors have suggested combining the QRS duration with bundle branch morphology to improve the distinction: a QRS duration > 0.14 s with right bundle branch pattern or a QRS duration > 0.16 s with left bundle branch pattern more strongly suggests VT [24,25].

QRS axis in frontal plane: In normal sinus rhythm, the normal QRS complex axis ranges from −30 degrees to +90 degrees, with an average of 60 degrees. In VT, the axis often changes to either a right or a left deviation, depending on the ventricular origin. Left-axis deviation (Figure 30.14) slightly favors VT over SVT, though right axis deviation (Figure 30.16) and extreme right axis deviation (Figure 17) strongly favor VT over SVT [23,30].

QRS morphologies in leads V1 and V6: Various QRS complex morphologies relate to BBB patterns, which help to sort out the diagnosis of WCT. Leads V1 and V6 are the most helpful in distinguishing these patterns. With a right BBB pattern, the presence of a qR or monophasic R complex in V1 and an rS (R : S ratio < 1) or QS complex in V6 strongly

favors VT (Figure 30.15) [10,24]. The rsR′ triphasic pattern in V1 (taller "right rabbit ear") (Figure 30.1) favors SVT with right BBB, whereas an Rsr′ pattern (taller "left rabbit ear") favors VT (Figure 30.17) [10,12].

When a left BBB pattern is present, if V1 shows an initial R wave > 30 ms and slurring or notching of the S wave > 70 ms (Figure 30.18), VT is more likely [33]. On the other hand, SVT with aberrant conduction is more likely when V1 shows a small R wave with a steep, downsloping S wave. V6 is not as helpful in distinguishing VT and SVT with the left BBB pattern, but when it shows a qR pattern, VT is very likely [12].

The most widely promoted morphology criteria that define SVT with aberrant conduction were proposed by Griffith and colleagues [34], with the default being VT if these criteria are *not* met. If a left BBB pattern is present (lead V1 is primarily negative), an SVT should have an rS or QS pattern in lead V1, a delay to S wave nadir of < 70 ms, and R waves without Q waves (monophasic R waves) in V6. If a right BBB pattern is present (lead V1 is primarily positive), an SVT should demonstrate rSR′ complexes in V1 and Rs or qRs complexes in V6 (R wave height greater than S wave depth) [34]. The sensitivity and specificity for SVT have been reported as 90–91% and 67–85%, respectively [34]. Therefore, these criteria still do not completely exclude the diagnosis of VT.

Concordance: Concordance refers to the polarity of the precordial leads. When they are all positive or negative, a diagnosis of VT is supported. Positive concordance is associated with the VT originating in the posterior ventricular wall [35]. Negative concordance correlates with an anterior wall or apical origin for VT [12,30].

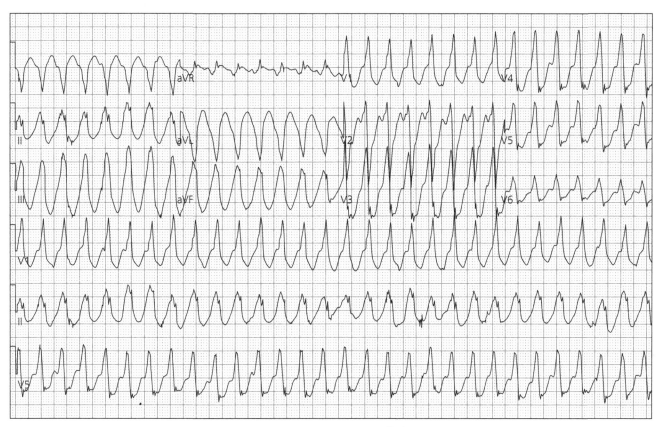

Figure 30.16 Ventricular tachycardia; rate, 180 bpm. Right axis deviation is present, a finding that strongly favors VT.

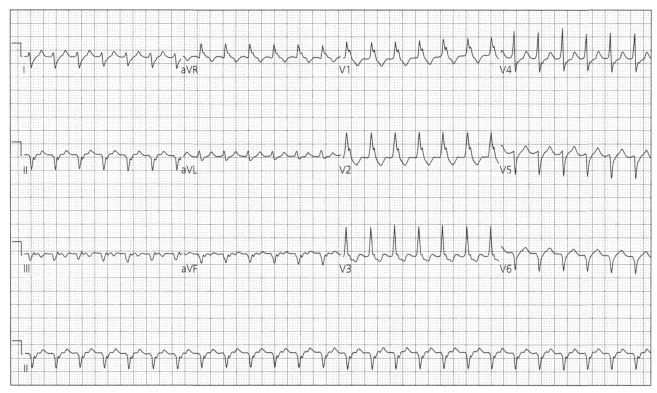

Figure 30.17 Ventricular tachycardia; rate, 160 bpm. Extreme right axis deviation is present, a finding that almost always proves the WCT is VT.

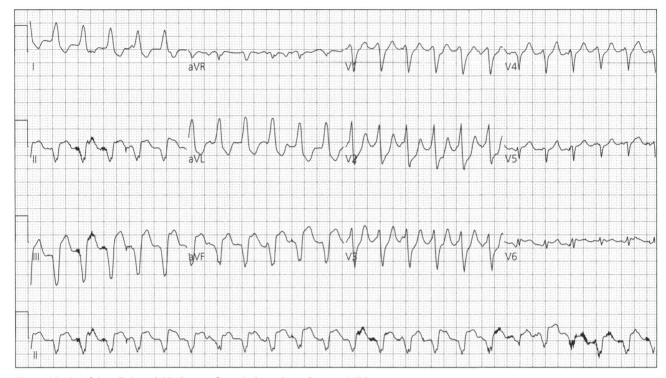

Figure 30.18 Left bundle branch block type of ventricular tachycardia; rate, 145 bpm.

Tachycardia QRS narrower than sinus QRS: The finding of a narrower QRS duration during tachycardia than during sinus rhythm on an old ECG suggests VT. This may occur when the VT origin is close to the intraventricular septum, resulting in faster activation of the ventricles and thus a more narrow appearance of the QRS complexes [12].

Presence of QR complexes: QR complexes are seen in approximately 40% of patients with VT after myocardial infarction [36]. This finding in association with WCT indicates scar in the myocardium.

Value of the Prior ECG: Acquisition of a baseline ECG is very helpful for correct interpretation of WCT. Changes in axis and QRS morphology, the presence of an old myocardial infarction, and evidence of preexisting ventricular pre-excitation or BBB are all very important in deciphering WCT in the emergent setting. Case 1 (Figures 30.1 and 30.2) demonstrates the value of baseline ECGs. If the baseline ECG had been available during initial management, it would have been apparent that the patient had a pre-existing right BBB with QRS complexes having identical morphology to the QRS complexes during WCT, as seen in Figure 30.1. This information would have likely led to early administration of adenosine. Similarly for Case 2, if a baseline ECG demonstrating a pre-existing WPW pattern had been available, the physician would likely have considered the diagnosis of atrial fibrillation with WPW syndrome earlier and avoided the cardiac arrest resulting from ventricular fibrillation.

Management of the patient with wide complex tachycardia

The first step in evaluating patients with WCT is determining the hemodynamic status: unstable or stable.

Hemodynamically unstable: If the patient is hemodynamically unstable, as defined by hypotension, ischemic chest pain, acute heart failure, or decreased mental status, then immediate synchronized cardioversion (if the patient has pulses) or defibrillation (if palpable pulses are lacking) should be strongly considered [21].

Hemodynamically stable: If the patient is hemodynamically stable, the next step is to obtain a 12-lead ECG and determine whether the rhythm is regular or irregular.

Regular: For regular WCT thought to be SVT, vagal maneuvers or adenosine is recommended. However, adenosine should not be used as a *diagnostic* maneuver because it can convert VT to sinus rhythm [37–39], which may mislead the unwary healthcare provider to assume that the arrhythmia was SVT. If VT is diagnosed, anti-arrhythmics may be considered. Based on current recommendations [40], the most appropriate treatment is intravenous procainamide. Intravenous amiodarone may be used if the rhythm is refractory to procainamide or electrical cardioversion. Intravenous lidocaine may still play a role in management, especially if the rhythm is thought to be secondary to myocardial ischemia [40]; however, no large randomized, controlled studies have been done to support its efficacy [41]. Regardless of the medication chosen, the physician should be prepared to electrically cardiovert the patient if signs of instability develop.

Irregular: When PVT is present and persistent, hemodynamic instability usually results. In the rare occasion when the patient is stable or if the arrhythmia is intermittent, intravenous beta-blockers, amiodarone, procainamide, or lidocaine may be used for treatment. If torsade de pointes is suspected based on a "twisting" QRS morphology or a pre-existent prolonged QT interval, electrical cardioversion is usually required. Patients with these signs are almost always hemodynamically unstable. If the arrhythmia is intermittent and the patient is hemodynamically stable, intravenous magnesium sulfate is indicated. Overdrive pacing and isoproterenol are also reasonable choices [40]. Following electrical or chemical cardioversion for PVT or torsade de pointes, management should focus on identifying and correcting the underlying cause (e.g. myocardial ischemia, electrolyte abnormalities, drug toxicities).

If the irregular WCT is suspected to be atrial fibrillation with WPW syndrome, AV nodal blocking agents such as adenosine, beta-blockers, calcium channel-blockers, and digoxin should be avoided [42]. These medications have been associated with accelerated conduction through the accessory pathway and rapid degeneration to ventricular fibrillation. Amiodarone should also be listed among the AV nodal-blockers to be avoided in the setting of rapid atrial fibrillation with WPW syndrome, because it has both beta-blocking and calcium channel-blocking effects [43]. When unstable, patients with atrial fibrillation and WPW syndrome are best treated with electrical cardioversion. For those who are stable, the first recommendation is also cardioversion, followed by IV flecainide, and, with less evidence to support them, intravenous procainamide or ibutilide [44].

Patients with irregular WCTs suspected to be atrial fibrillation with aberrant conduction (e.g. BBB) can be treated as patients with normal conduction atrial fibrillation are treated. Calcium channel-blockers, beta-blockers, digoxin, and amiodarone are all reasonable options in the stable patient.

Case conclusions

Cases 1 and 2 demonstrate the importance of using a baseline ECG, when available, to guide management of WCT. In Case 1, the patient, although elderly, was hemodynamically stable. Her ECG was appropriately assumed to indicate VT. The administration of amiodarone was effective, but adenosine could have been a reasonable first choice if the physician had the baseline ECG, showing BBB, for comparison. Case 2 nearly resulted in a disastrous outcome because of the administration of an AV nodal-blocking agent to a patient with atrial fibrillation and WPW syndrome. Consideration of the patient's age and differential diagnosis of the causes of irregular WCTs should have prompted a different approach to management. This case would have been more safely managed with electrical cardioversion, flecainide or procainamide.

Acknowledgment

The authors acknowledge the tremendous copyediting assistance provided by Linda J. Kesselring, MS, ELS.

References

1 Isenhour J, Craig S, Gibbs M, *et al.* Wide-complex tachycardia: continued evaluation of diagnostic criteria. *Acad Emerg Med* 2000; **7**(7):769–73.

2 Wrenn K. Management strategies in wide QRS complex tachycardia. *Am J Emerg Med* 1991;**9**(6):592–7.

3 Cummins R, editor. *ACLS Provider Manual.* Dallas, Texas: American Heart Association, 2004.

4 Morady F, Baerman JM, Dicarlo La Jr, *et al.* A prevalent misconception regarding tachycardia. *J Am Med Soc* 1985;**254**: 2790–2.

5 Goldman MJ. Definitions of electrocardiographic configurations. In: Goldman MJ, editor. *Principles of Clinical Electrocardiography.* Los Altos: Lange, 1973.

6 Brady W, Meldon S, DeBehnke D. Comparison of prehospital monomorphic and polymorphic ventricular tachycardia: prevalence, response to therapy, and outcome. *Ann Emerg Med* 1995; **25**:64–70.

7 Brady WJ, DeBehnke DJ, Laundrie D. Prevalence, therapeutic response, and outcome of ventricular tachycardia in the out-of-hospital setting: a comparison of monomorphic ventricular tachycardia, polymorphic ventricular tachycardia, and torsade de pointes. *Acad Emerg Med* 1999;**6**:609–17.

8 Clayton R, Murray R. Objective features of the surface electrocardiogram during ventricular tachyarrhythmias. *Eur Heart J* 1995;**16**:1115–9.

9 Dhurandhar RW, MacMillan RL, Brown DW. Primary ventricular fibrillation complicating acute myocardial infarction. *Am J Cardiol* 1990;**66**:1208–11.

10 Gupta A, Thakur RK. Wide QRS complex tachycardias. *Med Clin North Am* 2001;**85**(2):245–66.

11 Ray I. Wide complex tachycardia: recognition and management in the emergency room. *J Assoc Phys India* 2004;**52**:882–7.

12 Wellens H. Ventricular tachycardia: diagnosis of broad QRS complex tachycardia. *Heart* 2001;**86**:579–85.

13 Jackman W, Friday K, Anderson J, *et al.* The Long QT syndromes: a critical review, new clinical observations and a unifying hypothesis. *Prog Cardiovasc Dis* 1988;**31**:115–72.

14 Akhtar M. Electrophysiological bases for wide QRS complex tachycardia. *Pacing Clin Electrophysiol* 1983;**6**:81–98.

15 Atiga W, Calkins H. Catheter ablation of supraventricular tachycardia. In: Ganz L, editor. *Management of Cardiac Arrhythmias.* Totowa, New Jersey: Humana Press; 2002:56–9.

16 Hollowell H, Mattu A, Perron A, *et al.* Wide-complex tachycardia: beyond the traditional differential diagnosis of ventricular tachycardia vs supraventricular tachycardia with aberrant conduction. *Am J Emerg Med* 2005;**23**:876–89.

17 Singh N, Singh HK, Khan IA. Serial electrocardiographic changes as a predictor of cardiovascular toxicity in acute tricyclic antidepressant overdose. *Am J Therapeutics* 2002;**9**(1):75–9.

18 Gennari F. Disorders of potassium homeostasis: hypokalemia and hyperkalemia. *Crit Care Clin* 2002;**18**:273–88.

19 Persse DE, Zachariah BS, Wigginton JG. Managing the post-resuscitation patient in the field. *Prehosp Emerg Care* 2002;**6**(1): 114–22.

20 Schoenenberger RA, von Planta M, von Planta I. Survival after failed out-of-hospital resuscitation. *Arch Intern Med* 1994;**154**: 2433–7.

21 Part 7.3: Management of Symptomatic Bradycardia and Tachycardia. *2005 American Heart Association Guidelines for Cardiopulmonary Resuscitation and Emergency Cardiovascular Care* 2005;**112**(suppl IV): IV-67–IV-77.

22 Steinman RT, Herrara C., Schluger CD, *et al.* Wide QRS tachycardia in the conscious adult: ventricular tachycardia is the most frequent cause. *JAMA* 1989;**261**:1013–6.

23 Akhtar M, Shenasa M, Jazayeri M, *et al.* Wide QRS complex tachycardia: reappraisal of a common clinical problem. *Ann Intern Med* 1988;**109**:905–12.

24 Brugada P, Brugada J, Mont L, *et al.* A new approach to the differential diagnosis of a regular tachycardia with a wide QRS complex. *Circulation* 1991;**83**(5):1649–59.

25 Herbert ME, Votey SR, Morgan MT, et al. Failure to agree on the electrocardiographic diagnosis of ventricular tachycardia. *Ann Emerg Med* 1996;**27**:35–8.

26 Wellens H., Bar FW, Lie KI. The value of the electrocardiogram in the differential diagnosis of a tachycardia with widened QRS complex. *Am J Med* 1978;**64**:27–32.

27 Littman L, McCall MM. Ventricular tachycardia may masquerade as supraventricular tachycardia in patients with pre-existing bundle-branch block. *Ann Emerg Med* 1995;**26**:98–101.

28 Lobban JH, Schmidt SB, Rhodes LA, *et al.* Differential diagnosis of wide QRS tachycardias. *WV Med J* 1994;**90**:232–4.

29 Miller J, Mithilesh KD, Yadav AV, *et al.* Value of the 12-lead ECG in wide QRS tachycardia. *Cardiol Clin* 2006;**24**:439–51.

30 Hudson K, Brady WJ, Chan TC, *et al.* Electrocardiographic manifestations: ventricular tachycardia. *J Emerg Med* 2003;**25**(3): 303–14.

31 Brady W, Skiles J. Wide QRS complex tachycardia: ECG differential diagnosis. *Am J Emerg Med* 1999;**17**(4):376–81.

32 Meldon SW, Brady WJ, Berger S, Mannenbach M. Pediatric ventricular tachycardia: a review with three illustrative cases. *Pediatr Emerg Care* 1994;**10**:294–300.

33 Kindwall E, Brown J, Josephson ME. Electrocardiographic criteria for ventricular tachycardia in wide complex left bundle branch block morphology tachycardias. *Am J Cardiol* 1988;**61**:1279–83.

34 Griffith MJ, Garratt CJ, Mounsey P, Camm AJ. Ventricular tachycardia as default diagnosis in broad complex tachycardia. *Lancet* 1994;**343**:386–8.

35 Wellens HJJ, Brugada P. Diagnosis of ventricular tachycardia from the 12-lead electrocardiogram. *Cardiol Clin* 1987;**5**:511–25.

36 Wellens H. The electrocardiographic diagnosis of arrhythmias. In: Topol E editor. *Textbook of Cardiovascular Medicine*. Philadelphia: Lippincott, Raven, 1998:1591–609.

37 Hina K, Kusachi S, Takaishi A, *et al.* Effects of adenosine triphosphate on wide QRS tachycardia: analysis in 18 patients. *Jpn Heart J* 1996;**37**:463–70.

38 Lenk M, Celiker A, Alehan D, *et al.* Role of adenosine in the diagnosis and treatment of tachyarrhythmias in pediatric patients. *Acta Paediatr Jpn* 1997;**39**:570–7.

39 Lerman BB, Stein KM, Markowitz SM, *et al.* Ventricular arrhythmias in normal hearts. *Cardiol Clin* 2000;**18**:265–91.

40 Zipes DP, Camm AJ, Borggrefe M, *et al.* ACC/AHA/ESC 2006 Guidelines for management of patients with ventricular arrhythmias and the prevention of sudden cardiac death–executive summary. A report of the American College of Cardiology/American Heart Association Task Force and the European Society of Cardiology Committee for Practice Guidelines. *Circulation* 2006;**114**:1088–132.

41 Nasir N Jr, Taylor A, Doyle TK, Pacifico A. Evaluation of intravenous lidocaine for the termination of sustained monomorphic ventricular tachycardia in patients with coronary artery disease with or without healed myocardial infarction. *Am J Cardiol* 1994; **74**:1183–6.

42 Mattu A. *Myths and pitfalls in Advanced Cardiac Life Support*. www.eMedHome.com CME article: http://www.emedhome.com/features_archive-detail.cfm?FID=67, October 22, 2001. Accessed on February 18, 2008.

43 Tijunelis MA, Herbert ME. Myth: intravenous amiodarone is safe in patients with atrial fibrillation and Wolff-Parkinson-White syndrome in the emergency department. *CJEM* 2005;**7**:262–5.

44 Fuster V, Ryden L, Cannon DS, *et al.* ACC/AHA/ESC 2006 Guidelines for the management of patients with atrial fibrillation–Executive Summary. A report of the American College of Cardiology/American Heart Association Task Force on Practice Guidelines and the European Society of Cardiology Committee for Practice Guidelines. *Circulation* 2006;**114**(7):700–45.

Chapter 31 | Can the ECG guide management in the patient with bradydysrhythmias?

Joseph Shiber
Florida Hospital Emergency Medicine Residency, Orlando, FL, USA

Case presentation

A 56-year-old woman presents to the emergency department (ED) complaining of "feeling weak and dizzy" for the last 3 days. Her symptoms are worse when exerting herself. She denies chest pain but reports shortness of breath during these episodes; she denies syncope but reports severe lightheadedness. Her past medical history includes hypertension and diabetes mellitus.

Her vital signs are as follows: temperature 36.4 °C, pulse 40 beats per minute (bpm), blood pressure 95/50 mmHg, respiratory rate 22 breaths per minute, and oxygen saturation 95% on room air. She is pale, with cool, dry skin. She is awake and alert, and answers appropriately. No jugular venous distension is noted. Her lung fields are clear; her cardiac examination reveals a slow rate but regular rhythm. Her laboratory studies, including initial cardiac biomarkers, are unremarkable and her chest radiograph has no acute abnormalities. Her ECG shows sinus bradycardia but no ST segment elevation or depression (Figure 31.1).

The ECG and management of bradydysrhythmias

What is the differential diagnosis in this case? What are the indicated treatments in the ED? What is the appropriate disposition? These questions will be the focus of this chapter.

The normal resting heart rate parameters of 60–100 bpm were simply based on the convenience of ECG intervals of five 200-ms and three 200-ms intervals, respectively, on a standard ECG tracing [1,2]. There has not been any population sampling or study to support these limits, but there is evidence that more accurate guidelines are 50–90 bpm [1,3]. Adopting these new parameters will increase the sensitivity of recognizing tachycardia, as a resting heart rate of 95 is not normal physiology; it will also increase the specificity

for recognizing bradycardia, as a resting heart rate of 55 can certainly be normal in large segments of the population with even slower rates common while sleeping [1,3].

Under normal conditions, the primary cardiac pacemaker is the sinoatrial (SA) node located in the right atrium near the junction with the superior vena cava. Its blood supply is the SA nodal artery, a branch of the right coronary artery (RCA) in 55% of the population, a branch of the left circumflex artery (LCX) in 35%, and a dual supply from both arteries in 10% [2,4,5]. The impulse spreads through poorly defined interatrial pathways to the atrioventricular (AV) node located in the posterior-medial portion of the right atrium anterior to the coronary sinus and adjacent to the tricuspid annulus. It is supplied by the AV nodal artery, a branch of the RCA in 90% and a branch of the LCX in 10% [2,4,5]. The AV node connects to the His bundle, which enters the heart's fibrous skeleton and travels along the interventricular septum before branching into the bundle branches; the His bundle is supplied by the AV nodal artery and branches of the left anterior descending (LAD) artery. The right bundle branch is supplied by the AV nodal artery and branches of the LAD, while the left bundle branch splits into the anterior and posterior fascicles. The anterior fascicle is supplied by branches of the LAD, while the posterior fascicle receives dual supply from the LAD and the posterior descending artery [2,4,5].

Pathophysiology and electrocardiographic presentation

Depolarization of the SA node is not represented on a surface ECG recording but if the P wave, representing atrial depolarization, has a normal axis (upright P wave in limb leads I, II, III, and aVF and inverted in lead aVR), then it is inferred that the impulse originated in the sinus node [5,6]. When the impulse reaches the AV node, there is a designated delay, represented on the ECG as the PR interval. This delay allows for atrial contraction to contribute to ventricular filling (loss of atrial systole can reduce cardiac output by 20%) and limits too rapid transmission of impulses to the ventricles as in

Critical Decisions in Emergency and Acute Care Electrocardiography,
1st edition. Edited by W.J. Brady and J.D. Truwit. © 2009 Blackwell Publishing, ISBN: 9781405159067

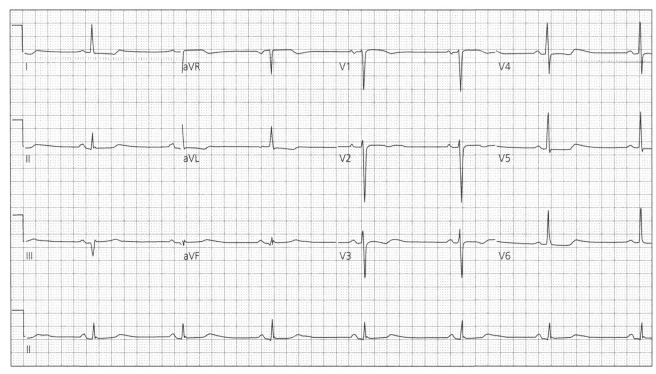

Figure 31.1 Sinus bradycardia with slight lateral ST depression in a middle-aged woman possibly an ischemic coronary syndrome; the QT is prolonged but when corrected for rate is acceptable. Sinus bradycardia in a middle-aged, non-athletic woman is not normal, but only requires immediate treatment if it is symptomatic.

supraventricular tachycardia or atrial fibrillation [3,5,7,8]. The impulse then travels through the common His bundle and into the right and left branches to depolarize the ventricular myocardium, represented by the QRS complex.

Bradycardia can result from decreased automaticity at the SA node or from conduction block at the SA or AV node. Bradycardia can also be separated into primary, or intrinsic etiologies versus secondary, or extrinsic etiologies (Table 31.1) [2,5,9,10]. Primary causes of bradycardia are less common in acute care patients, occur more often in elderly patients, and are less likely to respond to medical therapy with a permanent pacemaker as the definitive. Secondary causes are more common in the acute care arena and are more likely to be reversible with medical therapy [2,4].

Slowing of the sinus rate may be an appropriate physiologic response when the body is well conditioned or is at rest; it is considered to be clinically significant if the patient is symptomatic from hypoperfusion of vital organs (brain and heart) or if the heart rate fails to rise with activity [2,5]. Sinus node slowing may result from increased parasympathetic activity via the Vagus nerve and can be physiologic or pathologic, or it may result from pathologic sinus node failure [5]. A bradycardic rhythm may originate in the sinus node (sinus bradycardia, see Figure 31.1), in the atria (ectopic atrial rhythm or bradycardia, see Figure 31.2), in the AV node or His bundle (junctional rhythm), or from the ventricles (ventricular or idioventricular rhythm). These represent escape rhythms except sinus bradycardia, and are suppressed by the sinus node under normal conditions, only becoming the dominant pacemaker if the sinus node fails to conduct or if automaticity is increased in these other sites [5,6].

The conduction system is richly innervated by the autonomic nervous system. At rest, parasympathetic tone predominates at the SA node, while the sympathetic and parasympathetic

Table 31.1 Primary versus secondary causes of bradycardia

Primary/intrinsic	Secondary/extrinsic
Idiopathic-degenerative (Lenegre's)	Vagal tone
Cardiomyopathy	Medications
Myocarditis	Acute myocardial infarction (AMI)
Infiltrative diseases	Metabolic (hyperkalemia, acidosis)
Collagen-vascular diseases	Hypothyroidism, hypothermia
Hypertensive-heart disease	Infection (endocarditis, Lyme, Chagas)
Cardiac trauma/surgery	Sepsis

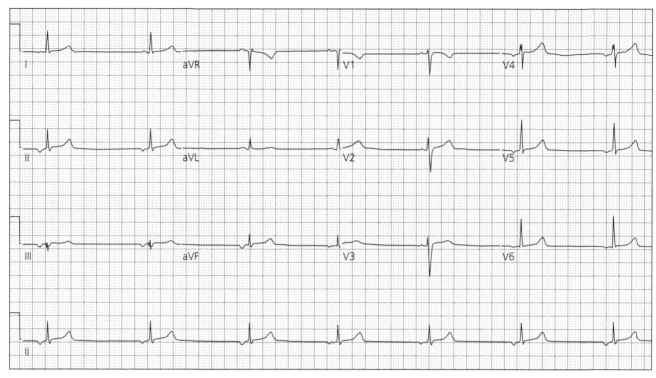

Figure 31.2 Ectopic atrial bradycardia in a young healthy man known to have a slow resting heart rate. Ectopic atrial bradycardia can occur in young healthy individuals with a high level of fitness, as this case likely illustrates, due to adaptive responses with a high level of vagal tone at the SA node allowing an atrial escape site to become the pacemaker site. There will be no symptoms and no therapy is indicated. This rhythm can possibly be abnormal if there are symptoms present, and may represent SA disease (sick sinus syndrome or myocarditis).

Table 31.2 Common vagal causes of bradycardia in the ED

Painful stimuli
Vomiting
Endotracheal intubation
Airway suctioning
Naso-gastric tube placement
Nasal packing
Increased intracranial pressure
Malignant hypertension

are balanced at the AV node [2]. Decreased automaticity of the sinus node can result from increased parasympathetic activity caused by neurologic reflexes, valsalva maneuvers, carotid sinus hypersensitivity, increased intracranial pressure, cervical spine injury with resultant loss of sympathetic tone, venous pooling, drugs that cause CNS depression and decrease sympathetic outflow (opiates, sedative-hypnotics, A2-agonists) and other causes (Table 31.2) [4,5]. Sinus bradycardia has also been reported to be associated with symptomatic hypoglycemia and the eating disorders anorexia and bulimia [10,11]. Acute intracranial pathology (subarachnoid hemorrhage, cerebrovascular accident, intracranial hemorrhage, meningitis, tumors, head trauma) is commonly complicated by bradydysrhythmias including sinus bradycardia, second- and third-degree AV block, and wandering atrial pacemaker [12].

Sinoatrial block occurs when an impulse is created but fails to emerge from the sinus node; a resultant atrial depolarization does not occur, thus no P wave is seen on the surface ECG. Sinoatrial block has the same four types as does AV block (first-, second- type 1, second- type 2, and third-degree), but only second-degree type 1 can be identified on ECG by a PP interval that is a multiple of preceding intervals [2,5,6]. If this mathematical pattern is not present, then a brief (2–3 s) period without P waves or QRS complexes cannot be determined to be from abnormal automaticity (i.e. sinus pause or arrest) versus abnormal conduction (i.e. SA block). Pauses less than 3 s in duration are common and typically not symptomatic; when such pauses are greater than 3 s and the patient is awake, this pause duration indicates sinus node pathology [2]. An early description of this syndrome, known as Stokes-Adams attacks was reported in 1909 in a patient with a slow pulse who had repeated syncope, and periods of asystole were present on a Mackenzie Polygraph (an early ECG) at the time of symptoms [13].

Sick sinus syndrome, also known in the United Kingdom by the more descriptive term "lazy sinus syndrome," has features of both abnormal automaticity and conduction (Figure 31.3) [13]. The clinical features of this syndrome include persistent bradycardia at rest without an appropriate response to sympathetic activity, absence of an escape rhythm when the sinus node slows or arrests, and SA suppression by atrial tachycardias (Table 31.3) [4,5]. This last feature of

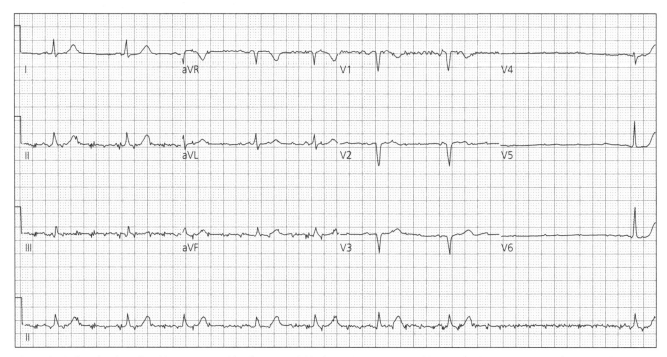

Figure 31.3 Sinus bradycardia with a 3 s pause either from SA exit block or a sinus pause possibly representing sinus node dysfunction/sick sinus syndrome in an elderly woman. Sinus bradycardia with a 3 s pause likely represents sick sinus syndrome in an elderly woman. The pause cannot be differentiated to be due to either SA exit block or sinus arrest, but the treatment doesn't differ; bridging medical therapy if the patient is acutely symptomatic while preparing for a temporary pacemaker followed by a permanent implanted pacer.

Table 31.3 Features of sick sinus syndrome

Persistent inappropriate bradycardia
Sinus pause/arrest or exit block with or without escape rhythms
AV node conduction abnormalities
Paroxysmal atrial tachycardias abruptly terminated by long pauses
(brady-tachy syndrome)

Table 31.4 Comparison of AV blocks

AV Nodal	Infra-nodal
PR prolongs prior to block	Sudden block w/o PR prolongation
Escape rate 40–60/min	Escape rate < 40/min
QRS < 120 ms	QRS > 120 ms
Stable hemodynamically	Often unstable hemodynamically
Responds to atropine	Poor response to atropine

atrial tachycardia (most commonly paroxysmal atrial tachycardia or atrial fibrillation) that abruptly terminates in a long pause resulting in syncope is known as the tachy-brady syndrome [2,4,5,7]. It has been proposed that it is not entirely accurate to blame the entire syndrome on the sinus node, as when the sinus rate is too slow or pauses a lower pacemaker site should take over as an escape rhythm. As this does not occur, it suggests that either heightened parasympathetic tone is affecting all of the pacemaker cells (not just the SA node) or there is an impairment of impulse formation in all pacemaker cells [5].

Atrioventricular block has the same etiologies as sinus bradycardia (Table 31.1). It is divided into four classifications: (1) first-degree, (2) second-degree type 1 (also known as Mobitz type 1 or Wenckebach, see Figure 31.4), (3) second-degree type 2 (see Figure 31.5), (4) third-degree (also known as complete heart block; see Figure 31.6) [2,4,5,6]. Conceptually, it may be helpful to rate the severity of the AV block as minor (first-degree: all impulses conducted but with a delay),

moderate (second-degree type 1 and 2: some impulses not conducted), or severe (third-degree: no impulses conducted) [5]. It may also be helpful to localize the level at which the block is occurring: the AV node, the common His bundle, or the right and left bundle branches. The second two levels – second-degree type 2 and third-degree – are referred to as *infra-nodal* block, with this distinction clinically significant (see Table 31.4) [4,5,6]. Infra-nodal block is less common than AV nodal block, but it has more associated morbidity and mortality due to the less reliable and slower escape rhythm of the ventricles. It typically occurs when a bundle branch block is already present and then an intermittent block occurs in the other bundle leading to non-conducted beats. If the block is continuous then a slow ventricular rate will be the only escape rhythm, but if no escape rhythm occurs, then asystole results [5].

First-degree AV block is defined as a PR interval greater than 210 ms, normal P wave morphology and axis, without

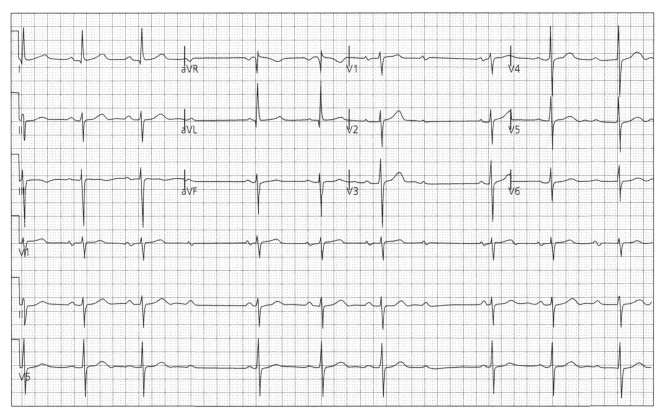

Figure 31.4 Second-degree type 1 AV block (Mobitz I, Wenckebach) in an elderly man. Second-degree type 1 AV block (Wenckebach) is an abnormal finding, but if not symptomatic requires only observation with cardiac monitoring to ensure that symptoms do no develop or that there is not progression of the AV block. If symptomatic, therapy is likely indicated.

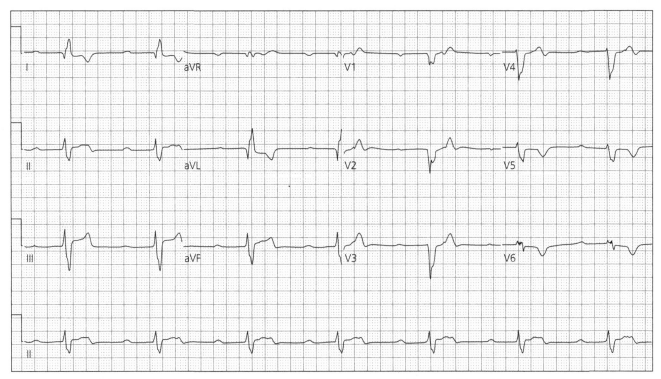

Figure 31.5 Second-degree AV block with 2 : 1 conduction in a middle-aged man. Second-degree AV block with 2 : 1 conduction should be managed as if type 2, and is particularly worrisome in this patient who reported acute lightheadedness and syncope.

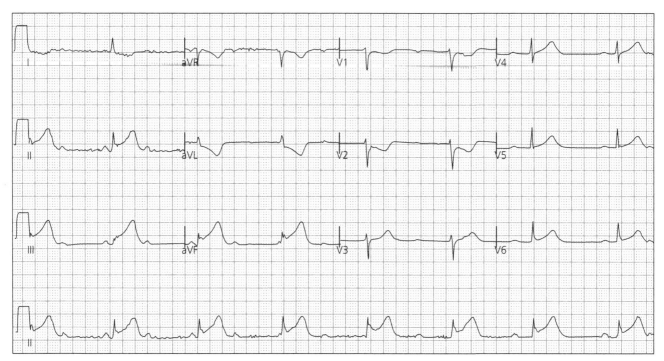

Figure 31.6 Third-degree block with a junctional escape during an inferior myocardial infarction. Third-degree (complete) heart block during an inferior ST segment elevation MI requires temporary transvenous pacer placement but atropine can be administered for acute symptomatic bradycardia while coronary reperfusion (via fibrinolysis versus percutaneous coronary intervention) is achieved; Of course, beta-blockers would be contraindicated.

any non-conducted atrial impulses; the delay almost always occurs at the AV node [2,4,6]. Second-degree type 1 AV block also typically occurs at the AV node. The pathognomonic feature is progressive lengthening of the PR interval prior to the non-conducted beat giving the ECG a pattern of grouped beats. Only the AV node can vary conduction time, while the His bundle and Purkinje cells cannot vary – conduction either occurs or it does not occur [5]. Second-degree type 2 AV block has no lengthening of the PR interval prior to the non-conducted atrial impulse; the intermittent block occurs at the His bundle or Purkinje system of the bundle branches [5,6]. When the ratio of atrial (P waves) to ventricular impulses (QRS complexes) is 2 : 1, there cannot be any determination of whether there is lengthening or not of the PR interval, therefore it should be assumed that it is second-degree type 2 block so that management is based on the worst of the two possibilities [4,5]. Third-degree AV block is due to continual infra-nodal block and will result in independent atrial and ventricular rates known as AV dissociation, but AV dissociation is not synonymous with complete heart block. If AV dissociation occurs due to third-degree heart block then the atrial rate must be faster than the ventricular rate with no AV capture [6]. If the atrial rate is slower than the ventricular rate then there may certainly be AV dissociation (Figure 31.7) but not complete AV block, as the ventricles may have become the dominant pacemaker site by increased automaticity. This usurpation of pacemaker status leads to refractoriness of the AV node that may block some of

the atrial impulses but not necessarily all, so that AV capture may still occur; ventricular tachycardia is an example of this phenomenon [5,6].

Premature atrial contractions should not be conducted if occurring early during the absolute refractory period of the AV node, therefore this is not considered to be AV block [5]. Likewise, if the atrial rate is very rapid (350–600 bpm) as with atrial fibrillation, then a degree of block is required to maintain a stable ventricular rate; this is regarded as the appropriate response and not pathologic unless the ventricular rate falls below 60 bpm. Atrial fibrillation with a slow ventricular response may be due to intrinsic disease of the AV node or may be iatrogenic due to the medications that are used to limit the rapid ventricular response or attempt to maintain sinus rhythm, such as beta-blockers, calcium channel-blockers, digoxin, procainamide, quinidine, or amiodarone; and can also be caused by metabolic abnormalities such as hyperkalemia (Figure 31.8) [5,8].

While intrinsic disease of the conduction system, such as the fibrosis and calcification associated with Lev's and Lenegre's diseases, is the most common cause of chronic complete heart block, acute complete heart block is more often due to extrinsic factors such as acute myocardial infarction (AMI), which causes 40% of all unstable third-degree AV block [4,5]. Acute myocardial infarction can cause bradycardia via multiple mechanisms including ischemia or necrosis of conduction tissue, altered autonomic balance, myocardial hyperkalemia, increased local production of

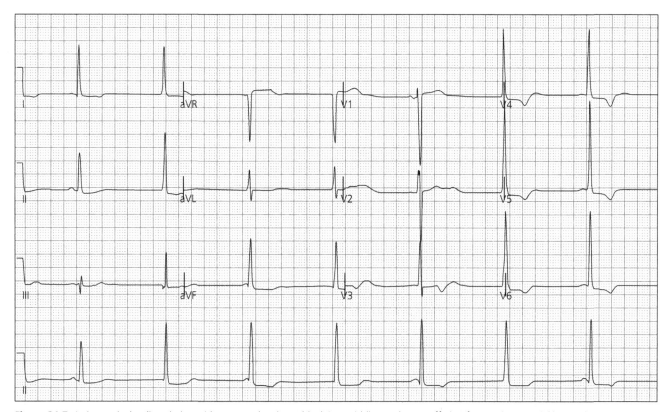

Figure 31.7 Atrioventricular dissociation without complete heart block in a middle-aged man suffering from an intracranial hemorrhage. Atrioventricular dissociation without complete heart block (there is at least one conducted P wave achieving AV capture) due to intracranial hemorrhage that is asymptomatic does not require any specific treatment except cardiac monitoring. In this case, the first QRS complex on the rhythm strip demonstrates a different morphology from the rest, and is preceded by a relatively normal PR interval, indicating that the P wave was conducted to the ventricle. Treating the underlying condition is vital, but atropine will rapidly reverse the high vagal tone responsible for the bradydysrhythmia.

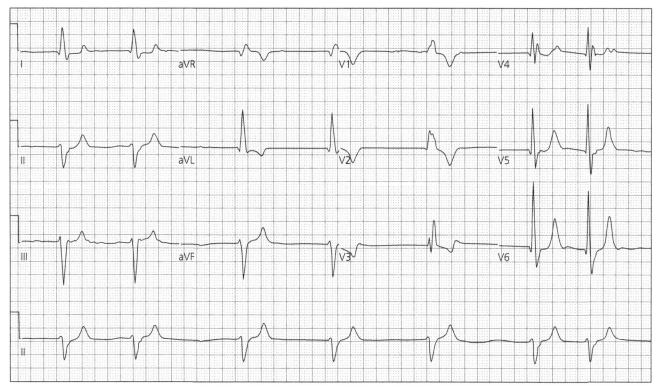

Figure 31.8 Atrial fibrillation with a very slow ventricular response in an elderly woman with renal insufficiency. Atrial fibrillation with a very slow ventricular response in a patient with known atrial fibrillation likely represents iatrogenic adverse effects from a rate-controlling medication (in this case digoxin toxicity with hyperkalemia).

Table 31.5 Bradycardia caused by AMI

Inferior MI	Anterior MI
Sinus bradycardia, sinus pauses, nodal AV block	Infra-nodal AV block
SA node and AV node ischemia, increased vagal tone	Ischemia of His-Purkinje system
First degree, second degree type I, and third degree AV block	Second degree type II and third degree AV block
Transient	Permanent
Good response to medications	Poor response to medications

SA = sino-atrial; AV = atrioventricular

adenosine, acidosis, hypoxia, or due to medical treatment (e.g. beta-blockers) [2,4]. Sinus bradycardia is found in 40% of AMI patients and causes 25% of the associated unstable bradydysrhythmias. First-degree AV block is seen in 15% of AMI cases, second-degree type 1 in 12%, second-degree type 2 is rare, but third-degree is found in 8% [4]. Junctional rhythm also occurs in 20% of AMI patients causing 20% of unstable bradydysrhythmias, while idioventricular rhythm occurs in 15% of cases and is responsible for 40% of unstable bradydysrhythmias [4].

Different bradydysrhythmias and clinical features are associated with different regions of myocardial infarction (Table 31.5) [4,5]. Inferior myocardial infarction more commonly has sinus bradycardia, sinus pauses/arrest, and so called "proximal" AV block occurring in the AV node due mostly to increased vagal tone which is transient and responds well to medical therapy. Anterior myocardial infarctions are associated with "distal" AV block occurring in the His-Purkinje pathways due to ischemic damage resulting in permanent block that responds poorly to medications. These unstable peri-infarct bradydysrhythmias have a 20% higher inpatient mortality believed to be attributed to the larger-sized area of myocardium involved [4].

Management

Treatment for acute symptomatic bradycardia can be divided into medications versus temporary external pacemakers. Medical therapy is often more readily available so should be

considered first, even as a so-called bridge when the underlying cause of the bradydysrhythmia is irreversible and a permanent pacemaker will be required eventually (Table 31.6) [2,4,14,15]. Atropine is the most commonly used agent for bradycardia in acute care. It increases SA automaticity and AV node conduction by inhibiting vagal input. The recommended initial dose in adults is 0.6–1 mg intravenously; dosages less than 0.5 mg should be avoided due to the possibility of paradoxical slowing of the heart rate. This dose can be repeated as necessary every 5 min until the full vagolytic dose of 0.04 mg/kg is reached. Atropine is indicated for asystole, symptomatic sinus bradycardia, bradycardia secondary to nitroglycerin administration, second-degree type 1 AV block, and nodal third-degree block (if the QRS complex is narrow). It may cause worsened bradycardia by increasing the AV block in second-degree type 2 and infra-nodal third-degree block (with a wide QRS complex) [2]. Atropine will not have an effect on denervated hearts after undergoing cardiac transplant, nor is it very effective on bradycardia due to cardioactive medications such as beta-blockers and calcium channel-blockers [2,14].

Isoproterenol is a non-specific beta-(1–2)-agonist that increases SA node rate as well as conduction velocity at the AV node and possibly in the His-Purkinje system [4]. It also increases contractility but can induce serious tachyarrhythmias including ventricular tachycardia. It is known to decrease coronary artery perfusion while increasing myocardial oxygen consumption, which may worsen infarct size if used during myocardial infarction. Theophylline (or aminophylline) increases SA automaticity but does not affect nodal conduction. It has been found to improve heart rates in patients after cardiac transplant, as well as after other cardiac surgery (coronary artery bypass grafting and valve replacement), reducing the need for permanent pacemaker insertion [14,16]. Glucagon increases SA and AV node automaticity but not conductivity, and is considered an antidote for beta-blocker or calcium channel-blocker induced bradycardia [4]. The bradycardic rhythms (sinus brady, junctional rhythm, atrial fibrillation with a very slow ventricular response) due to digoxin toxicity represent a special situation where standard medical therapy is most often not effective; digoxin binding antibody fragments are indicated for symptomatic bradycardia due to cardiac glycosides.

Temporary pacemakers can be placed transcutaneously or transvenously, and are indicated for symptomatic bradycardia causing hypoperfusion of the brain or heart (decreased

Table 31.6 Medications to treat symptomatic bradycardia

	SA node	AV node	His-Purkinje
Atropine	Increase SA activity	Decrease AVN block	No effect
Isoproterenol	Increase SA activity	Decrease AVN block	Decrease infra-nodal block?
Theophylline	Increase SA activity	No effect	No effect
Glucogon	Increase SA activity	Increase AV activity	No effect

level of consciousness, angina, congestive heart failure) or hemodynamic compromise if medical therapy is ineffective [2,7,17]. Transcutaneous pacing, first used by Zoll in 1952, is rapid, readily available, and easy to perform but has a lower rate of successful capture than transvenous pacing [2]. It should be attempted as a bridge to a more reliable means of pacing, but is recommended for only a short time period [4]. Temporary transvenous pacing can be done using the guidance of fluoroscopy, ultrasound, or even "blindly" with a high rate of success. The right internal jugular or left subclavian vein are the preferred access sites due to the relatively straight pathway to the heart. Complications occur in 4–20% of placements of a temporary transvenous pacemaker, including pneumothorax, cardiac perforation, and induced ventricular tachycardia. A prosthetic tricuspid valve is a contraindication to placement of a transvenous pacemaker [2].

Case conclusions

The initial ECG (Figure 31.1) demonstrated sinus bradycardia. This patient responded to intravenous fluid, atropine, and oxygen with an improved heart rate though her symptoms persisted. Approximately 1 h after presentation, the patient developed chest discomfort followed by recurrent bradycardia. A repeat 12-lead ECG (Figure 31.6) demonstrated ST elevation myocardial infarction of the inferior and lateral walls with possible posterior infarction as well. The rhythm was complete heart block. She received additional atropine with improvement in the heart rate. The patient was rapidly taken for percutaneous coronary intervention. An occluded right coronary artery was found and successfully stented. Her subsequent biomarkers were elevated, indicating AMI.

References

1 Spodick DH. Normal sinus heart rate: appropriates rate thresholds for sinus tachycardia and bradycardia. *Southern Med J* 1996;**89**: 666–7.

2 Kaushik V, Leon AR, Forrester JA *et al.* Bradyarrhythmias, temporary and permanent pacing. *Crit Care Med* 2000;**28**:121–8.

3 Abdon NJ, Landin K, Johansson BW. Athlete's bradycardia as an embolising disorder: symptomatic arrhythmias in patients aged less than 50 years. *Brit Heart J* 1984;**52**:660–6.

4 Brady WJ, Harrigan RA. Evaluation and management of bradyarrhythmias in the emergency department. *Emerg Med Clin N Am* 1998;**16**:361–88.

5 Wagner GS. Decreased automaticity and atrioventricular block. In: *Marriott's Practical Electrocardiography* 10th ed. Philadelphia: Lipincott Williams & Wilkins, 2001:397–426.

6 Navarro-Gutierrez S, Gonzalez-Martinez F, Fernandez-Perez MT *et al.* Bradycardia related to hypoglycemia. *Eur J Emerg Med* 2003;**10**:331–3.

7 Ferry DR. SA and AV nodal conduction abnormalities. In: *ECG in 10 Days* 2nd ed. New York: McGraw Hill Medical, 2007:94–150.

8 Moore CB, Bower PJ. The sick sinus syndrome: treatment by permanent transvenous atrial pacing. *Southern Med J* 1975;**68**: 580–3.

9 Aronow WS. Arial fibrillation. *Heart Dis* 2002;**4**:91–101.

10 Heitink-Polle KMJ, Rammeloo L, Hruda J *et al.* Rapid and full recovery after life-threatening complete atrioventricular block. *Eur J Pediatr* 2004;**163**:410–11.

11 Casiero D, Frishman WH. Cardiovascular complications of eating disorders. *Cardiol Rev* 2006;**14**:227–31.

12 Weintraub BM, McHenry LC. Cardiac abnormalities in subarachnoid hemorrhage: a resume. *Stroke* 1974;**5**:384–92.

13 Eraut D, Shaw DB. Sinus bradycardia. *Brit Heart J* 1971;**33**: 742–9.

14 Bertolet BD, Eagle DA, Conti JB *et al.* Bradycardia after heart transplant: reversal with theophylline. *J Am Coll Cardiol* 1996; **28**:396–9.

15 Swart G, Brady WJ, DeBehnke DJ *et al.* Acute myocardial infarction complicated by hemodynamically unstable bradyarrhythmia: prehospital and ED treatment with atropine. *Am J Emerg Med* 1999;**17**:647–52.

16 Chung MK. Cardiac surgery: postoperative arrhythmias. *Crit Care Med* 2000;**28**:136–44.

17 Ntalianis A, Nanan JN. Immediate relief of congestive heart failure by ventricular pacing in chronic bradycardia. *Cardiol Rev* 2006;**14**:e14–15.

Chapter 32 | What are the electrocardiographic indications for temporary cardiac pacing?

Michael Abraham[1], Michael C. Bond[2]
[1]Upper Chesapeake Medical Center, Bel Air, MD, USA
[2]University of Maryland School of Medicine, Baltimore, MD, USA

Case presentations

Case 1: A 55-year-old male comes into the emergency department (ED) due to chest pain that began about 1 h previously. The patient has a past medical history significant for diabetes and hypertension. He has been non-compliant with medications for 2 years. The patient describes the pain as dull and tugging in nature and the pain is associated with shortness of breath and a "clammy feeling." The pain feels like it is radiating to the left arm. The patient reports some nausea but no vomiting. On physical examination, the vital signs show a pulse of 88 beats per minute (bpm), blood pressure is 156/84 mmHg, respiratory rate is 22 per minute and slightly labored. The patient appears uncomfortable and diaphoretic. His rhythm is regular on cardiac examination and no murmurs are appreciated. His electrocardiogram (ECG) shows evidence of an ST segment elevation myocardial infarction (STEMI) in leads V1–V3 (Figure 32.1). While in the intensive care unit (ICU) later that day, the ECG shows the development of a conduction abnormality with the successive prolongation of the PR interval and then a dropped beat, suggesting a Mobitz I second-degree atrioventricular (AV) block, but a normal pulse rate.

Case 2: A 65-year-old male patient is brought in by ambulance after an episode of palpitations. The patient denies any chest pain, syncope or dyspnea. The patient has no significant past medical history. He last saw his primary care physician 1 year ago and was prescribed a medication for hypercholesterolemia. He also takes 81 mg of aspirin daily at the direction of his primary care physician. His family history is significant for coronary artery disease in his father who had a myocardial infarction (MI) at the age of 61, and paternal grandfather who also had a MI at the age of 55. The patient denies a history of smoking tobacco products, he does admit to social alcohol consumption with an average of two drinks daily. On physical examination, his vital signs show a heart rate of 50 bpm and regular, blood pressure 85/55 mmHg, respirations 16 per minute, and oxygen saturation of 99% on 2 L oxygen. The patient was in the process of being observed on a cardiac monitor when it was noted that his heart rate was 220. At this time, the patient again complained of palpitations and lightheadedness. While the nurse was preparing to perform the 12-lead ECG, the patient spontaneously converted to a sinus bradycardia with a rate of 48 bpm (Figures 32.2a and 32.2b).

Case 3: A 50-year-old male patient comes to the outpatient clinic for his yearly physical examination. In the review of symptoms, decreased exercise tolerance is noted. He denies chest pain, and dyspnea at rest. He usually runs two to three times per week, but has been unable to run for about 1 month due to dyspnea on exertion. He denies any chest pain or palpitations. He also denies paroxysmal nocturnal dyspnea and orthopnea. The remainder of his review of symptoms is negative. He does not take any medications with the exception of a daily vitamin supplement. He has never used tobacco products and only occasionally uses alcohol in social situations. His vital signs are all within normal limits with a pulse of 68 bpm, a blood pressure of 126/54 mmHg, and a respiratory rate of 14 breaths per minute. He is an athletic male, in no distress. He cardiac examination shows a regular rate and rhythm, with a physiologically split S2, without murmurs, rubs, or clicks. His pulmonary examination is also normal with symmetrical expansion, and clear lung sounds without evidence of wheezes, rhonchi, or rales. A plain radiograph of his chest shows no acute disease processes. A 12-lead ECG, however, shows complete heart block (Figure 32.3).

The patient is admitted to the ICU for further management. Soon after admission, the patient is noted to be unre-

Critical Decisions in Emergency and Acute Care Electrocardiography,
1st edition. Edited by W.J. Brady and J.D. Truwit. © 2009 Blackwell Publishing, ISBN: 9781405159067

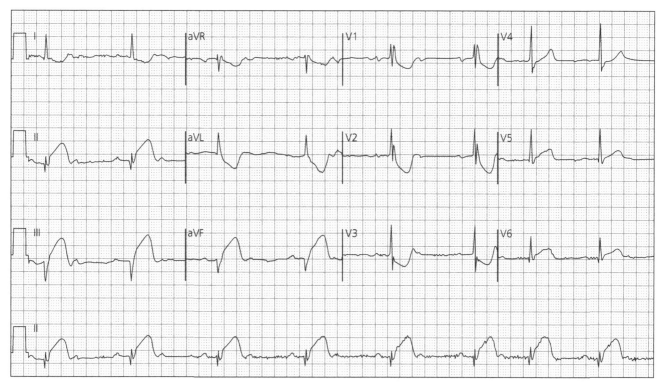

Figure 32.1 12-Lead ECG showing ST elevations in the inferior leads with reciprocal changes in V1 through V3, and a Mobitz I AV block. An ECG with this appearance would lead to the placement of temporary transcutaneous pacing pads, and pacing if the patient became bradycardic.

sponsive with a systolic blood pressure of 60 mmHg and a heart rate of 42 bpm. Atropine is given while endotracheal intubation is performed. With the atropine having limited response, a transcutaneous pacemaker is placed on the patient and activated with a palpable heart rate of 100 bpm and a blood pressure of 100/50 mmHg.

Electrocardiographic indications for temporary cardiac pacing

Emergency transcutaneous pacing was first described in 1952 by Zoll [1]. Zoll achieved this by attaching two electrodes to the chest wall with hypodermic needles and sending a pulsating current through them. This method of transcutaneous pacing was performed for ventricular standstill [2]. There is limited data on the benefits of pacing in certain situations; in the clinical setting of hemodynamic compromise, however, certain disease states can benefit from temporary cardiac pacing. For the sake of simplicity, hemodynamic instability can be described as hypotension (systolic pressure less than 90 mmHg), decreased mental status, ischemic chest pain, and/or cardiac pulmonary edema. It is important to note that temporary pacing is rarely, if ever, indicated for a patient, regardless of electrocardiographic findings if there is no evidence of hemodynamic instability. Prior to discussing the situations that would lead one to

consider temporary pacing; a brief review of the sinus node and its innervation may help in understanding the disease processes that can affect it.

In humans, the sinus node is a spindle-shaped structure composed of a fibrous tissue matrix with closely packed cells. It is 10–20 mm long and 2–3 mm wide. The blood supply to the sinus node is a branch of the right coronary artery 50–60% of the time; the remainder are supplied with a branch from the left circumflex coronary artery [3]. Due to the inherent pacemaking activity of the node, it is densely innervated. It has both postganglionic adrenergic and cholinergic nerve terminals. These pathways are crucial to the normal functioning of the node. The normal pacemaking cells in the sinoatrial (SA) node are designed to depolarize spontaneously. The ion channels of the SA node continually allow sodium to leak into the cell, making the net charge of the membrane less negative. At −40 to −50 mV, the cell automatically depolarizes and enters phase 0 of the action potential cycle. This depolarization is then transmitted to the remainder of the atria and the atrioventricular (AV) node. Due to the direct contact of the SA nodal cells with the atrial myocytes, the charge is transmitted through gap junctions and intercalated disks, which then causes the depolarization of the myocytes [4–6]. When the atrium depolarizes, it is seen on the electrocardiogram as a P wave. An important distinction must be made between the depolarization of the atria which appears on the ECG as the P wave, and the

(a)

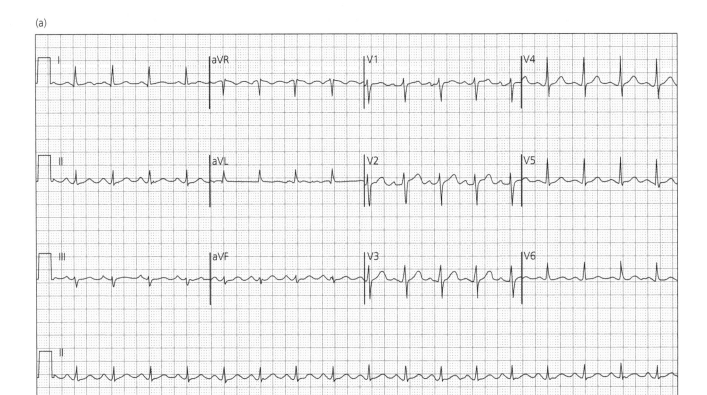

(b)

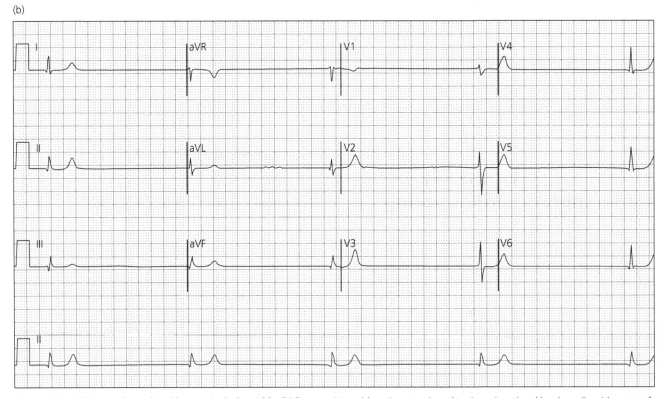

Figure 32.2 (a) Sinus tachycardia with a rate in the low 100s. (b) Same patient with no intervention, showing a junctional bradycardia with a rate of approximately 40 bpm.

(a)

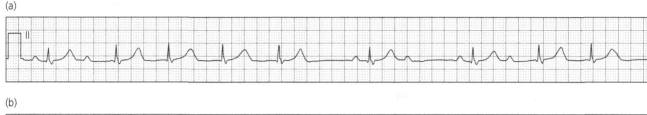

(b)

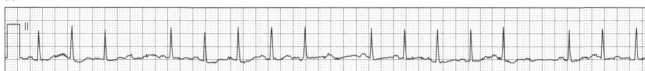

Figure 32.3 (a) Mobitz I AV block. Note the progressive PR prolongation followed by the absence of a QRS complex. The subsequent PR interval reverts to a normal interval. (b) Mobitz II AV block. In contrast to A, the PR interval is consistent throughout the tracing, with the occasional nonconduction of atrial depolarization.

depolarization of the SA node which cannot be detected on a surface ECG. A complex interplay between neurochemicals, ion channels, and action potentials is responsible for regulating the heart rate. Additional cardiac cells that have pacemaking capabilities such as the AV node, bundles of His, and the cardiac myocytes; however, their capabilities are suppressed by the higher inherent rate of SA node unless disease states are present. In the normal adult, the SA node will fire between 70 and 100 times per minute. This can change based on the health and overall conditioning of the patient. The maximal nodal discharge slowly decreases with age and can be estimated with a simple formula 220-age = maximal SA node discharge [7].

Indications for pacing in the patient with STEMI

Temporary cardiac pacing can be highly beneficial in many situations, especially in a patient with a STEMI. The American Heart Association/American College of Cardiology (AHA/ACC) published their recommendations on the management of STEMIs [8]. Using the ECG as a guide, they provide recommendations (Table 32.1) for the treatment of atrioventricular and intraventricular conduction disturbances due to STEMI. They classify their recommendations into two categories, anterior versus non-anterior, based on the anatomical location of the MI. For each anatomic location the recommendations are then based on the associated atrioventricular or intraventricular abnormality seen on the ECG. Temporary transcutaneous pacing is a Class I recommendation in normal AV nodal conduction or first-degree AV block when seen with an old or new fascicular block, old or new bundle branch block, or any fascicular block (left anterior or left posterior) with a right bundle branch block (RBBB). Transcutaneous pacing is also recommended when there is a Mobitz I or Mobitz II AV block combined with a bundle branch block that was present prior to the MI, or

Table 32.1 Indications for temporary cardiac pacing in the setting of an acute myocardial infarction

Class I recommendations for transcutaneous pacing

Any patient with normal AV conduction or first-degree AV block:
• Any old or new fascicular block in an anterior MI (Class I) non-anterior (Class IIb)
• Old or new bundle branch block
• Any fascicular block with a RBBB
• Mobitz I or Mobitz II heart block with an old bundle branch block, and a new or old fascicular block
• Mobitz I heart block with a new bundle branch or fascicular block

Class I recommendations for transvenous pacing
• Any AV node dysfunction with an alternating RBBB and LBBB block
• Mobitz II heart block with a fascicular block and RBBB
• Mobitz II heart block with a new bundle branch block

Adapted from Antman EM, Anbe DT, Armstrong PW, *et al.* ACC/AHA guidelines for the management of patients with ST-elevation myocardial infarction – executive summary: a report of the American College of Cardiology/American Heart Association Task Force on Practice Guidelines (Writing Committee to Revise the 1999 Guidelines for the Management of Patients With Acute Myocardial Infarction). *Circulation* 2004;**110**(5):588–636.

a new or old fascicular block. Other Class I indications for transcutaneous pacing are a new bundle branch block or a fascicular block with a RBBB in conjunction with a Mobitz I AV node block.

In addition to recommendations for transcutaneous pacing, there are also certain ECG criteria for transvenous pacing. Transvenous pacing is a Class 1 recommendation when there is AV node dysfunction or first-degree block with an alternating RBBB and left bundle branch block (LBBB). Transvenous pacing is also Class I with an alternating RBBB and LBBB in conjunction with any second-degree AV block, a Mobitz II AV block with a fascicular block and RBBB, or a Mobitz II AV block with a new bundle branch block.

All of these recommendations are based solely on the ECG findings. The situations described above are an exception to the rule that the patient's clinical status should dictate the need for temporary cardiac pacing.

Sinoatrial node dysfunction

Although ischemia and the resultant rhythm abnormalities are paramount, especially in the emergency physician's practice setting, there are other situations where the ECG can dictate the need for temporary pacing. One of these is the sick sinus syndrome (SSS), or sinus node dysfunction. Case 2 represents an example of SSS. The term SSS was first used by Lown in 1967 [9]; however, reports of syncopal episodes due to persistant bradycardia date back to Adams' article in 1827 [10]. Table 32.2 summarizes the multitude of ways in which SSS can present [11]. This syndrome can consist of persistent severe sinus bradycardia, a sinus arrest with no escape for short intervals, long periods of sinus arrest without the appearance of a new pacemaker and resulting in total cardiac arrest, chronic atrial fibrillation which is usually accompanied by a slow ventricular rate, inability of the heart to resume sinus rhythm following cardioversion for atrial fibrillation, and episodes of SA node exit block which are not related to drug therapy [12]. The tachycardia-bradycardia syndrome, as seen in the patient in Case 2, was initially reported by Short in 1954 [13]. This syndrome affects approximately 50% of the patients with sinus node dysfunction [14]. In a hemodynamically unstable patient, this syndrome

Table 32.2 Arrhythmias associated with sick sinus syndrome

Persistent and severe sinus bradycardia
Sinus arrest with no escape rhythm (sinus pause greater than 3 s)
Chronic atrial fibrillation with slow ventricular response
Inability of the heart to resume sinus rhythm following cardioversion for atrial fibrillation or flutter
Sinoatrial node block in the absence of drug effect
Tachycardia-bradycardia syndrome

Table 32.3 Indications for cardiac pacing in settings other than acute MI

Asystole
The following conditions should only be paced when the patient is also hemodynamically unstable:
Permanent pacemaker or AICD failure
Complete heart block
Sinus bradycardia
Sick sinus syndrome
Second-degree heart block
Slow ventricular response with atrial fibrillation or atrial flutter
Slow junctional escape rhythm

of alternating tachycardia and bradycardia would be a clear indication for temporary pacing. The exact form of pacing, whether transcutaneous or transvenous is dictated by the clinical scenario. For example, with an obese patient the clinician may encounter difficulty with transcutaneous pacing, and opt to initiate transvenous pacing.

There are other forms of sinus node disease; one of the first to appear clinically is persistent severe sinus bradycardia. As with all cardiac manifestations of disease, all cardioactive drugs should be excluded as a cause, prior to diagnosing a patient. The disease is described as bradycardia that does not increase with exertion and, in most cases, is the earliest manifestation of sinus node disease [15]. This diagnosis is difficult to make in the emergent setting and will most often be found in follow-up visits with primary care physicians. Thus, the diagnosis should be considered strongly in any patient with unexplained bradycardia at the time of evaluation, and the patient should be referred to a cardiologist or their primary physician for prompt evaluation. This early stage of sinus node dysfunction, if accompanied by hemodynamic instability would require placement of a permanent pacemaker to prevent hypotension. In the acute setting, as the sinus node is damaged, it does not respond to the normal physiologic stimuli, and atropine will have a limited effect. Therefore, in the acute setting, if the patient is experiencing hemodynamic compromise they must be paced temporarily until they can have a permanent pacemaker placed.

Another manifestation of SSS is a sinus arrest or sinus exit block. A sinus arrest will occur whenever the sinus node becomes so diseased that it ceases to fire impulses appropriately. A pause greater than 3 s is strongly suggestive of sinus node disease [16]. Due to the normal physiology of the sinus node, there is an inherent variability of firing rates. For example, in a very well-trained athlete, the conditioning leads to increased vagal tone. The parasympathetic actions on the SA node cause the rate of firing to decrease, and a sinus bradycardia with pauses of > 2 s have been documented. Conversely, a 3 s pause is very unusual even in a well-conditioned athlete. This is an example of a sinus exit block. In this case, the function of the heart is dependent on alternate pacemakers, as there is no transmission of the electrical charge from the SA node [17]. Sinoatrial exit block occurs whenever a conduction barrier within the SA node blocks exiting impulses directed to the atria, and is thought to involve the perinodal T cells. The node depolarizes but the charge is not transmitted to the myocytes. Therefore, no depolarization of the atria occurs, and no P wave is seen on the ECG. A sinus pause or arrest is defined as the transient absence of sinus P waves on the ECG that may last from 2 s to several minutes [18,19]. The pause or arrest often allows escape beats. As expected, as the episodes of the sinus arrest become longer, symptoms of dizziness, presyncope and syncope, and, ultimately, death may occur.

Sinoatrial node exit block, not to be confused with AV node block, can be classified just like AV block as first-, second-, and third-degree. It is very difficult to be able to distinguish these on the 12 lead surface ECG as the SA node depolarization is not seen, but rather the atrium response to the SA nodes firing. First-degree SA nodal exit block reflects a slowing of the impulse exit from the SA node, but there is still 1 : 1 conduction. This will be seen on surface ECG as sinus bradycardia. Second-degree SA nodal exit block has Type I (Wenckebach) and II classifications. Type I is described as increasing P-P intervals prior to a pause caused by a dropped P wave. The pause has a duration that is less than two P-P cycles of normal sinus rhythm. In Type II exit block, the P-P output remains constant before a pause. Both Type I and II second-degree SA node blockade should give a regularly irregular rhythm with ectopic beats and dropped P waves. Third-degree SA nodal exit block prevents pacemaker impulses from reaching the right atrium, giving the appearance of sinus arrest with escape beats. The ECG may show any number of rhythms from atrial fibrillation to a junctional escape rhythm depending on the underlying physiologic reason for the SA node exit block. Chronic atrial fibrillation with slow ventricular response can be another indication of sinus node disease. Unlike typical atrial fibrillation that responds to cardioversion by reverting to a sinus rhythm, attempts at cardioversion with sinus node disease typically produce a long sinus pause, followed by a slow unstable rhythm.

Atrioventricular node blocks

Progressing further down the cardiac conduction pathway, the next important step is the AV node. Just as SA node dysfunction can be responsible for hemodynamic instability, so can dysfunction of the AV node. The classification of AV node block is well described, as first-, second-, and third (complete)-degree AV block. As with the majority of the previous rhythms, the ECG findings alone cannot guide management; evidence of hemodynamic instability must be present. In this section, the findings of AV nodal block not in conjunction with MI are discussed.

The normal PR interval on the ECG, measured from the onset of the P wave to the beginning of the QRS complex, should range from 0.12–0.20 s at normal heart rates. First-degree AV block is defined as a PR interval exceeding 0.20 s. There are many causes of first-degree AV block, including congenital heart disease, idiopathic disease of the conduction system, ischemia, and conditioning. The overall incidence of

first-degree AV block is estimated to be anywhere from 0.65 to 1.1% of the general population, and is commonly found in asymptomatic individuals [20,21]. An intraventricular conduction delay, such as a bundle branch block, in conjunction with the first-degree AV block could very well result in symptomatic bradycardia. Occasionally, first-degree block can progress to a more profound AV block. Second-degree AV block was first reported in 1899 by Wenckebach, and further characterized by Hay in 1906. They identified the block by monitoring A, C and V waves seen in the jugular venous pulse. In 1924, Mobitz used the ECG to further classify the abnormal findings that make up second-degree AV node blockade [22].

Mobitz I AV block (see Figure 32.3a) is the most common form of second-degree AV block. The ECG shows progressive PR interval prolongation with a subsequent blocked sinus impulse (absence of QRS complex following the P wave). The greatest PR increment typically occurs prior to the dropped beat beats. Shortening of the PR interval occurs after the blocked sinus impulse, provided the P wave is conducted to the ventricle. Progressive PR interval shortening is crucial to the diagnosis of type I block. Unlike Mobitz I, Mobitz II AV block does not follow the systematic prolongation of the PR interval leading to the non-conducted P wave. The Mobitz II rhythm (see Figure 32.3b) is characterized by a stable PR interval with an occasional non-conducted P wave (absence of QRS complex following the P wave); the PR interval may or may not be prolonged, but, regardless of length, the PR interval remains constant in all conducted beats. Patients that have 2 : 1 AV conduction, with an absent QRS complex after every other P wave can only be classified as a Type II AV block. It is impossible to differentiate these patients as Mobitz I or Mobitz II AV block as one cannot see if the PR interval is lengthening prior to the non-conducted P waves [3,23].

The final AV nodal block is the most significant and is associated with the most emergent need for temporary and permanent pacing. Third-degree AV block, or complete heart block (see Figure 32.4) is the complete disassociation of the atria and the ventricles. The SA node depolarizes the atria at one rate and there is depolarization of the ventricles from a different pacemaker, usually at a slower rate. This results in the atria and ventricles working independently of each other. Hemodynamic compromise is encountered to a much greater extent in complete heart block when compared with either first- or second-degree heart block. Treatment of this rhythm with atropine often fails to improve the ventricular rate, as vagal stimulation of the AV node is not thought to be the

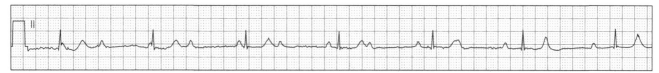

Figure 32.4 Complete heart block. Notice how the PP length and the QRS complexes are both stable. However, there is no correlation between P waves and the resultant QRS complexes.

cause of this finding. Atropine is generally successful only when an AV block is caused by excessive vagal tone. Early use of a pacemaker is generally the best course of action in patients with complete heart block and borderline or frank instability.

Permanent pacemaker malfunction

With the aging of our population, the number of individuals with pacemakers and automatic implantable cardioverter-defibrillators (AICD) will steadily increase. Fortunately, the technologic advances in battery development, software, and ventricular lead design have made them extremely reliable. With routine follow-up, there will be few patients that experience a pacemaker or AICD failure; however, should one fail it can be an indication for temporary cardiac pacing.

There are numerous problems that can occur with a pacemaker/AICD from lead oversensing or undersensing, failure to capture, and crosstalk (ventricular or atrial lead is picking up the pacing from the other chamber) [24]. Most of these conditions will require a 12-lead ECG along with interrogation of the pacemaker/AICD to diagnose the problem. One can check to see if oversensing is playing a role by placing a magnet over the device. This disengages the sensing amplifiers and puts most pacemakers in a fixed rate mode [25]. For AICDs, it will typically stop the device from defibrillating or overdrive pacing a patient.

Failure to capture can be noted on 12-lead ECG without interrogation of the device. Failure to capture can be due to lead failure, battery depletion, electrolyte abnormalities (i.e. hyperkalemia), MI or ischemia, drug therapy, and several other causes. This will generally be seen on the 12-lead ECG as pacer spikes with no subsequent P wave (if atrial-paced) or QRS (ventricular-paced) complex. If there is a problem with a lead or battery depletion, the pacer spike may not be seen at all. If there is failure to capture and the patient has symptomatic bradycardia or no escape rhythm, then temporary transcutaneous or transvenous pacing should be attempted.

Most newer pacemakers and AICDs will not be damaged by transcutaneous pacing or defibrillation as they have a diode that shunts excess energy away from the device. It is recommended that the pacer pads be placed as far away from the device as possible. Anterior-posterior lead placement is the preferred option [25].

Case conclusions

The 55-year-old male in Case 1 presented with an anterior STEMI, and then developed Mobitz I AV block. Any Mobitz I or Mobitz II second-degree AV block in the setting of a STEMI is an indication for temporary cardiac pacing. Transcutaneous pacing is recommended except if there is also an alternating RBBB and LBBB block, or if the patient has Mobitz II AV block plus a fascicular block plus RBBB, where transvenous pacing is recommended. It is NOT recommended that you wait for the patient to become hemodynamically unstable to initiate pacing; it should be in position and on demand mode to immediately start pacing should the patient become bradycardic or develop asystole. If the patient did not have a STEMI, then the decision to initiate pacing would depend on his hemodynamic status and symptoms.

The 65-year-old male in Case 2 presented with SSS as noted by his intermittent episodes of tachycardia and bradycardia. Patients with this condition are typically treated with a permanent pacemaker for the bradycardia and medication for the tachycardia. This patient should be treated with transcutaneous pacing, and, if unable to obtain capture, a transvenous pacer. It is recommended that you discuss the case with a cardiologist prior to placing a transvenous pacemaker so that the site of your temporary pacer does not affect the cardiologist's ability to place a permanent one.

The 50-year-old male in Case 3 presented to the outpatient clinic for a routine examination and was noted to have complete heart block on his 12-lead ECG. As this gentleman had been very active in the past, it would not be unusual for him to have a heart rate of 48 while at rest. However, because he was unresponsive with a systolic blood pressure of 60, he was, by definition, hemodynamically unstable. It would be reasonable to initiate resuscitation and administer atropine to this patient; however, it is not likely to be effective. The second treatment option is transcutaneous pacing, which was initiated successfully. A transvenous pacemaker was then placed without consequence via the right internal jugular vein. This patient ultimately required permanent pacemaker placement.

References

1 Zoll PM. Resuscitation of the heart in ventricular standstill by external electric stimulation. *N Engl J Med* 1952;**247**(20):768–71.

2 Zoll PM, Linenthal AJ, Gibson W, *et al.* Termination of ventricular fibrillation in man by externally applied electric countershock. *N Engl J Med* 1956;**254**(16):727–32.

3 Zipes DP, Jalife J. *Cardiac electrophysiology: from cell to bedside.* 3rd ed. Philadelphia: Saunders; 2000.

4 Boyett MR, Honjo H, Kodama I. The sinoatrial node, a heterogeneous pacemaker structure. *Cardiovasc Res* 2000;**47**(4):658–87.

5 Boyett MR, Dobrzynski H, Lancaster MK, *et al.* Sophisticated architecture is required for the sinoatrial node to perform its normal pacemaker function. *J Cardiovasc Electrophysiol* 2003;**14**(1): 104–6.

6 Joyner RW, van Capelle FJ. Propagation through electrically coupled cells. How a small SA node drives a large atrium. *Biophys J* 1986;**50**(6):1157–64.

7 James TN. The sinus node. *Am J Cardiol* 1977;**40**(6):965–86.

8 Antman EM, Anbe DT, Armstrong PW, *et al.* ACC/AHA guidelines for the management of patients with ST-elevation myocardial infarction – executive summary: a report of the American College of Cardiology/American Heart Association Task Force on Practice Guidelines (Writing Committee to Revise the 1999 Guidelines for

the Management of Patients With Acute Myocardial Infarction). *Can J Cardiol* 2004;**20**(10):977–1025.

9 Lown B. Electrical reversion of cardiac arrhythmias. *Br Heart J* 1967;**29**(4):469–89.

10 Keller KB, Lemberg L. The sick sinus syndrome. *Am J Crit Care* 2006;**15**(2):226–9.

11 Ferrer MI. The natural history of the sick sinus syndrome. *J Chronic Dis* 1972;**25**(6):313–15.

12 Adan V, Crown LA. Diagnosis and treatment of sick sinus syndrome. *Am Fam Physician* 2003;**67**(8):1725–32.

13 Short DS. The syndrome of alternating bradycardia and tachycardia. *Br Heart J* 1954;**16**(2):208–14.

14 Rubenstein JJ, Schulman CL, Yurchak PM, DeSanctis RW. Clinical spectrum of the sick sinus syndrome. *Circulation* 1972;**46**(1): 5–13.

15 Sutton R. Cardiac pacing for bradyarrhythmias in the elderly. *J R Soc Med* 1994;**87**(4):223–7.

16 Ector H, Rolies L, De Geest H. Dynamic electrocardiography and ventricular pauses of 3 seconds and more: etiology and therapeutic implications. *Pacing Clin Electrophysiol* 1983;**6**(3 Pt 1):548–51.

17 Jordan JL, Yamaguchi I, Mandel WJ. Studies on the mechanism of sinus node dysfunction in the sick sinus syndrome. *Circulation* 1978;**57**(2):217–23.

18 Hariman RJ, Krongrad E, Boxer RA, *et al.* Method for recording electrical activity of the sinoatrial node and automatic atrial foci during cardiac catheterization in human subjects. *Am J Cardiol* 1980;**45**(4):775–81.

19 Yamada T, Fukunami M, Shimonagata T, *et al.* Identification of sinus node dysfunction by use of P-wave signal-averaged electrocardiograms in paroxysmal atrial fibrillation: a prospective study. *Am Heart J* 2001;**142**(2):286–93.

20 Bexton RS, Camm AJ. First degree atrioventricular block. *Eur Heart J* 1984;**5** Suppl A:107–9.

21 Rardon DP MW, Zipes DP. Atrioventricular block and AV dissociation. In: Zipes DP JJ, ed. *Cardiac Electrophysiology: From Cell to Bedside.* 3 ed. Philadelphia: WB Saunders; 2000:935–42.

22 Silverman ME, Upshaw CB, Jr., Lange HW. Woldemar Mobitz and His 1924 classification of second-degree atrioventricular block. *Circulation* 2004;**110**(9):1162–7.

23 Lilly LS, Harvard Medical School. *Pathophysiology of heart disease: a collaborative project of medical students and faculty.* 2nd ed. Baltimore: Williams & Wilkins; 1998.

24 Reynolds J, Apple S. A systematic approach to pacemaker assessment. *AACN Clin Issues* 2001;**12**(1):114–26.

25 Hayes DL, Vlietstra RE. Pacemaker malfunction. *Ann Intern Med* 1993;**119**(8):828–35.

Chapter 33 | Can the ECG accurately diagnose pacemaker malfunction and/or complication?

Kevin C. Reed
Washington Hospital Center, Washington, DC, USA

Case presentations

Case 1: A 70-year-old male with a history of hypertension and congestive heart failure status-post pacemaker placement for third-degree heart block 3 weeks previously presents to the emergency department (ED) with fatigue for 1 week. He had a syncopal event that day while out playing with his grandchildren. On examination, he appears in mild distress with a blood pressure of 108/58, pulse of 44, respirations of 20 and oxygen saturation of 100% on 4 L nasal cannula. A rhythm strip is provided by emergency medical services (EMS) while the electrocardiogram (ECG) is obtained (Figure 33.1).

Case 2: A 75-year-old female with pacemaker placement 9 years previously presents to the ED with palpitations and dizziness with mild left-sided chest pain at onset 30 min prior to ED arrival. On examination, she is in acute distress. Her blood pressure is 98/60, respirations 28 and her pulse ox. is 98% on 100% non-rebreather. The ECG shows a wide complex tachycardia with pacer spike apparent at a rate of 210 (Figure 33.2).

The ECG and pacemaker malfunction/complication

The first implantable electronic pacemakers were introduced in the 1950s to prevent Stokes-Adams attacks [1]. Today, an estimated 112,000 to 121,000 new pacemakers are implanted annually with an additional 25,000 replacement procedures (majority due to approaching battery life) performed annually [2,3]. Over the past 20 years the development of new

Critical Decisions in Emergency and Acute Care Electrocardiography,
1st edition. Edited by W.J. Brady and J.D. Truwit. © 2009 Blackwell Publishing, ISBN: 9781405159067

technologies has significantly enhanced the sophistication, versatility, capability and effectiveness of the implanted pacemaker [4].

Current models are usually reliable, but malfunctions may arise. Patients with pacemaker malfunction often have vague and non-specific symptoms including palpitations, irregular heart beats, syncope, presyncope, dizziness, chest pain, dyspnea, orthopnea, paroxysmal nocturnal dyspnea, or fatigue [5]. Clinically significant abnormal pacemaker function arises from the following: sensing abnormalities, failure to pace, failure to capture, pacemaker-mediated tachycardias, and the pacemaker syndrome [5]. A 12-lead ECG is an essential part of the evaluation for pacemaker malfunction. The goal of this chapter is to educate clinicians regarding the basic components of pacers, the types of malfunctions and their associated ECG findings, and the initial management steps when abnormalities arise.

Basics of pacemakers

Pacemakers consist of a pulse generator and single or multiple electrical leads that are implanted into the heart muscle wall or coronary-sinus tract. The batteries are lithium-based and have lifespans approaching 10 years [3]. Pacemakers also contain a reed switch that can be activated by an externally placed magnet, allowing for testing of the pacemaker's pacing capacity [3]. Pacemakers may pace the atria, the ventricle or both sequentially; similarly, sensing of either atrial or ventricular activity is possible, and sensing may trigger or inhibit pacer activity [2]. Pacemakers are primarily implanted to treat symptomatic bradyarrythmias including bradycardia and various types of heart blocks [2]. A complete list of guidelines for implanting pacemakers was updated by the American College of Cardiology(ACA), the American Heart Association (AHA), and North American Society for Pacing and Electrophysiology (NASPE) in 2002 [6] and are available online at http://circ.ahajournals.org/cgi/content/full/112/16/2555

Figure 33.1 Failure of ventricular capture. This patient has underlying sick sinus syndrome and complete heart block. There is intermittent native atrial activity (*a*) and atrial pacing and capture (*p*) when no native activity is present. There is failure of ventricular capture, however, because no QRS complexes follow the ventricular pacing spikes (*arrow*). The QRS complexes on this tracing are slow ventricular escape beats (*v*). In the fourth QRS complex, the pacemaker generates a stimulus at the same time a ventricular escape beat occurs, yielding a type of fusion beat (*f*). Reprinted with permission from Chan TC, Cardall TY. Electronic pacemakers. *Emerg Med Clin N Am* 2006;**24**:179–94.

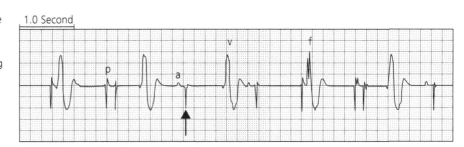

1.0 Second

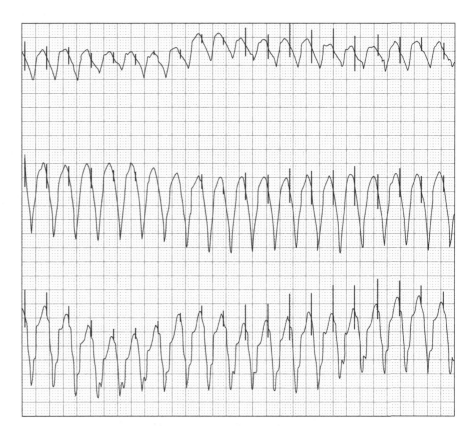

Figure 33.2 "Runaway pacemaker" from Harper RJ, Brady WJ, Perron AD, *et al*. The paced electrocardiogram: issues for the emergency physician. *Am J Emer Med* 2001;**19**:551–60.

Normal electrocardiographic findings: On the ECG, an electrical spike (a straight line or *pacemaker spike*) identifies a pacer stimulus (Figure 33.3). The pacing spike is typically 2 ms in duration [3]. Due to their low amplitude, they may not be visible in all leads, which is especially important to consider in the resuscitation setting where either a single-lead or three-lead rhythm strip is often used to guide management. Pacing spikes are much smaller with dual electrode systems (leads I, II, and III) than unipolar leads (leads aVr, aVl, aVf, and V1–V6), and consequently may be difficult to visualize [1].

The pacing leads used to pace the atrium are implanted in the appendage of the right atrium and the leads to pace the

ventricles are placed toward the apex of the right ventricle [1]. Atrial pacing appears as a small pacemaker spike just before the P wave and usually has normal morphology [1]. With the ventricular pacing lead placed in the right ventricle, the ventricles depolarize from right to left; the overall QRS morphology is similar to that of a left bundle branch block (LBBB), with widening of the QRS interval (Figure 33.3) [1]. This pattern occurs due to initiation of electrical activity in the right ventricle that spreads slowly to the left ventricle, similar to a right ventricular ectopic beat [4]. In contrast, in left ventricular epicardial placement, the QRS pattern resembles that of a right bundle branch block (RBBB), similar to a left ventricular ectopic beat. Occasionally, a pacemaker

(i)

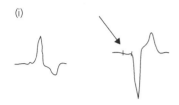

(ii)

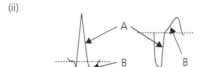

The rule of appropriate discordance is seen here, illustrating the normal relationship of the major, terminal portion of the QRS complex and the initial ST segment T wave

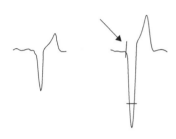

Note the pacer spikes (arrows) initiating atrial and ventricular depolarizations. The QRS complex is wide. In the upper left image (lead I or aVl), a monophasic R wave is seen. In this lead, the entire portion of the QRS complex is positive; in this instance with an entirely positive QRS complex, the rule of appropriate discordance states that the ST segment is depressed below the baseline with an inverted T wave. In the other leads (lower left, lead III; upper right, lead V1; and lower right, lead V6), the QRS complex is negative which is accompanied by an elevated ST segment with upright T wave

Figure 33.3 Schematic and tracings showing rule of appropriate discordance in pacemakers. From Mattu A, Brady W. *ECGs for the Emergency Physician*. London: BMJ Publishing Group, 2003.

is placed in the coronary sinus, a posterior structure of the heart. In this case, the ECG has a tall R wave in leads V1 through V6, stemming from activation in a posterior to anterior direction [4].

When considering the ST segments and T waves on the paced ECG, a guideline to remember is the need for appropriate discordance – namely, the major, terminal portion of the QRS complex is located on the opposite side of baseline from the ST segment/T wave complex. The ECG should have discordant ST segments and T waves with the QRS complex in contrast to the usual ECG pattern (Figure 33.3). Furthermore, the clinician must realize that the 12-lead ECG is largely invalidated in the evaluation of the chest pain patient suspected of ACS. These considerations must be integrated into the approach of the patient possible ACS and a paced ECG [1].

Pacing modes

Pacemakers are designated with up to a five-position code (I–V) as developed by the NASPE and the British Pacing and Electrophysiology Group (BPEG) to characterize pacemaker type and function [7] (Table 33.1). The indicator codes identify pacemaker lead location and functionality. Designations

include: (I) the chamber paced, (II) the chamber sensed, (III) the type of response, (IV) programmable functions, and (V) special tachyarrythmia functions for implanted cardiac defibrillators [4]. In the emergency department, intensive care unit (ICU) or clinic setting, the most commonly encountered pacemakers include AAIR, VVIR, DDD, DDDR or back-up pacing modes for defibrillator devices [1].

Single-chamber demand pacing (AAIR, VVIR): These pacemakers contain both sensing and pacing circuits. An AAI pacemaker paces the atrium, senses the atrium, and inhibits pacing activity if it senses spontaneous atrial activity (Figure 33.4) [1]. This is useful in patients with sinus node dysfunction and intact AV node conduction as it prevents the atrial rate from decreasing below a preset level [1]. In comparison to the AAI mode, VVI units pace and sense the ventricle. This is useful in patients with chronically ineffective atria, such as chronic atrial fibrillation or atrial flutter (Figure 33.5) [1]. VVI mode paces the ventricle if a QRS complex is not sensed within a predefined interval [2].

Dual chamber pacing (DDD): These pacing systems are capable of sensing, pacing, and inhibiting both the atrium and ventricles (Figure 33.6) [1]. DDD pacers are the most commonly encountered, as they preserve AV synchrony and

Table 33.1 NASPE/BPEG Codes for classification of pacing modes [7]

Position	I	II	III	IV	VI
	Chamber(s) paced	Chamber(s) sensed	Response to sensing	Programmability rate modulation	Anti-tachycardia (AICDs)
	O = none	O = none	O = none	O = none	O = none
	A = atrium	A = atrium	A = atrium	P = simple	P = pacing(anti-dysrhythmia)
	V = ventricle	V = ventricle	V = ventricle	M = multiprogrammable	S = shock
	D = dual chamber	D = dual chamber	D = dual chamber	C = communicating	D = dual (P + S)
				R = rate responsive	

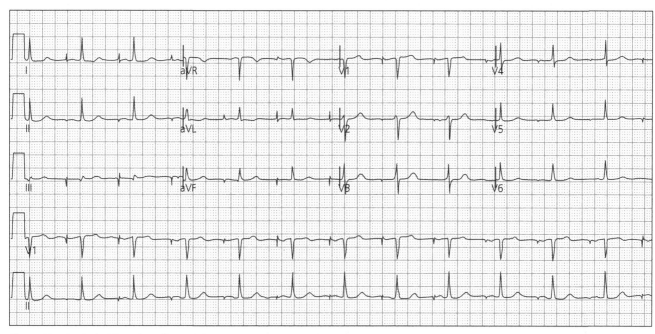

Figure 33.4 Typical ECG produced by complete AAI pacing. From Harper RJ, Brady WJ, Perron AD, *et al*. The paced electrocardiogram: issues for the emergency physician. *Am J Emer Med* 2001;**19**:551–60.

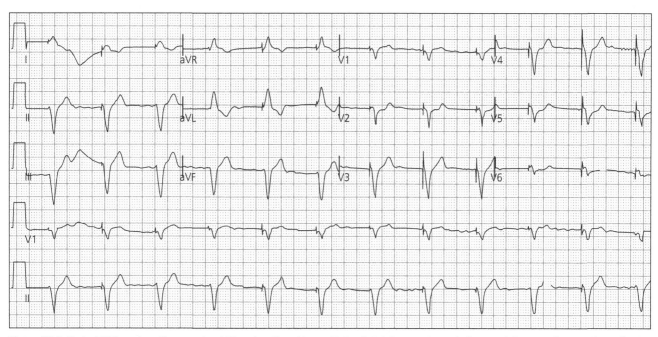

Figure 33.5 Typical ECG produced by complete VVI pacing. From Harper RJ, Brady WJ, Perron AD, *et al*. The paced electrocardiogram: issues for the emergency physician. *Am J Emer Med* 2001;**19**:551–60.

create a state similar to the physiology of normal AV conduction [1]. If the pacemaker does not sense any native atrial activity after a preset interval, it generates an atrial stimulus. Any atrial stimulus, either native or paced, initiates a period called the AV interval (AVI) [3]. This functions roughly as the PR interval. This is a refractory period during which the atrial channel of the pacemaker is inactive [1]. At the end of the AV interval, if no native ventricular activity is sensed by the

ventricular channel, the pacemaker generates a ventricular stimulus [1]. Following the AV interval, a postventricular atrial refractory period (PVARP) occurs, keeping the atrial channel inactive to prevent sensing the ventricular stimulus or resulting retrograde P waves as native atrial activity [1]. The total atrial refractory period (TARP) equals the AVI and the PVARP, which determines the upper rate of the pacemaker (upper rate, beats per minute [bpm] = 60/TARP) [1].

(a)
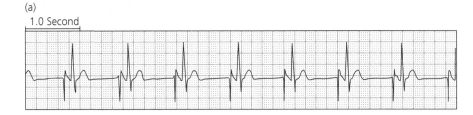

(b)
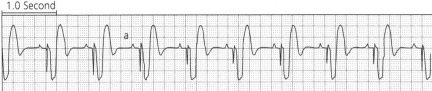

(c)
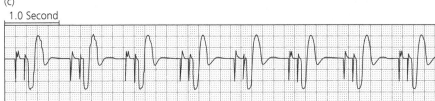

Figure 33.6 DDD pacing. (a) Atrial pacing with native ventricular QRS activity without ventricular pacing because of intact AV conduction. (b) There is atrial sensing of native P waves (a) that triggers subsequent ventricular pacing. (c) Atrial and ventricular pacing occur. Reprinted with permission from Chan TC, Cardall TY. Electronic pacemakers. *Emerg Med Clin N Am* 2006;**24**:179–94.

These periods are important in understanding certain types of pacemaker malfunctions.

Evaluation for suspected pacemaker malfunction

Patients with potential pacemaker failure will usually present with recurrent symptomatic bradyarrhythmias [2]. However, the most dangerous failures result from pacemaker-induced tachycardias [2]. Common conditions that predispose a pacemaker to complication include hyperkalemia, hypokalemia, hypoxemia, acute myocardial infarction, and cardioactive drugs [3]. In order to detect a malfunctioning pacemaker, it is crucial to identify the type and model of a pacemaker, as well as the site and status of pacing electrodes [4]. A 12-lead electrocardiogram, cardiac monitoring, and posterior-anterior (PA) and lateral chest radiographs are necessary in the initial evaluation.

Patients are requested to carry a card at all times (and most do) identifying the make and model of their implanted pacemaker, as well as the physician responsible for their pacer [2]. If this is unavailable, a chest radiograph can reveal useful information including a radio-opaque code from which the model number and manufacturer can be obtained [3]. Additional information such as lead dislodgement, migration, or fracture can also be seen on chest radiograph [1].

Patients may present with complaints potentially referable to pacemaker dysfunction, but with an intrinsic rhythm rapid enough to inhibit pacemaker function [2]. The presence or absence of a pacemaker spike on the ECG must be determined. If there is no pacemaker activity on the ECG, clinicians can attempt to obtain a paced ECG by applying a magnet. Application of a magnet allows for assessment of pacemaker capture (but not sensing), evaluation of battery life, treatment of pacemaker-mediated tachycardia, and assessment of pacemaker function when the native heart beat is greater than pacing threshold [1]. This typically switches the pacemaker to asynchronous pacing (a small minority exhibit a different preprogrammed effect or no effect). Atrial pacers will operate in AOO mode, ventricular pacers in VOO, and dual-chamber pacers in DOO mode (Figure 33.7) [2].

A completely paced ECG at a preset "magnet rate" (usually between 70 and 90 bpm) will result if the pacing suppresses the native rhythm [2]. Pacer spikes will be seen but capture may not occur if they are generated during the refractory period [2]. As the end of pacer life is entered (the elective replacement interval) the magnet rate slows [2]. Determining subtle rate changes requires additional information usually not available on the ECG, often requiring pacer interrogation for this diagnosis. One important clinical practice is to label the paced and non-paced ECG to avoid any confusion when formal ECG interpretation occurs at a later date [2].

Clinicians must be careful and methodical when evaluating the ECG in a patient with a pacemaker. National and international studies on the diagnostic accuracy of computer-based ECG rhythm interpretation have shown that the most common errors were related to patients with pacemakers. In this subgroup of patients (7–8% of the total study population),

Figure 33.7 Placement of magnet inhibits sensing and reverts the pacemaker to asynchronous pacing. The magnet allows for assessment of capture (but not sensing). The first four beats show native atrial activity inhibiting atrial pacing and triggering ventricular pacing. When the magnet is placed (*m*), atrial sensing is halted and asynchronous atrial and ventricular pacing occurs. This represents DOO pacing. Reprinted with permission from Chan TC, Cardall TY. Electronic pacemakers. *Emerg Med Clin N Am* 2006;**24**:179–94.

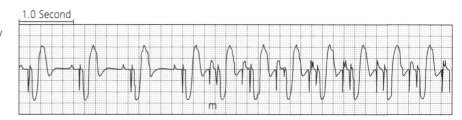

Figure 33.8 Atrial undersensing. In this patient with a DDD pacemaker, the native atrial events (*a*) are not sensed. If atrial sensing were occurring, atrial pacing (*e*) would be inhibited. Reprinted with permission from Chan TC, Cardall TY. Electronic pacemakers. *Emerg Med Clin N Am* 2006;**24**:179–94.

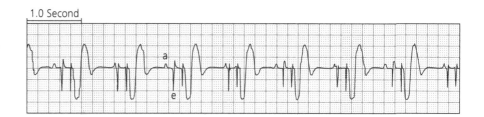

approximately 61–75% of the interpretations required revisions by a cardiologist [8–11]. The most common errors were due to failure to detect underlying rhythms or intrinsic beats, such as sinus rhythm with dual chamber pacing, underlying atrial, or premature atrial or ventricular contractions. Most important was the complete failure to identify pacemaker activity in 10–18% of the paced patients [8–11]. The clinical significance of these errors is not mentioned. However, these studies highlight the assertion that reliance on the computer-based ECG rhythm interpretation is not recommended, and that over-reading by the physician to identify any incorrect interpretations is mandatory.

Types of malfunction and associated electrocardiographic findings

Abnormal sensing: Abnormalities of sensing may occur due to undersensing, oversensing or failure to sense. Undersensing occurs when the pacemaker fails to sense or detect native cardiac activity [2]. This accounts for approximately 1.3% of pacemaker replacements [3]. In this setting the pacer will ignore any intrinsic rhythm and pace at a fixed rate, resulting in a pacemaker that is competitive with the intrinsic rhythm [3]. Anything that changes the amplitude, vector or frequency of intracardiac electrical signals can result in undersensing [1]. Causes of undersensing include new bundle branch blocks, premature ventricular contractions (PVCs), atrial or ventricular tachydysrhythmias, low current from a failing battery, magnetic resonance imaging (MRI) side effects, or exit block [1]. This is defined as an

elevation in the threshold voltage required for myocardial depolarization. Exit block can occur due to maturation of tissue at the electrode-myocardium interface following implantation, or from tissue damage at the interface due to external cardiac defibrillation [1].

Assessment for *undersensing* on the electrocardiogram is difficult, as there are no obvious findings on ECG [5]. Pacing artifacts may or may not be easily detectable; therefore, clinicians must infer from the surface ECG whether the pacemaker is sensing properly and responding with an appropriate output based on its internal program [1,5] (Figures 33.8 and 33.9). Pacer spikes that are seen may not result in capture if they are generated during the refractory period (TARP) [2]. An ECG with pacemaker spikes within native QRS complexes also suggests undersensing [2].

Oversensing can be defined as when the pacemaker unexpectedly senses a signal as a proper atrial or ventricular signal ventricular and does not fire [3]. This occurs when a pacer is too sensitive or has inappropriately set refractory periods [2]. It accounts for approximately 10% of pacemaker replacements [3]. Episodes can be intermittent, manifested by irregular pacemaker function including reoccurrence of the patients' underlying bradycardia [2]; alternatively, they can be constant, with either absent pacing or a decreased pacing rate [12]. Causes of oversensing include P, T, or large U waves, skeletal muscle myopotentials, or tremors that are incorrectly interpreted as QRS complexes [1,2,3]. Oversensing due to skeletal muscle myopotentials primarily occurs in unipolar pacing systems, rather than bipolar pacing systems [1].

The most common sources of myopotentials include the pectoralis, rectus abdominal, and the diaphragm muscles [1]. Oversensing can also occur due to electrical signals produced

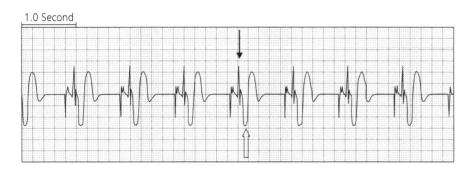

Figure 33.9 Ventricular undersensing. In this patient with a DDD pacemaker, intrinsic ventricular events are not sensed. A native, upright, narrow QRS complex (*narrow arrow*) occurs soon after each atrial stimulus, but these complexes are not sensed, and before ventricular repolarization has a chance to get started, ventricular pacing occurs, triggering the wider QRS complexes (*wide arrow*). Reprinted with permission from Chan TC, Cardall TY. Electronic pacemakers. *Emerg Med Clin N Am* 2006;**24**:179–94.

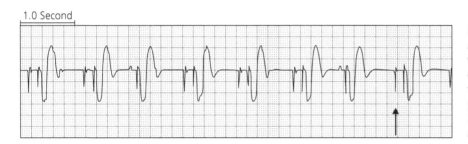

Figure 33.10 Failure of atrial capture. Atrial and ventricular pacing spikes are visible, but only the ventricular stimuli are capturing. There are no P waves following the atrial spikes (*arrow*). Reprinted with permission from Chan TC, Cardall TY. Electronic pacemakers. *Emerg Med Clin N Am* 2006;**24**:179–94.

by intermittent metal-to-metal contact, termed make-break signals [1]. Lead fracture, dislodgement, or loose connections within the pacemaker generator itself can cause these abnormal signals. Additional causes of oversensing include electrocautery, MRI, and extracorporeal shock wave lithotripsy [3,13,14]. On the ECG, inappropriate sensing of electrical signals that inhibit the pacemaker stimulus may or may not be seen during evaluation [1]. Clinicians can attempt to reproduce the oversensing by performing a 12-lead ECG rhythm strip while having the patient stimulate the rectus and pectoralis muscles [1]. Reprogramming of the pacemaker is usually required to eliminate oversensing [2].

Crosstalk is considered a type of oversensing in dual chamber pacemakers. It is defined as when the pacing stimulus in one chamber is sensed by the other chamber's sensors as that second chamber's own impulse [3]. A pacing spike is not generated by the ventricle leading to inadequate pacing, a potentially dangerous event for the pacemaker-dependent patient [3]. This is rectified by reprogramming the ventricular sensor to be refractory to a stimulus in the early period (12–25 ms) after atrial pacing begins [3].

Failure to sense usually represents an increase in resistance within the pacemaker circuit. Causes for this failure include fibrosis at the tip of the electrode, lead dislodgement, impending battery failure, as well as severe electrolyte abnormalities that widen the QRS and delay its upstroke [2]. In these cases where sensing is lost, competitive atrial or ventricular rhythms can be life-threatening [2].

Failure to pace: Pacemaker failure occurs when the pacemaker fails to deliver a stimulus in a situation where pacing

should occur [1]. This is due to numerous causes, including the above reviewed oversensing (most common), pacing lead problems (lead fracture or dislodgement), battery or pacemaker generator failure (rare), and electromagnetic interference (such as from MRI scanning or cellular telephones) [1]. Blunt trauma can cause pacemaker failure by damaging the pacemaker or its leads [1]. Failure to pace results in decreased or absent pacemaker function, with patients often presenting with dizziness, syncope, and lightheadedness [3].

The baseline ECG (without magnet) will have an absence of pacemaker spikes at a point at which the pacemaker spikes would be expected [1]. Malfunctions in dual-chambered pacing may be seen as isolated atrial or ventricular failure to pace [1]. In order to assess possible pacemaker output failure, the patient's heart rate must be below the preprogrammed pacer rate [2]. If the heart rate exceeds this rate, application of a magnet is useful in evaluating appropriate pacemaker function [1]. This application may also correct the problem [15].

Failure to capture: Failure to capture occurs when pacemaker output is generated but fails to depolarize myocardium [1,3]. The ECG typically shows a pacing spike without evidence of capture and depolarization (Figures 33.1, 33.10 and 33.11). This represents the malfunction in Case 1. The most common cause of failure to capture is due to exit block [1]. This usually occurs in the weeks following implantation due to maturation of tissues at the electrode-myocardium interface [1]. External cardiac defibrillation can also be responsible for exit block due to tissue damage at the electrode-myocardium interface [1]. Failure to capture may also occur due to inadequate energy generation, which is

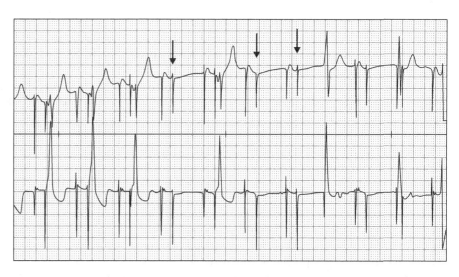

Figure 33.11 DDD pacing with intermittent loss of ventricular capture (*arrow*). After the third loss of capture event there is a junctional escape beat (*j*). In the next to last beat, a junctional escape beat is bracketed by two pacing spikes as a form of safety pacing. Rather than inhibiting ventricular pacing (and risk having no ventricular output if the sensed event were not truly a native ventricular depolarization), the AV interval is shortened and a paced output (*s*) occurs. Reprinted with permission from Chan TC, Cardall TY. Electronic pacemakers. *Emerg Med Clin N Am* 2006;**24**:179–94.

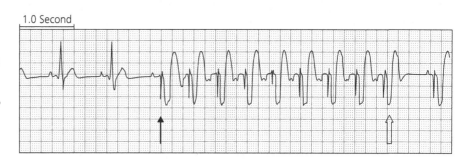

Figure 33.12 Pacemaker-mediated tachycardia. The third QRS complex is a paced beat (*narrow arrow*), and causes a retrograde P wave that triggers a run of PMT. In this case the pacemaker detects the PMT, and, in the penultimate beat (*wide arrow*), temporarily lengthens the PVARP, preventing atrial sensing of the retrograde P wave and breaking the re-entrant loop. Reprinted with permission from Chan TC, Cardall TY. Electronic pacemakers. *Emerg Med Clin N Am* 2006;**24**:179–94.

typically attributed to battery failure or from inappropriate pacemaker programming [2].

Additional sudden causes of failure to capture include lead fracture or dislodgement, electrolyte abnormalities, myocardial ischemia, insulation break, faulty connection of a lead to the pacemaker, or cardiac perforation by pacer leads (rare) [2,3]. A chest radiograph showing the lead tip out of the heart and an ECG with a paced complex with a new RBBB are suggestive of cardiac lead perforation [3]. In the setting of hyperkalemia, a progressive slowing of conduction can culminate in complete pacemaker exit block and failure to capture an isolated atrial or ventricular pacemaker, as well as a dual chamber pacemaker [16–19]. Twiddler's syndrome is a final cause of failure to capture due to a patient fidgeting with the pulse generator, resulting in the lead tip being pulled away from the myocardium [3].

Pacemaker-mediated dysrhythmias: Pacemakers usually treat or prevent dysrhythmias, but can also become a source of dysrhythmias [5]. These include pacemaker-mediated tachycardia (PMT), runaway pacemaker, dysrhythmias caused by lead dislodgement, and sensor-induced tachycardias [1]. These phenomena typically occur in dual chamber pacemakers [3].

Pacemaker-mediated tachycardia, also known as endless-loop tachycardia, results from interactions between native cardiac activity and the pacemaker [1,2]. It is a re-entry dysrhythmia that can occur where the pacemaker itself acts as a part of the re-entry circuit [1]. Initiation usually occurs by a PVC with retrograde atrial conduction, typically occurring after the pacemaker's PVARP [3]. The pacemaker senses this as a native atrial stimulus, leading to the generation of a ventricular stimulus and another retrograde P wave is produced [5]. The pacemaker acts as the antegrade conductor for the re-entrant rhythm, while the persistent retrograde conduction occurs through the intact AV node [5]. Additional triggers of PMT include oversensing of skeletal muscle myopotentials or the removal of an applied magnet [1]. The ECG will typically show a regular, ventricular paced tachycardia at a rate at or less than the maximum upper rate of the pacemaker (Figure 33.12) [1].

Fortunately, the maximum rate of PMT will not exceed the maximum tracking rate of the pacemaker (typically 160–180 bpm) [1,2]. As a result, hemodynamic instability is unlikely to occur, but tachycardia-induced ischemia may develop in the susceptible patient [2]. Treatment of PMT consists of applying the magnet to break the re-entry circuit by turning off all sensing, and then returning the pacemaker to the asynchronous mode of pacing [1]. Alternatively, PMT can be terminated by initiating ventricular-atrial conduction block with adenosine or judicious use of vagal maneuvers, which prolong retrograde and antegrade conduction through the AV node [1]. Advances in pacemaker programming that recognize and automatically terminate PMT are expected to significantly decrease the incidence of pacemaker-mediated tachycardia [1,2].

Sensor-induced tachycardias occur when pacemakers capable of rate-modulation (increase heart rate to meet physiologic demands, "R" in position IV) inappropriately pace when they are stimulated by non-physiologic parameters [1]. Non-physiologic parameters include abnormal vibrations or loud noises from the environment, sleeping on the side of the implant, fevers, hyperventilation, arm movement, or electrocautery [1]. The ECG typically shows a paced tachycardia that does not exceed the pacemaker's upper limit [1]. These are typically benign and can be terminated with the application of the magnet or cessation of the inciting event.

Runaway pacemaker is an exceedingly rare primary component failure in older-generation pacemakers [5]. Modern pacemakers typically have a preprogrammed upper rate limit that prevents this pathology [1]. Etiologies include end of the battery life or damage to the pacemaker generator from sources such as radiation [2]. This represents a true medical emergency during which inappropriately rapid stimuli can occur at rates up to 400 bpm, potentially inducing ventricular tachycardia or fibrillation [1]. The ECG typically shows a paced ventricular tachycardia as is illustrated in Case 2, often exceeding the expected maximum upper limit of an older pacemaker (Figure 33.2) [1]. Placement of a magnet may induce a slower pacing rate temporarily until interrogation and reprogramming can be achieved [1]. However, in cases where the magnet fails to slow the paced rate, the unstable patient will require emergent surgical intervention to disconnect or sever the pacemaker leads [1,2].

Pseudo-malfunction: Pacemakers have a number of normal adaptive responses that can be misinterpreted on the ECG as malfunctions [2]. *Pseudo-malfunction* can occur when pacing is actually occurring but no pacemaker spikes are seen, or when the clinician mistakenly expects the pacemaker to trigger when is it appropriately inactive [1]. The more common examples of pseudo-malfunction that have been captured on ECG include *heart blocks* mediated by the pacemaker, *hysteresis,* and *functional undersensing* [2,3].

A second-degree Type II AV block may occur with a DDD pacemaker in normal response to increasing native sinus rate [2]. The TARP is the period during which the atrium is refractory to depolarization after an atrial beat [5]. The TARP can be programmed to be longer than the upper rate-limit interval (the cardiac cycle duration at the pacemaker's maximum ventricular rate). As the native atrial rate approaches the preprogrammed upper rate limit, the duration of the cardiac cycle (P-P interval) shortens to less than the TARP [1,2].

Subsequently, every second atrial beat falls within the TARP, going undetected, resulting in a 2 : 1 block [1]. The ECG will show 2 : 1 AV block representing a normally functioning pacemaker in a patient with sinus tachycardia (Figure 33.13a) [2]. An abrupt drop in the heart rate due to the 2 : 1 block (ventricular rate is halved) may cause symptoms in active patients, requiring reprogramming for a smoother transition to a lower ventricular rate [2].

One way to help prevent the sudden reduction in ventricular pacing by DDD pacemakers as described above is to program the TARP to be shorter than the upper rate interval [5]. In this case, a second-degree Type I AV block (Wenckebach) response can occur. As the native atrial rate increases above the upper rate limit, the pacemaker senses the atrial activity. However, the pacer cannot release its ventricular stimulus faster than allowed by the upper rate interval, despite occurring after the TARP [1]. The pacemaker will wait to trigger the accompanying ventricular stimulus until the end of the upper rate limit interval [5]. On the ECG, an increasing AV delay will be seen with progressive lengthening of the PR interval until a dropped beat occurs, creating a pacemaker-mediated Wenckebach AV block (Figure 33.13b) [5]. This Wenckebach response is, once again, the result of a normally functioning pacemaker [5].

Hysteresis occurs when the interval between a sensed native QRS and paced QRS immediately following it exceeds the interval between two consecutive paced QRS complexes [3]. Hysteresis most commonly occurs in ventricular demand pacemakers [3]. Similar to oversensing, it is an attempt to allow the patient's own native rhythm to function at a rate slightly lower than the programmed pacing rate. This situation is preferred as sinus rhythm allows for atrial-ventricular synchrony and provides better physiologic function than the paced rhythm [2]. Clinicians can misinterpret this finding on the ECG as pacemaker malfunction, as the pacemaker triggers a stimulus at a rate slower than expected [2].

Functional undersensing, which is not considered a true malfunction, can occur in certain situations. If a P wave or QRS complex occurs during the pacemaker's refractory period, it will not be sensed and the pacer will fire earlier than expected [3]. Similarly, in dual chamber pacemakers, a functional complication known as "blanking" accounts for about 4% of undersensing malfunctions [3]. This refers to a period of ventricular component inactivity during the initial 12–125 ms of the AV interval, during which any intrinsic QRS complex will not be sensed [3].

Pacemaker syndrome: Classic *pacemaker syndrome* is a constellation of symptoms and signs in patients with normally functioning single chamber ventricular pacemaker systems with suboptimal pacing modes and programming [1,3]. Symptoms are vague, including shortness of breath, dizziness, fatigue, orthopnea, and confusion [2]. Signs include a drop in systolic blood pressure of 20 mmHg or greater when the patient changes from a spontaneous native rhythm to a

Figure 33.13 Pseudo-malfunction. AV block schematic for a normally functioning DDD pacemaker. (a) Sinus rate increases such that the native P-P interval is shorter than the TARP. Every other P wave occurs within the TARP and the paced QRS complex is dropped, resulting in a 2 : 1 AV block. (b) In this case, the native P-P interval is shorter than the preset upper rate-limit interval (minimum cardiac cycle duration for maximum pacemaker rate), but still longer than the TARP. Atrial activity is detected by the pacemaker, but the pacemaker cannot release its ventricular stimulus faster than the upper rate limit resulting in a progressive lengthening of the PR interval until a paced ventricular beat is dropped (Wenckebach). Reprinted with permission from Chan TC, Cardall TY. Electronic pacemakers. *Emerg Med Clin N Am* 2006;**24**:179–94.

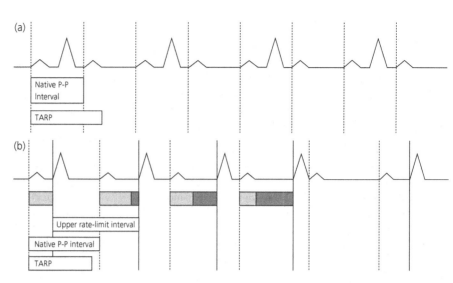

Figure 33.14 A patient with symptoms consistent with pacemaker syndrome. Note the presence of retrograde ventricular to atrial conduction (*arrows*). Inverted P waves occur after the QRS complex, suggesting AV dyssynchrony. From Harper RJ, Brady WJ, Perron AD, *et al.* The paced electrocardiogram: issues for the emergency physician. *Am J Emer Med* 2001;**19**:551–60.

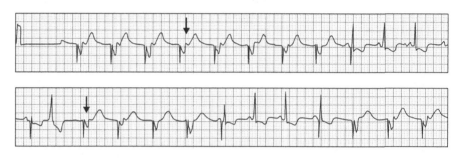

paced rhythm [1]. These occur due to loss of AV synchrony or AV dyssynchrony, resulting in unfavorable hemodynamics and decreased perfusion [1,20,21]. While this diagnosis cannot be made from the ECG alone, it can provide supporting evidence [2]. The presence of AV dyssynchrony as suggested by retrograde conduction (P waves) during ventricular pacing can result in atrial overload, which is part of the pacemaker syndrome in a symptomatic patient (Figure 33.14) [1,2].

In conclusion, clinicians with a basic understanding of pacemaker modes and function can use the ECG to assist with diagnosis of pacemaker malfunction and complications. In addition to a thorough history, physical exam and chest radiograph, the ECG is a valuable tool in evaluating and treating patients with symptoms giving concern for pacemaker malfunction in the emergency room, on the hospital floor, or in the ICU setting.

Case conclusions

In Case 1, the patient's underlying complete heart block is seen due to failure of ventricular capture from exit block. This is the most common cause of failure to capture in the weeks following implantation, due to maturation of tissues at the electrode-myocardium implantation site. A chest radiograph did not show signs of pacer lead fracture. The patient was urgently transferred to a tertiary-care facility with cardiothoracic surgery capabilities for lead repositioning and possible replacement.

In Case 2, "runaway pacemaker" is the source of this alarming presentation. Representing a true medical emergency, placement of a magnet in the ED induced a slower pacing rate temporarily until interrogation and reprogramming could be achieved. Urgent arrangements were made to transfer this patient to a tertiary-care facility with cardiothoracic surgery capabilities for possible surgical intervention to disconnect or sever the pacemaker leads if the magnet failed to keep a slow paced rate.

References

1 Chan TC, Cardall TY. Electronic Pacemakers. *Emerg Med Clin N Am* 2006;**24**:179–94.

2 Harper RJ, Brady WJ, Perron AD, *et al.* The paced electrocardiogram: issues for the emergency physician. *Am J Emer Med* 2001; **19**:551–60.

3 Sarko JA, Tiffany BR. Cardiac pacemakers: Evaluation and management of malfunctions. *Am J Emerg Med* 2004;**18**:435–40.

4 Lipman BS, Marvin D, Massie E. Arrhythmias. In: *Clinical Electrocardiography*, 7th ed. Meial, 1984.

5 Cardall TY, Chan TC. Pacemaker: abnormal function. In: *ECG in Emergency Medicine and Acute Care*. Philadelphia PA: Mosby, 2005: 136–42.

6 Gregoratos G, Abrams J, Epstein AE. ACC/AHA/NASPE 2002 Guideline Update for Implantation of Cardiac Pacemakers and Antiarrhythmia Devices: Summary Article A Report of the American College of Cardiology/American Heart Association Task Force on Practice Guidelines (ACC/AHA/NASPE Committee to Update the 1998 Pacemaker Guidelines) Committee Members. *Circulation* 2002;**106**:2145–61.

7 Bernstein AD, Camm AJ, Fisher JD, *et al.* North American Society of Pacing and Electrophysiology policy statement. The NASPE/BPEG Defibrillator Code. *Pacing Clin Electrophysiol* 1993;**16**:1776–80.

8 Poon K, Okin PM, Kligfield P. Diagnostic performance of a computer-based ECG rhythm algorithm. *J Electrocardiol* 2005;**38**: 235–8.

9 Laks MM, Sylvester RH. Computerized electrocardiography-an adjunct to the physician. *N Engl J Med* 1991;**325**:1803.

10 Guglin ME, Thatai D. Common errors in computer electrocardiogram interpretation. *Internat J Cardiol* 2006;**106**:232–7.

11 Guglin ME, Datwani N. Electrocardiograms with pacemakers: accuracy of computer reading. *J Electrocardiol* 2007;**40**:144–6.

12 Hayes DL, Vlietsstra RE. Pacemaker malfunction. *Ann Intern Med* 1993;**119**:828–35.

13 Thakur RK. Permanent cardiac pacing. In: Gibler WB, Aufderheide TP editors. *Emergency Cardiac Care*. St. Louis, MO: Mosby, 1994: 385–428.

14 Cooper D, Wilkoff B, Masterson M, *et al.* Effects of extracorporeal shock wave lithotripsy on cardiac pacemakers and its safety in patients with implanted pacemakers. *Pacing Clin Electrophysiol* 1998;**11**:1607–16.

15 Barold SS, Falkoff MD, Ong LS, *et al.* Oversensing by single-chamber pacemakers: mechanisms, diagnosis, and treatment. *Cardiol Clin* 1985;**3**:565–85.

16 Kahloon MU, Aslam AK, Aslam AF, *et al.* Hyperkalemia induced failure of atrial and ventricular pacemaker capture. *Int J Card* 2005;**105**:224–6.

17 Barold SS, Faloff MD, Ong LS, Heinle RA. Hyperkalemia induced failure of atrial capture during dual chamber cardiac pacing. *J Am Coll Cardiol* 1987;**10**:467–9.

18 Bashour TT. Spectrum of ventricular pacemaker exit block owing to hyperkalemia. *Am J Cardiol* 1986;**57**:337–8.

19 Sathyamurthy I, Krishnaswami S, Sukumar IP. Hyperkalemia induced pacemaker exit block. *Indian Heart J* 1984;**36**:176–7.

20 Ellenbogen KA, Gilligan DM, Wood MA, *et al.* The pacemaker syndrome-a matter of definition [editorial]. *Am J Cardiol* 1997; **79**:1226–9.

21 Ellenbogen KA, Stambler BS. Pacemaker syndrome. In: Ellenbogen KA, Gay GN, Wilkoff BL, editors. *Clinical Cardiac Pacing*. Philadelphia: WB Saunders, 1995:419–31.

Chapter 34 | How can the ECG guide acute therapy in the Wolff Parkinson White (WPW) patient?

Michael C. Bond
University of Maryland School of Medicine, Baltimore, MD, USA

Case presentations

Case 1: A-25-year-old male presents to the emergency department (ED) with intermittent palpitations. He is currently asymptomatic. He denies shortness of breath or chest pain when he has the palpitations, and he has not noted anything that is more likely to bring them on. He does report that they never occur during his 5-mile daily runs. He has no significant medical history, medications, or allergies. He does not smoke or chew tobacco, drink alcohol, or use illicit drugs. He is not taking anabolic steroids. His physical exam is completely normal. His 12-lead electrocardiogram (ECG) is shown in Figure 34.1.

Case 2: A 26-year-old male presents to the ED complaining of a racing heartbeat and lightheadedness, which started while he was watching television 2 h previously. The lightheadedness gets worse when he stands. His family called 911 when he had a syncopal episode while walking to the bathroom. He notes some chest tightness but denies severe pain or pressure sensation. He has no significant medical problems, has never been hospitalized, but recently had an annual examination, during which he was told there was "something wrong" with his ECG. He has not yet had an appointment with a cardiologist. He does not use alcohol, tobacco, or illicit drugs. His vital signs are remarkable for a pulse of 140 beats per minute (bpm), blood pressure of 110/60 mmHg, respiratory rate of 18 breaths/min, and oxygen saturation of 98% on room air. His examination is remarkable only for irregularly irregular tachycardia. His mental status is normal, his lungs are clear, and no jugular vein distention (JVD) is seen or murmur heard. His 12-lead ECG is shown in Figure 34.2. Laboratory studies and chest film are all normal. His cardiac enzymes are at normal levels.

Case 3: An 18-year-old male presents to the ED via ambulance after having a syncopal episode at home. Emergency medical services (EMS) personnel noted a wide complex tachycardia on the initial rhythm strip. His vital signs are as follows: blood pressure 124/76 mmHg, pulse 130 bpm, respiratory rate 18 breaths/min, and oxygenation saturation 98%. He denies chest pain and shortness of breath. He has never had hypertension, diabetes mellitus, or cardiac disease. Physical examination is remarkable only for regular tachycardia. His mental status is normal, his lungs are clear, and there is no pedal edema. His 12-lead ECG is shown in Figure 34.3. While in the ED, he has another episode of unresponsiveness and is electrically cardioverted. His 12-lead ECG after the cardioversion shows a normal sinus rhythm with a shortened PR interval, delta wave, and mildly prolonged QRS complex, consistent with the Wolff-Parkinson-White (WPW) pattern.

The ECG and acute therapy in the patient with WPW syndrome

These three patients all have evidence of pre-excitation syndrome on their ECGs. Do these patients require medical intervention? If so, can you treat them all the same? How can the ECG help you optimize treatment for each patient appropriately?

Wolff, Parkinson, and White, in their initial article published in 1930, described 11 patients with recurrent tachycardia that had a "bundle branch block with short PR interval" [1]. In 1933, Holzmann and Scherf correctly reported the mechanism of the WPW pattern as an acceleration of conduction from the atria to the ventricle, rather than a block [2]. During the past century, our understanding of WPW syndrome has continued to grow through histologic study of bypass tracts and detailed electrophysiologic studies of accessory pathways

Critical Decisions in Emergency and Acute Care Electrocardiography,
1st edition. Edited by W.J. Brady and J.D. Truwit. © 2009 Blackwell Publishing, ISBN: 9781405159067

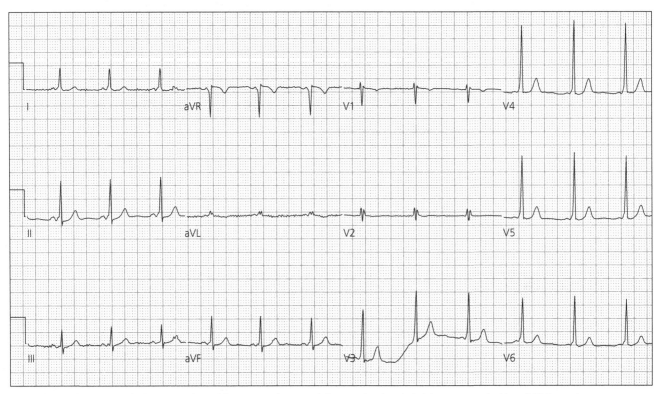

Figure 34.1 Normal sinus rhythm in a patient with WPW syndrome and shortened PR interval, delta wave, and widened QRS complex. (ECG courtesy of Amal Mattu, MD.)

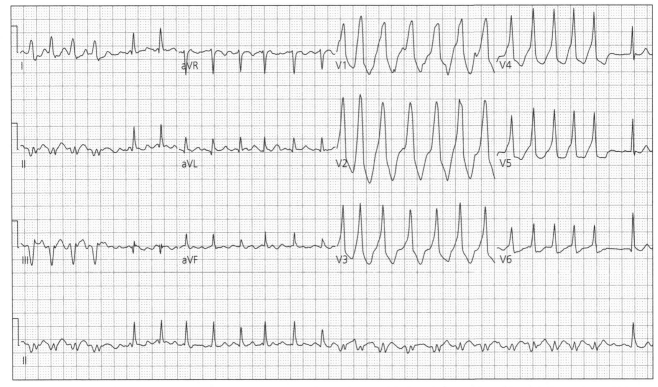

Figure 34.2 Atrial fibrillation in a patient with WPW syndrome. Note the rapid rate and the irregularly irregular, widened QRS complexes with beat-to-beat variation in the QRS complex morphology. (ECG courtesy of Amal Mattu, MD.)

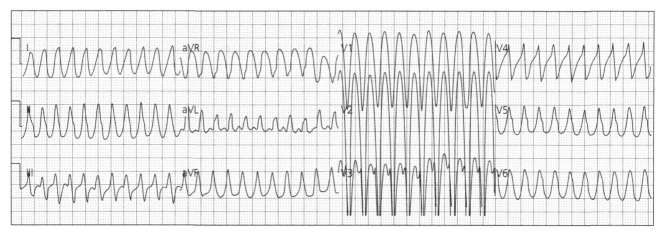

Figure 34.3 Wide QRS complex tachycardia (antidromic AVRT) in a patient with WPW syndrome. Note the widened QRS complex, very rapid rate, and delta wave. (ECG courtesy of William Brady, MD.)

and epicardial mapping techniques. The current definition of the WPW pattern is the electrocardiographic tetrad of: (1) PR interval < 0.12 s, (2) slurring and slow rise of the initial QRS complex (delta wave), (3) a widened QRS complex with a total duration > 0.10 s, and (4) secondary ST segment–T wave changes directed opposite the major delta wave and QRS complex changes. The electrocardiographic definition also includes the presence of dysrhythmia [3–5].

The 12-lead ECG has proven to be extremely important in directing the care of patients with WPW syndrome. For the acute care clinician, it can help direct which medications would be the safest for aborting an episode of paroxysmal supraventricular tachycardia (PSVT). For the electrophysiologist, the 12-lead ECG can localize the bypass tract and direct whether studies and ablation could be curative for a particular patient, whether the patient can be treated safely with medication in order to prevent episodes of PSVT, or whether the patient can be observed safely with no medical treatment.

To understand WPW syndrome, one must understand accessory pathways and the ways they can alter the normal conduction of the heart. Conduction through the accessory pathway can be antegrade (toward the ventricle) or retrograde (away from the ventricle). Most accessory pathways can conduct in both directions, but a small percentage of accessory pathways can conduct only antegrade (rare) or retrograde (approximately 15% of all pathways). Retrograde accessory pathways are considered "concealed pathways," as their effect on the conduction of the heart is not apparent on a surface 12-lead ECG [6].

In a general sense, when a patient is in sinus rhythm, accessory pathways lead to pre-excitation of the ventricle, which can be seen on the 12-lead ECG as the presence of a delta wave or shortening of the PR interval (Figure 34.4). The presence of a delta wave and the degree of shortening of the PR interval depend on two factors [4]:

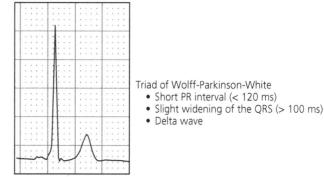

Triad of Wolff-Parkinson-White
- Short PR interval (< 120 ms)
- Slight widening of the QRS (> 100 ms)
- Delta wave

Figure 34.4 Single ECG P-QRS-T cycle in a patient with WPW syndrome. Note the shortened PR interval, delta wave, and widened QRS complex. (ECG courtesy of Amal Mattu, MD.)

(1) The location of the accessory pathway. Pathways on the left side of the AV node tend to be associated with less pre-excitation and minimal PR shortening. Bypass tracts on the right side tend to have more apparent pre-excitation.

(2) Relationship of conduction times and refractory periods of the AV node and the accessory pathway. Increases in sympathetic tone (e.g. high stress states) or decreases in vagal tone (e.g. after atropine administration) will increase conduction through the AV node and decrease the amount of pre-excitation seen on the ECG. When the patient is in a high vagal state or if the AV node is preferentially blocked by drugs such as verapamil, diltiazem, digoxin, beta-blockers, or adenosine, conduction through the accessory pathway will be relatively greater than the conduction through the AV node. In this case, pre-excitation is more pronounced. Therefore, the effect of the accessory pathway on ventricular depolarization is minimized as conduction through the AV node increases.

It is not uncommon to see intermittent pre-excitation on serial 12-lead ECGs. This intermittent finding can occur even with minimal changes in the underlying heart rate, but it is more commonly seen with changes in vagal tone or the effects of drug blockade on the AV node. Intermittent pre-excitation with minimal heart rate variability suggests that the accessory pathway has a long refractory period. An accessory pathway with a long refractory period is unlikely to be able to provoke ventricular tachycardia/fibrillation in a patient in whom atrial fibrillation develops [7].

Tachycardias can occur in patients with WPW syndrome via several mechanisms, not all of which involve use of the accessory pathway. Atrial tachycardia, sinus tachycardia, junctional tachycardia, and ventricular tachycardia can all occur with the accessory pathway as an innocent bystander. The most common tachycardias in which the accessory pathway plays a role can be more broadly classified as atrioventricular re-entrant tachycardias (AVRTs), subclassified as antidromic and orthodromic.

Antidromic AVRT occurs when the atrial impulse travels antegrade down the accessory pathway, causing ventricular depolarization, and is then conducted retrograde through the AV node to the atrium. In this condition, the ventricles are not depolarized by the normally highly efficient His-Purkinje system; therefore, antidromic AVRT is associated with regular wide complex tachycardias that are virtually indistinguishable from ventricular tachycardia. Antidromic AVRT is rare in WPW syndrome, occurring in only 5–10% of patients.

Over 90% of the AVRTs associated with WPW syndrome are orthodromic: conduction travels antegrade through the AV node to the ventricles and retrograde through the accessory pathways to the atrium. Therefore, as ventricular activation occurs through the normal conduction system, orthodromic AVRT results in a regular narrow complex tachycardia that resembles a normal PSVT. During an orthodromic AVRT, there will be no delta wave or shortened PR interval, because the accessory pathway is carrying impulses to the atrium rather than to the ventricle [2,4,8].

Atrial fibrillation (AF) occurs in approximately 20% of patients with WPW syndrome. The mechanisms are not completely clear. One theory postulates that retrograde activation of the atrium occurs during its vulnerable phase through the accessory pathway [2].

The acute care clinician must use extreme caution in treating a patient with a history of WPW syndrome who presents with tachyarrhythmia, particularly AF. In these patients, administration of a medication that preferentially blocks the AV node (calcium channel-blocker, digoxin, adenosine, beta-blocker) can increase conduction through the accessory pathway, resulting in paradoxic acceleration of the ventricular rate and induction of ventricular tachycardia or ventricular fibrillation. This response is especially true for patients with AF related to WPW syndrome. Amiodarone, which has calcium channel-blocking and beta-blocking effects, is also best avoided in patients with AF and WPW syndrome.

Electrocardiographic findings suggestive of WPW syndrome

Wolff-Parkinson-White syndrome should be considered in any patient who has a short PR interval (< 0.12 s), a slurred upstroke of the QRS complex (the delta wave), and a QRS complex duration > 0.10 s. This condition should also be considered in any patient who presents with narrow complex supraventricular tachycardia (SVT) with a rate greater than 140 bpm. The AV node will generally limit SVT to less than 180 bpm. If the rate greatly exceeds this value, one must consider AVRT. The rate of SVT caused by WPW syndrome is usually between 140 and 250 bpm. One electrocardiographic finding in narrow complex tachycardia that strongly suggests an accessory pathway and orthodromic conduction is an inverted P wave buried in the late part of QRS complex, the ST segment, or the T wave [4,9]. As the accessory pathway is being used for retrograde conduction to the atrium, classic electrocardiographic signs of pre-excitation will not be found reliably (Figure 34.5). Having the luxury of a baseline ECG that shows classic signs of a WPW pattern would support the diagnosis. This form of AVRT is difficult to distinguish from AVNRT, the typical PSVT; fortunately, management strategies are similar for both dysrhythmias.

The wide complex tachycardias seen in patients with WPW syndrome (antidromic conduction) can be extremely difficult to differentiate from ventricular tachycardia (VT) and, more importantly, polymorphic VT (PVT). Polymorphic VT and AF associated with WPW syndrome can appear very similar, with alternating wide QRS complexes and variable R-R intervals. However, AF associated with WPW syndrome will generally have a stable electrocardiographic axis compared with the changing axis found in PVT. Table 34.1 summarizes the differences between the three major causes of irregular, wide complex tachyarrhythmias: PVT, AF associated with WPW, and AF associated with a bundle branch block.

Depending on the location of the accessory pathway, WPW syndrome can produce electrocardiographic changes similar to left ventricular hypertrophy and myocardial infarction. Table 34.2 lists the changes seen on the ECG depending on the site of the accessory pathway [10,11]. Figure 34.6 shows an ECG with a pseudo-inferior wall infarction pattern. In the setting of chest pain, these electrocardiographic changes need to be assumed to be ischemic, and serial enzymes should be obtained at a minimum.

How to predict whether the patient is at low risk for sudden death?

One of the greatest concerns is the patient's risk for sudden cardiac death due to arrhythmia. The 12-lead ECG can help

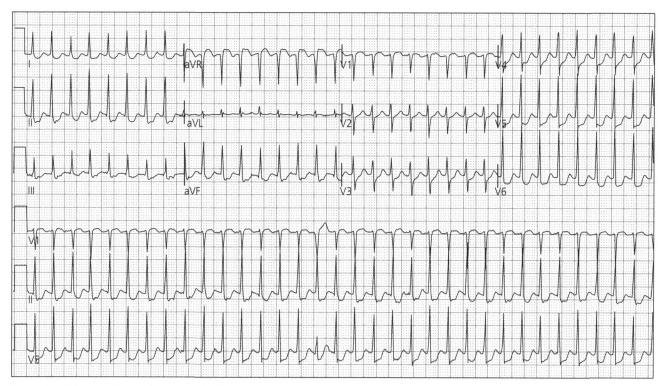

Figure 34.5 Narrow QRS complex tachycardia (orthodromic AVRT) in a patient with WPW syndrome. (ECG courtesy of Amal Mattu, MD.)

Table 34.1 Comparison of irregular wide complex tachycardias

Atrial fibrillation with WPW syndrome	Polymorphic ventricular tachycardia	Atrial fibrillation with bundle branch block (BBB)
Rapid rate (> 200 bpm)	Rapid rate (180–280 bpm)	Rate usually < 180 bpm
Irregular rhythm (variable R-R interval)	Irregular rhythm	Irregular rhythm
Wide bizarre* QRS complexes	Wide bizarre QRS complexes	Wide QRS complexes consistent with BBB; complexes demonstrate minimal, if any, changes in morphology
Stable axis	Undulating axis	Stable axis

*Bizarre, changing in shape and morphology

Table 34.2 Electrocardiographic changes depending on location of the accessory pathway

Accessory pathway location	Change seen on ECG
Right-sided	Increased R-wave amplitude in left-side limb leads, simulating left ventricular hypertrophy
Left-sided	Increased R waves in right precordial leads, simulating right ventricular hypertrophy
Right lateral	Prominent Q waves in right precordial leads, simulating an anteroseptal infarction
Left lateral	Prominent Q waves in lateral limb leads, simulating a high lateral infarction
Posteroseptal	Prominent Q waves in inferior limb leads, simulating inferior infarction

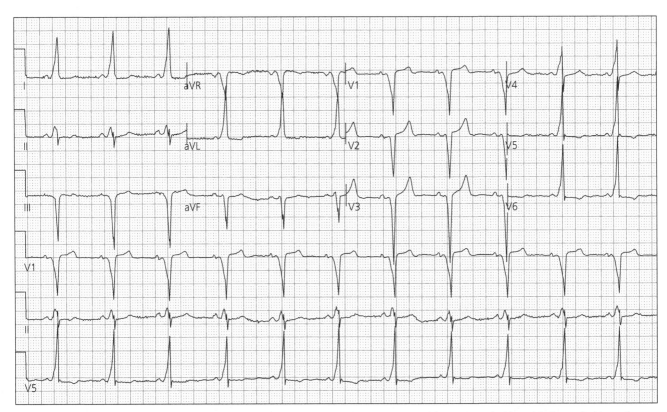

Figure 34.6 Normal sinus rhythm in a patient with WPW syndrome and shortened PR interval, delta wave, and widened QRS complex. Note the "pseudo-infarction" findings, including ST segment and T wave changes as well as Q waves caused by abnormal repolarization, not by coronary ischemia or infarction. (ECG courtesy of Amal Mattu, MD.)

to determine the risk. Patients who have intermittent pre-excitation with minimal heart rate variation are considered low risk, as this constellation of findings predicts a long refractory period for the accessory pathway. The same is true for pre-excitation that disappears with exercise and an increased heart rate. A final non-invasive test that can be performed, but not likely by a physician who is not an electrophysiologist, is the administration of intravenous procainamide (10 mg/kg over 5 min). Complete block of the accessory pathway by the procainamide suggests a long refractory period; in contrast, failure to produce a complete block in the accessory pathway suggests a short anterograde refractory period and an increased risk of sudden death. Intravenous procainamide testing is not recommended in the ED, because it can lead to complete heart block that could require temporary cardiac pacing [12].

Can the ECG guide acute therapy in the patient with WPW syndrome?

Any patient presenting with tachydysrhythmia associated with hemodynamic instability, as evidenced by ischemic chest pain, respiratory distress due to pulmonary edema, syncope, or altered mental status, should be considered for synchronized direct current cardioversion.

When assessing a hemodynamically stable patients with tachydysrhythmias and WPW syndrome, the acute care clinician should separate rhythms possibly related to WPW syndrome into three basic groups: regular, narrow QRS complex tachycardia; irregular, wide QRS complex tachycardia; and regular wide QRS complex tachycardia.

Patients with regular, narrow QRS complex tachycardia are experiencing orthodromic AVRT. Three basic treatment options are available for hemodynamically stable patients with this type of rhythm: vagal maneuvers can be attempted first; if they are not successful, medication can be administered; last, direct current cardioversion remains an option. Atrioventricular nodal blocking agents (e.g. adenosine, beta-blocking agents, and calcium antagonists) are all reasonable treatment options for the stable patient. The concern regarding the use of AV nodal blocking agents for patients with WPW syndrome and an orthodromic AVRT does not exist to any significant extent; this concern is greatest in patients with WPW syndrome who present with atrial flutter, atrial fibrillation, or the antidromic form of AVRT.

The treatment of patients with wide QRS complex tachycardia, either regular or irregular, should follow similar, initial strategies as with the narrow complex AVRT. If the patient is unstable, immediate electrical therapy is indicated.

If the patient is stable, then further rhythm distinction is necessary. If the rhythm is regular, then antidromic AVRT is likely and parenteral procainamide or amiodarone is indicated. Atrial fibrillation with WPW is the likely dysrhythmia in a patient presenting with a wide QRS complex and irregularly irregular rhythm. Intravenous procainamide or ibutilide is the best treatment. Of course, in either presentation, if the patient does not respond to the initial medical therapy or becomes unstable, electrical cardioversion should be considered. In most wide complex rhythms, regardless of regularity, AV nodal blocking agents (adenosine, beta-blocking agents, and calcium antagonists) should be avoided in that ventricular fibrillation has been reported in these patients.

Adenosine is generally safe and is an ideal drug to treat AVNRT (i.e. the non-WPW PSVT) and AVRT (the WPW PSVT). However, it has been responsible for inducing ventricular fibrillation in patients with WPW syndrome, particularly in the setting of wide complex tachycardia and atrial fibrillation [13]. Adenosine should be used with caution if there is any evidence of pre-excitation on the initial 12-lead ECG. It is not recommended in the diagnosis or treatment of any irregularly irregular or wide QRS complex tachycardias if the patient is known to have, or is suspected of having, WPW syndrome.

The safest drugs to use in patients with WPW syndrome, whether there is a narrow complex, a wide complex, or an irregular tachycardia, are procainamide and ibutilide. Atrial fibrillation and the wide complex form of AVRT are best managed with either of these agents. The intravenous procainamide dose is 50–100 mg every 2 min to a maximum dose of 17 mg/kg; the ibutilide dose is 0.01 mg/kg (maximum, 1 mg) over 10 min [14,15]. Ibutilide may be the ideal drug for AF associated with WPW syndrome in the acute setting because it has a short half-life (4 h), it does not require hepatic or renal dosing adjustments, it does not interact with other medications typically used for rate control, and it significantly prolongs the refractory period of the accessory pathway and decreases the ventricular response [16]. The main concern with ibutilide is that it has been associated with torsade de pointes due to QT prolongation, a complication that may occur in up to 5% of patients. Patients who are young and have a normal ejection fraction are at low risk for this potentially fatal arrhythmia.

Amiodarone is recommended by the American Heart Association in its 2005 ACLS guidelines [17] for the control of rapid ventricular rate caused by accessory pathway conduction in pre-excited atrial arrhythmias (Class IIB). However, parenteral amiodarone has its greatest effect on the SA and AV nodes and little effect on the accessory pathway [14]. Numerous case reports have shown that IV amiodarone has also been associated with ventricular fibrillation or an increase in the ventricular rate [18]. Parenteral amiodarone is best avoided in patients with WPW syndrome with AF and the wide complex form of AVRT.

Case conclusions

The 25-year-old in Case 1 with a history of intermittent palpitations has evidence of pre-excitation on his ECG. His report that he never experienced any episodes while exercising hints at a short refractory period in his accessory pathway, which is protective against fatal arrhythmias. The patient was discharged from the ED and referred to an electrophysiologist for further evaluation.

The 26-year-old in Case 2 presented to the ED with a history of palpitations and syncope. His ECG (Figure 34.2) showed AF associated with Wolff-Parkinson-White syndrome. This patient was treated with procainamide and admitted for catheter ablation therapy, which was successful. Had he become unstable, he would have been treated immediately with direct current cardioversion.

The 18-year-old in Case 3 presented to the ED after having a syncopal episode at home. His ECG showed wide complex tachycardia that responded to direct current cardioversion after he had another episode of unresponsiveness in the emergency department. A repeat ECG showed normal sinus rhythm (NSR) with WPW syndrome. Due to the severity of his symptoms, this patient was admitted to the hospital for an electrophysiology study and catheter ablation of his accessory pathway. In consultation with cardiology, he was started on procainamide while in the ED, with the goal of preventing further recurrences.

Acknowledgment

The author thanks Linda J. Kesselring, MS, ELS, for copyediting the manuscript.

References

1 Wolff L, Parkinson J, White PD. Bundle-branch block with short PR interval in healthy young people prone to paroxysmal tachycardia. *Am Heart J* 1930;**5**:685–704.

2 Al-Khatib SM, Pritchett EL. Clinical features of Wolff-Parkinson-White syndrome. *Am Heart J* 1999;**138**(3 Pt 1):403–13.

3 Dovgalyuk J, Holstege C, Mattu A, Brady WJ. The electrocardiogram in the patient with syncope. *Am J Emerg Med* 2007;**25**(6): 688–701.

4 Jayam VKS, Calkins H. Supraventricular tachycardia: AV nodal reentry and Wolff-Parkinson-White syndrome. In: Fuster V *et al.*, editors. *Hurst's the Heart.* 11th ed. New York: McGraw-Hill, 2004.

5 Rosner MH, Brady WJ Jr, Kefer MP, Martin ML. Electrocardiography in the patient with the Wolff-Parkinson-White syndrome: diagnostic and initial therapeutic issues. *Am J Emerg Med* 1999; **17**(7):705–14.

6 Ross DL, Uther JB. Diagnosis of concealed accessory pathways in supraventricular tachycardia. *Pacing Clin Electrophysiol* 1984;**7** (6 Pt 1):1069–85.

7 Klein GJ, Gulamhusein SS. Intermittent preexcitation in the Wolff-Parkinson-White syndrome. *Am J Cardiol* 1983;**52**(3): 292–6.

8 Keating L, Morris FP, Brady WJ. Electrocardiographic features of Wolff-Parkinson-White syndrome. *Emerg Med J* 2003;**20**(5):491–3.

9 Keating GM, Goa KL. Nesiritide: a review of its use in acute decompensated heart failure. *Drugs* 2003;**63**(1):47–70.

10 Khan IA, Shaw IS. Pseudo ventricular hypertrophy and pseudo myocardial infarction in Wolff-Parkinson-White syndrome. *Am J Emerg Med* 2000;**18**(7):807–9.

11 Khan IA, Shaw IS. Pseudo myocardial infarction and pseudo ventricular hypertrophy ECG patterns in Wolff-Parkinson-White syndrome. *Am J Emerg Med* 2000;**18**(7):802–6.

12 Wellens HJ, Rodriguez LM, Timmermans C, Smeets JP. The asymptomatic patient with the Wolff-Parkinson-White electrocardiogram. *Pacing Clin Electrophysiol* 1997;**20**(8 Pt 2):2082–6.

13 Gupta AK, Shah CP, Maheshwari A, *et al.* Adenosine induced ventricular fibrillation in Wolff-Parkinson-White syndrome. *Pacing Clin Electrophysiol* 2002;**25**(4 Pt 1):477–80.

14 Fengler BT, Brady WJ, Plautz CU. Atrial fibrillation in the Wolff-Parkinson-White syndrome: ECG recognition and treatment in the ED. *Am J Emerg Med* 2007;**25**(5):576–83.

15 Fuster V, Ryden LE, Asinger RW, *et al.* ACC/AHA/ESC guidelines for the management of patients with atrial fibrillation: executive summary. A Report of the American College of Cardiology/American Heart Association Task Force on Practice Guidelines and the European Society of Cardiology Committee for Practice Guidelines and Policy Conferences (Committee to Develop Guidelines for the Management of Patients with Atrial Fibrillation): developed in Collaboration with the North American Society of Pacing and Electrophysiology. *J Am Coll Cardiol* 2001;**38**(4):1231–66.

16 Glatter KA, Dorostkar PC, Yang Y, *et al.* Electrophysiological effects of ibutilide in patients with accessory pathways. Circulation 16 2001;**104**(16):1933–9.

17 2005 American Heart Association Guidelines for Cardiopulmonary Resuscitation and Emergency Cardiovascular Care. *Circulation* 13 2005;**112** (24 Suppl):IV1–203.

18 Tijunelis MA, Herbert ME. Myth: intravenous amiodarone is safe in patients with atrial fibrillation and Wolff-Parkinson-White syndrome in the emergency department. *CJEM* 2005;**7**(4):262–5.

Chapter 35 | What is the role of the ECG in PEA cardiac arrest scenarios?

Colin G. Kaide
The Ohio State University, Columbus, OH, USA

Case presentations

Case 1: A 38-year-old female presents to the emergency department (ED), via paramedics, in cardiac arrest. She was found by a clinic nurse sitting in her car in the parking lot of her orthopedic doctor's office after a follow-up appointment for an ankle fracture. On arrival of emergency medical services (EMS), the patient is minimally responsive with a blood pressure (BP) of 40/P and a heart rate of 120. Her respiratory rate is about 30 and shallow. She is not able to give any additional information. She is orotracheally intubated with IV placement through which she receives a 500 cc bolus of normal saline. Shortly after arrival to the ED, a 12-lead ECG is obtained (Figure 35.1). A few minutes later the patient becomes pulseless with the monitor showing a heart rate of 140 bpm; cardiopulmonary resuscitation (CPR) is initiated. The patient appears to be in pulseless electric activity (PEA) arrest. A transient pulse is regained after 1 mg of epinephrine is given. A bedside ultrasound shows a rapidly beating heart with a dilated right ventricle. No pulse is palpable and the ultrasound shows no pulsation in the aorta both with and without CPR in progress.

Case 2: A 29-year-old female with a history of systemic lupus erythematosus arrives in the ED after a syncopal event. She complains of shortness of breath and lightheadedness. She has been experiencing a severe lupus flare, and is under the care of her rheumatologist who placed her on prednisone. She is alert and oriented times three with a BP of 100/85 mmHg, a pulse of 140 bpm and a respiration rate of 40 breaths/min. The patient is diaphoretic and complains primarily of shortness of breath, which has been getting worse over the last few days. During the course of her extended ED visit, her condition deteriorates and she becomes unconscious. Her most recent set of vital signs show a BP of 50/40 mmHg, a pulse of 160 bpm and a respiratory rate of 40 breaths/min. An ECG was done on arrival to the ED. Leads I and II are demonstrated in Figure 35.2.

Case 3: A 65-year-old male presents to the ED by EMS, confused and lethargic, after he was found on the floor of his home by a neighbor who said that she had not seen him in the last few days, and he did not answer his phone or the doorbell. She entered his home and found him on the kitchen floor, where it appears that he may have fallen from a step stool. On ED arrival his initial blood pressure was noted at 200/125 mmHg with a pulse of 30 bpm and a respiratory rate of 22 breaths/min. The patient is intubated using the rapid sequence induction (RSI) technique with succinylcholine. Within 2 min of the intubation, the patient develops cardiac arrest with no detectable pulse; however, a wide complex bradycardia is seen on the monitor (Figure 35.3). Cardiopulmonary resuscitation is initiated.

The ECG in the PEA arrest scenario

These cases all represent PEA arrest with different causes and different manifestations. In at least one of the cases, a bedside ultrasound was available to document a clearly beating heart, despite any detectable perfusion. The ECG findings in each case should help to narrow the differential diagnosis and suggest a possible cause for the PEA arrest.

Pulseless electric activity is characterized by co-ordinated electrical activity generated by the endogenous cardiac pacemaker with no detectable evidence of perfusion. The overall prognosis for patients with PEA is poor, unless a rapidly reversible cause is identified and corrected. The detection of PEA prompts the need for a rapid search for possible causes, and the goals of therapy are aimed at correcting a reversible cause while attempting to maintain perfusion. In some cases of PEA, the ECG can help to identify a precipitating cause that may suggest a specific therapy. These ECGs most likely will have been obtained prior to the PEA arrest and have certain findings that may imply an underlying etiology.

Critical Decisions in Emergency and Acute Care Electrocardiography, 1st edition. Edited by W.J. Brady and J.D. Truwit. © 2009 Blackwell Publishing, ISBN: 9781405159067

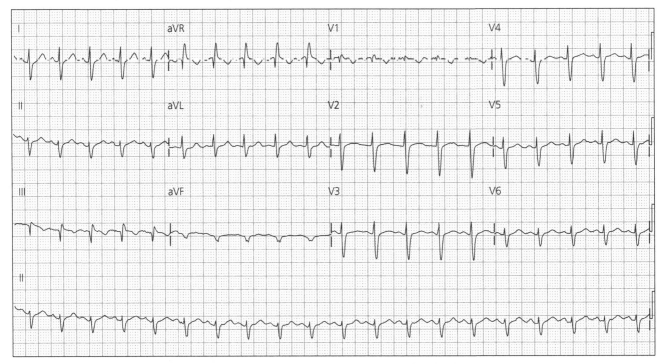

Figure 35.1 Sinus tachycardia. The ECG also demonstrates a rightward axis.

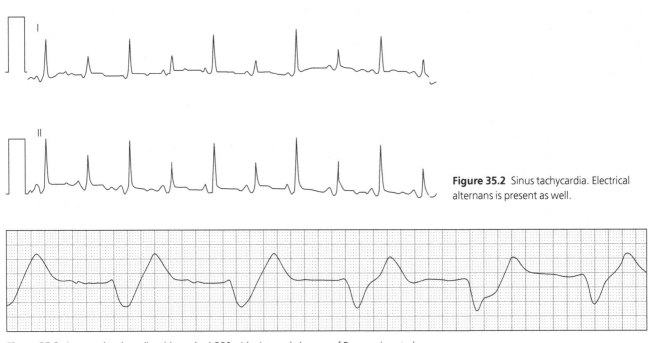

Figure 35.2 Sinus tachycardia. Electrical alternans is present as well.

Figure 35.3 A severe bradycardia with marked QRS widening and absence of P waves is noted.

Pathophysiology

Understanding the underlying mechanisms that can produce PEA is very useful in that it will allow one to consider the potential causes, predict ECG abnormalities, and understand possible treatments. Pulseless electric activity was originally termed electromechanical dissociation (EMD), indicating that the heart showed no mechanical activity during this type of arrest situation despite an electrical rhythm. Studies using echocardiography along with intravascular manometry have demonstrated, in certain patients, the presence of limited cardiac wall and valve motion, along with small arterial pulse pressures during PEA arrest [1–3]. This presentation may practically be called pseudo-PEA. The differentiation between pseudo-PEA and true PEA may be very useful in that it allows one to understand the cause and direct therapy.

Pseudo-PEA occurs in the absence of true electromechanical uncoupling of myocardial cells [4]. In this case, the causes may be related to inadequate preload to fill the heart or some type of mechanical obstruction that interrupts the flow of blood into or out of the heart. Pseudo-PEA causes may include profound hypovolemia, pericardial tamponade, tension pneumothorax or pulmonary embolism. Additionally, rupture of the myocardial wall or of a papillary muscle may produce the same pulselessness, despite preserved electrical activity. In general, the ECG complexes will usually be narrow with a fast rate in cases of pseudo-PEA. Eventually, with continued arrest, the pseudo-PEA becomes true PEA when the depleted myocardium ceases to contract; the ECG likely will demonstrate a slower, wide QRS complex rhythm – essentially, a premortal event.

True EMD represents an uncoupling of the electrical activity and contraction of the myocardial cells such that contraction ceases. The mechanism is not well understood but may represent profound energy depletion of the myocardium [4]. Causes include hypothermia, hyper/hypokalemia, hypoxia/ischemia, acidosis, and certain drug overdoses. Owing to global myocardial dysfunction, including conduction abnormalities, the ECG complexes will usually be wide and mostly bradycardic.

There is, of course, a connection between true and pseudo-PEA. This connection can be described as the PEA feedback loop [5]. Decreased preload or obstruction to forward flow decreases perfusion to the coronary arteries and the remainder of the body. This hypoperfusion in turn leads to ischemia and acidosis, causing worsening myocardial function and decreased perfusion, and so on. Thus, pseudo-PEA will transform into true PEA if the process is not interrupted.

PEA differential diagnosis

The importance of having a limited differential diagnosis in the PEA scenario (Tables 35.1 and 35.2) is to rapidly identify any treatable causes for the PEA and make an attempt to reverse the process as rapidly as possible.

Table 35.1 Common etiologies of PEA arrest scenario

The "5Hs and 5Ts" of PEA	
Hypoxia	Tension
Hypovolemia	Tamponade
Hypothermia	Thrombus
Hyperkalemia	Toxin
Heart attack	Test other pulses

*Make sure that other pulses are also absent

Table 35.2 Mnemonic for etiologies of PEA

ME HATTTE ODs	
M	Massive MI
E	Electrolytes
H	Hypovolemia/Hypoxia
A	Acidosis
T	Tension
T	Tamponade
T	Temperature (Hypothermia)
E	Embolism
ODs	Overdoses

Specific causes of PEA

In this section, different causes of PEA will be presented along with ECGs that represent common findings that may be seen in the various conditions. Certain ECG changes when coupled with the correct clinical scenario can point the clinician toward or away from a particular diagnosis. Additionally, the presence of certain findings on the ECG rhythm strip obtained during PEA correlated with outcome. In a large series of over 500 patients with out-of-hospital PEA arrests, certain findings on the field and ED ECGs correlated with the ability to regain spontaneous circulation. Faster initial rates, the presence of P waves (organized atrial activity) and shorter QRS and QT intervals predicted a higher likelihood of resuscitation. Patients in PEA showing second- or third-degree AV block, atrial fibrillation or slow, wide complex rhythms without atrial activity were least likely to have a return to spontaneous circulation [6].

True PEA

Massive myocardial infarction: Myocardial infarctions (MIs) cause substantial ischemia to the myocardium and can result in significant damage to impair the ability of the affected segment to contract effectively. If a large enough portion of the heart is affected, PEA may result [5]. A study, reviewing the postmortem examination of patients dying of a PEA arrest, identified myocardial ischemia as the cause in 44% [7].

Additionally, malignant arrhythmias such as ventricular fibrillation (VF) are highly metabolically active, rapidly consuming the limited supply of energy substrate and ATP [8]. If there is a considerable delay in restoring a normal electrical rhythm, the heart muscle may experience severe dysfunction, impairing contraction – classically called myocardial stunning. Pulseless electric activity has been reported in up to 60% of patients who were defibrillated to an organized rhythm [9].

Electrolyte abnormality: Various electrolyte abnormalities, when at their extremes, can produce PEA. When this happens, there may be a relatively long period of time in which progressive, characteristic ECG changes occur. Eventually, the ability of the myocardium to contract becomes compromised and PEA may result.

Often, the interplay between the various electrolyte derangements plays an important role in the various pathologic arrhythmias that may develop. Multiple electrolyte problems are especially problematic in the face of certain drug toxicities (digoxin, tricyclic anti-depressants, calcium channel-antagonists, and beta-adrenergic-blocking agents). The most notable electrolyte problems that can lead to PEA are hypokalemia and hyperkalemia. The presence of other electrolyte problems (calcium and magnesium) can exacerbate the problem.

Potassium extremes – hypokalemia and hyperkalemia: The more common of the potassium derangements that can result in profound inability of the heart to contract is hyperkalemia. There is a classic progression of ECG findings that strongly suggest hyperkalemia (see Table 35.4 and Figures 35.6 and 35.7). The classic electrocardiographic findings of hyperkalemia include peaked T waves, flattened P waves, prolonged PR interval (first-degree heart block), widened QRS complex, deepened S waves, merging of S and T waves, sine-wave pattern, idioventricular rhythm, ventricular tachycardia and fibrillation, and asystole. These changes represent a progression that roughly parallels the rise in potassium. Aggressive treatment to reverse hyperkalemia is indicated.

Pulseless electric activity can result from hypokalemia; however, extremely low levels of potassium would be necessary [10]. The effects of hypokalemia on the ECG are listed in Table 35.3 and demonstrated in Figures 35.4 and 35.5.

Table 35.3 ECG changes in hypokalemia

Ventricular arrythmias
Prolongation of the QT interval
ST segment depression
T wave flattening
Appearance of U waves
TU wave fusion

Table 35.4 ECG changes of hyperkalemia

Peaked T waves
Flattened P waves
Prolonged PR interval (first-degree heart block)
Widened QRS complex
Deepened S waves
Merging of S and T waves
Sine-wave pattern
Idioventricular rhythms
Asystole

The various electrocardiographic findings in the patient with significant hypokalemia include prolongation of the QT interval, ST segment depression, T wave flattening, appearance of U waves, T-U wave fusion, and ventricular arrhythmias. These ECG abnormalities, as well as the hypokalemic effects on the heart, are exacerbated in patients using digoxin.

Hypoxia: Pulmonary causes resulting in respiratory failure and hypoxia may be the cause of PEA in 20–53% of cases [7,11]. Respiratory etiologies represent the most frequent class of PEA causes. Respiratory failure, leading to tissue hypoxia and acidosis, can frequently be reversed by aggressive intervention. Electrocardiogram findings in hypoxia

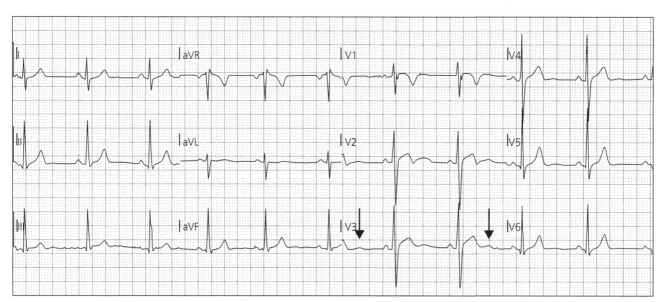

Figure 35.4 Hypokalemia with U waves (arrows).

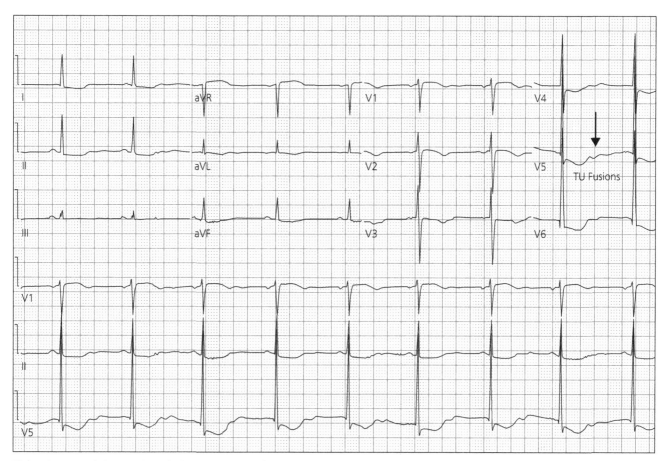

Figure 35.5 Hypokalemia with TU fusions. The U wave of hypokalemia may sometimes blend or "fuse" to the end of the T wave, a finding often referred to as "T-U fusion."

Table 35.5 Possible ECG findings in hypoxia

Sinus tachycardia
Progressive sinus bradycardia
Evidence of myocardial ischemia
COPD findings
Changes possibly seen in PE

depend heavily on the underlying cause. Findings can range from simple sinus tachycardia initially, to changes indicative of chronic obstructive pulmonary disease (COPD), to evidence of myocardial ischemia (see Table 35.5). As hypoxia worsens, profound bradycardia develops. Findings which may support the diagnosis of pulmonary embolism may be seen in some cases. Pulmonary embolism is discussed in a separate section.

Acidosis: Profound metabolic or respiratory acidosis has been shown to produce decreases in myocardial contractility [5]. Changes in the ECG seen in acidosis may reflect the underlying pathology which is producing the acidosis – in other words, there are no specific electrocardiographic findings suggestive of profound acidosis.

Hypothermia: Hypothermia is defined as a core temperature less than 95 °F or 35 °C. As the core temperature drops below 90 °F/32 °C, the hypothermic patient goes from an excitatory stage of sinus tachycardia to a bradycardic rate. At 82 °F/28 °C, the heart rate may drop by as much as 50%. Additionally, slow atrial fibrillation becomes common below 90 °F. As the core temperature continues to fall, the PR interval, QRS complex, and QT interval all become progressively prolonged. At temperatures below 77 °F/25 °C, ventricular fibrillation, asystole, and PEA are possible.

Along with the widening of the ECG complexes, a classic finding in hypothermia is the Osborn wave, or J wave, which appears in up to 80% of patients at core temperatures below 95 °F/35 °C (Figure 35.8). The Osborn wave becomes larger with decreasing temperature and can be seen in all ECG leads if the patient is very cold – body temperatures less than 95 °F/35 °C [12]. Studies suggest that the Osborn wave results from cold-induced delayed closing of the outward potassium channel current of the heart's epicardium [13]. This abnormality resolves as the patient warms. The Osborn wave is not pathognomonic for hypothermia as it can also appear in hypercalcemia, cerebral injury, and autonomic dysfunction.

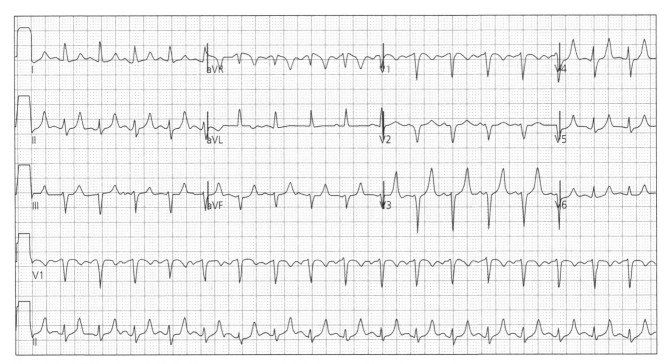

Figure 35.6 Mild hyperkalemia. Peaked T waves are present, but the P waves and intervals are normal.

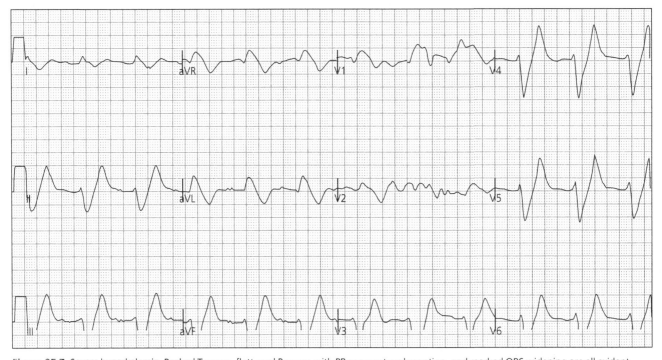

Figure 35.7 Severe hyperkalemia. Peaked T waves, flattened P waves with PR segment prolongation, and marked QRS widening are all evident.

Medication overdose

Tricyclic anti-depressants (TCA): Patients who overdose on TCAs are well known to develop rapid neurologic and hemodynamic decompensation: they may be alert and talking one moment and may develop status epilepticus or complete cardiovascular collapse moments later. Pulseless electric activity may be the result of profound vasodilation along with direct toxic effects on the myocardium.

Tricyclic anti-depressants have many complex pharmacologic actions, many of which have cardiovascular implications. The most important for this discussion are anti-cholinergic effects, and blockade of cardiac fast sodium channels. These

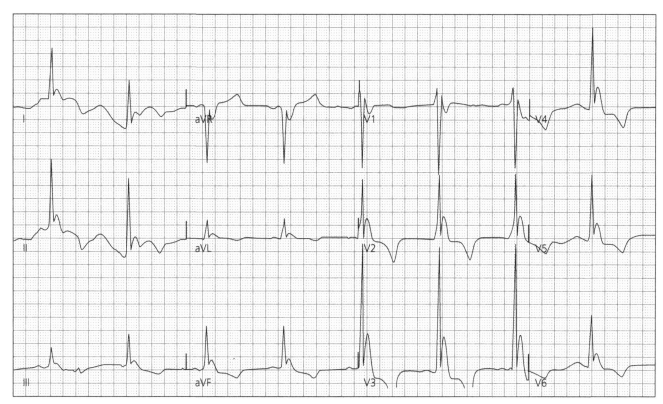

Figure 35.8 Hypothermia. Upward deflections at the terminal portion of the QRS complexes, termed Osborn waves or J waves, are noted. These Osborn waves are most obvious in the precordial leads and resolve with warming.

effects create the ECG changes seen in TCA poisoning [14] (Table 35.6 and Figure 35.9). The most specific ECG finding in TCA overdose is the presence of a rightward deviation of the vector of the terminal 40 ms of the QRS complex; this rightward shift occurs between 130° and 207°. This right-ward shift produces an R or R′ wave in the terminal 40 ms of the QRS in lead aVr and an S wave in lead I. It is postulated that the right ventricular conduction system is more suscep-tible than the left to TCA effects. The presence of this finding had shown a sensitivity for TCA toxicity ranging from 83 to 100% and a specificity of 63 to 98% [15]. The treatment of TCA overdose with sodium bicarbonate leads to fairly rapid reversal of many of the ECG findings and their clinical conse-quences [16]. The presence of a wide QRS complex, rather than tachycardia, is the indication for sodium bicarbonate administration.

Digoxin: Although death from massive digoxin (and other digitalis preparations and plant sources) overdose is usually from conduction system impairment and ventricular arrhy-thmias, approximately 10% of deaths result from acute left ventricular dysfunction – resulting in PEA arrest. Owing to its primary inhibition effect of the Na/K-ATPase on myocardial calcium channels, potassium moves to the extracellular space resulting in hyperkalemia. Electrocardiogram changes characteristic of hyperkalemia may also be seen, further

Table 35.6 Possible ECG findings in TCA Overdose

Rhythm problems
Sinus tachycardia
Atrial dysrhythmias
   Atrial and AV junctional tachycardias
   Atrial fibrillation
   Atrial flutter
   Bradycardia
Ventricular dysrhythmias
   PVCs
   Idioventricular rhythm
   Ventricular tachycardia
   Ventricular fibrillation
   Torsade de pointes
Asystole

Other ECG findings
Non-specific ST or T wave changes
PR, QRS, QT interval prolongation
Right bundle branch block
Right axis deviation
   R wave in AVR with S wave in I
AV nodal block
Brugada-type changes (ST elevation in V1–V3 and right bundle branch block)

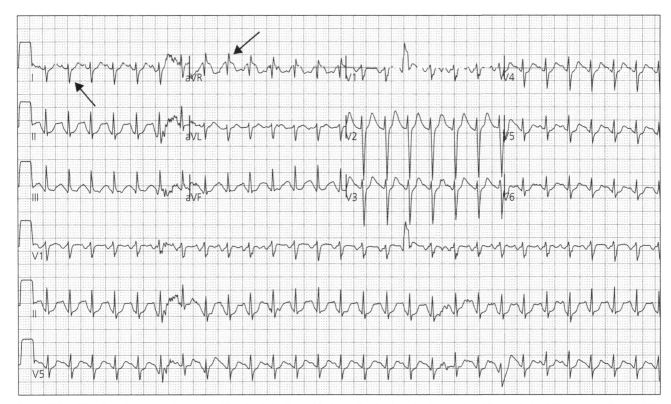

Figure 35.9 Tricyclic antidepressant overdose. The classic findings of tachycardia, rightward axis, prominent S wave in lead I (large arrow) and tall R wave in aVR (small arrow) are present.

complicating the cardiovascular toxicity. Treatment of the resultant hyperkalemia with calcium in the face of digoxin toxicity may result in increased calcium influx intracellularly. There have been two human cases of reported myocardial tetany producing asystole – the so-called stone heart – with calcium boluses in digoxin toxicity. The cause of death in these cases was unclear and inconclusive. "Stone heart" as a cause of PEA, if it occurs at all, is extremely rare and has been highly inconsistent in studies looking at the interaction of digoxin and calcium, likely relegating this issue to the myth category [17].

Any arrhythmia is possible with digoxin toxicity [18] (see Table 35.7). The most common abnormal finding on the ECG in digoxin overdose is premature ventricular contractions, and the most common arrhythmias are an accelerated junctional rhythm (often in the presence of atrial fibrillation and complete heart block; Figure 35.10) and paroxysmal atrial tachycardias with variable AV block. Multiple different arrhythmias can occur simultaneously. The combination of conduction blockade with enhanced automaticity clearly describes the rhythm disturbances seen in digoxin toxicity. Digoxin immune Fab (antigen binding fragments) should be considered in patients with PEA and digoxin toxicity.

Beta-adrenergic and calcium channel-blockers: Beta-adrenergic and calcium channel-blockers can be considered together because of similar effects on the cardiovascular

Table 35.7 ECG findings in digoxin overdose

ECG findings with digoxin use

PR interval prolongation

QT interval shortening

Inverted/flattened T waves with "scooped" ST segments (often referred to as the "Salvador Dali" or "digoxin effect" appearance at the terminal portion of the QRS complex.

Arrhythmias

PVCs, PACs, PJCs

Any arrhythmia (increased automaticity + increased vagal tone lead to both tachy and bradyarrhythmias)

Paroxysmal atrial tachycardia with variable AV block

Accelerated junctional rhythm

Other findings

Bundle branch blocks

Varying AV nodal blocks

system – hypotension and bradycardia with minimal impact on the QRS complex and QT intervals [19]. Ventricular tachydysrhythmias are uncommon, with the exceptions occurring with bepridil and sotalol. These agents have additional anti-arrhythmic effects, which, in overdose, can be pro-arrhythmic: sotalol has both Class II and Class III effects, while bepridil has Class I anti-arrhythmic effects. Ventricular conduction disturbances are more likely to occur in patients who have beta-blocker poisoning, because the drugs are able

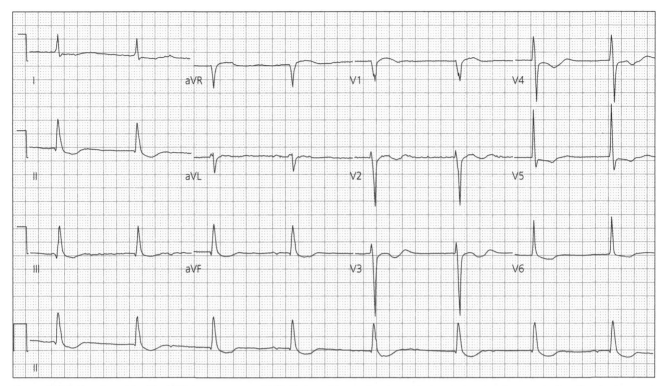

Figure 35.10 Digoxin toxicity. The ECG demonstrates atrial fibrillation with complete heart block and a junctional escape rhythm. The classic "digoxin effect" appearance at the terminal portion of the QRS complexes is present as well. (ECG courtesy Amal Mattu, MD.)

to block myocardial sodium channels, whereas high-degree AV blocks are more likely to occur in patients who have calcium channel-blocker poisoning. Certain calcium channel-blockers have effects primarily on vascular tone (nifedipine, nicardipine, amlodipine), and others cause impairment of contractility and AV nodal blocking effects. Beta-blockers lose most of their beta-1 and beta-2 selectivity in overdose.

Although most of the toxic effects associated with overdose of these agents are related to bradycardia, AV nodal blocks and resultant hypotension, the impairment of contractility, resultant profound hypotension and subsequent lactic acidosis can produce PEA presentations. The arrest scenario may be a true PEA or a pseudo-PEA resulting from profound hypotension. Although a reflex tachycardia may occur with the vasodilating calcium channel-blockers, typical ECG manifestations of both beta-blockers and calcium channel-blockers include bradycardia, AV nodal blockade, escape rhythms, and asystole [19].

Therapy must be prompt in the patient with PEA. For PEA related to beta-blockers, glucagon should be administered. Intravenous calcium should be provided to patients with PEA related to calcium channel-blockers.

Pseudo-PEA

Hypovolemia: Profound hypovolemia such as that occurring from trauma or major hemorrhagic events can produce

pseudo-PEA. A profound drop in preload does not allow enough cardiac filling to generate a pulse. When an ultrasound probe is placed on the chest, a beating heart is usually seen, at least initially. Eventually, if adequate perfusion is not restored, electrical activity will cease. The most common initial ECG finding is sinus tachycardia, followed in the terminal stages by bradycardia and asystole. Profound hypovolemia is an extremely important cause of PEA to identify immediately, because aggressive therapy may be able to reverse the pulselessness.

Tension pneumothorax: Pulseless electric activity arrest from a tension pneumothorax is likely the most reversible of all causes. The development of a tension pneumothorax causes progressive compression of the vena cava along with distortion of the cavoatrial junction and compression of the opposite lung. Rising intrathoracic pressure retards venous return and leads to progressive hypotension. Severe respiratory distress and hypoxia typically develops before hypotension. Electrocardiogram changes may represent hypoxia and or ischemia. Additionally, depending on the hemithorax that is affected, shifting of the mediastinum may distort the 12-lead findings (Table 35.8), occurring due to rotation or distortion of the position of heart, air in the chest cavity, and right ventricular dilation [20]. Chest tube insertion is imperative.

One process that shares a similar physiologic abnormality is the inadvertent application of positive pressure ventilation

Table 35.8 ECG changes in tension pneumothorax

Left-sided tension PTX

Sinus tachycardia
Decreased QRS voltage
Poor R wave progression
T wave inversion in precordial leads
Electrical alternans

Right-sided tension PTX

Sinus tachycardia
$S_1Q_3T_3$
S wave in V_1
Decreased QRS voltage
Anterior or posterior MI pattern (rare)

Table 35.9 ECG findings of pericardial tamponade*

Sinus tachycardia
Low voltage QRS complexes
Electrical alternans
PR depression
Diffuse ST segment elevation
ST segment depression in aVR and V_1

*The absence of these findings cannot rule out significant effusion or tamponade

resulting in a substantially elevated level of auto-PEEP. An end-expiratory pressure that is associated with a higher than resting lung volume is called intrinsic or auto-PEEP. Similar to a tension pneumothorax, this high pressure can retard cardiac return and produce progressive hypotension. Cases of PEA have been reported as the result of aggressive ventilation during resuscitation [21]. Simply disconnecting the patient from the ventilator or Ambu Bag will result in restoration of pulse and blood pressure.

Pericardial tamponade: Pericardial tamponade prevents normal ventricular filling and severely decreases cardiac output. As the pressure in the pericardium increases, the pulse pressure narrows and a palpable pulse can be lost. The development of this degree of tamponade is usually not sudden unless a traumatic injury is involved. If tamponade is the result of pericarditis, some of the typical ECG changes of pericarditis may be seen – diffuse ST segment elevation with PR depression.

Electrical alternans is a beat-to-beat variation in the amplitude of electrical complexes on the ECG. While very specific for the diagnosis of pericardial effusion, its sensitivity is only around 30%. Likewise, the "classic" presentation of electrical alternans, low voltage QRS complexes and PR depression, is very insensitive (1–17%), but highly specific for diagnosing effusion and tamponade [22] (Table 35.9 and Figure 35.11).

Sinus tachycardia and low voltage QRS complexes are the most common findings in pericardial tamponade as the heart rate increases to try to compensate for the low cardiac output. Any of these findings in the appropriate clinical scenario

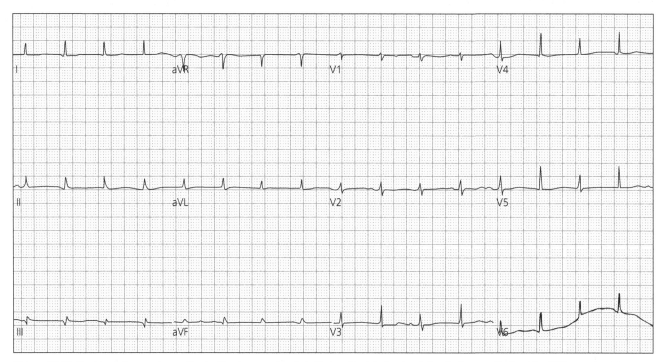

Figure 35.11 Electrical alternans in a patient with a large pericardial effusion. Beat-to-beat variation in the amplitude of the QRS complexes is noted. Other findings typical of a large pericardial effusion include sinus tachycardia and low QRS voltage.

should prompt a rapid echocardiographic examination to look for effusion/tamponade as the cause of PEA arrest. Bedside pericardiocentesis is indicated when PEA is a result of cardiac tamponade.

Pulmonary embolism (PE): A study in 2001 by Courtney and colleagues concluded that patients suffering a witnessed arrest with primary PEA had a high probability of having had a massive PE [23]. For a PE to produce PEA, it would have to either completely obstruct flow between the right and left ventricles or decrease the left ventricular filling enough to decrease cardiac output, cause shock and pulselessness. This cascade of events may occur suddenly with a saddle embolus or develop over a few minutes. Increasing right ventricular stain and a bulging of the intraventricular septum into the left ventricle contribute to progressive reduction of left ventricular filling and cardiac output, and LV failure ultimately resulting in PEA arrest [24].

In 2004, Richman and colleagues considered 49 patients with PE and 49 who ruled out for PE. Although new ECG changes were found more frequently in PE patients, there were no specific findings that differentiated reliably between those with PE and those who were ruled out [25]. Further, a "Best Evidence Topic Report" from 2005 also concluded that, although ECG changes are more common in patients with PE, the ECG alone is not sensitive or specific enough to rule in or rule out the diagnosis of PE [26]. The best role of the ECG in PE is to rule out other diagnoses.

The most common finding unfortunately is non-specific ST segment-T wave changes, followed by sinus tachycardia. When present, specific ECG findings in PE reflect acute or subacute pulmonary hypertension – sinus tachycardia, right bundle branch blocks, T wave inversions in V1–V4, and the $S_1Q_3T_3$ pattern (Table 35.10) [27]. Practically speaking, in the setting of PEA, an ECG with any of the classic findings should trigger one to suspect PE. Thrombolytic therapy would be indicated in patients with PEA in whom the clinician has a high suspicion for PE based on clinical and ECG parameters.

Table 35.10 ECG findings in pulmonary embolism*

Non-specific ST-T wave changes
Sinus tachycardia
$S_1Q_3T_3$ (acute cor pulmonale)
Right heart strain pattern
   QR in V1
   Asymmetrical T wave inversion or ST depression in V_1
   R wave in V1
   rSR' in V1
   Right axis deviation
P pulmonale: P wave > 2.5 mm in lead II

*May not be reliably present in PE.

Conclusion

Pulseless electric activity can result from direct interference with the contractile function of the heart (true PEA), or by either depriving the heart of preload or obstructing flow from the right heart to the left (pseudo-PEA). In PEA arrest, the goal is to identify the precipitating cause as quickly as possible and reverse it in time to preserve brain and heart function. In some cases, the ECG can help to identify the cause of PEA and thereby suggest a potentially effective treatment strategy. The reader is cautioned to view the ECG in terms of the clinical context to best interpret the findings and their significance.

Case conclusions

In Case 1, the patient suffered a massive PE. The ECG demonstrated $S_1Q_3T_3$ pattern, suggestive of PE. The ECG along with the clinical scenario of immobilization and sudden collapse prompted the bedside ED ultrasound. Upon finding a beating heart despite pulselessness (complete obstruction to flow), the presumptive diagnosis of PE was made. Despite aggressive resuscitation including fibrinolysis, the patient expired.

In Case 2, the patient developed a pericardial effusion during the course of her lupus flare. Electrical alternans is evident on her ECG. Immediately prior to cardiac arrest, the pulse pressure was very narrow. These findings strongly suggest a pericardial effusion with tamponade physiology. During the PEA arrest, an ultrasound-guided pericardiocentesis was performed using the subxiphoid approach. A large amount of fluid was withdrawn and the patient developed a pulse with measurable blood pressure. She was transferred to the operating room for a formal pericardial window. The patient was discharged neurologically intact 7 days later.

This patient in Case 3 was "found down" for a prolonged period of time. His ECG demonstrated a wide complex bradycardic rhythm, approaching a sine-wave pattern. During the course of the resuscitation, a dialysis shunt was discovered. The diagnosis of hyperkalemia was made. The patient received one amp. of calcium chloride after which he regained pulses. He was treated with sodium bicarbonate, insulin, glucose, and albuterol. He was transferred for emergent dialysis. The missed dialysis, along with potassium release from muscle damage (rhabdomyolysis from prolonged immobilization on the ground), likely caused hyperkalemia. The use of succinylcholine in this case may have contributed to his already elevated potassium, precipitating the PEA arrest.

References

1 Paradis N, Martin G, Goetting M, *et al.* Aortic pressure during human cardiac arrest: Identification of pseudo-electromechanical dissociation. *Chest* 1992;**101**(1):123–8.
2 Bocka J, Overton D, Hauser A. Electromechanical dissociation in human beings: an echocardiographic evaluation. *Ann Emerg Med* 1988;**17**:450–2.

3 Blaivas M, Fox J. Outcome in cardiac arrest patients found to have cardiac standstill on bedside emergency department echocardiogram. *Acad Emerg Med* 2001;**8**:616–21.

4 Ward K. Resuscitation. In: Marx J, Hockberger R, Walls R, *et al.* editors. *Rosen's Emergency Medicine: Concepts and Clinical Practice.* 6th ed. Philadelphia: Mosby/Elsevier, 2006.

5 Aufderheide T. Etiology, Electrophysiology, and Myocardial Mechanics of Pulseless Electrical Activity. In: Paradis N, Halperin H, Kern K, Volder W, Chamberlain D, editors. *Cardiac Arrest: The Science and Practice of Resuscitation Medicine.* 2nd ed. Cambridge: Cambridge University Press, 2007:426–46.

6 Aufderheide TP, Thakur RK, Stueven HA, *et al.* Electro-cardiographic characteristics in EMD. *Resuscitation* 1989;**17**(2):183–93.

7 Pirolo JS, Hutchins GM, Moore GW. Electromechanical dissociation: pathologic explanations in 50 patients. *Hum Pathol* 1985; **16**(5):485–7.

8 Angelos MG, Torres CA, Rath DP, *et al.* In-vivo myocardial substrate alteration during perfused ventricular fibrillation. *Acad Emerg Med* 1999;**6**(6):581–7.

9 Warner LL, Hoffman JR, Baraff LJ. Prognostic significance of field response in out-of-hospital ventricular fibrillation. *Chest* 1985;**87**(1):22–8.

10 Part 10.1: Life-Threatening Electrolyte Abnormalities. *Circulation* 2005;**112**(24 Suppl):IV-121-5.

11 Stueven HA, Aufderheide T, Waite E, Mateer J. Electromechanical Dissociation: Six Years Prehospital Experience. *Resuscitation* 1989;**17**:173–82.

12 Cheng D. The ECG of Hypothermia. *J Emerg Med* 2002;**22**(1): 87–91.

13 Brunson C, Abbud E, Osman K, *et al.* Osborn (J) Wane Appearance on the Electrocardiogram in Relation to Potassium Transfer and Myocardial Metabolism During Hypothermia. *J Invest Med* 2005;**53**(8):434–47.

14 Thanacoody HKR, Thomas SHL. Tricyclic antidepressant poisoning: cardiovascular toxicity. *Toxicologic Rev* 2005;**24**(3):205–14.

15 Niemann J, Bessen H, Rothstein R, *et al.* Electrocardiographic criteria for tricyclic antidepressant cardiotoxicity. *Am J Cardiol* 1986;**57**:1154–9.

16 Hoffman JR, McElroy CR. Bicarbonate therapy for dysrhythmia and hypotension in tricyclic antidepressant overdose. *West J Med* 1981;**134**(1):60–4.

17 Suchard J. Common Myths and Practice in Toxicology: Conference Powerpoint Presentation. In: *American College of Emergency Physicians Scientific Assembly, 2007.* Seattle, Washington, 2007.

18 Moorman JR, Pritchett EL. The arrhythmias of digitalis intoxication. *Arch Intern Med* 1985;**145**(7):1289–92.

19 Kaide CG. Beta Blocker and Calcium Channel Blocker Toxicity. In: Hoekstra JW, ed. *Handbook of Cardiovascular Emergencies.* 2nd ed. Lippincott Williams & Wilkins, Philadelphia, 2001; pp. 363–72.

20 Hedayati T, Swadron S. The ECG in Selected Noncardiac Conditions. In: Mattu A, Tabas J, Barish R, editors. *Electrocardiography in Emergency Medicine.* Dallas: American College of Emergency Physicians, 2007.

21 Mehrishi S, George L, Awan A. Intrinsic PEEP: An Underrecognized Cause of Pulseless Electrical Activity. *Hospital Physician* 2004;**3**:30–6.

22 Eisenberg MJ, de Romeral LM, Heidenreich PA, *et al.* The diagnosis of pericardial effusion and cardiac tamponade by 12-lead ECG. A technology assessment. *Chest* 1996;**110**(2):318–24.

23 Courtney D, Sasser H, Pincus C, Kline J. Pulseless electrical activity with witnessed arrest as a predictor of sudden death from massive pulmonary embolism in outpatients. *Resuscitation* 2001; **49**:265–72.

24 Goldhaber S. Pulmonary Embolism. In: Braunwald E, editor. *Heart Disease: A Textbook of Cardiovascular Medicine.* 5th ed. London: W.B. Saunders, 1997:1582–603.

25 Richman PB, Loutfi H, Lester SJ, *et al.* Electrocardiographic findings in Emergency Department patients with pulmonary embolism. *J Emerg Med* 2004;**27**(2):121–6.

26 Mackway-Jones K. Towards evidence based emergency medicine: best BETs from the Manchester Royal Infirmary. *Emerg Med J* 2005;**22**(10):729.

27 Kline J, Runyon M. Pulmonary Embolism and Deep Venous Thrombosis. In: Marx J, Hockberger R, Walls R, *et al.*, editors. *Rosen's Emergency Medicine: Concepts and Clinical Practice.* 6th ed. Philadelphia: Mosby/Elsevier, 2006:1368–81.

Part 5 | **The ECG in Critical Care**

Chapter 36 | What is the role of the ECG in the critically ill, non-coronary patient?

Clay A. Cauthen, Ajeet Vinayak
University of Virginia, Charlottesville, VA, USA

Case presentations

Case 1: An 82-year-old female with known atrial fibrillation is admitted to the intensive care unit (ICU) for monitoring after a large upper gastrointestinal bleed. After endoscopic resolution of a bleeding peptic ulcer and hemodynamic, the patient becomes aphasic and is unable to move her left upper and lower extremities. Neuroimaging demonstrates a large ischemic stroke of the middle cerebral artery. Admission electrocardiogram (ECG) is notable for only atrial fibrillation (Figure 36.1) and postischemic stroke demonstrates persistent T wave inversions in the lateral leads. Cardiac biomarkers and nuclear stress test are negative for cardiac ischemia.

Case 2: A 58-year-old male with past medical history significant for chronic obstructive pulmonary disease and coronary artery disease is admitted for respiratory failure. Admission ECG demonstrates low voltage QRS complexes across the frontal leads and poor R wave progression (Figure 36.2) raising concerning for an anterior myocardial infarction. The patient denies chest pain. No left ventricular wall motion abnormalities are present on echocardiogram. Cardiac biomarkers remain normal. The clinical course improves with antibiotics and steroids.

Case 3: A 42-year-old male is admitted to the intensive care unit for severe pancreatitis that has been complicated by hypotension. Admission ECG demonstrates sinus tachycardia and ST segment elevations in II, III, and aVF (Figure 36.3). Cardiac biomarkers are not elevated and cardiac catheterization demonstrates minimal non-occlusive coronary disease. No intervention is performed. After the resolution of the pancreatitis, a repeat ECG is performed that demonstrates normal sinus rhythm in the absence of T wave or ST segment abnormalities.

Critical Decisions in Emergency and Acute Care Electrocardiography,
1st edition. Edited by W.J. Brady and J.D. Truwit. © 2009 Blackwell
Publishing, ISBN: 9781405159067

The role of the ECG in the critically ill, non-coronary patient

These clinical scenarios represent common case presentations in the ICU setting with significant and worrisome ECG findings due to non-ischemic pathologies. Non-cardiac admissions to the ICU often present with either symptoms or ECG findings, or both, that can be seen with cardiac dysfunction. As an intensivist, what role does the ECG have in the diagnostic approach to patients without known coronary disease?

The ECG is an invaluable tool for the diagnosis and monitoring of ischemic and non-ischemic cardiac dysfunction in the cardiac care unit (CCU). Routine acquisition of ECGs occurs in other multidisciplinary intensive care unit (ICU) settings; however, the role is less defined. In this chapter, we will discuss the advantageous use of the ECG and the detection of specific ECG patterns in a selection of non-coronary diseases common to the ICU setting. Coronary etiologies of ECG abnormalities must never be disregarded, but the goal of this chapter is to provide a systems-based approach highlighting common ECG findings for the critically ill, non-coronary patients to assist with diagnosis and management. When possible, we will provide information regarding the prognostic value of the specific ECG patterns in specific clinical scenarios.

The role of the ECG and acute central nervous system events

The inter-relation of cardiovascular dysfunction and central nervous system (CNS) pathology has been well established. It is believed that normal cardiac function is modulated not only by the excitatory and inhibitory actions of the autonomic nervous system, but also through CNS-mediated regulation of electrolyte and fluid balance [1]. Acute CNS events have been described to present various ECG abnormalities including bradyarrhythmias, tachyarrhythmias, abnormal ST-T segment abnormalities, prominent U waves,

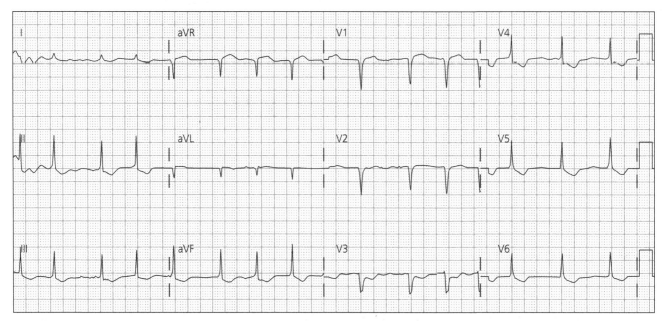

Figure 36.1 Admission ECG demonstrating atrial fibrillation and new inferolateral T wave inversion.

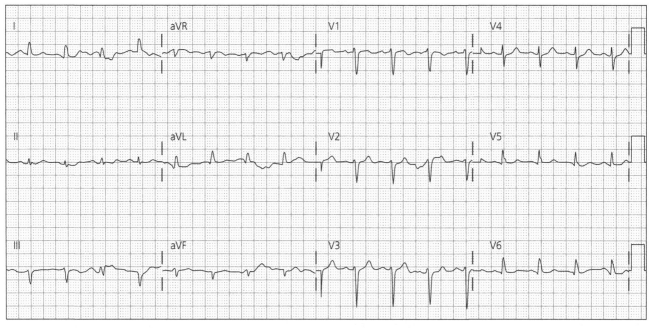

Figure 36.2 Admission ECG of patient with severe COPD with an exacerbation demonstrating sinus tachycardia, low voltage QRS complexes in the frontal leads, and poor R wave progression.

QT prolongations, and tall, inverted or notched T waves [2]. The original descriptions by Cushing described several cases of intracranial hemorrhages that were complicated by both bradyarrhythmias and tachyarrhythmias [3]. Electrocardiogram findings in acute CNS events were later observed when Byer and colleagues described inverted T waves and prolonged QT intervals in patients with subarachnoid hemorrhages (SAH) [4]. Since then, the ECG has gained more prominent attention in the literature in the management of acute CNS events.

Most of the ECG abnormalities in patients with acute CNS events are thought to be primarily associated with the increase of intracranial pressure (ICP). Characteristic findings of increased ICP include bradycardia, U waves, non-specific T wave abnormalities, and QT interval disturbances [2,3]. Early studies by Jachuk demonstrated pressure-dependent ECG patterns: prominent U waves and notched T waves with ICP > 30 mmHg; QTc shortening with ICP 30–65 mmHg and QT prolongation with ICP > 65 mmHg [2]. Even though these observations have not been well validated in large clin-

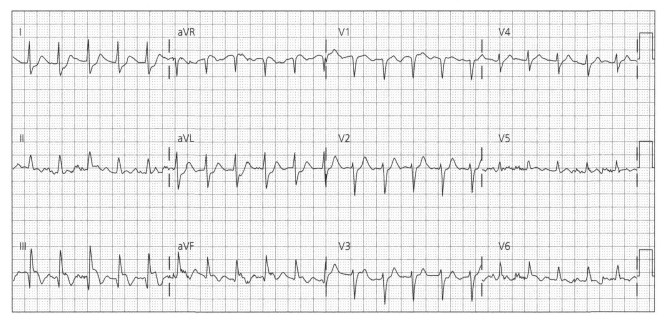

Figure 36.3 Admission ECG of patient with acute pancreatitis demonstrating sinus tachycardia at 127 bpm and ST segment elevations in II, III, and aVF.

ical trials, the evolutionary nature of these ECG patterns may provide further evidence of, and alert the intensivist, to the degree and severity of rising ICP.

Patients presenting with SAH frequently have ECG abnormalities. While studies have demonstrated the negative effect of left ventricular dysfunction on mortality in patients with SAH [5], the impact of ECG changes on prognosis in SAH have been widely studied with inconsistent results. Pathologic Q waves, peaked P waves, peaked T waves, large U waves, QT prolongation [6], and ST segment depressions [7] have been associated with increased mortality by some studies, whereas others have found no correlation between these ECG changes and mortality [8].

The role of the ECG in ischemic strokes is less well established; however, patients with ischemic strokes are more likely to present with abnormal ECG [8]. Reasons for these observations are thought to be twofold: most patients with ischemic strokes have pre-existing ischemic cardiac diseases. As 14% of all strokes are embolic in origin, the presence of ECG abnormalities, specifically atrial fibrillation, is not unexpected [8]. In the absence of increased ICP or the conversion of an ischemic to a hemorrhagic stroke, the presence of QT prolongation, T wave abnormalities, and the presence of U waves are uncommon. The ECG may provide prognostic information as studies have demonstrated that patients presenting with ischemic strokes and abnormal ECGs (most commonly ischemic patterns and atrial fibrillation) have a twofold increased 6-month mortality [9].

Electrocardiogram abnormalities in acute CNS events occur commonly (Table 36.1). As demonstrated in the first

Table 36.1 Common ECG findings in acute CNS events

Common ECG findings in acute CNS events		
Increased intracranial pressure (ICP)	**Subarachnoid hemorrhage**	**Ischemic strokes**
Sinus bradycardia or tachycardia	Peaked P waves	Atrial fibrillation
U waves	Peaked T waves	Atrial flutter
Non-specific T wave abnormalities	T wave inversion	T wave inversion
Qtc abnormalities	J wave or Osborn wave	ST segment depression
ICP < 30 mmHg	Prominent U waves	
Prominent U waves	Pathologic Q waves	
Notched T waves	ST segment elevation and depression	
ICP 30–65 mmHg	QTc prolongation	
QTc Interval Shortening		
ICP > 65 mmHg		
Qtc prolongation		

case, the presence of the ECG changes further reflects the CNS and cardiovascular inter-relation. Recognition of specific ECG patterns as seen with increased ICP and SAH may raise the clinical suspicion of an acute CNS event allowing for early diagnosis. The prognostic value of the ECG should be interpreted with a high level of clinical discretion as these observations have yet to be validated.

The role of the ECG in pulmonary conditions

Critically ill patients with pulmonary conditions commonly present to acute care settings with severe dyspnea. The role of the ECG in these patients is vast. Along with clinical history and radiographic data, awareness of specific ECG patterns may help exclude primary cardiac diagnoses or suggest co-existing pulmonary conditions such as chronic obstructive pulmonary disease (COPD), restrictive pulmonary disease, pulmonary hypertension (PH) or pulmonary embolism (PE).

Restrictive and obstructive lung diseases have a number of ECG findings. Both processes may lead to right-sided strain, chamber dilation, and/or hypertrophy. In both restrictive and obstructive disease, right atrial depolarization, which normally occurs slightly before the left atrium, can be delayed. As a result, simultaneous activation of both atria can occur. In this scenario, the ECG will demonstrate tall P waves (> 2.5 mm) most notably in lead II (also in III, AVF, and the initial portion of V1) and is termed P pulmonale. Hypertrophy and dilation of the right atrium can further contribute to larger P wave amplitudes. Right atrial enlargement can exist with-out right atrial hypertrophy, and vice versa. As both atrial anatomic abnormalities are associated with increased P wave amplitude, it is expected that ECG evidence of P pulmonale lacks the diagnostic accuracy in identifying clinically significant right ventricular failure or cor pulmonale.

Cor pulmonale is the clinical diagnosis of right ventricular failure due to right-sided pressure overload. Over time, both obstructive and restrictive lung disease, especially in the presence of hypoxemia, can lead to pulmonary hypertension. This consequence brings along additional ECG abnormalities as discussed below.

In COPD, hyperinflation of the lungs is common and can lead to additional specific ECG findings [10,11]. As a result of diaphragmatic downward displacement resulting in the narrow, "tear drop" heart, cardiac axis rotation can be observed. The ECG pattern common in this scenario may demonstrate delayed transition from rS to qR along the precordial leads, resulting in poor R wave progression. Awareness of this phenomenon may avoid an erroneous diagnosis of anterior infarct as the cause of this finding. Hyperinflation can also lead to an overall decrease in QRS amplitude due to increased distance between the electrode and the heart. Additionally, the P wave axis, which lies between 0 and +70°, can also be rotated rightward (> +70°). This seems to occur more commonly with obstructive lung disease than the restrictive processes [12]. While seen as a normal variant also, $S_1S_2S_3$ patterns have been described in patients with severe emphysema and PE (Figure 36.4).

Pulmonary hypertension may be encountered in a variety of clinical settings, including severe COPD, severe restrictive lung disease, severe left ventricular dysfunction, PE, or other

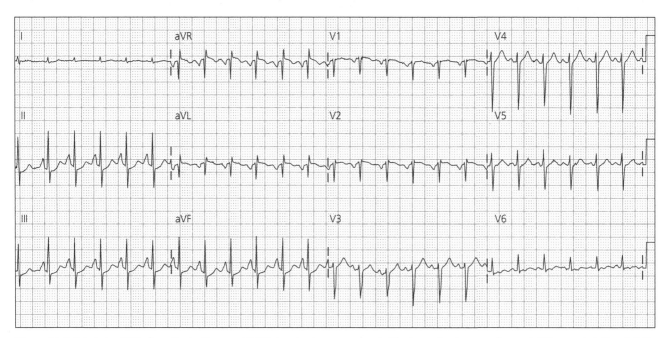

Figure 36.4 Admission ECG of a patient with severe COPD showing many exaggerated features of pulmonary disease: tall P waves in II, III and AVF; late R wave progression across the horizontal leads; an $S_1S_2S_3$ pattern; and a P wave axis greater than 70°.

Table 36.2 Electrocardiographic criteria of right ventricular hypertrophy

Criteria for right ventricular hypertrophy	
Right axis deviation > 100°	Exclusion of other causes of tall V1R:
RV1 > 7 mm	Wolff-Parkinson-White syndrome
RV1 + SV5 (or SV6) > 10 mm	Right bundle branch block
R/S ratio V1 > 1	Posterior infarct
R/S ratio V6 < 1	Normal variants, especially in the very young
P pulmonale	
RSR′ in V1 or V2	
Strain pattern in inferior leads (ST depression, T wave inversion)	

miscellaneous and idiopathic causes. Given its association with severe disease, it is commonly encountered in the ICU. The diagnosis of PH is best confirmed by a right heart catheterization that demonstrates mean pulmonary artery pressure (PAP) > 25 mmHg at rest or > 30 mmHg with exercise. As the disease progresses, PH leads to increasing hypoxemia, RV dilation, hypertrophy, and eventually cor pulmonale. Electrocardiogram findings in PH reflect the burden of right ventricular dysfunction and commonly demonstrate tachycardia, increased P wave amplitude in II, III, and aVF, qR in V1, and RVH criteria. Commonly cited ECG criteria for RVH are listed in Table 36.2. Interestingly, the amplitude of the P wave and the presence of qR in V1, and RVH by WHO criteria in patients with PH has been significantly associated with increased mortality where every mm increase in P wave amplitude, the presence of qR and RVH were associated with 4.5-, 3.6-, and 4.3-times increased risk of death, respectively [13]. In addition, ECG patterns focusing on R and S amplitudes in V1 and right axis deviation with a QRS > 110° have been shown to offer excellent positive predictive values for the presence and severity of PH [14].

The role of the ECG in distinguishing RV failure from other causes of heart failure will be discussed in Chapter 38.

Pulmonary emboli, another cause of RV overload, frequently complicate care in the ICU. As this topic will be thoroughly discussed in a subsequent chapter, we will only briefly mention significant abnormal ECG patterns and their predictive value when determining massive versus non-massive PE. As the $S_1Q_3T_3$, incomplete or complete right bundle branch (RBBB) patterns are prevalent and well described in PE, these patterns have been shown to present frequently (50%, 22%, and 21%, respectively). However, they provide little predictive value for determining massive versus non-massive PE [15]. Identification of PE and other causes of RV failure have specific consequences in medical management of critically ill patients.

Role of the ECG in sarcoidosis

Sarcoidosis is an idiopathic, systemic disease characterized by non-caseating granulomatous inflammation. While pul-

monary involvement typically dominates, multisystemic disease occurs frequently. Identified cardiac involvement is found in 20–30% of patients at necropsy [16]. Many cases of cardiac sarcoidosis likely go undiagnosed. While echocardiogram, holter monitoring, exercise ECG, and magnetic resonance imaging (MRI) provide superior diagnostic accuracy, the 12-lead ECG plays a paramount role as an initial, cost-effective screening tool. In this section, we will briefly discuss frequent ECG abnormalities encountered and the utility of the ECG in routine monitoring for cardiac involvement.

Cardiac sarcoidosis may occur asymptomatically. The prevalence of ECG abnormalities increases with the severity of cardiac involvement (Table 36.3). Grossly observable myocardial involvement, the pathologic definition of severe disease, results in ECG abnormality in up to 75% of cases [17].

Electrocardiography abnormalities range between atrial tachycardia, ventricular tachycardia, atrioventricular (AV) block, bundle branch block, and bradycardia. Additional ECG patterns that occur include those related to consequent hypercalcemia or PH. The ECG can play a diagnostic role in looking for these associated manifestations of sarcoidosis. Patterns of pericardial disease are infrequent. Finally, sudden death, while not a common initial presentation of the disease, may occur in up to 50% of all cardiac sarcoidosis [18]. Most of these events are thought to be related to fulminant ventricular arrhythmia.

The finding of ECG abnormalities in a patient with likely or diagnosed sarcoidosis should immediately prompt further diagnostic steps. In a minority of cases, histologic diagnosis may require proceeding to endomyocardial biopsy. Cardiac sarcoidosis treatment ranges from systemic steroids to anti-arrhythmic treatment to implantable cardioverter-defibrillator placement.

Role of ECG in gastrointestinal disorders: acute pancreatitis and biliary disease

As acute pancreatitis is diagnosed by clinical, radiographic and biochemical findings suggestive of pancreatic damage, the role of the ECG is less established. Acute pancreatitis has

ECG abnormalities in cardiac sarcoidosis*

Incidence by stage (%)	Conduction abnormalities (% incidence)	Other commonly seen findings
Stage 0 (0%)	Supraventricular arrhythmias (16–28%)	T wave inversions ST-T segment changes
Stage I (13%)	Atrioventricular block	
Stage II (50%)	Complete heart block (22%)	
Stage III (4.7%)	Intraventricular conduction delays Bundle branch blocks (22–38%) Premature ventricular contractions (29%) Ventricular tachycardia	

Table 36.3 Electrocardiographic abnormalities found with cardiac sarcoidosis

*Table generated from data by Caner et al. (52).

ECG abnormalities in acute pancreatitis	ECG abnormalities in acute gallbladder disease
Bradyarrhymias Tachycardia* T wave inversion	T wave inversion ST segment depressions ST segment elevations Brugada-type ST shift:
ST segment depressions* ST segment elevations*	(1) right bundle branch block (2) coved ST segment elevations in the precordial leads
PQ interval prolongation* Left hemi-block† Repolarization abnormalities (flat or inverted T waves)†	

Table 36.4 Electrocardiographic abnormalities associated with acute pancreatitis and acute gallbladder disease

*Associated with increased severity.
†Most common ECG findings not significantly associated with electrolyte abnormalities.

been associated with abnormalities such as bradyarrhythmias, tachyarrhythmias, interval prolongation, non-specific T wave abnormalities, T wave inversions, ST segment depressions, and ST segment elevations in the absence of coronary disease [19–21]. Specific ECG patterns worrisome for coronary ischemia or infarct have been described, as illustrated in Case 3. Some authors suggest that specific ECG patterns may provide valuable prognostic information and may reflect the severity of the disease [22].

Electrocardiogram abnormalities can be seen in up to 50–80% of patients presenting with acute pancreatitis [19,23,24]. Many of the electrographic changes are non-specific and can be attributed to secondary causes such as electrolyte abnormalities commonly associated with acute pancreatitis: hypocalcemia, hypokalemia, hyponatremia, and hypomagnesemia [25]. As most ECG abnormalities described in the literature are non-specific and may demand less attention from the physician, ECG findings mimicking myocardial ischemia or infarction are of great concern. ST segment elevations [25–29], de novo left bundle branch block [24], as well as

T wave inversion and ST depressions [21,25,30–32] have been reported in the absence of significant coronary artery disease. Interestingly, concomitant regional wall motion abnormalities have been described with these ischemic ECG patterns. Both the wall motion and ECG abnormalities normalized with the resolution of the acute pancreatitis [21,25,31]. In addition, one of these studies reported the administration of thrombolytics when a presentation of acute pancreatitis was mistakenly diagnosed as myocardial infarction [27].

An abnormal ECG may play a prognostic role for patients with acute pancreatitis. In a prospective study of 333 patients admitted with acute pancreatitis, Tomulic and colleagues demonstrated that heart rate, PQ interval duration, and ST segment elevations or depressions were significantly associated with the severity of acute pancreatitis [22]. As tachycardia and a shortened PQ interval can be readily attributed to the dramatic sympathetic surge associated with acute pancreatitis [33], the etiology of the ST segment abnormalities is less clear [34]. Smaller studies of acute pancreatitis patients without a previous history of heart disease demonstrated an increased incidence of abnormal ECG on presentation, where the most frequent ECG findings were non-specific changes in repolarization (flat or inverted T waves) in 20% of patients, sinus tachycardia (12%), and left hemi-block (10%) [19]. In a secondary analysis, they demonstrated that non-specific changes of repolarization were not significantly associated with electrolyte abnormalities, but did tend towards higher levels of potassium and lower levels of phosphorous. Sinus tachycardia, however, was significantly associated with higher concentrations of potassium and lower calcium and phosphorous. In conflict with previous reports, these ECG abnormalities were not associated with increased cardiac mortality or severity of acute pancreatitis [19]. As the prognostic value of an abnormal ECG is still controversial, the clinical application remains unclear until large clinical trials can be performed.

Gallbladder disease is a common ailment in the critically ill and may present with abnormal ECG findings. Acute cholecystitis and symptomatic cholelithiasis are typically associated with non-specific ECG findings of ST segment depressions and T wave inversions which, in the correct clinical context, may be suggestive of myocardial ischemia [35–37]. However, patients have been reported to present with more ominous ECG findings suggestive of myocardial infarction. To date, there have been five reported cases of acute cholecystitis presenting with ST segment elevations with no evidence of coronary disease [36,38–41]. Three of the patients underwent cardiac catheterization demonstrating no coronary disease and two received thrombolytics with no therapeutic benefit. Interestingly, all of the ST segment elevations electrographically corresponded to a single coronary artery domain and resolved after appropriate therapy. In another case report, Furuhashi and colleagues described the development of a Brugada-type ST shift, defined by a right bundle branch block with coved (or saddle-back) ST segment elevations in the precordial leads, in a patient with acute cholecystitis [42]. Again, the ECG findings normalized with resolution of the disease process. A vagally mediated biliary-cardiac reflex has been proposed to account for ECG changes seen in acute gallbladder disease.

As the differential of ECG abnormalities suggestive of myocardial infarction rarely includes acute pancreatitis or biliary disease, the intensivist should use caution when interpreting these data. There is little role for the ECG establishing or confirming diagnosis of gastrointestinal pathologies in the ICU. While coronary syndromes are being excluded in cases of ambiguity, simultaneous medical investigation should continue when other clinical data suggest abdominal pathology.

Role of ECG in endocrinopathies

Endocrinopathies embody another large subset of systemic disorders that often complicate the management of critically ill patients. Prompt assessment of glycemic homeostasis,

as well as thyroid and adrenal function, is often obtained in critically ill patients. Glucose, thyroid, and adrenal dysfunction can commonly present with specific ECG findings.

Electrocardiogram abnormalities have been described in both hyper- and hypoglycemic states. Most common for both hyper- and hypoglycemia are rhythm disturbances, T wave changes, and the presence of QT interval lengthening. Cardiac autonomic neuropathy resulting in an imbalance of left and right heart sympathetic tone has been proposed as the underlying mechanism for cardiac dysfunction and ECG abnormalities in diabetics [43]. Prolongation of the corrected QT interval (QTc) has been reported in both the presence and absence of autonomic dysregulation [44]. Thus, it is believed that the systemic response to hyperglycemia, including hyperinsulinemia and the accompanying hyperadrenergic state, may account for this finding. The clinical significance of QTc prolongation is well established and includes the development of ventricular dysrhythmias, torsade de pointes, ventricular tachycardia, sudden cardiac death as well as increased all-cause mortality in the absence of ventricular arrhythmias. However, the significance of a transient QTc prolongation in the presence of hyperglycemia still remains unclear.

In addition, patients who present with hyperosmolar hyperglycemic states (HHS) and diabetic ketoacidosis (DKA) commonly experience electrolyte abnormalities such as hypokalemia and hypophosphatemia. Despite normal to slightly elevated serum potassium concentrations, patients with HHS or DKA have a net potassium deficit that manifests with adequate hydration and insulin therapy. Electrocardiogram manifestations of hypokalemia include broad, flat T waves, ST depression, QT interval prolongation and ventricular arrhythmias [45]. These ECG findings are typically absent in mild to moderate hypokalemia and seen only when serum potassium falls below 2.7 mmol/L. However, ventricular extrasystoles are not uncommon in patients with potassium 2.5–3.0 mmol/L [45].

Hypoglycemia is a common, potentially life-threatening complication in the critically ill that may present with transient non-specific ECG features. Bradycardia, changes in repolarization, QTc prolongation as well as supra- and ventricular tachyarrhymias have been reported, and resolve with restoration to euglycemia [46–48]. For the intensivist, it is important to recognize these atypical manifestations of hypoglycemia during the evaluation of the critically ill patient.

Increased circulating thyroid hormone results in increased cardiac output and heart rate. In hyperthyroidism and thyrotoxicosis, ECG findings are common; sinus tachycardia, atrial fibrillation, increased QRS voltage, and shortened PR interval are the most prevalent [45,49]. As sinus tachycardia can be seen in up to 40% of those with hyperthyroidism, atrial fibrillation, commonly with a rapid ventricular response, occurs in 15–20% of patients with hyperthyroidism. The incidence appears to increase in patients over 60 years old [45,49,50]. Atrial flutter, paroxysmal SVT, and ventricular tachycardia appear to be uncommon, and these findings in a hyperthyroid patient should raise the suspicion of underlying cardiac disease.

Despite shortening of the PR interval suggestive of enhanced AV conduction, intra-atrial and intraventricular conduction abnormalities have been reported in patients with hyperthyroidism. Increased P wave duration or notching is the most common intra-atrial conduction abnormality. Increased P wave duration has been associated with the development of atrial fibrillation. A P wave duration > 130 ms has a sensitivity, specificity, and positive predictive value of 79%, 85% and 83%, respectively, for paroxysmal atrial fibrillation in hyperthyroidism [51]. Intraventricular conduction delays have also been reported with the development of RBBB up to 15% of the time, and, paradoxically, advanced AV blocks have been reported [49].

Electrocardiographic abnormalities in hypothyroidism are common and can be attributed to global slowing of metabolic rate and organ function. Sinus bradycardia, prolonged QT interval, and flat or inverted waves are common ECG findings in hypothyroidism. Patients with hypothyroidism have a three times increased risk of developing atrial, intraventricular, and ventricular conduction disturbances [50]. Severe hypothyroidism has, not infrequently, been associated with the development of advanced heart block and BBB [45]. Additionally, pericardial effusions can be seen in up to 30% of patients with hypothyroidism, giving rise to electrical alternans [50].

In summary, ECG abnormalities in endocrinopathies are common and non-specific. As the role of the ECG is limited in endocrinopathies, awareness of specific ECG abnormalities may provide insights underlying endocrine disorders of the critically ill.

Case conclusions

The cases detailed above are intended to represent those found in many medical, surgical, or neurological ICUs. In these patients, hemodynamic and respiratory instability often leads to clinical assessments including ECG evaluation. Abnormal findings on ECG are common, and, while coronary pathology should not be overlooked, additional information can be used to assist in diagnosis, to evaluate co-existent cardiac dysfunction, uncover additional electrolyte abnormalities, and provide assistance with prognosis. Specific ECG findings and implications of hypothermia, PH and PE are discussed in later chapters in this section.

References

1 Arab D, Yahia AM, Qureshi AI. Cardiovascular manifestations of acute intracranial lesions: pathophysiology, manifestations, and treatment. *J Intensive Care Med* 2003;**18**(3):119–29.

2 Jachuck SJ, Ramani PS, Clark F, Kalbag RM. Electrocardiographic abnormalities associated with raised intracranial pressure. *Br Med J* 1975;**1**(5952):242–4.

3 Cushing HW. Some experimental and clinical observations concerning the state of increased intracranial tension. *Am J Med Sci* 1902;**124**:375–400.

4 Byer E, Ashman R, Toth LA. Electrocardiograms with large, upright T waves and long Q-T intervals. *Am Heart J* 1947;**33**:796–806.

5 Pollick C, Cujec B, Parker S, Tator C. Left ventricular wall motion abnormalities in subarachnoid hemorrhage: an echocardiographic study. *J Am Coll Cardiol* 1988;**12**(3):600–5.

6 Cruickshank JM, Dwyer GN. Proceedings: Electrocardiographic changes in subarachnoid haemorrhage: role of catecholamines and effects of beta-blockade. *Br Heart J* 1974;**36**(4):395.

7 Hersch C. Electrocardiographic changes in head injuries. *Circulation* 1961;**23**:853–60.

8 Davis TP, Alexander J, Lesch M. Electrocardiographic changes associated with acute cerebrovascular disease: a clinical review. *Prog Cardiovasc Dis* 1993;**36**(3):245–60.

9 Bozluolcay M, Ince B, Celik Y, *et al*. Electrocardiographic findings and prognosis in ischemic stroke. *Neurol India* 2003;**51**(4):500–2.

10 Harrigan RA, Jones K. ABC of clinical electrocardiography. Conditions affecting the right side of the heart. *BMJ* 2002;**324**(7347):1201–4.

11 Shah NS, Velury S, Mascarenhas D, Spodick DH. Electrocardiographic features of restrictive pulmonary disease, and comparison with those of obstructive pulmonary disease. *Am J Cardiol* 1992;**70**(3):394–5.

12 Ikeda K, Kubota I, Takahashi K, Yasui S. P-wave changes in obstructive and restrictive lung diseases. *J Electrocardiol* 1985;**18**(3):233–8.

13 Bossone E, Paciocco G, Iarussi D, *et al*. The prognostic role of the ECG in primary pulmonary hypertension. *Chest* 2002;**121**(2):513–8.

14 Al-Naamani K, Hijal T, Nguyen V, *et al*. Predictive values of the electrocardiogram in diagnosing pulmonary hypertension. *Int J Cardiol* 2008;**127**(2):214–8.

15 Ferrari E, Imbert A, Chevalier T, *et al*. The ECG in pulmonary embolism. Predictive value of negative T waves in precordial leads – 80 case reports. *Chest* 1997;**111**(3):537–43.

16 Schulte W, Kirsten D, Drent M, Costabel U. Cardiac involvement in sarcoidosis. *Eur Respir J Monogr* 2005;**10**:130–49.

17 Silverman KJ, Hutchins GM, Bulkley BH. Cardiac sarcoid: a clinicopathologic study of 84 unselected patients with systemic sarcoidosis. *Circulation* 1978;**58**(6):1204–11.

18 Ghosh P, Fleming HA, Gresham GA, Stovin PG. Myocardial sarcoidosis. *Br Heart J* 1972;**34**(8):769–73.

19 Rubio-Tapia A, Garcia-Leiva J, Asensio-Lafuente E, *et al*. Electrocardiographic abnormalities in patients with acute pancreatitis. *J Clin Gastroenterol* 2005;**39**(9):815–8.

20 Wang K, Asinger RW, Marriott HJ. ST-segment elevation in conditions other than acute myocardial infarction. *N Engl J Med* 2003;**349**(22):2128–35.

21 Yu AC, Riegert-Johnson DL. A case of acute pancreatitis presenting with electrocardiographic signs of acute myocardial infarction. *Pancreatology* 2003;**3**(6):515–7.

22 Tomulic V, Radic M, Haefeli WE, *et al*. Electrocardiographic changes in patients with acute pancreatitis. *Gut* 2005;**54**(Suppl vii):A224.

23 Faintuch JJ, Abrahao MM, Giacaglia LR, *et al*. [Electrocardiographic changes in pancreatitis]. *Arq Bras Cardiol* 1989;**52**(5):259–60.

24 Pezzilli R, Barakat B, Billi P, Bertaccini B. Electrocardiographic abnormalities in acute pancreatitis. *Eur J Emerg Med* 1999;**6**(1): 27–9.

25 Patel J, Movahed A, Reeves WC. Electrocardiographic and segmental wall motion abnormalities in pancreatitis mimicking myocardial infarction. *Clin Cardiol* 1994;**17**(9):505–9.

26 Albrecht CA, Laws FA. ST segment elevation pattern of acute myocardial infarction induced by acute pancreatitis. *Cardiol Rev* 2003;**11**(3):147–51.

27 Cafri C, Basok A, Katz A, *et al.* Thrombolytic therapy in acute pancreatitis presenting as acute myocardial infarction. *Int J Cardiol* 1995;**49**(3):279–81.

28 Hung SC, Chiang CE, Chen JD, Ding PY. Images in cardiovascular medicine: pseudo-myocardial infarction. *Circulation* 2000;**101**(25): 2989–90.

29 Korantzopoulos P, Pappa E, Dimitroula V, *et al.* ST-segment elevation pattern and myocardial injury induced by acute pancreatitis. *Cardiology* 2005;**103**(3):128–30.

30 Ro TK, Lang RM, Ward RP. Acute pancreatitis mimicking myocardial infarction: evaluation with myocardial contrast echocardiography. *J Am Soc Echocardiogr* 2004;**17**(4):387–90.

31 Shah A. Electrocardiographic and segmental wall motion abnormalities in pancreatitis mimicking myocardial infarction. *Clin Cardiol* 1995;**18**(2):58.

32 Spritzer HW, Peterson CR, Jones RC, Overholt EL. Electrocardiographic abnormalities in acute pancreatitis: two patients studied by selective coronary arteriography. *Mil Med* 1969; **134**(9):687–93.

33 Whitcomb DC. Clinical practice. Acute pancreatitis. *N Engl J Med* 2006;**354**(20):2142–50.

34 Stimac D, Tomulic V, Hauser G, *et al.* Is there any connection between severity of acute pancreatitis and electrocardiographic changes? *J Clin Gastroenterol* 2006;**40**(6):559; author reply 559–60.

35 Krasna MJ, Flancbaum L. Electrocardiographic changes in cardiac patients with acute gallbladder disease. *Am Surg* 1986;**52**(10): 541–3.

36 Durning SJ, Nasir JM, Sweet JM, Cation LJ. Chest pain and ST segment elevation attributable to cholecystitis: a case report and review of the literature. *Mil Med* 2006;**171**(12):1255–8.

37 Dickerman JL. Electrocardiographic changes in acute cholecystitis. *J Am Osteopath Assoc* 1989;**89**(5):630, 635.

38 Ryan ET, Pak PH, DeSanctis RW. Myocardial infarction mimicked by acute cholecystitis. *Ann Intern Med* 1992;**116**(3):218–20.

39 Doorey AJ, Miller RE. Get a surgeon, hold the cardiologist: electrocardiogram falsely suggestive of myocardial infarction in acute cholecystitis. *Del Med J* 2001;**73**(3):103–4.

40 Clarice N. Electrocardiographic changes in active duodenal and gall bladder disease. *Am Heart J* 1945;**29**:628–32.

41 Cohen O. Electrographic ST-segment elevation in cholecystitis. *Hosp Physician* 1991;**27**:15–8.

42 Furuhashi M, Uno K, Satoh S, *et al.* Right bundle branch block and coved-type ST-segment elevation mimicked by acute cholecystitis. *Circ J* 2003;**67**(9):802–4.

43 Veglio M, Borra M, Stevens LK, *et al.* The relation between QTc interval prolongation and diabetic complications. The EURODIAB IDDM Complication Study Group. *Diabetologia* 1999; **42**(1):68–75.

44 Marfella R, Nappo F, De Angelis L, *et al.* The effect of acute hyperglycaemia on QTc duration in healthy man. *Diabetologia* 2000; **43**(5):571–5.

45 Slovis C, Jenkins R. ABC of clinical electrocardiography: Conditions not primarily affecting the heart. *BMJ* 2002;**324**(7349): 1320–3.

46 Lee SP, Yeoh L, Harris ND, *et al.* Influence of autonomic neuropathy on QTc interval lengthening during hypoglycemia in type 1 diabetes. *Diabetes* 2004;**53**(6):1535–42.

47 Navarro-Gutierrez S, Gonzalez-Martinez F, Fernandez-Perez MT, *et al.* Bradycardia related to hypoglycaemia. *Eur J Emerg Med* 2003;**10**(4):331–3.

48 Robinson RT, Harris ND, Ireland RH, Macdonald IA, Heller SR. Changes in cardiac repolarization during clinical episodes of nocturnal hypoglycaemia in adults with Type 1 diabetes. *Diabetologia* 2004;**47**(2):312–5.

49 Fadel BM, Ellahham S, Ringel MD, *et al.* Hyperthyroid heart disease. *Clin Cardiol* 2000;**23**(6):402–8.

50 Wald DA. ECG Manifestations of Selected Metabolic and Endocrine Disorders. *ECG Emerg Med* 2006;**24**(1):145–57.

51 Montereggi A, Marconi P, Olivotto I, *et al.* Signal-averaged P-wave duration and risk of paroxysmal atrial fibrillation in hyperthyroidism. *Am J Cardiol* 1996;**77**(4):266–9.

52 Caner M, Demirci S, Gunes Y, *et al.* ECG Abnormalities in Turkish Patients with Sarcoidosis. *Int J Cardiol* 2006;**3**(2):3.

Chapter 37 | Can the ECG distinguish between coronary and non-coronary etiologies in the critically ill patient?

Michael J. Lipinski[1], D. Kyle Hogarth[2]
[1]University of Virginia, Charlottesville, VA, USA
[2]University of Chicago, Chicago, IL, USA

Case presentations

The included cases occur in a large community hospital with a medical intensive care unit (ICU) and 24-h invasive cardiology support for percutaneous coronary intervention (PCI).

Case 1: A 74-year-old male with chronic obstructive pulmonary disease (COPD), tobacco abuse, and hypertension is admitted for severe COPD exacerbation and intubated for hypercapnic respiratory failure. During initial evaluation, the patient has a normal electrocardiogram (ECG). He is admitted to the medical ICU for respiratory care. Following an uncomplicated intubation, the patient becomes hypotensive, requiring vasoactive medications. The patient becomes difficult to ventilate and chest x-ray demonstrates pulmonary edema. An ECG was performed and is shown in Figure 37.1. He is rushed for coronary angiography, which shows a 99% stenosis of the proximal left anterior descending artery that is revascularized with stent placement.

Case 2: A 52-year-old male is found unresponsive by his wife and is initially hypertensive (systolic blood pressure, BP, of 190 mmHg) and tachycardic (with a pulse of 130 beats per minute, bpm) per rescue squad. Per the wife, he has no known medical problems, is not currently taking any medications, smokes one pack of cigarettes daily, and drinks three to five beers daily; she denies he uses drugs. On physical examination, he is afebrile, has a heart rate of 92 bpm, respiratory rate of 28 per minute, blood pressure of 78/40 mmHg, and oxygen saturation of 94% on room air. He is obtunded, pale, and diaphoretic with jugular venous

distension, bibasilar crackles, and an S3 gallop. Electrocardiogram was performed as seen in Figure 37.2. The patient undergoes emergent coronary angiography, which demonstrates normal coronaries. During angiography, coronary spasm is visualized in the distal left main coronary artery and the patient develops ventricular fibrillation, which recurs despite cardioversion, sodium bicarbonate infusion, intracoronary nitrate administration, and intracoronary thrombolytic therapy. Following his death, the wife admitted to earlier cocaine use, having been too afraid to mention this for fear of legal prosecution.

Case 3: A 96-year-old female is transferred to the emergency department (ED) from a nursing facility with altered mental status that has progressed over 3 days. The patient has known coronary artery disease, ischemic left ventricular dysfunction, and hypertension. A prior ECG demonstrated left ventricular hypertrophy, anteroseptal Q waves and intraventricular conduction delay. On physical examination, she has a heart rate of 152 bpm, respiratory rate of 42, BP of 112/45 mmHg, temperature of 35.9°C, and oxygen saturation of 92% on room air, jugular venous distension, tachycardia, and bibasilar crackles. Laboratory studies reveal an elevated serum creatinine, blood urea nitrogen, and potassium. The anion gap is calculated at 18, with a white blood cell count of 15,000, beta-natiuretic peptide of 1256 pg/mL, and troponin I of 0.25 ng/mL. An ECG was performed and is found in Figure 37.3. Chest radiograph demonstrates cardiomegaly and pulmonary vascular congestion, and urinalysis demonstrates large leukesterase, negative nitrites, 56 white blood cells, and many bacteria. A central venous line is inserted, early goal-directed therapy is initiated, and a stat echocardiogram demonstrates global left ventricular dysfunction with no isolated segmental wall motion defects and an ejection fraction of 35%.

Case 4: A 67-year-old female is transferred to the ICU following an episode of melena and subsequent hematochezia.

Critical Decisions in Emergency and Acute Care Electrocardiography, 1st edition. Edited by W.J. Brady and J.D. Truwit. © 2009 Blackwell Publishing, ISBN: 9781405159067

(a)

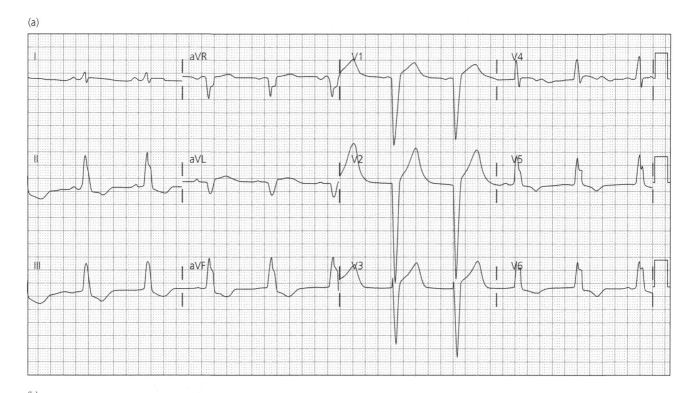

(b)

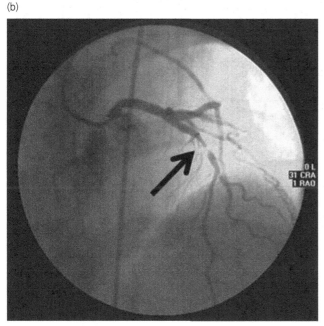

Figure 37.1 (a) Given the initial ECG was normal, this ECG represents interval development of a new left bundle branch block with QRS prolongation (> 120 ms), poor R wave progression in V1–V4 with T waves in the opposite direction to the QRS vector. The characteristic "rabbit ears" (rsR pattern) is present in V5 and V6. (b) The patients accompanying left coronary angiogram demonstrates a 99% stenosis of the left anterior descending coronary artery (arrow).

She recently lost her job following a back injury, for which she had been taking large doses of ibuprofen. While receiving fluid resuscitation and blood transfusions, the patient developed 8/10 crushing substernal chest pressure with dyspnea lasting 45 min. Electrocardiogram was performed during the episode of pain and can be seen in Figure 37.4. Cardiac troponins peak at 4.2 ng/mL and the patient is later taken for coronary angiography, which demonstrates no significant coronary stenoses; however, left ventriculography demonstrates an estimated ejection fraction of 25% with anterior, anterolateral, and apical akinesis with apical dilatation.

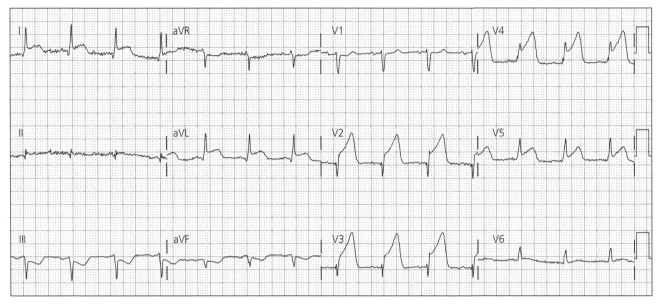

Figure 37.2 ECG demonstrating significant ST segment elevation in leads I, aVL, and V2–V5 with reciprocal ST segment depression in leads III and aVF consistent with a large anterior MI.

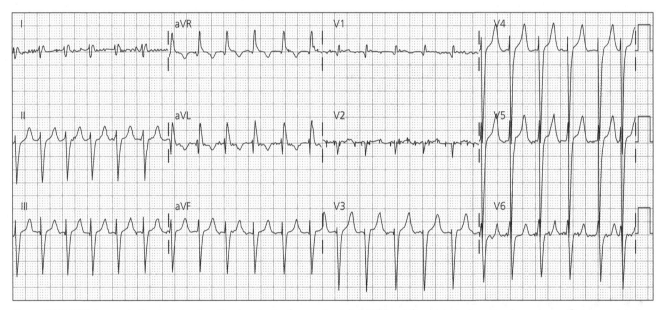

Figure 37.3 ECG demonstrating tachycardia with a heart rate of approximately 140 bpm, left ventricular hypertrophy, non-specific intraventricular conduction delay, poor R wave progression, and Q waves in V1 and V2. Upon closer examination with calipers, irregularity is noted in the R to R interval, consistent with atrial fibrillation with rapid ventricular response. Following fluid resuscitation, the patient's heart rate slowed and demonstrated clear atrial fibrillation.

The diagnostic use of electrocardiography in the evaluation of coronary versus non-coronary diagnoses in the critically ill

These four cases illustrate a sampling of scenarios that can present to ICUs and, either on presentation or during their care, may have clinical evidence suggestive of an acute coronary syndrome (ACS). While coronary events are a major concern, alternate diagnoses can often present with similar features. Given the variety of pathologies that may produce ECG abnormalities, how can the ECG be used to distinguish coronary from non-coronary etiologies in the ICU?

The ECG has become a powerful diagnostic tool in the management of critically ill patients. Since its introduction by Willem Einthoven [1], the ECG has consistently demonstrated its utility in providing information regarding the heart

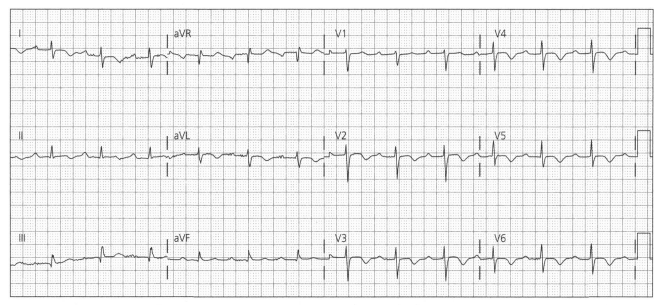

Figure 37.4 ECG demonstrating first-degree AV block with PR interval of 280 ms and diffuse T wave inversions in leads I, aVL, and V2–V6.

and other organ systems. Additionally, prognostic information can be provided and incorporated into risk assessment and clinical decision-making. Obtaining an ECG of high quality is also extremely important as simple issues such as lead placement are frequently overlooked by clinicians. A detailed patient history, physical examination, laboratory values, and radiographic studies are extremely important not only to the management of critically ill patients in general but also for ECG interpretation. As is often the case in the ICU, the patient may be unable to answer questions due to intubation or severity of illness so every effort should be made to obtain these data from the patient, the patient's family members, or the medical records. If available, obtaining previous ECGs is a basic, yet invaluable, tool in ECG interpretation. It is with these fundamentals that we review the characteristic findings on the ECG suggestive of ischemia and how these findings may affect clinical management in critically ill patients.

Myocardial ischemia and injury: As cardiomyocytes achieve 90% of their energy through aerobic metabolism, maintenance of adequate blood flow to the myocardium is crucial as infarction begins after 15 min without blood flow. With the development of ischemia, massive shifts occur in cellular transmembrane ion concentrations, especially an increase in extracellular potassium, due to inadequate ATP. This alteration results in loss of resting membrane potential and development of intracellular gradients between ischemic and normal myocardial cells, and leads to injury current development. The first ischemic sign seen due to these changes is the development of T wave inversion. While ST segment depression and T wave abnormalities are both associated with ischemia, recent data suggest T wave abnormalities are a stronger predictor of cardiovascular mortality than ST segment depression [2].

Subendocardial injury causes depression of the ST segment and elevation of the electrocardiographic baseline, while epicardial injury results in elevation of the ST segment and depression of the baseline. Alternatively, the ECG represents electrical vectors and, therefore, it is important to realize that ST segment depression on an electrode (subendocardial injury) may actually represent ST segment elevation on the other side of the heart (epicardial injury) and vice versa. Typically, horizontal or downward sloping ST segment depression represents ischemic change and often is accompanied by inverted T waves. However, the location of ST segment depression does not accurately correlate with the ischemic region. Findings of PR segment displacement can also be representative of atrial infarction. The inversion or increased amplitude of the U wave may also suggest ischemia. Finally, QRS prolongation can occur due to prolonged conduction through the ischemic myocardium and may eventually lead to bundle block formation, a finding consistent with AMI.

An acute injury pattern is defined as abnormal ST segment elevation in two or more adjacent leads among the standard 12 leads, except in aVR which is derived from an injury current flowing between an injured or depolarized tissue and normal polarized tissue. Electrocardiogram lead patterns demonstrating acute injury and the corresponding myocardial regions (i.e. II, II, and aVF for inferior myocardial infarction, MI) are discussed in greater detail elsewhere [3]. A worrisome sign is the development of frequent premature ventricular complexes during myocardial ischemia, which may lead to the sudden onset of ventricular fibrillation or other fatal arrhythmias. During the progression of AMI, Q waves may develop on the ECG between 6 to 14 h after symptom onset with a mean of 9 h [4] and represent a larger MI than non-Q wave MI [5]. Finally, while these findings may represent myocardial ischemia due to ACS, it is

Table 37.1 Conditions associated with ST segment changes and T wave inversions

ST segment elevation	ST segment depression and T wave abnormalities
Normal variant	Normal variant
AMI	Ischemia
Coronary embolism	Coronary spasm
Coronary spasm	Reciprocal ST elevation
Coronary dissection	Tako-tsubo cardiomyopathy
Aortic dissection	Left ventricular hypertrophy
Reciprocal ST depression	Bundle branch block
Tako-tsubo cardiomyopathy	Ventricular beat (PVC, Pacer)
Left ventricular hypertrophy	Wolff-Parkinson-White syndrome
Bundle branch block	CNS injury
Left ventricular aneurysm	Acute pulmonary embolism
Ventricular beat (PVC, pacer)	Pericarditis
CNS injury	Myocarditis
Acute pulmonary embolism	Pancreatitis
Pericarditis	Kawasaki disease
Myocarditis	Digitalis
Pancreatitis	Sepsis
Hyperkalemia	Abdominal pathology
Hypercalcemia	Tachycardia
Sepsis	Anemia
Cardiac malignancy	
Tricyclic anti-depressant poisoning	
Organophosphate poisoning	
Duchenne muscular dystrophy	
Friedreich ataxia	
Brugada syndrome and ARVD	

important to remember that these patterns represent an injury pattern which may be produced by alternative causes. Table 37.1 provides examples of conditions that may produce ECG findings consistent with ischemia. The ability to assess ischemic changes on the ECG is made extremely challenging when the patient has a bundle branch block, left ventricular hypertrophy, Wolff-Parkinson-White syndrome, or a ventricular rhythm due to a cardiac pacemaker. These conditions frequently have baseline ST segment deviation or T wave changes due to strain pattern or the repolarization pattern [6–9]. Therefore, to investigate for active ischemia, a baseline ECG should be compared with an ECG during chest pain to look for significant ST segment and T wave changes. Additionally, bedside echocardiography can be performed to assess for segmental LV wall motion abnormalities.

Cardiogenic shock: In the critically ill patient, the ability to differentiate between ischemic and non-ischemic findings on the ECG remains of vital importance. For example, identification of acute injury patterns consistent with ST segment elevation myocardial infarction (STEMI) or equivalent may enable institution of early optimal medical therapy and emergent revascularization strategies such as PCI [10]. Acute

myocardial infarction (AMI) complicated by cardiogenic shock, which occurs in approximately 2% of patients with non-ST-segment elevation myocardial infarction (NSTEMI) and 7–8% presenting with STEMI [11], is associated with an extremely poor outcome. While the incidence of cardiogenic shock following ACS has remained stable, mortality from cardiogenic shock has improved from 60.3% in 1995 to 47.9% in 2004 [12]. It is important to consider other causes of sudden cardiogenic shock such as severe mitral regurgitation, acute decompensated heart failure, ventricular septal rupture, cardiac tamponade, or non-cardiac etiologies of shock. Therefore, the combination of the ECG along with clues from the history, physical examination, laboratory values, and imaging studies may help determine the etiology of hemodynamic compromise in critically ill patients and enable appropriate management.

The SHOCK (SHould we emergently revascularize Occluded Coronaries in cardiogenic shocK) investigators randomized 152 patients with acute MI and cardiogenic shock to early revascularization and 150 patients to initial medical therapy. While there was no significant difference in 30-day mortality between the early revascularization and medically stabilized groups (53.3 versus 44.0%), early revascularization significantly improved 6-month (49.7 versus 36.9%), 1-year (46.7 versus 33.6%), and 6-year survival (32.8 versus 19.6%) compared with initial medical stabilization [13,14]. These benefits were found to apply, even in elderly patients, though these patients were less likely to be taken to PCI [15]. In hospitals without PCI capability, thrombolytic therapy with intra-aortic balloon pump offers a reasonable alternative [16]. Finally, patients with NSTEMI and cardiogenic shock had similar mortality compared with STEMI and cardiogenic shock (62.5 versus 60.4%), demonstrating the need to institute an early revascularization strategy upon identification of NSTEMI in patients with cardiogenic shock [17]. Despite the proven importance of early revascularization, a recent large study demonstrated only 52.4% of patients with cardiogenic shock underwent coronary angiography [11]. As was seen in Case 1, the patient developed MI as evidenced by the development of new left bundle branch block on ECG. The physical exam was suggestive of cardiogenic shock as the patient suddenly developed hypotension with pulmonary edema. Cardiac troponins should be checked and intra-aortic balloon pump placement should be considered for blood pressure support to decrease oxygen demand rather than use of vasoactive medications which may further increase myocardial ischemia. If the ECG had demonstrated ST segment depression or T wave inversions, coronary angiography could be considered appropriate in the setting of high clinical suspicion for AMI.

Cocaine and coronary spasm: Cocaine is derived from the *Erythroxylon coca* plant and is an alkaloid with potent effects on the cardiovascular system. It has anesthetic effects that block sodium and potassium channels, which blocks initiation and conduction of electrical impulses (prolongation of QT and QRS intervals), leading to a pro-arrhythmic effect [18]. It also is a neurotransmitter reuptake inhibitor of dopamine and norepinephrine, which leads to increases in heart rate, blood pressure, and contractility but decreases vagal tone. Acute myocardial infarction occurs secondary to alpha-sympathetic stimulation causing coronary spasm, thrombus formation in 24% of cases [19] due to a combination of the coronary spasm and increased platelet aggregatability [20], and increased myocardial oxygen demand. The onset of AMI following use can range from minutes to 24 h later, with onset being faster with intravenous use, followed by crack cocaine, and then nasal insufflations [19]. Cocaine can induce not only MI but can also lead to aortic dissection, myocarditis, endocarditis with intravenous use, hypertensive emergency and intracranial hemorrhage (the ECG findings are discussed later), arrhythmias, and cardiomyopathy. The toxic effects of cocaine can induce global myocyte dysfunction and hypokinesis. These patients should be managed with optimal medical therapy such as nitroglycerin, oxygen, aspirin, benzodiazepines, calcium channel-blockers or phentolamine for spasm (use with care in cardiogenic shock), and sodium bicarbonate to reverse QRS prolongation. The patient in Case 2 presented with AMI as demonstrated by the profound ST elevation in I, aVL, V2–V5, and ST segment depression with T wave inversion likely representing reciprocal changes in III and aVF. Upon presentation, there would be no way without an accurate history to differentiate between STEMI with cardiogenic shock and cocaine-induced AMI and the patient was appropriately taken for coronary angiography. This example demonstrates the importance of the patient history in ECG interpretation and the limitations of medicine despite optimal care.

Atrial fibrillation: Atrial fibrillation is characterized by the absence of P waves and the presence of disorganized electrical activity in the atrium with ventricular conduction dependent on the time-dependent refractoriness of the AV node and the voltage-dependent refractoriness of the His-Purkinje system. The disorganized electrical activity can appear as fine or coarse fibrillation. Atrial fibrillation with rapid ventricular response can be difficult to differentiate from sinus tachycardia and other supraventricular tachycardias such as AV node re-entrant tachycardia and atrial flutter. When the AV node is bypassed by accessory AV pathways, atrial fibrillation may result in rapid transmission of electrical impulses that may lead to ventricular fibrillation and death. This stresses the importance of identifying conditions such as Wolff-Parkinson-White syndrome, which may become fatal if the patient develops atrial fibrillation. The prevalence of atrial fibrillation increases drastically with age [3]. While multiple conditions are associated with atrial fibrillation, conditions such as cor pulmonale, rheumatic heart disease, and ischemic heart disease are thought to cause atrial fibrillation through atrial stretch. As seen in Case 3, the patient has atrial fibrilla-

tion which appears fairly regular until the area circled in Figure 37.3. As the patient has known coronary disease and heart failure, it is not clear whether the development of the atrial fibrillation is due to ischemia, decompensated heart failure, or the stress associated with sepsis. Recent evidence provides a link between atrial fibrillation and the inflammation associated with sepsis [21]. Therefore, the first priority in these patients is identification of their major medical problem as atrial fibrillation is likely a complicating disease. Therefore, therapy should be directed at treating the underlying condition, which, in this case, involved initiation of early goal-directed therapy and ruling out ischemia as an etiology. The presence of ST segment and T wave abnormalities was due to left ventricular hypertrophy with strain pattern. The loss of the atrial contraction and development of rapid ventricular response can pose a challenge in patients with hypotension and sepsis. As electrical cardioversion frequently fails to achieve long-term sinus rhythm in acute atrial fibrillation [22], rate control and, potentially, chemical cardioversion remain the better options. Rate control with beta-blockade and calcium channel-blockers can be dubious in the setting of hypotension, especially with need for vasoactive medications. Digoxin may also be useful in the setting of atrial fibrillation and heart failure as it may slow ventricular response and help increase contractility. Intravenous anti-arrhythmics can exacerbate hypotension but potentially terminate the atrial fibrillation, which may increase cardiac output through restoration of sinus rhythm and potentially restoring atrial contraction. Anti-coagulation should also be considered. A more detailed management strategy is reviewed elsewhere [23].

Tako-tsubo cardiomyopathy: Tako-tsubo cardiomyopathy, also known as stress cardiomyopathy, apical ballooning syndrome, or the broken heart syndrome, is characterized by reversible left ventricular dysfunction with apical ballooning, non-obstructive coronary arteries, and, frequently, elevation in cardiac enzymes. Controversy currently exists as to the cause of this condition but one of the leading hypotheses is that the condition arises as a result of catecholamine surge during stressful situations [24]. The most frequent findings on ECG are deep T wave inversion, ST segment depression, ST segment elevation, QT interval prolongation, and normal ECG. This condition can be challenging to diagnose in the setting of the ICU as patients are frequently unable to communicate and the diagnosis is typically made based on coronary angiogram, which is prompted by elevation of cardiac enzymes and changes on ECG [25]. The characteristic apical balloon seen with cardiac imaging may lead clinicians to suspect this diagnosis but coronary angiography should be performed to rule out flow-limiting stenoses. Case 4 presented in typical fashion with characteristic ECG findings (T wave inversions), which later resolved, and had elevated cardiac enzymes. The concern is that this patient is having demand ischemia or AMI in the setting of her gastrointestinal

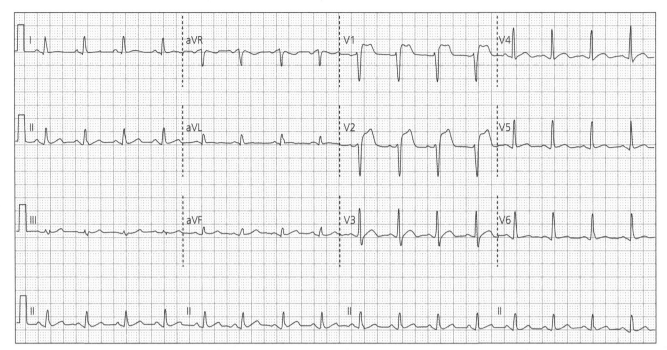

Figure 37.5 ECG demonstrating right bundle branch block (QRS interval ≥ 120 ms, "rabbit ears" (rsR pattern), in V1 and V2, and R wave greater than S wave in V1 with T wave vector in the opposite direction to the QRS vector) and characteristic high takeoff ST segment elevation in the early precordial leads with coved or saddle-back morphology.

bleed. Her diagnosis was ultimately determined by the presence of apical ballooning and clean coronary arteries. The stressor for this patient could be either the stress of her recent job loss, the gastrointestinal bleed, or a combination. Mortality typically occurs from arrhythmias (ventricular fibrillation and torsade de pointes from QT prolongation) and from acute decompensated heart failure. These patients should be aggressively treated for heart failure with ACE inhibition and beta-blockade.

Brugada syndrome: Brugada syndrome was described in 1992 by Pedro and Josep Brugada [26]. They described eight patients with right bundle branch block, normal QT interval, and ST elevations in V1 through V2 or V3 on ECG. These findings are seen in Figure 37.5 and are characteristic for the syndrome. In this case, a 34-year-old man was resuscitated with the assistance of an automatic external defibrillator (AED) in an airport. Cardiac catheterization was unrevealing and an automated implantable cardioverter-defibrillator was placed without complication. The ECG findings were not due to ischemia, electrolyte abnormalities, structural heart disease, and no histologic abnormalities were found on ventricular biopsy. Following a short coupled ventricular extrasystole, these patients developed a rapid polymorphic ventricular tachycardia [26]. The ECG demonstrates a characteristic high takeoff ST segment elevation in the early precordial leads with either a coved or saddle-back morphology. A multitude of other conditions can cause ST segment elevation in the early precordial leads and are listed elsewhere

[27]. This syndrome may account for 40–60% of cases of idiopathic ventricular fibrillation [28]. Brugada syndrome has been shown to result from a missense mutation in the cardiac sodium channel gene SCN5A [28]. While very similar, Brugada syndrome is different from arrhythmogenic right ventricular dysplasia, which was described by Volta as early as 1961 [29]. However, the disease was later coined arrhythmogenic right ventricular dysplasia [30] and is characterized by progressive fibrofatty replacement of the right ventricular free wall with propensity to develop ventricular arrhythmias. Electrocardiogram can present with right bundle branch block and ST segment elevation, which is similar to Brugada syndrome. However, management is the same and requires implantation of automated implantable cardioverter-defibrillator.

Summary

It is noteworthy to acknowledge ECG reader reliability is a variable in accurately identifying ischemic states. In an ICU population, Lim and colleagues found that ECG interpretation was moderately reliable and bolstered considerably by knowledge of additional clinical variables, in particular, troponin values [31]. While ischemic findings on the ECG are frequently encountered in the ICU setting, it is important to follow a systematic method to determine whether the changes are due to ACS or other serious cardiac pathology. ST segment changes are often dismissed as demand ischemia and these cases serve to stress to the reader to always keep a broad differential diagnosis and incorporate all available clinical data when determining how to manage the critically ill patient. Electrocardiogram interpretation reliability is also bolstered with addition clinical data. An ECG diagnosis alone of ACS in the ICU patient should not prompt definitive action until clinical variables are assessed with coronary intervention sometimes being inappropriate.

Case conclusions

Cases 1 and 2 sharply contrast similar clinical situations with widely discordant cardiac catheterization findings. Paramount to the accuracy of the ECG, as with any diagnostic test, is the pretest probability. The omission of cocaine use in the initial patient intake in Case 2 significantly impacts the role of the ECG. Little difference may have ensued with the choice to proceed to cardiac catheterization, but alternate pharmacologic management may have initially been implemented.

Cases 3 and 4 serve as reminders that numerous preexisting conditions, both frequent and rare, may present with ECG features of an ACS. The point of emphasis remains the use of clinical acumen along with laboratory data to detect these alternate diagnoses. In Case 3, early identification of sepsis led to correct resuscitation. Cardiac catheterization was required in Case 4 to exclude myocardial injury in the face of elevated troponins and concerning ECG findings. The coronary catheterization along with the echocardiographic evaluation assisted in the final diagnosis of a Takotsubo cardiomyopathy.

Acknowledgments

We would like to acknowledge the generous contributions of Drs Victor Froelicher, David Winchester, and Raj Subramanian who provided ECG and coronary angiographic images.

References

1 Einthoven W, Fahr G, De Waart A. Über die richtung und die manifeste grosse der potentialschwankungen in menschlichen herzen und über den einfluss der herzlage auf die form des elektrokardiograms. *Arch Physiol* 1913;**150**:275–315.

2 Beckerman J, Yamazaki T, Myers J, *et al.* T-wave abnormalities are a better predictor of cardiovascular mortality than ST depression on the resting electrocardiogram. *Ann Noninvasive Electrocardiol* 2005;**10**:146–51.

3 Surawicz B, Knilans TK. Chou's Electrocardiography in Clinical Practice: Adult & Pediatric. 5th edition ed. Philadelphia, PA: Saunders, 2001.

4 Essen R, Merx W, Effert S. Spontaneous course of ST-segment elevation in acute anterior myocardial infarction. *Circulation* 1979;**59**:105–12.

5 Krone RJ, Greenberg H, Dwyer EM, Jr., *et al.* Long-term prognostic significance of ST segment depression during acute myocardial

infarction. The Multicenter Diltiazem Postinfarction Trial Research Group. *J Am Coll Cardiol* 1993;**22**:361–7.

6 Greenland P, Kauffman R, Weir EK. Profound exercise-induce ST segment depression in a patient with Wolff-Parkinson-White syndrome and normal coronary arteriograms. *Thorax* 1980;**35**:559–60.

7 Nimura Y. A vectorcardiographic analysis of left ventricular strain pattern comparatively studied with ST-T change of left bundle branch block and ventricular premature beat of right ventricular origin. *Am Heart J* 1959;**57**:552–77.

8 Okin PM, Devereux RB, Nieminen MS, *et al.* Relationship of the electrocardiographic strain pattern to left ventricular structure and function in hypertensive patients: the LIFE study. Losartan Intervention For End point. *J Am Coll Cardiol* 2001;**38**:514–20.

9 Brady WJ, Chan TC, Pollack M. Electrocardiographic manifestations: patterns that confound the EKG diagnosis of acute myocardial infarction-left bundle branch block, ventricular paced rhythm, and left ventricular hypertrophy. *J Emerg Med* 2000;**18**:71–8.

10 Antman EM, Anbe DT, Armstrong PW, *et al.* ACC/AHA guidelines for the management of patients with ST-elevation myocardial infarction; A report of the American College of Cardiology/American Heart Association Task Force on Practice Guidelines (Committee to Revise the 1999 Guidelines for the Management of patients with acute myocardial infarction). *J Am Coll Cardiol* 2004;**44**:E1–E211.

11 Iakobishvili Z, Behar S, Boyko V, *et al.* Does current treatment of cardiogenic shock complicating the acute coronary syndromes comply with guidelines? *Am Heart J* 2005;**149**:98–103.

12 Babaev A, Frederick PD, Pasta DJ, *et al.* Trends in management and outcomes of patients with acute myocardial infarction complicated by cardiogenic shock. *JAMA* 2005;**294**:448–54.

13 Hochman JS, Sleeper LA, Webb JG, *et al.* Early revascularization in acute myocardial infarction complicated by cardiogenic shock. SHOCK Investigators. Should We Emergently Revascularize Occluded Coronaries for Cardiogenic Shock. *N Engl J Med* 1999;**341**:625–34.

14 Hochman JS, Sleeper LA, Webb JG, *et al.* Early revascularization and long-term survival in cardiogenic shock complicating acute myocardial infarction. *JAMA* 2006;**295**:2511–5.

15 Dzavik V, Sleeper LA, Cocke TP, *et al.* Early revascularization is associated with improved survival in elderly patients with acute myocardial infarction complicated by cardiogenic shock: a report from the SHOCK Trial Registry. *Eur Heart J* 2003;**24**:828–37.

16 Sanborn TA, Sleeper LA, Bates ER, *et al.* Impact of thrombolysis, intra-aortic balloon pump counterpulsation, and their combination in cardiogenic shock complicating acute myocardial infarction: a report from the SHOCK Trial Registry. SHould we emergently revascularize Occluded Coronaries for cardiogenic shocK? *J Am Coll Cardiol* 2000;**36**:1123–9.

17 Jacobs AK, French JK, Col J, *et al.* Cardiogenic shock with non-ST-segment elevation myocardial infarction: a report from the SHOCK Trial Registry. SHould we emergently revascularize Occluded coronaries for Cardiogenic shocK? *J Am Coll Cardiol* 2000;**36**:1091–6.

18 Bauman JL, Grawe JJ, Winecoff AP, Hariman RJ. Cocaine-related sudden cardiac death: a hypothesis correlating basic science and clinical observations. *J Clin Pharmacol* 1994;**34**:902–11.

19 Hollander JE, Hoffman RS. Cocaine-induced myocardial infarction: an analysis and review of the literature. *J Emerg Med* 1992;**10**:169–77.

20 Rezkalla SH, Mazza JJ, Kloner RA, *et al.* Effects of cocaine on human platelets in healthy subjects. *Am J Cardiol* 1993;**72**:243–6.

21 Boos CJ, Lip GY, Jilma B. Endotoxemia, inflammation, and atrial fibrillation. *Am J Cardiol* 2007;**100**:986–8.

22 Hemels ME, Van Noord T, Crijns HJ, *et al.* Verapamil versus digoxin and acute versus routine serial cardioversion for the improvement of rhythm control for persistent atrial fibrillation. *J Am Coll Cardiol* 2006;**48**:1001–9.

23 European Heart Rhythm Association and the Heart Rhythm Society, Fuster V, Ryden LE, *et al.* ACC/AHA/ESC 2006 Guidelines for the Management of Patients With Atrial Fibrillation: A Report of the American College of Cardiology/American Heart Association Task Force on Practice Guidelines and the European Society of Cardiology Committee for Practice Guidelines (Writing Committee to Revise the 2001 Guidelines for the Management of Patients With Atrial Fibrillation). *J Am Coll Cardiol* 2006;**48**: e149–246.

24 Lyon AR, Rees PS, Prasad S, *et al.* Stress (Takotsubo) cardiomyopathy – a novel pathophysiological hypothesis to explain catecholamine-induced acute myocardial stunning. *Nat Clin Pract Cardiovasc Med* 2008;**5**:22–9.

25 Haghi D, Fluechter S, Suselbeck T, *et al.* Takotsubo cardiomyopathy (acute left ventricular apical ballooning syndrome) occurring in the intensive care unit. *Intensive Care Med* 2006;**32**:1069–74.

26 Brugada P, Brugada J. Right bundle branch block, persistent ST segment elevation and sudden cardiac death: a distinct clinical and electrocardiographic syndrome. A multicenter report. *J Am Coll Cardiol* 1992;**20**:1391–6.

27 Gussak I, Antzelevitch C, Bjerregaard P, *et al.* The Brugada syndrome: clinical, electrophysiologic and genetic aspects. *J Am Coll Cardiol* 1999;**33**:5–15.

28 Chen Q, Kirsch GE, Zhang D, *et al.* Genetic basis and molecular mechanism for idiopathic ventricular fibrillation. *Nature* 1998; **392**:293–6.

29 Dalla Volta S, Battaglia G, Zerbini E. "Auricularization" of right ventricular pressure curve. *Am Heart J* 1961;**61**:25–33.

30 Frank R, Fontaine G, Vedel J, *et al.* [Electrocardiology of 4 cases of right ventricular dysplasia inducing arrhythmia]. *Arch Mal Coeur Vaiss* 1978;**71**:963–72.

31 Lim W, Qushmaq I, Cook D, *et al.* Reliability of electrocardiogram interpretation in critically ill patients. *Crit Care Med* 2006;**34**(5): 1338–43.

Chapter 38 | What is the role of the ECG in therapeutic considerations/medical management decisions in the critically ill patient?

Billie Barker[1], Adam Helms[2], Ajeet Vinayak[2]
[1]University School of Medicine, Detroit, MI, USA
[2]University of Virginia, Charlottesville, VA, USA

Case presentations

Case 1: A 70-year-old male is admitted to the hospital with a community-acquired pneumonia and started on intravenous (IV) moxifloxacin. Over the first 24 h of his hospital course, he develops progressive respiratory distress and is found to have an empyema. He is transferred to the intensive care unit (ICU) and a chest tube is placed. He stabilizes but continues to have hypoxia, requiring 4 L/min oxygen by nasal cannula. On hospital day #3, he becomes hypotensive with a blood pressure of 86/50 mmHg and is found to have new-onset atrial fibrillation with a rapid ventricular response. He begins an amiodarone intravenous load over the following 24 h and converts to sinus rhythm. However, the next day his monitoring alarm triggers, and the telemetry monitoring strip (Figure 38.1) shows polymorphic ventricular tachycardia (VT). Because he lacks a pulse, defibrillation is performed, and he converts to sinus rhythm only briefly. He goes through several doses of epinephrine and repeated cardioversions. Magnesium is given intravenously, followed by isoproterenol. A transvenous pacing wire is placed, and, following another cardioversion, he is successfully paced at 100 beats per minute (bpm).

Case 2: A 54-year-old male is admitted to the medical floor with complaints of chest pain and cough and is given the diagnosis of pneumonia. He carries no prior medical diagnoses as he has had little prior health maintenance. He is treated with IV moxifloxacin and normal saline. Over the first 12 h he reports some worsening dyspnea and increased

chest pain. That night he is found stuporous and more hypoxic, requiring 100% oxygen. The decision for ICU transfer is made. Admission data, including an electrocardiogram (ECG), are reviewed, leading to concern for prior myocardial infarction (MI) (Figure 38.2a). Given his acute worsening, chest pain, and hypoxia, the concern for an acute coronary syndrome (ACS) prompts orders for heparin and cardiology consultation. A repeat ECG on ICU admission shows normal findings, with the notable absence of concerning prior findings of possible infarct (Figure 38.2b). Initial cardiac enzymes return as normal. A repeat chest radiograph demonstrates interval worsening of a left lobar pneumonia and development of pleural effusion. Heparin orders are cancelled, and cardiology deems the discordant ECG data related to lead reversal/misplacement on the initial tracing.

Case 3: A 75-year-old male is admitted with cough, dyspnea, and clear sputum production. His past medical history is notable for severe emphysema, and coronary artery disease with bypass surgery 5 years prior. His initial ECG is reported as atrial fibrillation (AF) with aberrancy and rapid ventricular response at 110 bpm. Initial cardiac biomarkers are normal. Chest radiograph reveals a lobar pneumonia. He has a modest 4 L fluid resuscitation, given concerns of underlying heart disease. He remains mildly hypotensive with a blood pressure of 87/49 mmHg, irregularly tachycardic at 115 bpm, and develops marked hypoxia. He is started on a norepinephrine drip and IV antibiotics upon admission to the ICU. That first night he becomes unresponsive and gets intubated. By 11 pm his norepinephrine dose has doubled to maintain mean arterial pressures of 60 mmHg. An ECG is obtained as part of his evolving shock assessment (Figure 38.3a). An interpretation of right bundle branch block (RBBB) and atrial fibrillation is initially made. These findings are all thought to be consistent with his known diagnosis of emphysema, and coronary artery disease complicated by

Critical Decisions in Emergency and Acute Care Electrocardiography,
1st edition. Edited by W.J. Brady and J.D. Truwit. © 2009 Blackwell Publishing, ISBN: 9781405159067

(a)

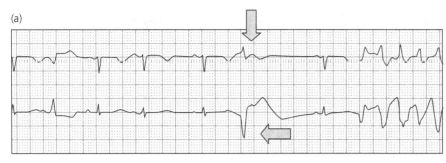

(b)

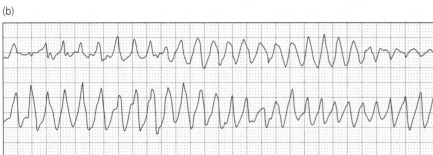

Figure 38.1 Initiation of ventricular tachycardia (VT) and continuation into a torsade de pointes pattern. (a) The top rhythm strip shows initiation of VT. The green arrows identify a premature ventricular contraction occurring during the repolarization phase in a patient with a long QT. (b) The sustained VT has polymorphic QRS morphology that appears to have phasic variations consistent with torsade de pointes.

pneumonia. Discussion of adenosine or amiodarone administration is debated initially until repeat assessment of his admission ECG (Figure 38.3b) is compared with the most recent ECG (Figure 38.3a) and the wide complex rhythm is re-identified as VT. He is cardioverted back into a sinus tachycardia with aberrancy (left bundle branch block, LBBB). Given that norepinephrine may have contributed to the VT, further management includes adjustment of vasoactive drugs and more aggressive fluid administration. Hemodynamic management is guided with the placement of a right heart catheter. His further ICU course involves pneumonia therapy, eventual ventilator removal, and initiation of amiodarone therapy for recalcitrant VT before being transferred to the medical floor.

How the ECG affects medical management in the critically ill patient

These three cases exemplify how the ECG can have marked impact on diagnosis and therapy in the ICU. A number of different ECG-driven management and therapy choices are worth noting in the ICU patient. As evident in the second and third cases, management decisions may change dramatically after complete and proper application and interpretation of the ECG. We will also review the use of the ECG in hemodynamic measurements and its assistance in the diagnosis of particular states of shock. To begin, we will address general therapeutic considerations in the dysrhythmic ICU patient and then characterize common ICU medication therapy-related iatrogenesis presenting as arrhythmia.

General management considerations in the dysrhythmic ICU patient

As many as one in five patients are thought to have an episode of symptomatic arrhythmia during their ICU stay [1]. Detailed diagnostic and management features in the dysrhythmic patient are discussed in the prior section, but certain aspects as they pertain to therapy and the critically ill patient are worth re-attention. Initial assessment beyond laboratory (electrolytes, myocardial damage markers) and prior echocardiography studies looking for structural heart disease, includes a 12-lead ECG and the telemetry data at the time of arrhythmia origination.

Supraventricular tachycardias (SVTs) are the most common variety of ICU arrhythmia [1]. Initial diagnostic differentiation based on the QRS feature of narrow versus wide VT remains the most likely cause of wide complex tachycardias in the ICU, but awareness of aberrancy, paced rhythms and hyperkalemia as causes of wide complex morphology in an underlying SVT are important considerations for the intensivist. Additionally, acute hemodynamic instability and tachycardia should lead to synchronized electrical cardioversion. Adenosine can be administered if a supraventricular origin is evident and there is hemodynamic stability. This agent should be avoided in VT as atrioventricular (AV) node blockade can potentiate continued VT.

Electrocardiogram identification of atrial fibrillation, the most common arrhythmia in the ICU, deserves additional therapeutic attention. As electrical cardioversion frequently fails to achieve long-term sinus rhythm in acute atrial fibril-

(a)

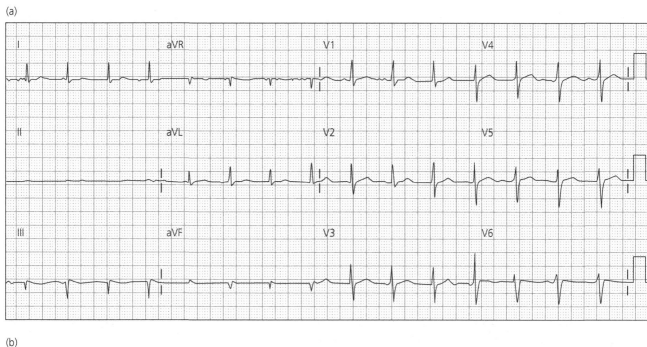

(b)

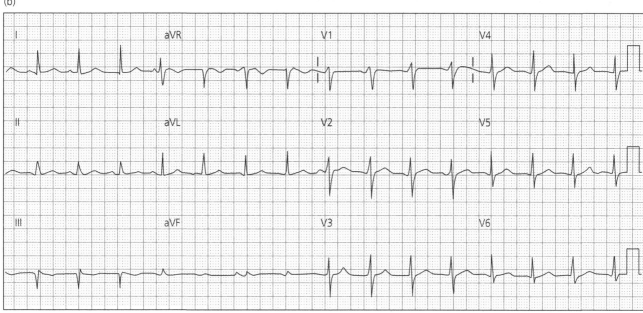

Figure 38.2 Precordial lead reversal ECGs. (a) The large R wave in V1 and Q waves inferiorly are suggestive of an inferior-posterior infarction. This is seen if the precordial leads have been flipped completely V6 ≥ V1. (b) Correct positioning of the precordial leads results in a normal ECG tracing.

lation [2], rate control and, potentially, chemical cardioversion remain the better options. Rate control with beta-blockade and calcium channel-blockers should be avoided in the setting of hypotension, especially with need for vasoactive medications. Digoxin may also be useful in the setting of atrial fibrillation and heart failure as it may slow ventricular response and help increase contractility. Intravenous anti-arrhythmics can exacerbate hypotension, but potentially terminate the atrial fibrillation that may increase cardiac output

through restoration of sinus rhythm and restoration of atrial contraction. Anti-coagulation should also be considered.

Stable wide complex tachycardia of ventricular origin is most often managed with amiodarone, but procainamide and lidocaine have also been used. Consideration of an implantable cardioverter-defribillator (ICD) placement, at a later date, should occur if cardiomyopathy and lack of a reversible cause of VT are found. When refractory to magnesium and lidocaine, torsade de pointes may be managed with transvenous

(a)

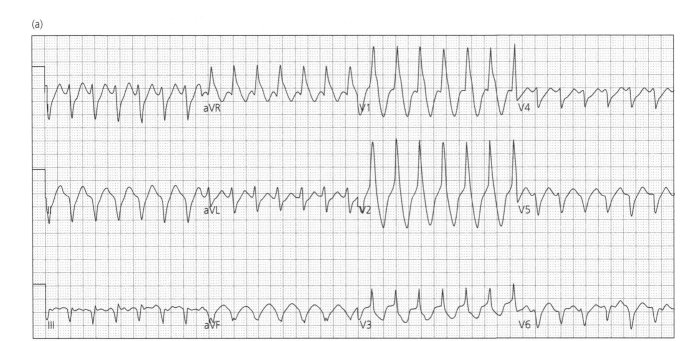

(b)

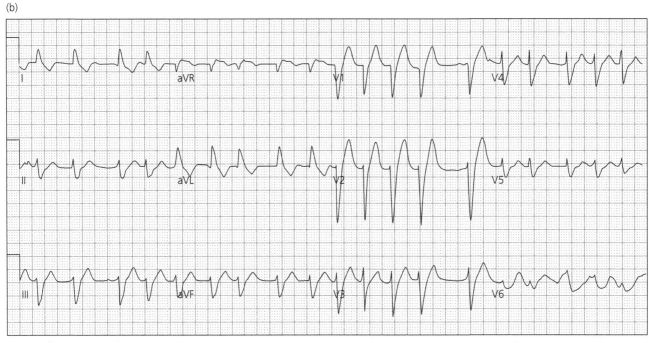

Figure 38.3 (a) The ECG read at the time of the initial decline shows a wide complex tachycardia with a ventricular rate just above 150 bpm. Rightward QRS axis, terminal S waves in I, AVL, and V6 directed rightward were suggestive of right bundle branch block (RBBB). Given the irregular on strip, this rhythm was initially read as atrial fibrillation with RBBB aberrancy. (b) Admission ECG shows wide complex tachycardia with a left bundle branch pattern. The rhythm is irregularly irregular and read as atrial fibrillation with aberrancy.

cardiac pacing with a goal rate of 80–100 bpm (as in Case 1). This override pacing can assist in curtailing the QT interval [3].

Significant bradycardia accounts for 10% of ICU arrhythmias [3]. Atropine administration is the initial pharmacologic approach if bradycardia is deemed unstable, but its action is short-lived. Pacing strategies are also used for hemodynamically significant bradycardias or high-degree block. Temporary pacing options include transcutaneous and transvenous approaches, with the latter considered for anticipated lengthy therapy given discomfort associated with the prior. Initial transcutaneous pacing settings include: current (40–100 mA) and rate (60–70 bpm). When the transvenous pacer is available, initial current can be dropped to 3–5 mA

[4]. These settings should be adjusted to maintain capture and assure hemodynamic stability.

Often, while the underlying disease process is being treated, persistent hypotension associated with an arrhythmia can be managed with vasoactive drug infusions. Many of these agents have intrinsic adrenergic activity or reflex mechanisms that promulgate tachycardia or risk further ventricular ectopy (as in Case 3). Norepinephrine, epinephrine, dobutamine, and dopamine all stimulate alpha- and beta-adrenergic receptors. Again, the adrenergic effects of these agents also make them pro-arrhythmic and lead to atrial and ventricular arrhythmias. The phosphodiesterase inhibitor, milrinone is theoretically more appealing due to its lack of adrenergic action, though it, too, has been associated with tachycardia and ventricular arrhythmias [5]. Often, the management of septic or cardiogenic shock mandates the use of one or more of these agents and continuous ECG monitoring.

In these patients with sepsis, SVTs occur frequently. Choice of alternative vasoactive drug choices may be directed by hemodynamic instability caused by worsening tachycardia or persistent ectopy with one of the above beta-adrenergic agents. Phenylephrine, a potent primarily alpha-adrenergic agonist, has been shown to lead to favorable blood pressure response with less tachycardia mediated by baroreflex inhibition of chronotropy [6]. Vasopressin has also been increasingly used in vasodilated states. Administered at hormone replacement doses (0.01–0.04 U/min), it has virtually no direct effect on heart rate via the vasopressin (V1) receptor.

In theory, coronary ischemia has been postulated at higher doses of vasopressin, yet limited investigations have shown no ischemia at this low dose. In fact, stable coronary perfusion variables have been seen when vasopressin is used in treatment of myocardial ischemia [7,8]. We acknowledge there is little evidence to advocate clear recommendations of specific agents. Yet, in the treatment of refractory atrial tachyarrhythmias after volume resuscitation, we often rely on phenylephrine and/or vasopressin infusion in the face of persistent hypotension associated with sepsis.

Polymorphic ventricular tachycardia and medications

Case 1 describes a patient with polymorphic VT associated with a baseline prolonged QT interval (i.e. torsade de pointes). Case 1 represents a typical scenario in the ICU, in which complex medical care can be confounded by interacting treatments. In this case, an ill patient is administered two medications (moxifloxacin and amiodarone) that both prolong the QT interval without following the QT interval with serial ECGs.

Both monomorphic and polymorphic VT are frequently encountered in the ICU. Monomorphic VT (Figure 38.4) is typically a result of scar within the left or right ventricle, around which develops a re-entry circuit creating uniform-appearing QRS complexes on the ECG. Monomorphic VT is

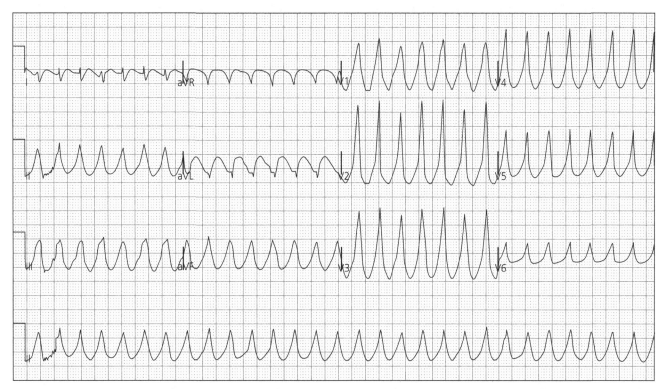

Figure 38.4 Monomorphic ventricular tachycardia is appreciated as a wide QRS complex tachycardia with consistent QRS morphology and polarity across the precordium – the so-called positive concordant precordial pattern.

Medications	Other conditions
Antibiotics	**Electrolyte disturbance**
Fluoroquinolones (e.g. ciprofloxacin)	Hypokalemia
Macrolides (e.g. azithromycin)	Hypomagnesemia
Pentamidine	Hypocalcemia
Chloroquine	
Psychiatric and pain medications	**Physiologic states**
Phenothiazines (e.g. haloperidol, risperidal)	Bradycardia
Tricyclic anti-depressants (e.g. amitriptyline)	Recent conversion from atrial fibrillation
Methadone	Increased adrenergic tone (e.g. sepsis)
Anti-arrhythmics	**Heart disease**
Class IA (quinidine, procainamide)	Congestive heart failure
Class IB (disopyramide)	Myocardial ischemia
Class III (sotalol, dofetilide, amiodarone)	

Table 38.1 Partial list of medications and other factors that predispose to QT prolongation and thus contribute to polymorphic ventricular tachycardia in the intensive care unit

typically caused by prior MI that has created the scar, or by non-ischemic cardiomyopathy, in which remodeling and fibrosis create the wound. Polymorphic VT, by contrast, is a result of chaotic re-entry circuits that develop due to repolarization abnormalities in the ventricles and result in QRS complexes whose morphologies vary from one to the next. Polymorphic VT is of particular concern in the critical care unit, where a confluence of multiple risk factors including medications and electrolyte disarray occurs.

Polymorphic ventricular tachycardia is categorized depending on the baseline QT interval. When the QT interval is normal, polymorphic VT most likely arises from acute coronary ischemia (other causes, such as catecholaminergic VT, are much less common). When the QT interval is prolonged, polymorphic VT is due to either a hereditary long QT syndrome or from acquired conditions, primarily medications or electrolyte disturbances (Table 38.1) [9].

Medications that contribute to QT prolongation are particularly common in the ICU. Quinolone or macrolide antibiotics are both commonly used to treat pneumonia, among other types of infection. Anti-psychotics are often used in the setting of ICU-related delirium, and anti-arrhythmic agents are used when supraventricular or ventricular arrhythmias develop. The degree of QT prolongation roughly correlates with the risk of torsade de pointes, and, therefore, the QT interval should be monitored in patients who are on one or more drugs known to increase the QT interval. An equation can be used to estimate risk, $R = 1.052X$, where X is a 10 ms increase in the QT interval [10]. A notable exception to this general rule is amiodarone, which significantly increases the QT interval but is associated with only a small risk (< 1%) of torsade de pointes [11].

Another important consideration is concurrent medications that inhibit the metabolism of QT-prolonging medications. For example, the anti-fungal azoles (e.g. fluconazole) and ranitidine, both used in the ICU, do not prolong the QT interval. However, they do inhibit the cytochrome P450 CYP3A system, which metabolizes the macrolide antibiotics (except azithromycin) and amiodarone – thus the levels of these medications are increased [11].

Other risk factors for developing acquired QT prolongation should be assessed prior to starting medications that prolong the QT interval. These factors include female sex, electrolyte disturbances, increased adrenergic tone, congestive heart failure, left ventricular hypertrophy, myocardial ischemia, recent conversion from atrial fibrillation, and bradycardia [11]. Continuous electrocardiographic monitoring should be performed routinely in the ICU and, where available, should include QT monitoring on patients started on QT prolonging medications or with significant electrolyte abnormalities [12].

The ECG and sedative drugs

Many additional medication-associated ECG findings can occur in the ICU. One particular category of agents unique to the ICU environment is the sedative drug. The sedative propofol has been associated with case reports of myocardial failure since early 1990. Bradycardia is a well-recognized effect of the agent. A more concerning clinical entity, propofol infusion syndrome (PIS), has since been identified in which prolonged propofol infusions have been associated with bradycardia that is refractory to treatment and may progress to asystole. Bradycardia is required for the diagnosis, along with at least one other feature including lipemia, hepatomegaly secondary to fatty infiltration, severe metabolic acidosis, and the presence of muscle involvement with evidence of rhabdomyolysis or myoglobinuria [13]. While not part of the diagnostic criteria, severe hyperkalemia may also be noted with additional ECG abnormalities. Co-administration of analgesic agents, such as opiates, has been shown to reduce propofol dose requirements. Whether this effect might attenuate PIS incidence is unknown. Close monitoring is recommended in patients with propofol infusion, and consideration of discontinuation of the agent should be made if the patient develops arrhythmia or metabolic acidosis.

Opiates and benzodiazepines are also commonly utilized in ICU sedative regimens, and are also not without accompanying risk. Bradycardia and hypotension are the most commonly seen effects associated with these medications. As a patient nears extubation or requires less sedation, the clinician must also be cognizant of the possibility of withdrawal from these medications, which most often presents with hypertension and tachycardia and necessitates partial re-institution of the drug. Electrocardiogram monitoring and evidence of autonomic instability often is the first alarm for ill effect or withdrawal from these agents. One caveat exists with the administration of methadone. This opiate, often used for chronic opiate withdrawal or prolonged analgesic needs, has been associated with QT interval prolongation and associated VT [14].

Recently, dexmetomidine, a selective alpha-2 adrenergic receptor agonist, is experiencing a greater role in ICU sedation [15]. Its effects on the sympathetic nervous system make it a theoretically more desirable agent where more of an anxiolytic effect is desired over pure sedation. However, given these same adrenergic actions, the use of this drug may result in hypotension and bradycardia. Continuous electrocardiographic monitoring is important when using this drug, and we recommend that it be used for limited durations of sedation.

Fluctuations in catecholamine levels during sedative limiting practices have been suggested to be a risk factor for ischemia. While ischemia does occur with ventilator management, a recently published study suggests no correlation with ECG-determined ischemia to proximal sedative discontinuation in a cohort of patients with coronary risk factors [16].

ECG data acquisition and artifact

A common tenet in ICU care that overlaps with the basic ECG interpretation is the need to critically analyze the validity of available data. Erroneous interpretations can occur by mistakes in acquisition or failure to recognize changes from prior ECG data. Case 2 illustrates a problem with ECG lead placement. Lead misplacement can easily occur, but, fortunately, this results in easily recognizable patterns (Figure 38.2). The inversion of all precordial leads as in Case 2 may lead to a posterior infarction diagnosis that has implications in the differential of shock. Other notable lead placement errors can result in low voltage (RA–RL), other infarction patterns (RA-LA or RA-LL), or nonsensical aberrations in QRS progression across the precordium [17,18]. Also paramount to accurate ECG interpretation is the addition of prior ECG data. Case 3 illustrates the role of prior baseline abnormalities that can lead to correct identification of a malignant rhythm (Figure 38.3).

Pre-existing pacemakers and implanted cardioversion devices in the ICU

While ICD indications and pacemaker dysfunction have been discussed in the last section, several important ICU management points are noteworthy when these devices accompany course of critical illness. Persistent ICD discharges associated with reversible conditions (electrolyte abnormalities, sepsis, drugs) may need to be addressed by temporarily disabling the device while implemented pharmacologic therapies take effect. Low battery charge may lead to recurrent firings. Emergent discontinuation of shocks can be achieved by placing a magnet over the ICD until experienced electrophysiology personnel arrive [4,19]. Also, external cardioversion in the ICU setting can cause these devices to be damaged, requiring follow-up device interrogation.

Hemodynamic monitoring and ECG

Common invasive hemodynamic measurements, such as right atrial pressure and pulmonary capillary wedge pressure (PCWP), are made with significant therapeutic consequences dependent on their accuracy. Several key points are tied to the role of the ECG in this evaluation. Variations in these waveforms occur with variation associated with both the respiratory and cardiac cycle. In practice, the mean of the A wave at end-expiration is the accurate point for identification and comparative assessments. In theory the mean of the A wave is a close approximation to end-diastolic pressures. The A wave occurs immediately after the P wave (in the PR interval) on the ECG tracing. This temporal relationship between P wave to A wave widens on PCWP measurement, given the longer distance and, therefore, longer time of pressure transmission from the left atrium to the tip of the right heart catheter where this value is measured. The A wave coincides with the QRS complex on the ECG. At times, in particular when the prominent left atrial V waves exist, this fact is a guide that can help distinguish a wedged catheter from a pulmonary artery tracing (Figure 38.5).

Identification of acute right heart syndromes in the ICU and implications on management

Shock requiring this type of hemodynamic monitoring is often the criterium for ICU admission. Among causes of shock, low cardiac output states are frequently identified. While the vast majority of these "pump failure" shocks are

(a)

(b)

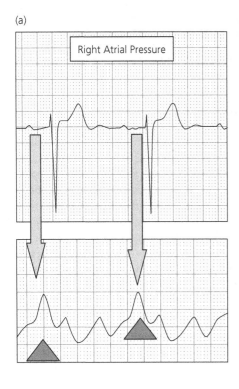
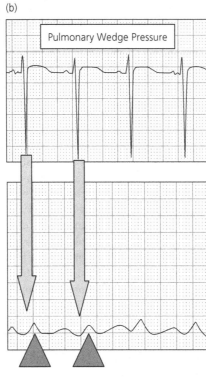

Figure 38.5 Correct hemodynamic monitoring assessment based on ECG. Correct identification of the A wave (green arrows) occurs in conjunction with the ECG. The red arrows in (a) show A waves occurring just after the P wave. In (b), the A wave is associated with the QRS complex. (Image courtesy of Steven Koenig, MD.)

related to left ventricular dysfunction, right heart dysfunction occurs and marked differences in therapy and management are significant. As their incidence appears to be increasing, a high degree of clinical vigilance is required in their identification [20,21]. The acutely failing right ventricle (RV), also termed acute cor pulmonale or acute right heart syndrome (AHRS) [4], occurs for a number of reasons, with acute pulmonary embolism being the prototypical and most recognized event. Right ventricular infarction or many conditions associated with acute deterioration of patients with chronic pulmonary hypertension also comprise AHRS. Unique experiences in the ICU such as acute respiratory distress syndrome, excessive positive pressure ventilation, pericardial disease, certain toxins, and sepsis, are often the inciting events leading to this pressure overload of the RV.

Therapeutic considerations in ARHS differ from goals of left ventricular failure management. The RV has a less impressive contractile functionality than the left ventricular pump. Therefore, fluid removal aimed at decreasing preload can cause underfilling of the RV which requires the adequate pressure to oppose its elevated afterload, the pulmonary arterial hypertension. Furthermore, the coronary supply of the right-sided myocardium is far more limited than the left. It is for this reason that therapies aimed at decreasing systemic afterload can threaten the balance of this tenuous coronary perfusion in the setting of increased myocardial demand of the failing right heart.

Clinical signs of right heart dysfunction include elevated jugular veins, pulsatile liver, peripheral edema (more prominent than pulmonary edema), chest radiographic evidence

and suggestive ECG findings. These ECG findings most commonly reflect the overloaded pressure of the right side, but may also be diagnostic of RV infarction. Subsequent echocardiogram can rapidly confirm clinically suspected ARHS.

Electrocardiogram findings of right heart disease include right axis deviation, signs of right atrial enlargement (p pulmonale) and pulmonary hypertension. P pulmonale, described in Chapter 36, is defined as tall P waves (> 2.5 mm) especially in lead II but also often present in III, aVF, and the initial portion of V1. Right ventricular hypertrophy occurs when chronic pulmonary hypertension over time leads to remodeling (ECG characteristics are outlined in Table 36.2, first chapter of section) (Figure 38.6). Addition patterns of RV strain include ST segment depression and T wave inversions in right precordial leads or an $S_1Q_3T_3$ pattern. The prognostic implications of these findings in pulmonary hypertension and pulmonary embolism are also discussed elsewhere in this section.

Right ventricular infarction occurs frequently with inferior MI and also may be seen in anterior infarction. The occurrence of RV infarct increases mortality likelihood above isolated left ventricular infarction [22,23]. Rarely, sepsis and specific toxins can mimic a RV infarct scenario. Rather than increased pulmonary vascular afterload, RV dilatation due to myocardial injury leads to increased right atrial pressure.

The ECG findings of RV infarct include evolving ST-T wave changes or Q waves in II, III, and aVF. Confirmation of right-sided infarct requires right-sided precordial leads (similar to left-sided leads and labeled V1R to V6R). ST segment elevations over 1 mm in these leads, especially in V4R, are the

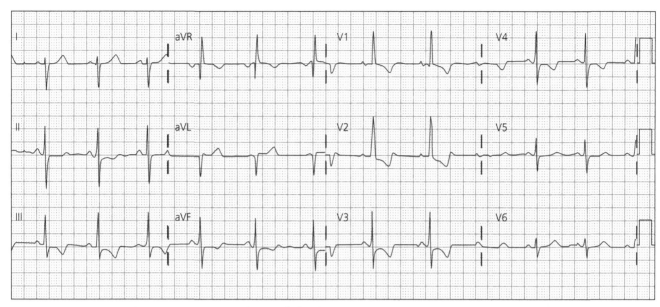

Figure 38.6 Right ventricular overload. ECG with significant right-sided findings including right axis deviation, right atrial enlargement (tall P waves inferior lead > 2.5 mm), right ventricular hypertrophy (prominent R wave in V1 > 7 mm), and strain pattern inferiorly and across early precordial leads (ST depressions and T wave inversions in leads II, III, aVF, and V1–V4).

characteristic findings [24]. This finding is highly specific and 70% sensitive, yet may be transient in nature. It is suggested that right-sided ECG be done within 10 h to assure diagnosis. Common arrhythmias that accompany right-sided infarct include RBBB and complete heart block.

Low cardiac output states commonly occur as a consequence or result of critical illness. Correctly, management is directed toward optimization [21] of left-sided systolic dysfunction. When this pump dysfunction is primarily due to an ARHS, conventional strategies such as diuresis and afterload reduction may be deleterious. In addition, specific vasoactive drug management must be tailored to optimizing RV function [4,20]. The diagnosis of ARHS is dependent on clinical suspicion and confirmed with the use of echocardiogram. Clinical suspicion further aids in appropriate and correct ECG testing in cases of RV ischemia. Identification can be aided with rapid application of specific ECG patterns along with other clinical findings.

Case conclusions

The cases described show how proper ECG evaluation can avoid erroneous diagnoses or detect potentially avoidable iatrogenesis and guide proper therapy in the ICU. In Case 1, overdrive-pacing assisted in control of torsade de pointes that may have been identified earlier if QT prolongation had been recognized or followed with serial ECGs. Even when ECG is routinely employed, error in interpretation can occur if improper ECG acquisition techniques are employed as in Case 2. The diagnostic concern for coronary disease is rapidly decreased when proper ECG evaluation occurs. Case 3 emphasizes the role of the prior ECG data for comparison and its impact on management. Differentiating a VT, rather than a SVT, leads to a host of alternative therapies and diagnostic steps. Other applications of 12-lead ECGs and tracings that impact management in the ICU include accuracy of frequent hemodynamic measurements and assistance in the proper diagnosis of complex cases of shock.

References

1 Reinelt P, Karth GD, Geppert A, *et al.* Incidence and type of cardiac arrhythmias in critically ill patients: a single center experience in a medical-cardiological ICU. *Intensive Care Med* 2001;**27**(9):1466–73.

2 Hemels ME, Van Noord T, Crijns HJ, *et al.* Verapamil versus digoxin and acute versus routine serial cardioversion for the improvement of rhythm control for persistent atrial fibrillation. *J Am Coll Cardiol* 2006;**48**(5):1001–9.

3 Reising S, Kusumoto F, Goldschlager N. Life-threatening arrhythmias in the intensive care unit. *J Intensive Care Med* 2007;**22**(1): 3–13.

4 Hall JB, Schmidt GA, Wood LDH. *Principles of critical care*. 3rd ed. New York: McGraw-Hill, 2005, xxvii, 1778 pp.

5 Bayram M, De Luca L, Massie MB, *et al.* Reassessment of dobutamine, dopamine, and milrinone in the management of acute heart failure syndromes. *Am J Cardiol* 2005;**96**(6A):47G–58G.

6 Leitch JW, Basta M, Fletcher PJ. Effect of phenylephrine infusion on atrial electrophysiological properties. *Heart* 1997;**78**(2): 166–70.

7 Jolly S, Newton G, Horlick E, *et al.* Effect of vasopressin on hemodynamics in patients with refractory cardiogenic shock complicating acute myocardial infarction. *Am J Cardiol* 2005; **96**(12):1617–20.

8 Palmaers T, Albrecht S, Heuser F, *et al.* Milrinone combined with vasopressin improves cardiac index after cardiopulmonary resuscitation in a pig model of myocardial infarction. *Anesthesiology* 2007;**106**(1):100–6.

9 Woosley R, ACA Board. *Drugs That Prolong the QT Interval and/or Induce Torsades de Pointes.* www.qtdrugs.org

10 Webster R, Leishman D, Walker D. Towards a drug concentration effect relationship for QT prolongation and torsades de pointes. *Curr Opin Drug Discovery Dev* 2002;**5**(1):116–26.

11 Chiang C-E. Congenital and acquired long QT syndrome. Current concepts and management. *Cardiol Rev* 2004;**12**(4):222–34.

12 Drew BJ, *et al.* Practice standards for electrocardiographic monitoring in hospital settings: an American Heart Association scientific statement from the Councils on Cardiovascular Nursing, Clinical Cardiology, and Cardiovascular Disease in the Young: endorsed by the International Society of Computerized Electrocardiology and the American Association of Critical-Care Nurses. [Erratum appears in Circulation. 2005 Jan 25;111(3):378.] *Circulation* 2004;**110**(17):2721–46.

13 Kang TM. Propofol infusion syndrome in critically ill patients. *Ann Pharmacother* 2002;**36**(9):1453–6.

14 Ehret GB, Desmeules JA, Broers B. Methadone-associated long QT syndrome: improving pharmacotherapy for dependence on illegal opioids and lessons learned for pharmacology. *Expert Opin Drug Saf* 2007;**6**(3):289–303.

15 Pandharipande PP, Pun BT, Herr DL, *et al.* Effect of sedation with dexmedetomidine vs lorazepam on acute brain dysfunction in mechanically ventilated patients: the MENDS randomized controlled trial. *JAMA* 2007;**298**(22):2644–53.

16 Kress JP, Vinayak AG, Levitt J, *et al.* Daily sedative interruption in mechanically ventilated patients at risk for coronary artery disease. *Crit Care Med* 2007;**35**(2):365–71.

17 Harrigan RA. Electrode misconnection, misplacement, and artifact. *Emerg Med Clin North Am* 2006;**24**(1):227–35, viii.

18 Peberdy MA, Ornato JP. Recognition of electrocardiographic lead misplacements. *Am J Emerg Med* 1993;**11**(4):403–5.

19 Chow AWC, Buxton AE. *Implantable Cardiac Pacemakers and Defibrillators: All You Wanted to Know.* Malden, Mass.: Blackwell Pub./BMJ Books, 2006, vii, 176 pp.

20 Piazza G, Goldhaber SZ. The acutely decompensated right ventricle: pathways for diagnosis and management. *Chest* 2005;**128**(3): 1836–52.

21 Mebazaa A, Karpati P, Renaud E, *et al.* Acute right ventricular failure – from pathophysiology to new treatments. *Intensive Care Med* 2004;**30**(2):185–96.

22 Goldstein JA. Pathophysiology and management of right heart ischemia. *J Am Coll Cardiol* 2002;**40**(5):841–53.

23 Mehta SR, Eikelboom JW, Natarajan MK, *et al.* Impact of right ventricular involvement on mortality and morbidity in patients with inferior myocardial infarction. *J Am Coll Cardiol* 2001; **37**(1):37–43.

24 Kinch JW, Ryan TJ. Right ventricular infarction. *N Engl J Med* 1994;**330**(17):1211–7.

Chapter 39 | Can the ECG predict risk in the critically ill, non-coronary patient?

Clay A. Cauthen, Ajeet Vinayak
University of Virginia, Charlottesville, VA, USA

Case presentations

Case 1: A 64-year-old male is admitted to the intensive care unit (ICU) with sepsis from a bacterial pneumonia. His course is complicated by hypotension requiring pressors and by renal failure. A pulmonary artery catheter is placed to assess volume status. Over the next several hours, increased ectopy is noted on continuous electrocardiographic monitoring. A 12-lead electrocardiogram (ECG) is obtained (Figure 39.1). The catheter is removed with resolution of ventricular bigeminy.

Case 2: A 62-year-old female smoker with chronic obstructive pulmonary disease receives a tracheostomy. During weaning trials, the ECG demonstrates ST depressions and T wave inversions (Figure 39.2) in the anterior leads that resolve when the patient is placed by on pressure support.

Case 3: A 42-year-old male with hepatitis C cirrhosis presents with spontaneous bacterial peritonitis that is complicated by septic shock. The patient receives appropriate antibiosis and a 22-L volume resuscitation. As a result of the large volume resuscitation, the patient developed anasarca. In reviewing his chart, the physician notes that the 12-lead ECG obtained on admission demonstrated tachycardia with a prolonged QRS of 126 ms (Figure 39.3a), consistent with an intraventricular conduction delay (IVCD) that had been noted on previous admissions. However, the most recent 12-lead ECG demonstrated a decrease in the QRS amplitude and resolution of the IVCD (89 ms) (Figure 39.3b). As the patient clinically improves, he receives appropriate diuresis to his dry body weight and plans are made for discharge. An ECG prior to discharge demonstrates normalization of the QRS amplitude and the return of the IVCD.

Critical Decisions in Emergency and Acute Care Electrocardiography,
1st edition. Edited by W.J. Brady and J.D. Truwit. © 2009 Blackwell Publishing, ISBN: 9781405159067

The ECG and risk prediction in the critically ill, non-coronary patient

For many non-coronary, critically ill patients, the majority of time is spent in the ICU after accomplishment of initial resuscitative and diagnostic phases. The focus of this remaining time is supportive care and minimization of complications while monitoring recovery. Each case above highlights specific causative or consequential aspects of ICU care that introduce risk and threaten this recovery: Sepsis syndrome is common and accounts for the largest proportion of ICU mortality and morbidity; During resuscitation, vasoactive drugs are used and fluid administration may lead to an edematous state; key tools in the supportive care arsenal of the modern ICU include the mechanical ventilator and initiation of hemodialysis. The intensivist applies clinical data daily for early recognition of complication. In this chapter we will outline the role of the ECG in this daily risk assessment as patients are subjected to the perils of ICU care.

ICU complications

In certain circumstances, the ECG may provide the initial sign of complication. In fact, continuous electrocardiography is indicated in all patients admitted to the ICU [1]. Continuous electrocardiographic monitoring is important to identify increased ventricular ectopy in these patients, as it indicates a higher risk of ventricular tachycardia. By earlier identification of this dangerous arrhythmia, rapid steps toward management can be taken. In addition, polymorphic ventricular tachycardia from QT-prolonging medications is a not infrequent complication of medical care in the intensive care unit, and is discussed separately.

New-onset atrial tachyarrhythmias are seen frequently, followed by ventricular rhythms, and are often the first presenting symptom of ICU care complications. Their presence,

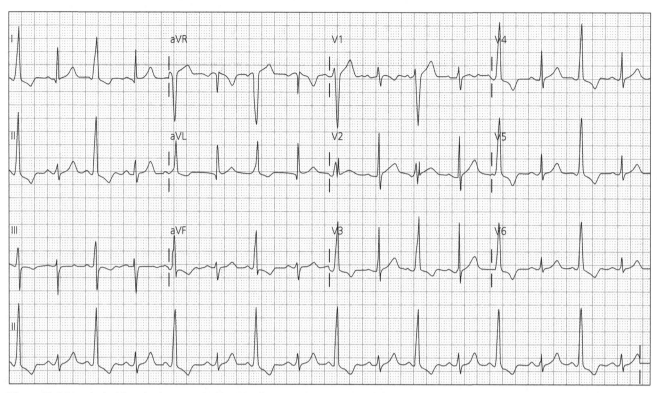

Figure 39.1 Ventricular bigeminy is present in this ECG. Alternating beats are identified as ventricular by their longer QRS duration and by their different axis and morphology.

(a)

(b)

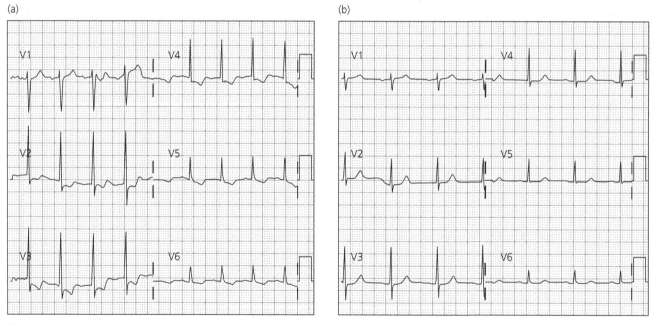

Figure 39.2 (a) ST depressions in anterior and lateral precordial leads that occur during liberation trials from mechanical ventilation, and (b) resolve upon resumption of supported ventilator breaths.

appropriately, prompts an investigation for occult ischemia, and anxiety or pain, especially in the critically ill patient who is unable to communicate additional symptomatology. After this initial pass, if several alternate diagnoses are not considered, significant morbidity may ensue. These conditions include nosocomial sepsis (see below), thromboembolic disease, or gastrointestinal disease (ileus, small bowel obstruction, pancreatitis).

The ECG may also be the first clue that a complication is directly related to interventions performed in the ICU.

(a)

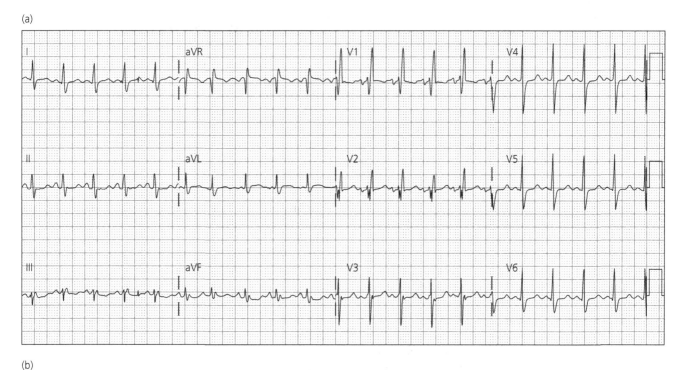

(b)

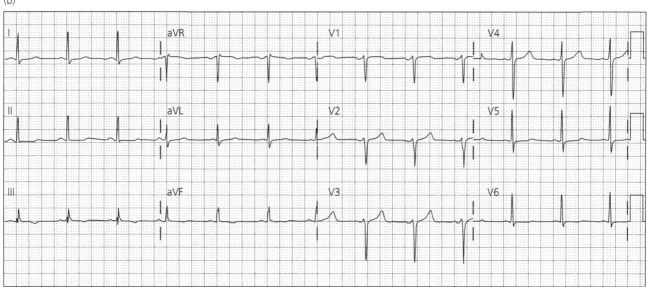

Figure 39.3 (a) Baseline intraventricular conduction delay presents with a QRS duration (QRSd) of 126 ms. After the development of anasarca (b), there is an apparent loss of IVCD (QRSd 89 ms) with changes in precordial QRS morphology due to lead placement.

Common procedures include central line placement, thoracentesis, and nasogastric tube insertion. Pneumothorax and conduction system abnormalities are the most common complications during central line placement. Conduction system abnormalities range from sinus tachycardia and atrial arrythmia to ventricular excitability (Figure 39.1). Pneumothorax, which has been reported to occur in 0 to 4.5% of patients [2], will be discussed separately at the end of this section along with other deadly non-acute coronary syndrome (ACS) ECG findings.

The role of the ECG in sepsis

Sepsis is the systemic inflammatory response to infection characterized by perturbations in vital signs and peripheral leukocyte counts. The syndrome is defined along a spectrum that goes on to involve organ dysfunction, and then persistent hypotension despite resuscitation. These latter states are termed severe sepsis and septic shock, respectively. Despite innovations in management, such as early goal-directed therapy, identification of safer ventilatory strategies, and optimal endocrine management, sepsis still remains the leading cause of mortality in the ICU with mortality rates of 30% and over 215,000 deaths annually [3]. Mortality may even approach 50% in cases of septic shock.

The most common finding on ECG with sepsis is tachycardia, most often atrial in nature. A heart rate greater than 90 beats per minute (bpm) defines the heart rate criteria for systemic inflammatory response syndrome (SIRS). Other non-specific ECG abnormalities have been reported to occur frequently in ICU patients and there remains no pathognomonic ECG finding. Rich and colleagues hypothesized that loss of myocardial excitability resulted in decreased QRS amplitude and increased QRS duration, which were observed 82% and 47% of the time, respectively, in patients with severe sepsis and septic shock [4]. Other reports have demonstrated the presence of J waves in patients with sepsis-induced hypothermia [5,6]. The clinical significance of these findings remains unclear.

Compelling evidence supports the notion that in the ICU ECG is quite insensitive for detecting myocardial injury in the absence of an acute infarct. Arlati and colleagues demonstrated that the ECG failed to identify myocardial injury in 78% of patients with abnormally high cardiac enzymes [7]. In this study, non-cardiac patients who developed elevated cardiac enzymes were found to more frequently be hypotensive, requiring vasoactive drug support, and to require mechanical ventilation. They believed the elevation in cardiac enzymes to be a direct result of myocardial necrosis due to these transient hypotensive events.

The role of the traditional 12-lead ECG may be limited in the initial diagnosis of sepsis, but ECG-derived analysis such as heart rate variability (HRV) has been implicated in the early detection of the deteriorating septic patient. Heart rate variability analyzes the variation in RR intervals from beat to beat or over a period of time. A number of calculations and statistical results have been characterized by observing variations in RR intervals.

Recent studies have demonstrated that HRV can be used as an early marker for multi-organ dysfunction syndrome [8], as a potential forecaster of morbidity and mortality in the emergency department [9], and as a predictor of progression to septic shock in patients presenting with sepsis [10]. Low, or decreasing, HRV may reflect a greater severity of illness, as well as portend a worse prognosis in the ICU. Mechanisms accounting for this observation in septic patients include decreased myocardial responsiveness to catecholamines, increased parasympathetic tone, the negative impact of nitrous oxide and endotoxin on the central nervous system (CNS), and the uncoupling of the cardiovascular system and other organs [9]. At this time HRV remains a research tool, but acquisition of ECG data over a short period of time while in the emergency room, medical floor, or ICU may help assist triage or assign risk in patients with the diagnosis of sepsis in the near future.

Mechanical ventilation

Mechanical ventilation (MV) is a common measure instituted in the critically ill patient. It is employed when a patient is deemed to need support during periods of respiratory insufficiency, cardiovascular collapse or inability to protect the airway. Yet myocardial ischemia has been noted to occur, both during use and removal of the ventilator. Up to a 10% rate of arrhythmia has been identified during the intubation process itself [11]. Routine ECG monitoring may help identify these events and even portend outcome.

Positive pressure ventilation has several salutary effects on cardiac function, including reducing oxygen consumption by unloading stressed respiratory muscles, decreasing preload and, therefore, myocardial demand in a overworked heart, and reducing the afterload seen by the left ventricle. It stands to reason that the time period of returning back to spontaneous breathing would be the period at greatest risk for ischemic events. Yet, in ICU patients with cardiac risk factors, ischemia has been shown to occur in 21% of patients when continuous 12-lead ECG monitoring was employed [12]. In this study of a general medicine population, nearly 70% of the patients were undergoing MV. Both MV and the presence of troponin elevation were associated with increased mortality risk. Frazier and colleagues [13] also showed ECG evidence for ST depression or elevation in 70% of mechanically ventilated patients. The majority of these events were noted before attempts to remove ventilatory assistance. Likely explanations for a link between ischemia and MV include excessive drops in preload leading to exacerbation of coronary insufficiency or adrenergically driven ischemia from anxiety or dysynchronous breathing efforts associated with MV. In these instances, continuous ECG monitoring may be the first line in identifying sedative requirement or adjusting ventilator parameters.

As mentioned above, during the attempt to return to spontaneous breathing there is a considerable risk for ischemia. Electrocardiogram evidence of ischemia during ventilator weaning has been reported in anywhere from 6 to 35% patients [14–16]. The presence of this finding has led to two to three times the likelihood of failure of spontaneous breathing trials, and has been associated with longer duration of MV and ICU length of stay. In at least one study, the incidence of observed ECG ischemia was not linked to the decrease of sedatives during the weaning process. Even though catecholamines, heart rate, and heart rate-blood pressure product were all significantly increased after sedative drug decline, ST segment deviation occurred haphazardly before and after sedative drug adjustment [17]. The cause-effect relationship of weaning failure and ischemia in current practice is not clear. It is possible that ischemia is the cause of weaning failure just as much as the observed consequence of removal of the beneficial effects of positive pressure. Regardless, it is clear that ECG monitoring can add information to the clinical assessment when attempting to remove MV from patients in the ICU. Its analysis in the patient with recurrent ventilatory failure of failed weaning attempts may help identify previously undiagnosed coronary disease in need of correction.

Hemodialysis

Like MV, hemodialysis (HD) frequently occurs as part of ICU care. Familiarity of ECG changes and their temporal relationship to HD administration can be useful knowledge for the intensivist. Electrocardiogram changes have been best characterized in patients with chronic renal disease. Given co-existing conditions, such as hypertension and diabetes, and a high incidence of cardiovascular mortality, ECG findings are common [18].

Among a group of 221 patients receiving ongoing HD for chronic renal failure, 143 (65%) had 12-lead ECG findings excluding sinus arrhythmia, sinus bradycardia, or sinus tachycardia [19]. Risk factors for ECG findings included hypertension, diabetes and increasing age. Left ventricular hypertrophy (LVH) (29%) was most common, followed by ventricular (12%) and supraventricular premature contractions (7%). Ischemic changes were captured in 7.2% of ECGs while non-specific ST-T changes occurred 5.9% of the time.

The temporal relationship of ECG abnormalities to HD administration was explored with 24-h holter monitor by these investigators [19]. Arrhythmias and ST-T wave changes were common, with a large proportion occurring during dialysis and resolving a few hours after HD termination. This finding was echoed by the observation of ventricular ectopy occurring in 90% of another cohort during HD and up to 4 h after the conclusion of HD conclusion [20].

Circumstantial evidence for the cause of these arrhythmias has been made by specific changes noted in the QT interval during dialysis. QT dispersion is defined as the difference between minimum and maximal QT intervals on an ECG. Lorincz and colleagues [21] showed that significant changes in potassium and calcium levels before and after dialysis were associated with increases in QT interval and QT dispersion (Figure 39.4). The implications being that changes in ventricular repolarization attributed to dialysis may explain ventricular arrhythmia. QRS prolongation following HD-assisted edema removal has also been reported and will be discussed further below.

The ischemic changes and arrhythmias mentioned above, related to electrolyte shifts, have been well characterized in patients with chronic renal failure. In these patients, risk factors and consequent hormonal changes explain observed LVH, abnormal coronary blood flow, and perturbations in calcium and glucose homeostasis. The institution of HD in the ICU occurs for acute and chronic causes of renal failure. In a general medicine ICU population, arguably some of the same risk factors, hypertension and diabetes, routinely exist in the acute renal failure population. Yet very few data exist detailing the experience of ICU patients on HD.

Furthermore, continuous renal replacement techniques are increasingly being used in the critically ill population. More gradual volume removal and subtler solute shifts may avoid the negative arrhythmic effects listed above. There has been a singular case report of continuous veno-venous

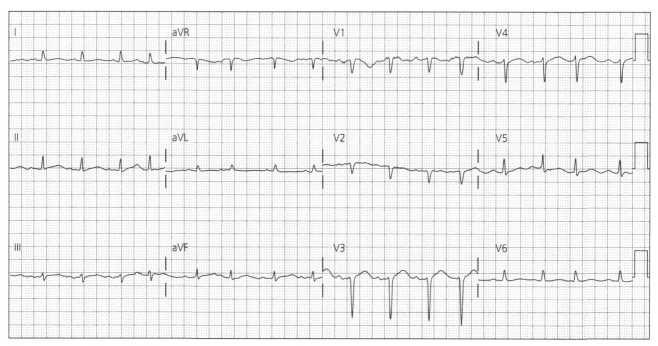

Figure 39.4 ECG obtained following intermittent hemodialysis in the ICU given change in rhythm. Notable new findings include sinus tachycardia with a variable rate between 80 and 127 bpm, QTc increased to 495 ms, and T wave flattening in anterior and lateral leads.

(a)

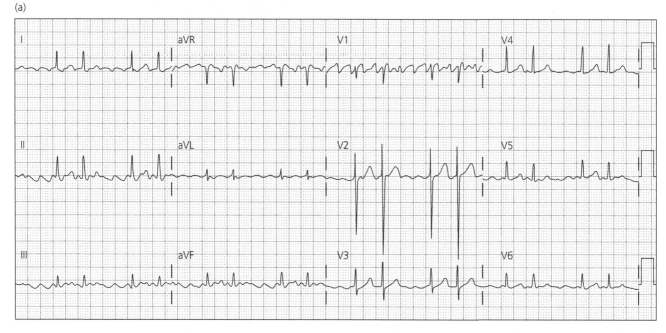

(b)

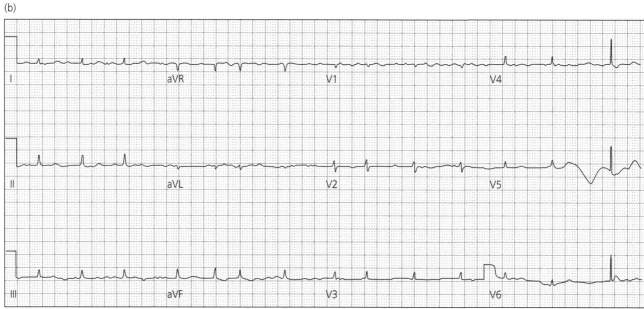

Figure 39.5 (a) Admission ECG of elderly female with pulmonary embolism and respiratory distress. Fibrinolytics were withheld in part due to contraindications. Atrial flutter and left ventricular hypertrophy are present. (b) ECG after massive fluid resuscitation reveals low voltage. Atrial arrhythmia persists and QRS duration has reduced from 84 ms to 58 ms.

hemodialysis mimicking atrial flutter on ECG. Interruption of the HD circuit revealed that the observed flutter wave was related to electrical phenomena reflected in the ECG. Given the known association of atrial arrhythmia with HD, the authors caution avoidance of erroneous interpretations [22].

The ECG in edematous states and anasarca

Edematous states are characterized by palpable swelling due to increased interstitial fluid accumulation. Edema occurs with peripheral localization to gravity-dependent areas of the body. Anasarca describes a generalized and more widespread fluid accumulation. Edematous states are commonly seen in critically ill patients, and, more specifically, those with a poor nutritional status, heart failure syndromes, cirrhosis, and nephrosis. They occur frequently in the absence of any of these risk factors when massive resuscitation occurs with either blood products or synthetic colloid, or crystalloid, solutions. It has been well established that edematous states typically demonstrate low-voltage ECG (LVE), but recent studies have further described alterations in P wave and QRS amplitude as well as interval durations. For patients

Table 39.1 Conditions commonly associated with low-voltage electrocardiogram (LVE). LVE is defined by QRS < 5 mm in the limb leads or < 10 mm in the precordial leads

Various conditions associated with LVE
Edematous states
Obesity
Cardiac disease
Infiltrative heart disease
Pericardial effusions
Constrictive pericarditis
Heart failure
Pulmonary diseases
Chronic obstructive pulmonary disease
Pneumothorax
Pleural effusion

with edematous states, the ECG can serve a role in detecting changes in the patient's volume status during times of accumulation, diuresis, and hemodialysis, as well as in providing valuable information with respect to conduction and wave abnormalities.

Low-voltage ECG can be seen with edematous states, obesity, infiltrative heart disease, emphysema, pulmonary infiltrates, pneumothoraces, pleural effusions, pericardial effusions, and constrictive pericarditis (Table 39.1) [23]. Low-voltage ECG is defined by QRS < 5 mm in the limb leads or < 10 mm in the precordial leads. Electrocardiogram potentials are resultant of current generation by the myocardium, electrode placement, and the resistance generated by fluid- and air-filled spaces between the myocardium and electrodes. Furthermore, determinants of the QRS amplitude are a result of the size and contractility of the ventricular chambers, as well as the proximity of the electrodes to the chamber. In a series of prospective studies evaluating LVE in anasarca, Madias and colleagues analyzed the sum of the QRS amplitudes (ΣQRS) to correlate QRS amplitude changes to fluid weight gains and losses [23,24]. They demonstrated that attenuation of ΣQRS corresponded well with increasing weight and peak weight gain. Similarly, they observed that increased ΣQRS correlated to weight loss. In comparison of different ECG systems (12-, 6-, 2-lead ECGs), non-inferiority between the three systems indicated that ΣQRS$_2$ and ΣQRS$_6$ may be employed instead of the ΣQRS$_{12}$ [24].

In addition to LVE, patients with edematous states also demonstrate QRS interval shortening. The QRS duration (QRSd) reflects the time for left and right ventricular activation. A normal QRSd is < 100 ms; values > 100 ms represent IVCD [25]. Madias and colleagues have demonstrated a dramatic shortening of the QRSd in patients with anasarca and peripheral edema [26]. It appears that shortening of QRSd best correlates with peak weight gain and not dynamic changes such as ΣQRS measurements. Madias conjectures that the shortened QRSd reflects apparent, rather than actual, changes in conduction velocity due to alterations in the extracardiac medium [26]. This hypothesis has been sup-

ported in a case series of nine patients with admission ECGs demonstrating either IVCD or bundle branch block (BBB) whose clinical course was complicated by the development of anasarca [27]. After gaining average of 50 lbs, all QRSd shortened and 44% of the patients demonstrated an apparent resolution of IVCD or BBB [27]. Furthermore, once admission weight had been re-established, the QRSd increased with return of the IVCDs and BBBs. The presence of a prolonged QRSd is a clinically important observation to make as increased QRSd is associated with the development of lethal arrythmias, reflects intra- and interventricular mechanical dyssynchrony, portends a worse prognosis in patients with systolic heart failure, and is a major criterium for the initiation of cardiac resynchronization therapy [27]. Thus, the degree of QRSd may be underestimated in patients with edematous states and conclusions regarding the level of mechanical dyssynchrony in the critically ill may be of less value.

With such dramatic changes in the QRS amplitude and duration, it would be expected that similar changes would be observed in P wave morphology and duration. However, while attenuation of P wave amplitude corresponds with QRS amplitudes, changes in P wave duration may predictably trend with changes of QRS duration [29–31]. Alterations in P wave amplitude correspond well with QRS amplitude in patients with anasarca and patients undergoing HD [29]. These changes have been shown to mask characteristic P wave abnormalities associated with atrial and valvular pathologies such as p pulmonale, p mitrale, and biatrial enlargement [30]. In addition, an apparent loss of P wave activity, suggestive of atrial fibrillation, has been demonstrated in the absence of atrial dysrhythmias [29,32]. Again, attenuation and the loss of the P wave amplitude is an apparent change rather than an actual one.

Alterations of P wave duration are controversial in the literature. P wave duration appears to lengthen with aggressive fluid challenges, which can be attributed to acute hemodynamic changes within the atria [33], but P wave duration does not appear to change in the development of edematous states [31]. Thus, accurate measurement of P wave morphology and interval is best performed once an edematous state or volume overload state has been resolved [29]. In the ICU, recognition of P wave alterations in patients with dynamic changes in volume status, either in edematous states or aggressive fluid challenges, may allow for more accurate ECG interpretation.

Changes in QRS amplitude, QRSd and P wave amplitude offer many practical roles of the ECG for the intensivist in managing patients with edematous states, during aggressive fluid challenges, and during fluid removal therapy with diuretics or renal replacement devices. Diagnostic implications are involved when considering the differential diagnosis of LVE and several important clinical implications must be considered. Also, ΣQRS can be used as an additional marker of volume status [34]. Recognition of changes in the QRS and the P wave can assist the intensivist's management in recognizing an underlying atrial rhythm in patients demonstrating an apparent loss of P wave activity, in differentiating atrial and ventricular dysrhythmias when the QRS is prolonged or shortened, and in monitoring the development or resolution of an evolving edematous state [33].

Case conclusions

In Case 1, the proximal relationship to the procedure and ECG findings allowed the care team to identify the arrhythmia as a complication. Rapid removal of the device led to reversal of the condition. Ischemia during spontaneous breathing trials likely occurs more often than is identified. While many patients in multidisciplinary ICUs have no prior history of myocardial ischemia, they often have several risk factors. In this case, the ECG may lead to further diagnostic testing for ischemia or medical management of heart disease. All too often, persistent failure during spontaneous breathing trials is attributed to the inciting need for ventilation and addition days are accrued with MV without ischemia identified. Finally, in the last case, identification of IVCD was masked by superimposed edema. The lack of acknowledgment that this was due to artifact could have had implications in care if the patient had developed arrhythmias while in the ICU.

Paramount to the mission of intensive care is the fastidious monitoring of complications that can lead to delays or setbacks in patient recovery. Electrocardiogram monitoring is routinely done throughout ICU care and provides a first line in terms of identification of potential risks. Many conditions (i.e. sepsis), procedures, therapeutics (i.e. HD) and routine care in the ICU can cause changes appreciated in the ECG. Many of these alterations are non-specific. As we continue to have technology gains and computerized automation in the ICU, other potential analyses besides HRV and QT dispersion may be shown to assist in the ongoing risk assessment.

References

1 Drew BJ, Califf RM, Funk M, et al. Practice standards for electrocardiographic monitoring in hospital settings: an American Heart Association scientific statement from the Councils on Cardiovascular Nursing, Clinical Cardiology, and Cardiovascular Disease in the Young: endorsed by the International Society of Computerized Electrocardiology and the American Association of Critical-Care Nurses. Circulation 2004;**110**(17):2721–46.

2 Hall JB, Schmidt G, Wood L. Principles of Critical Care. 3rd edition. McGraw-Hill, New York 2005.

3 Jones AE, Focht A, Horton JM, Kline JA. Prospective external validation of the clinical effectiveness of an emergency department-based early goal-directed therapy protocol for severe sepsis and septic shock. Chest 2007;**132**(2):425–32.

4 Rich MM, McGarvey ML, Teener JW, Frame LH. ECG changes during septic shock. Cardiology 2002;**97**(4):187–96.

5 Cardenas GA, Ventura HO, Francis JE. Osborn waves in sepsis. South Med J 2006;**99**(11):1302–3.

6 Salerno D, Vahid B, Marik PE. Osborn wave in hypothermia from Vibrio vunificus sepsis unrelated to exposure. Int J Cardiol 2007;**114**(3):e124–5.

7 Arlati S, Brenna S, Prencipe L, et al. Myocardial necrosis in ICU patients with acute non-cardiac disease: a prospective study. Intensive Care Med 2000;**26**(1):31–7.

8 Pontet J, Contreras P, Curbelo A, et al. Heart rate variability as early marker of multiple organ dysfunction syndrome in septic patients. J Crit Care 2003;**18**(3):156–63.

9 Barnaby D, Ferrick K, Kaplan DT, et al. Heart rate variability in emergency department patients with sepsis. Acad Emerg Med 2002;**9**(7):661–70.

10 Chen WL, Kuo CD. Characteristics of heart rate variability can predict impending septic shock in emergency department patients with sepsis. Acad Emerg Med 2007;**14**(5):392–7.

11 Jaber S, Amraoui J, Lefrant JY, et al. Clinical practice and risk factors for immediate complications of endotracheal intubation in the intensive care unit: a prospective, multiple-center study. Crit Care Med 2006;**34**(9):2355–61.

12 Landesberg G, Vesselov Y, Einav S, et al. Myocardial ischemia, cardiac troponin, and long-term survival of high-cardiac risk critically ill intensive care unit patients. Crit Care Med 2005;**33**(6):1281–7.

13 Frazier SK, Brom H, Widener J, et al. Prevalence of myocardial ischemia during mechanical ventilation and weaning and its effects on weaning success. Heart Lung 2006;**35**(6):363–73.

14 Chatila W, Ani S, Guaglianone D, et al. Cardiac ischemia during weaning from mechanical ventilation. Chest 1996;**109**(6):1577–83.

15 Hurford WE, Favorito F. Association of myocardial ischemia with failure to wean from mechanical ventilation. Crit Care Med 1995;**23**(9):1475–80.

16 Abalos A, Leibowitz AB, Distefano D, et al. Myocardial ischemia during the weaning period. Am J Crit Care 1992;**1**(3):32–6.

17 Kress JP, Vinayak AG, Levitt J, et al. Daily sedative interruption in mechanically ventilated patients at risk for coronary artery disease. Crit Care Med 2007;**35**(2):365–71.

18 Selby NM, McIntyre CW. The acute cardiac effects of dialysis. Semin Dial 2007;**20**(3):220–8.

19 Abe S, Yoshizawa M, Nakanishi N, et al. Electrocardiographic abnormalities in patients receiving hemodialysis. Am Heart J 1996;**131**(6):1137–44.

20 Wald DA. ECG manifestations of selected metabolic and endocrine disorders. ECG Emerg Med 2006;**24**(1):145–57.

21 Lorincz I, Zilahi Z, Kun C, et al. ECG abnormalities in hemodialysis. Am Heart J 1997;**134**(6):1138–40.

22 Kostis WJ, Cohen L, Dominiecki SM. Continuous veno-venous hemodialysis pseudoflutter. J Electrocardiol 2007;**40**(4):316–8.

23 Madias JE, Bazaz R, Agarwal H, et al. Anasarca-mediated attenuation of the amplitude of electrocardiogram complexes: a description of a heretofore unrecognized phenomenon. J Am Coll Cardiol 2001;**38**(3):756–64.

24 Madias JE. A comparison of 2-lead, 6-lead, and 12-lead ECGs in patients with changing edematous states: implications for the employment of quantitative electrocardiography in research and clinical applications. Chest 2003;**124**(6):2057–63.

25 Chou TC. Electrocardiography in clinical practice. 3rd Edition. Philadelphia: W.B. Saunders Company, 1991.

26 Madias JE. Significance of shortening of the mean QRS duration of the standard electrocardiogram in patients developing peripheral edema. Am J Cardiol 2002;**89**(12):1444–6.

27 Madias JE. Apparent amelioration of bundle branch blocks and intraventricular conduction delays mediated by anasarca. *J Electrocardiol* 2005;**38**(2):160–5.

28 Kearney MT, Zaman A, Eckberg DL, *et al.* Cardiac size, autonomic function, and 5-year follow-up of chronic heart failure patients with severe prolongation of ventricular activation. *J Card Fail* 2003;**9**(2):93–9.

29 Madias JE. P waves in patients with changing edematous states: implications on interpreting repeat P wave measurements in patients developing anasarca or undergoing hemodialysis. *Pacing Clin Electrophysiol* 2004;**27**(6 Pt 1):749–56.

30 Madias JE. Peripheral edema masks the diagnoses of P pulmonale, P mitrale, and biatrial abnormality: clinical implications for patients with heart failure. *Congest Heart Fail* 2006;**12**(1):20–4.

31 Madias JE. P-wave duration and dispersion in patients with peripheral edema and its amelioration. *Indian Pacing Electrophysiol J* 2007;**7**(1):7–18.

32 Madias JE, Narayan V, Attari M. Detection of P waves via a "saline-filled central venous catheter electrocardiographic lead" in patients with low electrocardiographic voltage due to anasarca. *Am J Cardiol* 2003;**91**(7):910–4.

33 Madias JE. Reversible attenuation of voltage of QRS complexes and P waves and shortening of QRS duration and QTc interval consequent to large perioperative intravenous fluid infusions. *J Electrocardiol* 2006;**39**(4):415–8.

34 Madias JE, Song J, White CM, *et al.* Response of the ECG to short-term diuresis in patients with heart failure. *Ann Noninvasive Electrocardiol* 2005;**10**(3):288–96.

Chapter 40 | What is the proper role of the ECG in the evaluation of patients with suspected PE?

Peter M. Pollak[1], Joseph E. Levitt[2]
[1]University of Virginia, Charlottesville, VA, USA
[2]Stanford University Medical Center, Stanford, CA, USA

Case presentations

Case 1: A 23-year-old woman who is 27 weeks pregnant arrives at the emergency department (ED) with a sudden-onset sharp chest pain, non-productive cough, and shortness of breath. She has had multiple visits documented in the ED involving substance abuse. She admits to recent ingestion of cocaine. She has significant hypertension and tachycardia and the decision is made to admit her to the intensive care unit (ICU) for closer monitoring. Upon arrival at the ICU she is requiring oxygen at 6 L/min and looks uncomfortable. Vitals are significant for a blood pressure of 140/95 mmHg and a pulse rate of 127 beats per minute (bpm). Initial ED 12-lead electrocardiogram (ECG) (Figure 40.1a) shows sinus tachycardia at a rate of 144, an S wave in lead I, a subtle Q wave in lead III, and an inverted T wave in lead III ($S_1Q_3T_3$). On examination, she has notable jugular venous distension, a palpable parasternal lift, and left leg swelling. Given her thromboembolic risk, pregnancy, she has a computed tomography pulmonary angiogram (CTPA) performed with her gravid abdomen shielded. It reveals massive bilateral pulmonary embolism (PE) (Figure 40.1b). Heparin is started immediately.

Case 2: An 83-year-old woman is admitted to the ICU from the general medicine floor with new-onset atrial fibrillation and increased dyspnea. She has been hospitalized for 6 days with a diagnosis of *Clostridium difficile* diarrhea complicating treatment of a urinary tract infection at the assisted living center where she resides. She has a medical history notable for longstanding hypertension and diabetes. She has an extensive smoking history but no formal diagnosis of emphysema. Overnight she has her rate controlled with continuous IV calcium channel-blockade. The next morning her physical exam reveals a healthy appearing woman with clear lungs and no peripheral edema. Her pulse is noted to be irregular and tachycardic at a rate of 101 and a blood pressure of 144/85. A chest roentgenogram reveals large lung fields and no infiltrate. Her ECG demonstrates atrial fibrillation and a rightward QRS axis (Figure 40.2). The diagnosis of PE as the cause of her atrial fibrillation is suggested by the cardiology consultant. Computed tomography pulmonary angiogram and full digital subtraction pulmonary angiogram were both negative. Her eventual diagnosis was emphysema with an exacerbation.

Case 3: An otherwise healthy 45-year-old female presents at the ED with left leg swelling and mild dyspnea and pleuritic chest pain. She has had two prolonged car rides in the last 48 h. She denies any prior history of blood clots, and has two healthy children following uncomplicated pregnancies. She reports an excellent baseline functional status and is very active. Vitals are significant for a blood pressure of 110/65 mmHg and a pulse rate of 105 bpm. A CTPA shows extensive bilateral clot with near occlusion of each main pulmonary artery bilaterally with diffuse extension (Figure 40.3a). Dilation of the right ventricle is commented on in the radiologist's preliminary report. She is admitted to the ICU late that evening. She is comfortable and has minimal supplemental oxygen requirement, saturating 98% on only 2 L/min via nasal cannula. An echocardiogram will only be available in several hours. She desires to return to her active lifestyle. The role of thrombolysis for PE with significant acute right ventricular (RV) strain is considered. Her admission ECG is available and is notable for a clear $S_1Q_3T_3$ and some T wave inversions (Figure 40.3b). An echocardiogram the next morning confirms moderate RV dilation and a pulmonary artery systolic pressure estimated at 42 mmHg. The patient, after a discussion of risks and benefits of thrombolysis, opts for anti-coagulation alone.

The proper role of the ECG in the evaluation of patients with suspected PE

These three cases illustrate patients with possible or known acute pulmonary thromboembolism. The evaluation and

Critical Decisions in Emergency and Acute Care Electrocardiography,
1st edition. Edited by W.J. Brady and J.D. Truwit. © 2009 Blackwell
Publishing, ISBN: 9781405159067

(a)

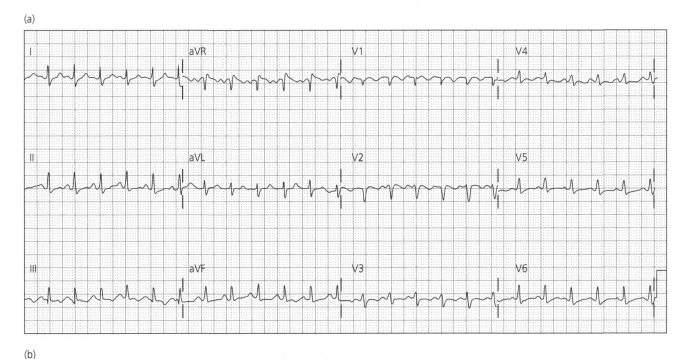

(b)

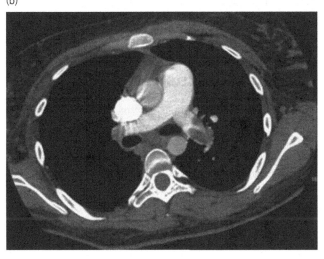

Figure 40.1 (a) Sinus tachycardia at a rate of 144. Significant S wave in I, small Q wave in III, and inverted T waves in III ($S_1Q_3T_3$). Additional leads with T wave abnormalities include aVF, V1–V4. (b) Computed tomography image with bilateral main stem pulmonary arteries with extensive filling defects.

management for each patient will differ. How should the ECG findings of each patient be used in their evaluation and management?

Pulmonary embolism remains a significant source of morbidity and mortality. Incidence estimates vary around one in 1000, with most studies highlighting the caveat of probable underdiagnosis. In one autopsy study of almost 52,000 patients over 21 months, 70% of patients in whom PE was the proximal cause of death were *not* suspected of having a PE [1]. Others have reported that less than 50% of PE are diagnosed at presentation [2]. The mortality rate even when PE is diagnosed also remains very high, around 10%. Early diagnosis and treatment decreases the morbidity and mortality of PE significantly [3].

The basis for early diagnosis is a high clinical suspicion. Unfortunately, the signs and symptoms of PE are highly vari-

able and indistinct from other acute cardiopulmonary processes. It is useful to remember, however, that sudden-onset dyspnea, chest pain, or fainting alone or in combination are present in 96% of patients who go on to be diagnosed with PE [4]. While this information raises the concern of PE in a tremendous number of patients, it also allows the clinician to minimize the likelihood of PE in patients without one of those complaints.

Unfortunately, a good screening test does not exist. The D-dimer assay, in its most sensitive form, functions as a highly sensitive test, but its low specificity limits its use to ruling out deep vein thrombosis (DVT) in patients with low (< 5%) pretest probability of clot (i.e. a patient without chest pain, dyspnea, or syncope). Similarly, the duplex U/S of the leg veins is useful if a clot is seen, but does little to eliminate PE from the differential if negative.

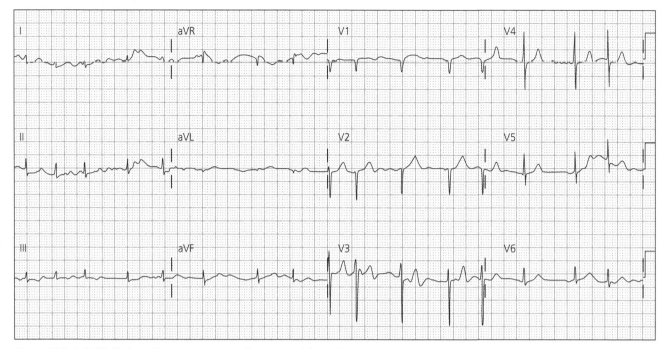

Figure 40.2 Atrial fibrillation with a ventricular rate of 101–116. Rightward QRS axis at 110 degrees.

Also problematic, the diagnostic test of choice today, the helical CTPA, is expensive, requires use of nephrotoxic contrast dye, and still only has a sensitivity of 83% based on recent data [5]. Alternative methods are also limited. Magnetic resonance pulmonary angiography can no longer be safely used in patients with renal insufficiency for fear of nephrogenic sclerosing dermopathy. The clinician is left with a constant need to expeditiously and safely deal with the nearly ubiquitous presence of PE on the list of differential diagnoses in any patient with new cardiopulmonary symptoms.

Appropriate evaluation of the patient with suspected PE

A number of strategies and algorithms have been devised to assist the clinician in the expeditious evaluation of suspected PE [6]. In nearly all of these, following the history and physical exam, the patient must receive a chest radiograph and 12-lead ECG, neither of which can "make the diagnosis" of PE. This early step serves primarily to evaluate for alternative

Table 40.1 Revised Geneva and Wells prediction rules for pulmonary embolism*

Revised Geneva score	Points	Wells score	Points
Previous pulmonary embolism or deep vein thrombosis	+3	Previous pulmonary embolism or deep vein thrombosis	+1.5
Active malignancy or cure (< 1 year)	+2	Heart rate > 100 bpm	+1.5
Age > 65	+1	Recent surgery or immobilization	+1.5
Surgery (general anesthesia) or fracture (lower extremity) < 1 month	+2	Clinical signs of deep vein thrombosis	+3
Heart rate		Alternative diagnosis less likely than pulmonary embolism	+3
75–94	+3	Cancer(within 6 months or palliative)	+1
≥ 95	+5	Hemoptysis	+1
Lower limb tenderness and unilateral edema	+4		
Complaint of unilateral lower limb pain	+3		
Complaint of hemoptysis	+2		
Clinical probability		Clinical probability	
Low	0–3	Low	0–1
Intermediate	4–10	Intermediate	2–6
High	≥ 11	High	≥ 7

*Adapted from refs [7,8].

(a)

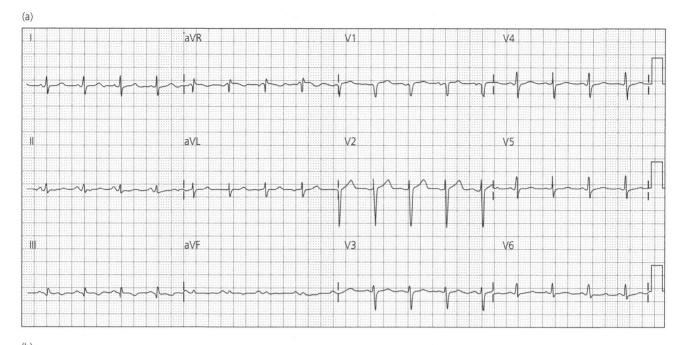

(b)

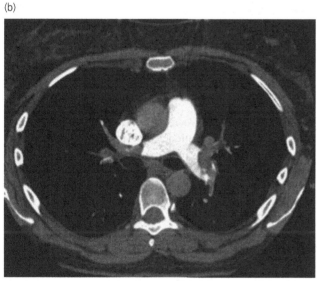

Figure 40.3 (a) Sinus tachycardia at a rate of 105. Significant S wave in I, small Q wave in III, and inverted T waves in III ($S_1Q_3T_3$). Additional leads with T wave abnormalities include aVF. (b) Computed tomography image with bilateral main stem pulmonary arteries with extensive filling defects.

processes that could cause similar signs and symptoms, but which can be readily diagnosed by these methods, such as myocardial infarction, spontaneous pneumothorax, pneumonia, etc.

As mentioned above, the degree of pretest probability guides the direction and extent of further investigation. A number of scoring systems based on clinical variables have been derived to facilitate and standardize this estimation. They include those put forward by Wells (including the more ubiquitous simplified Wells criteria) and the Revised Geneva scoring system (Table 40.1) [7,8]. The "gestalt" estimation of experienced physicians has been studied and shown to approximate the same accuracy as the Wells criteria in at least one study, but the scoring systems remain objective, easier to study, and useful for less experienced clinicians [9].

The utility of the ECG can be improved by using a scoring system of ECG findings, such as that proposed by Daniel and colleagues (Table 40.2) [10]. Unfortunately, combining an ECG scoring system with the Wells scoring system did not improve diagnostic accuracy [11].

Variety of ECG findings in acute PE, their basis and usefulness

There is almost as much variability in ECG changes associated with PE as in clinical presentations. In 1935, McGinn and White first described the $S_1Q_3T_3$ changes seen in Cases 1 and 3 (a deep S wave in lead I, Q wave and inverted T wave in lead III) in ECGs of patients with acute cor pulmonale

Table 40.2 The 21 electrocardiographic scoring system*

Tachycardia > 100 bpm	+2
Incomplete right bundle branch block	+2
Complete right bundle branch block	+3
S wave in I	0
T wave inversion in III	+1
Q wave in III	+1
S1Q3T3	+2
T wave inversion in V1–V4	+4
T wave inversion in V1	
< 1 mm	0
1–2 mm	+1
> 2 mm	+2
T wave inversion in V2	
< 1 mm	+1
1–2 mm	+2
> 2 mm	+3
T wave inversion in V3	
< 1 mm	+1
1–2 mm	+2
> 2 mm	+3
Total score possible	21

*Adapted from ref. [10].

Table 40.3 ECG abnormality frequency with pulmonary embolism*

Finding	%
Normal	9–30
Abnormal rhythm	
Sinus tachycardia	8–69
PACs and PVCs	4–23
Atrial fibrillation and flutter	0–35
Axis deviation	
Right	3–66
Left	2–14
Indeterminate	9–31
P pulmonale	2–31
QRS disturbance	
$S_1Q_3T_3$	11–50
Right bundle branch block	6–67
Low voltage	4–29
Late transition	7–51
Q in III and aVF	14–49
S in I and aVL	28–73
ST and T wave changes	
T wave inversions	10–51
T wave inversions in III and aVF	17–35
T wave inversions in V1 and V2	27–68
ST elevations or depressions	14–50
ST or T wave changes	49–77

*Adapted from ref. [13].

resulting from PE [12]. Soon thereafter, a number of other ECG changes were associated with PE, and, in 1940, the first systematic review showed sinus tachycardia to be the most common ECG change associated with PE and cast doubt on the utility of the ECG in establishing the diagnosis of PE.

Since then, our ability to diagnose PE accurately has improved. A number of studies have investigated the actual incidence of various ECG findings in PE and have been summarized (Table 40.3) [13]. The most common findings on ECG are changes in rhythm, conduction, P wave morphology, QRS axis, and T wave direction. The most frequent rhythm disturbance remains sinus tachycardia, though a high percentage of patients (up to one in four or one in three) will have a normal ECG. Changes in ST segments and T wave morphology are more common in larger PE, which cause hemodynamic effects. This relationship is discussed below.

The pathophysiology of these ECG changes in PE remains poorly understood and multiple explanations exist. Many physiologic changes accompany PE, including hemodynamic, anatomic, metabolic (hypoxia), and autonomic (elevated catecholamines) [14]. Hemodynamic changes include acute pulmonary hypertension (increased RV afterload), causing RV dilation and increased wall tension, both of which increase myocardial workload and oxygen demand leading to possible myocardial ischemia. Anatomic changes include bronchoconstriction and pulmonary ischemia. From the interplay of these physiologic changes, arises the changes on the ECG.

It is felt that in cases of acute PE, the strain placed on the heart is responsible for many of the ECG findings. The right ventricle is especially prone to relative ischemia given its non-dominant coronary supply and usually low myocardial work constraints. The sudden rise in pulmonary vascular resistance increases RV afterload. This has been shown to occur in many cases on echocardiogram. The consequent reduction to left-sided preload further exacerbates any ischemia by decreasing resultant coronary perfusion.

Atrial arrhythmia and PE

One area of particular interest is the association of PE with new-onset atrial fibrillation, as in the Case 3. The frequency with which atrial fibrillation (AF) occurs in patients with PE is difficult to accurately quantify. Many studies muddy the question by lumping all atrial arrhythmias together, while others include atrial flutter and AF together. The variation in published papers is tremendous with some citing numbers as low as 0–3%, and others reporting as much as 18–35% [15,16]. In one echocardiographic study of patients with PE, only two out of 63 patients with PE had AF and two out of 27 patients with right-sided clot had atrial fibrillation, but only one of those had PE [17]. Other studies have placed the association between AF and PE between 8 and 31% [18].

Atrial fibrillation is thought to most often arise from the left atrium, which is much less affected by the acute hemodynamic changes of PE [19]. The surge in catecholamines that accompanies PE, largely driven by pain and dyspnea, could certainly increase the irritability of the atria in general and increase the likelihood of fibrillation. It is more likely that acute cor pulmonale would perturb the right atrium leading to a right-sided arrhythmia such as atrial tachycardia, atrial flutter, or right ventricular ectopy. One electrophysiology study noted that over half the cases of atrial flutter over a 3-year period were associated with the clinical diagnosis of PE [20]. Nevertheless, acute right atrial stretch could feasibly effect the appropriate substrate within the atria for fibrillation to propagate. Unfortunately, given the low incidence of atrial arrhythmia in PE, few studies have distinguished between them. Little evidence exists, therefore, to accurately estimate the risk of PE with new-onset AF.

Classical wisdom has held that AF in the setting of PE is caused by the PE (or its hemodynamic effects). On the contrary, some have postulated PE could be a presenting symptom of underlying AF [21]. In this scenario of primary PE, the clot arises in the appendage (auricle) of the right atrium due to stasis, and embolizes into the pulmonary arterial system in the same way systemic emboli commonly arise from the left atrium. As it is nearly impossible to tell reliably from where a clot in the pulmonary artery arose, this is a difficult question to study directly. Nevertheless, there is evidence supporting the idea. In an autopsy study of 693 patients who died with AF, 12.6% had clot in their left atrium while 7.5% had clot in their right atrium [22]. In more recent studies, spontaneous echo contrast (thought to be a precursor to clot formation) has been found in the right atria of patients with AF [23].

Prognostic utility of the ECG in acute PE

Despite its shortcomings in establishing the diagnosis of PE, the ECG may be useful in identifying those patients who bear closer monitoring, may have worse outcomes, or may benefit from thrombolytics. Some have suggested expanding the use of thrombolytics from those with PE and shock to include patients at high risk of poor outcome [24]. Right ventricular dysfunction accompanying a PE has been shown to identify patients with greater morbidity and mortality. In one study, echocardiographic evidence of RV dysfunction was found in 31% of normotensive patients with PE, and 10% of those went on to develop PE-related shock, while 5% died in hospital [25].

It is postulated that the inversion of T waves precordially stems from acute increases in RV afterload, increased RV wall tension, and resulting RV ischemia. Elevation of troponin I (TnI) in the setting of PE lends evidence of acute myocardial ischemia. A positive TnI has been shown to be associated with RV dysfunction on echocardiogram [26]. A detectable cardiac troponin T (TnT > 1 ug/L) is associated with prolonged hypotension and cardiogenic shock, and it is an independent predictor of 30-day mortality [27]. A similar relationship exists with RV pressure, PE, B-type natriuretic peptide

levels, and mortality, supporting the accepted concept of RV dysfunction in PE as an independent predictor of morbidity [28].

In a study of patients with PE and treated with thrombolytics, the finding of inverted precordial T waves, especially when present on admission, was shown to correlate with increased severity of PE and higher pulmonary artery pressures (PAP > 30 mmHg) [29]. Resolution before the hospital day #6 portends a favorable outcome. Underscoring this relationship, the greater number of leads with T wave inversion has been more recently associated with a higher risk of requiring catecholamine support, mechanical ventilation, or cardiopulmonary resuscitation [30].

Right ventricular dysfunction identified echocardiographically may be a physiologic surrogate for clot burden and may manifest with a number of ECG findings (Figure 40.4). In fact, using an ECG scoring system that assigns points for various changes associated with PE (Table 40.2) has been shown to accurately correlate with patients who have greater degree of perfusion defects on V/Q testing [31], RV dysfunction and poorer hospital outcomes [32]. Geibel showed that patients with PE who had at least one of the following, atrial arrhythmia, complete RBBB, peripheral low voltage, pseudo-infarction pattern (Q waves in III and aVF), or ST changes over the left precordial leads, had a 29% in-hospital mortality rate as opposed to only 11% in patients who did not [33].

One fundamental flaw in the literature that correlates ECG findings with outcomes and severity remains the frequent exclusion of patients with known pre-existing cardiopulmonary disease. The sensitivity and predictive value of ECG findings for PE outcome would likely decrease in cardiac patients with abnormal baseline ECGs and chronic lung disease patients at higher risk for chronic pulmonary hypertension.

Case conclusions

The high rate of missed diagnoses of PE and its staggering overall mortality, punctuate the importance of early and accurate diagnosis of the disease. The elusiveness of the diagnosis in the face of ever-expanding diagnostic technologies may also be a signal as to why ECG contribution to correct identification is not good. The largest role of the ECG in patients with acute cardiopulmonary symptomatology is in the exclusion of alternative processes, in particular, acute coronary syndromes. An ECG should be obtained for every patient where PE is suspected. It can point to an alternative diagnosis, such as myocardial infarction or arrhythmia, but there is no ECG change that can establish the diagnosis of PE. Unfortunately, ECG scores in addition clinical prediction tools have not augmented diagnostic clarity.

In Case 1, the presence of certain ECG findings was helpful in bolstering the clinical suspicion for PE already raised by the patient's later stage pregnancy and acute presentation. If she had not been pregnant, identification of the $S_1Q_3T_3$

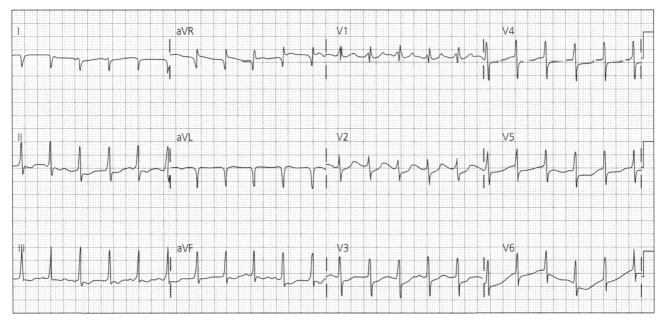

Figure 40.4 Electrocardiogram in a patient with PE with many features present in ECG scoring system in addition to others. While there is no evidence of significant conduction delay, morphology of QRS in V1 shows a right bundle pattern; prominent S waves in leads I and AVL; transition zone shifted to V5; QRS axis is rightward at 120 degrees; T wave inversions are noted in leads III, aVF, V3, and V4. The underlying rhythm is atrial tachycardia at a rate of 129 bpm.

may have helped avoid attributing the symptoms of the presentation to the cocaine use.

In Case 2, the findings of AF and right axis deviation prompted extensive investigation for PE. The final diagnosis of chronic obstructive pulmonary disease (COPD) exacerbation was made. Given recent correlations between COPD and PE incidence, the diagnostic work-up was not unreasonable [34]. The case does highlight the lack of diagnostic ECG findings for PE.

There may be a role for ECG assessment of hemodynamic effects of PE. In Case 3, the findings of T wave inversions inferiorly and $S_1Q_3T_3$ eventually were shown to be accurate in identifying RV strain on echocardiogram. It was applicable in this situation, particularly given the absence of suspicion for other pre-existing pulmonary or cardiac disease. Yet, given the lack of clear outcomes data and scant data, the ECG has not replaced the echocardiogram in this role, but may help identify those at highest need for further investigation and management.

References

1 Stein PD, Henry JW. Prevalence of acute pulmonary embolism among patients in a general hospital and at autopsy. *Chest* 1995; **108**(4):978–81.

2 Donnamaria V, Palla A, Giuntini C. Gender, age and clinical signs in patients suspected of pulmonary embolism. *Respiration* 1994;**61**(1):1–7.

3 Silverstein MD, Heit JA, Mohr DN, *et al.* Trends in the incidence of deep vein thrombosis and pulmonary embolism: a 25-year population-based study. *Arch Intern Med* 1998;**158**(6):585–93.

4 Miniati M, Prediletto R, Formichi B, *et al.* Accuracy of clinical assessment in the diagnosis of pulmonary embolism. *Am J Respir Crit Care Med* 1999;**159**(3):864–71.

5 Stein PD, Fowler SE, Goodman LR, *et al.* Multidetector computed tomography for acute pulmonary embolism. *N Engl J Med* 2006;**354**(22):2317–27.

6 Wells PS, Anderson DR, Rodger M, *et al.* Excluding pulmonary embolism at the bedside without diagnostic imaging: management of patients with suspected pulmonary embolism presenting to the emergency department by using a simple clinical model and d-dimer. *Ann Intern Med* 2001;**135**(2):98–107.

7 Wells PS, Anderson DR, Rodger M, *et al.* Derivation of a simple clinical model to categorize patients probability of pulmonary embolism: increasing the models utility with the SimpliRED D-dimer. *Thromb Haemost* 2000;**83**(3):416–20.

8 Le Gal G, Righini M, Roy PM, *et al.* Prediction of pulmonary embolism in the emergency department: the revised Geneva score. *Ann Intern Med* 2006;**144**(3):165–71.

9 Chunilal SD, Eikelboom JW, Attia J, *et al.* Does this patient have pulmonary embolism? *JAMA* 2003;**290**(21):2849–58.

10 Daniel KR, Courtney DM, Kline JA. Assessment of cardiac stress from massive pulmonary embolism with 12-lead ECG. *Chest* 2001;**120**(2):474–81.

11 Kanbay A, Kokturk N, Kaya MG, *et al.* Electrocardiography and Wells scoring in predicting the anatomic severity of pulmonary embolism. *Respir Med* 2007;**101**(6):1171–6.

12 McGinn SWP. Acute cor pulmonale resulting from pulmonary embolism. *JAMA* 1935;**104**:1473–80.

13 Chan TC, Vilke GM, Pollack M, *et al.* Electrocardiographic manifestations: pulmonary embolism. *J Emerg Med* 2001;**21**(3):263–70.

14 Spodick DH. Electrocardiographic responses to pulmonary embol-

ism. Mechanisms and sources of variability. *Am J Cardiol* 1972; **30**(6):695–9.

15 Sreeram N, Cheriex EC, Smeets JL, *et al.* Value of the 12-lead electrocardiogram at hospital admission in the diagnosis of pulmonary embolism. *Am J Cardiol* 1994;**73**(4):298–303.

16 Weber DM, Phillips JH, Jr. A re-evaluation of electrocardiographic changes accompanying acute pulmonary embolism. *Am J Med Sci* 1966;**251**(4):381–98.

17 Wiener I. Clinical and echocardiographic correlates of systemic embolization in nonrheumatic atrial fibrillation. *Am J Cardiol* 1987;**59**(1):177.

18 Szwast A, Hanna B, Shah M. Atrial fibrillation and pulmonary embolism. *Pediatr Emerg Care* 2007;**23**(11):826–8.

19 Haissaguerre M, Jais P, Shah DC, *et al.* Spontaneous initiation of atrial fibrillation by ectopic beats originating in the pulmonary veins. *N Engl J Med* 1998;**339**(10):659–66.

20 Johson JC, Flowers NC, Horan LG. Unexplained atrial flutter: a frequent herald of pulmonary embolism. *Chest* 1971;**60**(1):29–34.

21 Klein HO, Bakst A, Kaplinsky E. Pulmonary embolism and atrial fibrillation. *Am J Cardiol* 1988;**61**(6):498–9.

22 Aberg H. Atrial fibrillation. I. A study of atrial thrombosis and systemic embolism in a necropsy material. *Acta Med Scand* 1969; **185**(5):373–9.

23 Flegel KM. When atrial fibrillation occurs with pulmonary embolism, is it the chicken or the egg? *CMAJ* 1999;**160**(8):1181–2.

24 Cannon CP, Goldhaber SZ. Cardiovascular risk stratification of pulmonary embolism. *Am J Cardiol* 1996;**78**(10):1149–51.

25 Grifoni S, Olivotto I, Cecchini P, *et al.* Short-term clinical outcome of patients with acute pulmonary embolism, normal blood pressure, and echocardiographic right ventricular dysfunction. *Circulation* 2000;**101**(24):2817–22.

26 Meyer T, Binder L, Hruska N, *et al.* Cardiac troponin I elevation in acute pulmonary embolism is associated with right ventricular dysfunction. *J Am Coll Cardiol* 2000;**36**(5):1632–6.

27 Giannitsis E, Muller-Bardorff M, Kurowski V, *et al.* Independent prognostic value of cardiac troponin T in patients with confirmed pulmonary embolism. *Circulation* 2000;**102**(2):211–7.

28 ten Wolde M, Tulevski II, Mulder JW, *et al.* Brain natriuretic peptide as a predictor of adverse outcome in patients with pulmonary embolism. *Circulation* 2003;**107**(16):2082–4.

29 Ferrari E, Imbert A, Chevalier T, *et al.* The ECG in pulmonary embolism. Predictive value of negative T waves in precordial leads – 80 case reports. *Chest* 1997;**111**(3):537–43.

30 Kosuge M, Kimura K, Ishikawa T, *et al.* Prognostic significance of inverted T waves in patients with acute pulmonary embolism. *Circ J* 2006;**70**(6):750–5.

31 Iles S, Le Heron CJ, Davies G, *et al.* ECG score predicts those with the greatest percentage of perfusion defects due to acute pulmonary thromboembolic disease. *Chest* 2004;**125**(5):1651–6.

32 Toosi MS, Merlino JD, Leeper KV. Electrocardiographic score and short-term outcomes of acute pulmonary embolism. *Am J Cardiol* 2007;**100**(7):1172–6.

33 Geibel A, Zehender M, Kasper W, *et al.* Prognostic value of the ECG on admission in patients with acute major pulmonary embolism. *Eur Respir J* 2005;**25**(5):843–8.

34 Tillie-Leblond I, *et al.* Pulmonary embolism in patients with unexplained exacerbation of chronic obstructive pulmonary disease: Prevalence and risk factors. *Ann Intern Med* 2006;**144**:390–6.

Chapter 41 | What is the role and impact of the ECG in the patient with hyperkalemia?

Steve Herndon, Benjamin Holland, Ajeet Vinayak
University of Virginia, Charlottesville, VA, USA

Case presentations

Case 1: A 51-year-old man with diabetes and chronic renal failure presents to the emergency department (ED) with dyspnea after reportedly undergoing hemodialysis that day. He reports non-compliance with his insulin therapy and admits to recent cocaine use. Physical examination is remarkable for an afebrile, middle-aged man in mild distress; the vital signs are blood pressure (BP) 195/105 mmHg, pulse 115 beats per minute (bpm), and respiration 25 breaths a minute. The serum chemistry panel reveals potassium 6.7 mmol/L, glucose 1239 mg/dL, sodium 127 mEq/L and an anion gap of 30 with a serum bicarbonate of 8 mEq/L. Evaluation for possible myocardial injury by electrocardiogram (ECG) shows peaked T waves, with conduction delay initially thought to be a bifasicular block with an indeterminate P wave morphology (Figure 41.1a). Chest x-ray is unremarkable. The patient is subsequently admitted to the intensive care unit (ICU) for insulin infusion. Heparin infusion is initiated empirically for concerns of ketoacidosis exacerbated by cocaine-induced coronary syndrome. Dialysis is planned as definitive therapy for hyperkalemia. Upon arrival to the ICU there had been a substantial change in the rhythm (over an hour) (Figure 41.1b). The patient then has a pulseless arrest and responds to cardioversion and epinephrine administration. Intravenous calcium is administered and he is emergently dialyzed. His discharge ECG is also shown (Figure 41.1c). He admits to having missed two of his last three dialysis runs. He has a negative work-up for infection or coronary event.

Case 2: A 67-year-old man with a known history of atrial fibrillation, recently in good health, presents to the ED with the chief complaint of rapid-onset abdominal discomfort. Past medical history is significant for hypothyroidism, for which he is being treated with levothyroxine. The patient does not otherwise complain of chest pain or shortness of

breath. Physical examination shows an afebrile, middle-aged man in mild distress. He is markedly hypotensive with a blood pressure of 75/55 mmHg and tachycardic with a heart rate of 115 bpm. His mucous membranes are dry. His physical examination is otherwise unremarkable. Initially, a complete blood count is normal, though the chemistry panel shows elevated serum potassium of 6.6 mmol/L. He is also found to have normal kidney function and no evidence of liver abnormality. Evaluation for possible myocardial injury by ECG shows atrial fibrillation with moderately peaked T waves and non-specific ST changes (Figure 41.2a). The patient is subsequently admitted to the ICU and at that time that he requires both vasopressors and fluids to maintain a mean arterial pressure above 65 mmHg. His serum cortisol level returns at 2.9 μg/dL which, in the context of his clinical presentation, supports the diagnosis of acute adrenal insufficiency. Discharge ECG shows atrial fibrillation with T wave inversion in inferior leads and lead V5, which had been normal at admission. This is attributed to "pseudo-normalization" on initial presentation.

Case 3: An 83-year-old female with a prior coronary bypass surgery presents with increased shortness of breath and syncope. She is transported to the ED via emergency medical services (EMS). En route, EMS records a slow initial rhythm; she has been given 2 mg of atropine in the field. She has had progressive symptoms for a week. She recently saw her cardiologist and had her medications adjusted, including an addition of angiotensin converting enzyme blocker. Transcutaneous pacing is initiated as lab. work is obtained. On examination, she is afebrile with a respiratory rate of 26 and a paced pulse at 60 bpm, a blood pressure of 128/78 mmHg and an oxygen saturation of 95% on 100% oxygen. The remainder of her examination is notable for bilateral crackles on lung examination. Initial rhythm strips from the EMS staff are shown in Figure 41.3a. Her serum creatinine returns at 2.9 mg/dL and her initial potassium is 7.1 mmol/L. She is given insulin, glucose, and calcium as more definitive correction of her potassium is initiated in the ICU. Temporary pacing (Figure 41.3b) is continued with poor response in potassium levels to clearance therapeutics. The patient

Critical Decisions in Emergency and Acute Care Electrocardiography, 1st edition. Edited by W.J. Brady and J.D. Truwit. © 2009 Blackwell Publishing, ISBN: 9781405159067

(a)

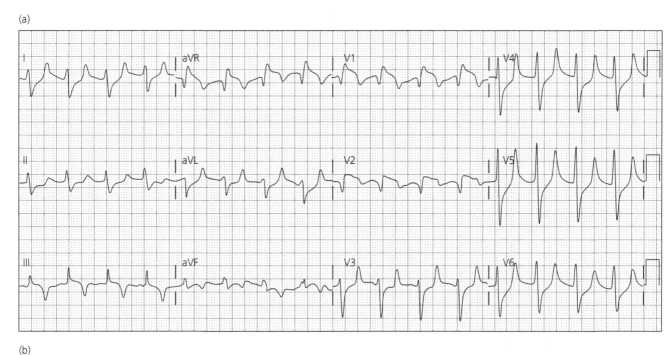

(b)

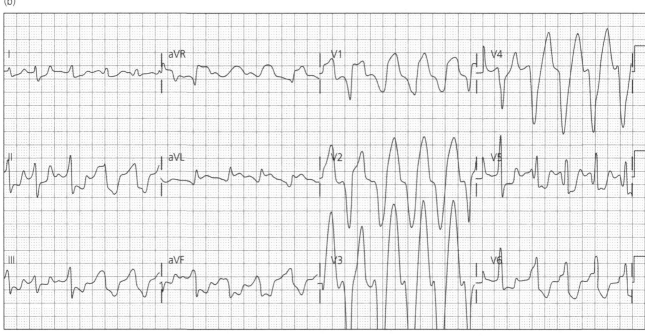

Figure 41.1 (a) Wide complex rhythm with tall tented T waves in leads V3–V6; absent P wave. Initially thought to be bifascicular block. (b) Sine wave pattern prominent.

undergoes hemodialysis with subsequent resolution of brad-yarrhythmia (Figure 41.3c).

The role and impact of the ECG in the critically ill patient with hyperkalemia

The three cases above are common acute-care presentations with hyperkalemia. The ECG and rhythm strip information can provide essential clues to the correct diagnosis and initial management. What is the role of the ECG in the care of the hyperkalemic patient?

Of the common electrolyte abnormalities affecting the ECG, disorders of potassium, in particular, hyperkalemia is most often associated with life-threatening arrhythmia. It has been reported in 1–10% of hospitalized patients [1]. The ECG manifestations of this disorder can be used for early recognition and subsequent evidence of resolution in the critically ill patient. It is also important to note that ECG

(c)

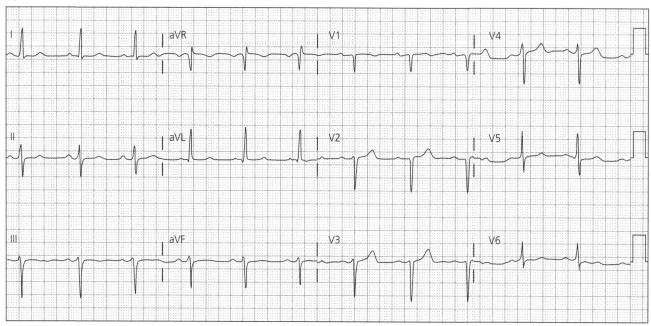

Figure 41.1 (*cont'd*) (c) At discharge ECG shows normal sinus rhythm.

findings are not always so obvious and may mimic alternative diagnoses.

Hyperkalemia must be considered in many different presenting scenarios and its physical signs (parasthesias, respiratory distress) and symptoms (weakness, fatigue) are frequently difficult to interpret without laboratory values [2,3]. Any historic suggestion of elevated serum potassium requires an immediate ECG to ascertain whether ominous signs of electrolyte imbalance are present, because their presence can lead to sudden death from cardiac arrhythmias. Given this urgency, the ECG should be obtained immediately, as it is easier and quicker to acquire than laboratory values. Knowledge of potassium homeostasis and a brief review of the normal electrophysiology can assist in the clinical diagnosis and management of this disorder.

Hyperkalemia and the myocyte

Normal serum potassium is 3.5–5.0 mmol/L in a healthy individual. This concentration is continuously maintained at the cellular level by the exchange of sodium and potassium that is primarily regulated by insulin, β2 adrenergic receptors and mineral corticosteroids. Potassium regulation is globally affected by the balance that occurs between gastrointestinal intake and renal excretion. The overall body store of potassium is 50 mmol/kg, 3500 mmol in a 70-kg person. In health, the kidney contributes to 90% of all potassium removal. In the face of chronic renal dysfunction, the gastrointestinal tract can help make up for the loss of excretion from the kidney by increasing its share of elimination from

5 to 10%, to up to 25% of all losses [2]. Medications that effect renal excretion and function or mineralocorticoid effect can lead to hyperkalemia. In addition, excessive potassium loads from enteral sources or cell breakdown can overload excretion and cause elevated serum potassium levels. In the ICU, patients are also exposed to conditions that lead to sudden release of cellular potassium (succinylcholine use, acidosis) or causes of pseudo-hyperkalemia (Table 41.1).

The majority of potassium in the body is located within cells (~98%) [2,4]. This concentration gradient is maintained by the sodium- and potassium-activated adenosine triphosphatase (Na^+/K^+–ATPase) pump. The concentration gradient is the major determinant of resting membrane potential (RMP) of the myocyte. The passive efflux of potassium out of the cell is offset by competing actions of sodium attempting to enter the cell across its gradient and anions trying to leave the intracellular milieu, both opposed by an impermeable membrane. At equilibrium, the cellular concentration differences of ions are balanced by an electrical gradient that leaves the intracellular environment of a ventricular myocyte 90 mV lower than its outside environment [5]. The RMP level influences the ensuing action potential. Small changes in the ratio of potassium inside and outside the cell effect RMP level and action potential generation and thereby have great effects on the excitability of cardiovascular system.

Electrolyte imbalances affect both the depolarization and repolarization phases of the cardiac cycle action potential by altering potentials across cardiac myocyte cellular membranes [4,5]. Figure 41.4 provides an overview of the altered myocyte electrophysiology in question with hyperkalemia. When extracellular potassium rises, the transmembrane

(a)

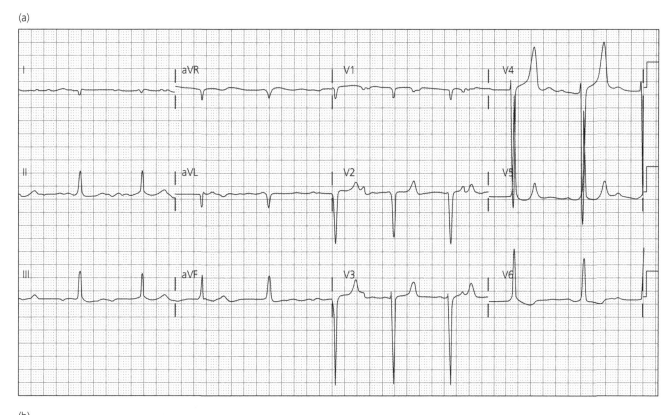

(b)

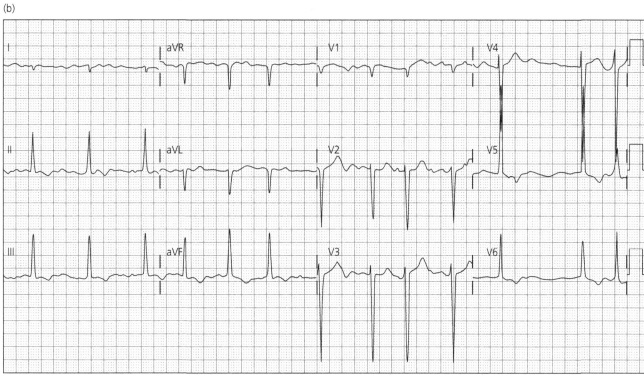

Figure 41.2 (a) Normal sinus rhythm with small P waves, and tall (tented T waves) in V4 and V5. (b) T wave changes include loss of tall waves and now the presence of T wave inversions in V5, II, III, aVF.

(a)

(b)

(c)

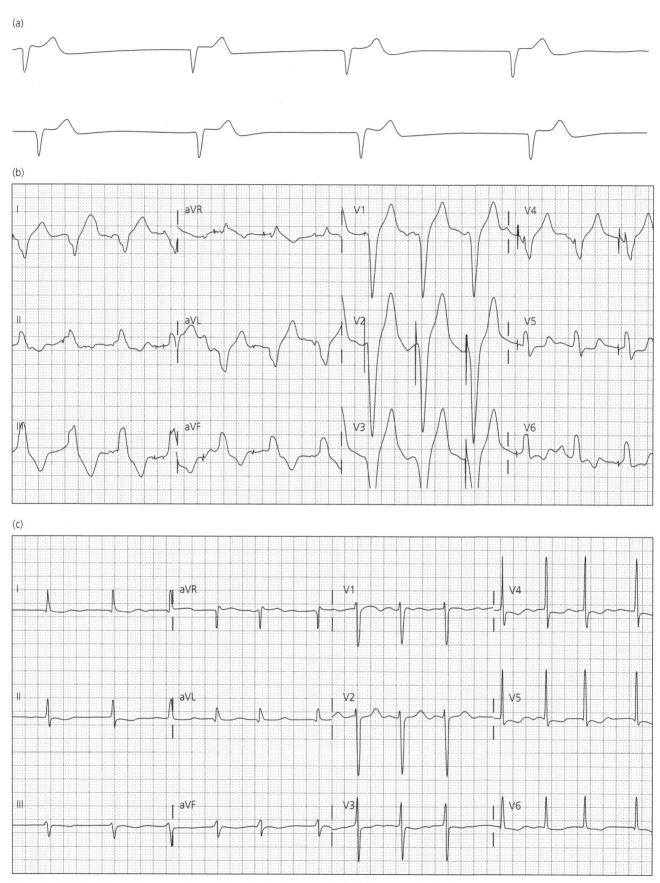

Figure 41.3 (a) Junctional rhythm at a rate of 30 bpm. (b) Paced rhythm. (c) At discharge atrial fibrillation is at normal rate.

Table 41.1 Hyperkalemia causes

Pseudo-	Increased intake	Cellular shift	Decreased excretion
Phlebotomy	Oral	Hypoinsulinemia	Renal insufficiency
Hemolysis	Dietary	Acidemia	Volume depletion
Leukocytosis	K supplement	Digitalis toxicity	Congestive heart failure
Thrombocytosis	Parenteral	Succinylcholine	NSAID use
	TPN	β-blockers	Decreased aldosterone
	Fluids	Cellular breakdown	Type IV RTA
	Old blood transfusions	Ischemia	ACE inhibitor
	Penicillin	GI hemolysis	Adrenal insufficiency
		Rhabdomyolysis	Ketoconazole
		Tumor lysis	Heparin
			Trimethoprim
			Cyclosporine A
			Tacrolimus
			Spironolactone

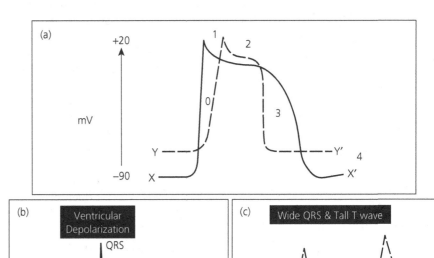

Figure 41.4 (b) Action potentials of cardiac myocyte. Solid line (X → X′) shows normal state with resting membrane potential of –90 mV. Dashed line (Y → Y′) shows a hyperkalemic state. Resting membrane potential is elevated given decreased gradient of potassium concentration across the cell membrane. Phase 0 (depolarization) with slower slope, Phase 3 (repolarization) with steeper slope (see text). (b) ECG normal state. (c) Stylized consequence of hyperkalemia.

gradient level for potassium is significantly decreased. Potassium efflux is not as brisk and RMP at baseline is consequentially increased (X → Y). Phase 0 rise in the atrium affects the P wave, and in the ventricle will alter the QRS complex. The resultant decrease in slope and magnitude in phase 0 (depolarization) leads to the widening and loss of P waves and increase of the QRS interval. The increased slope of phase 3 (repolarization) correlates with the T wave. Phase 3's more rapid return in the hyperkalemic patient leads to the characteristic prominent T waves. In between, the shorter phase 2 duration leads to preservation and shortening of the QT interval. Automaticity is decreased in hyperkalemia

and is related to the loss of the upward slope in phase 4 in pacemaker myocytes [2,5–7].

Levels of hyperkalemia and ECG findings

The classic ECG changes are due to the physiologic effect of the electrolyte on myocardial cells at different levels of potassium. Mild increases of serum potassium (5.5–6.5 mmol/L) can first alter and accelerate terminal repolarization (increased slope in terminal phase 3) leading to T wave abnormalities.

Resultant peaked T waves are considered to be the earliest abnormalities seen in the ECG [7,8]. These waves are often called "tented," referring to the increase in amplitude without an increase in duration [5]. As the QT duration has not changed dramatically this may result in a different morphology in the QT and T wave in hyperkalemia versus other disorders such as an acute coronary syndrome or subarachnoid hemorrhage. These other conditions are associated with widened QT intervals and a broad T wave (Figure 41.5). While this classic thin, tall T is expected, it has been suggested that only a minority of peaked T waves from hyperkalemia are distinguishable from T wave abnormalities seen in these other disorders [2,5].

The T wave abnormalities are typically seen in the lateral precordial and inferior leads as in Figure 41.5. Another recognized change in the T wave is pseudo-normalization. This refers to baseline inverted T waves that now have a positive deflection due to the effect of rapid terminal repolarization in the associated myocytes [4]. Case 2 shows an example of this phenomenon (Figure 41.2). At this early, mild level of hyperkalemia (5.5–6.5 mmol/L), rapid repolarization of atrial myocytes is expressed by a shortened PR interval [5]. As other parts of the action potential are about to be affected, loss of rapid conduction is about to occur as potassium continues to increase.

Moderate hyperkalemia (6.6–8.0 mmol/L) causes depression of conduction between adjacent cardiac myocytes, resulting in prolongation of the PR and QRS intervals [2,5]. These changes are consequences of further elevations of RMP as extracellular potassium rises. These are direct manifestations of decrements in the phase 0 slope (slower depolarization of atria and ventricles). Case 1 offers an example of this ECG change (Figure 41.1a).

Atrial myocytes are particularly sensitive to elevated potassium and, as a result, ECG findings include P wave prolongation followed by P wave depression or absence. The widened QRS and blunted P wave expression can often help identify the moderately hyperkalemic ECG and avoid confusion with bundle branch blocks. The ventricular myocytes are next in the order of hyperkalemia sensitivity and QRS prolongation is evidenced. At this time, QT interval length appears to have increased given this QRS change. The sinoatrial (SA) node is thought to be more refractory than these other cell types [2]. It has been demonstrated in dogs that while P waves are absent, the SA node may still be orchestrating ventricular depolarization, albeit with a widened QRS as predicted by the effect on phase 0 of the ventricular myocyte [9].

At even higher levels of potassium (severe hyperkalemia, > 8.0 mmol/L), progressive SA nodal blockage results in junctional beats and then (atrioventricular) AV nodal blockade with resultant degrees of heart block and escape rhythms. This explains the presenting rhythm and need for pacing in Case 3. Eventually, the widened QRS complexes without P waves result in the classic "sine wave," which is a harbinger of critical myocardial instability [10]. This is represented in Figure 41.1b and 41.6. At this point, hyperkalemic myocardium is at highest risk for ventricular fibrillation or asystole [1,4,7,11].

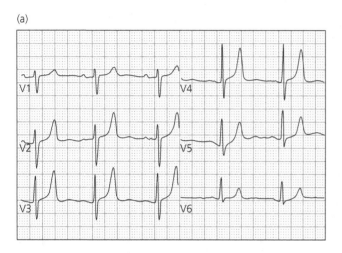

(a)

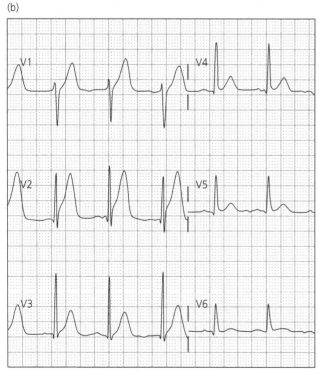

(b)

Figure 41.5 Frontal leads shown only (a) Hyperkalemia with narrow, tall, tented T waves and normal QT interval. (b) Acute myocardial injury with tall T waves that appear broad and associated with a prolonged QT interval.

Special ECG considerations in hyperkalemia

While the progression of ECG findings with serum potassium levels described above holds true, in many clinical situations variability in this correlation exists. Rarely, severe hyperkalemia can present without ECG signals. The lack of ECG

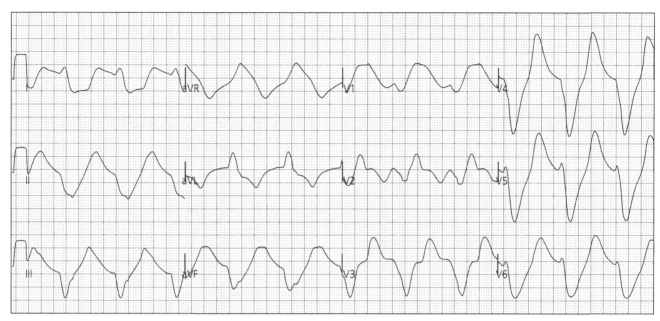

Figure 41.6 Sine wave seen in severe hyperkalemia.

changes even at high levels of serum potassium should arouse suspicion for pseudo-hyperkalemia. Common scenarios in the ICU include conditions associated with intravascular hemolysis (disseminated intravascular coagulation, thrombotic thrombocytopenia, sickle cell crisis, etc.), most commonly from blood-drawing technique. Profound leukocytosis (> 70,000) or thrombocytosis (> 600,000) has also been associated with false elevations of potassium.

Yet ECG changes, on rare occasions, have been reported to be absent with true severe hyperkalemia (> 8 mmol/L) [12,13]. Certain clinical features may alter the possibility of ECG manifestations and arrhythmia. Hypernatremia, normal or elevated pH, hypercalcemia, and slow rate of hyperkalemia development all may attenuate the effects on ECG abnormality formation. The latter two variables have been implicated in the absence of ECG findings in patients on chronic hemodialysis [14–16]. Conversely, metabolic acidosis, rapid hyperkalemia, and hypocalcemia should be causes for concern for accentuated cardiac sensitivity [17].

An additional confounding ECG pattern reported with hyperkalemia can mimic myocardial infarction. Thought to be due to uneven regional depolarization, ST segment elevation has been illustrated most often in the anteroseptal precordial leads. Potassium levels are usually severely elevated above 7.5 mmol/L [18,19]. This phenomenon has been shown to resolve with dialysis alone, yet has been known to incur cardiac catheterization on occasion [18,20].

Several special ICU situations in the care of the hyperkalemic patient deserve mention. It has been commented that resuscitation from hyperkalemic cardiac arrest may have better outcomes with recovery even in cases requiring prolonged resuscitation [17]. Furthermore, typical pharmacologic therapy with calcium should be cautioned if hyper-

kalemia is thought due to digitalis toxicity. In this situation, intracellular calcium elevation may be augmented with exogenous administration and promulgate further arrhythmia. Proper therapy should include digoxin FAB in these situations.

In the critically ill patient requiring neuromuscular blockade, succinylcholine administration has been associated with hyperkalemia. Conditions that predispose to this result include underlying myopathic diseases and situations with significant tissue damage such as burn, trauma, and prolonged immobility. The myopathic patients risk rhabdomyolysis when succinylcholine is used. In general, refractory hyperkalemia in the critically ill patient should prompt investigation for rhabdomyolysis of any etiology or cellular necrosis that has gone undiagnosed (tumor lysis, necrotic bowel).

Case conclusions

Although ECG changes are not present in all patients with elevated serum potassium, the ECG is a useful diagnostic tool that may allow the clinician to quickly assess the critically ill patient with a potentially life-threatening serum potassium abnormality and employ a timely and appropriate therapeutic intervention. In an ED study evaluating the predictive accuracy for hyperkalemia in patients at risk, the sensitivity of ECG analysis was poor (~40%) with significantly better specificity (~85%) [21]. Awareness of ECG findings is imperative, as it is often available before laboratory values have been sent.

The presence of hypercalcemia and chronic elevations in potassium have been found to be associated with poorer correlation between hyperkalemia and ECG findings in a patient chronically receiving hemodialysis. Yet, as seen in Case 1, a rapid response to the presence of ECG findings is required to avoid hemodynamic instability. In this case, the recent dialysis and moderate elevation in serum potassium levels accounted for delays in calcium and insulin administration. Complicating this case was the concomitant metabolic acidosis from diabetic ketoacidosis and dialysis non-compliance. The presence of this acidosis and hypoinsulinemia may explain the rapidity of electrical conversion to an unstable rhythm. Initial ECG interpretation with bundle branch block along with T wave prominence fueled concerns for a coronary syndrome. Examination of the initial ECG (Figure 41.1a) shows loss of P waves and normal QT intervals when QRS prolongation is accounted. These clues can help clinicians with the diagnosis of significant hyperkalemia.

Case 2 illustrates characteristic tented T waves laterally, and pseudo-normalization of T waves in other leads. Resolution of hyperkalemia was limited to medical management with calcium, insulin, and treatment of the underlying disorder, mineralocorticoid deficiency. While detailed treatment algorithms for severe hyperkalemia are beyond the scope of this chapter, Case 3 brings up specific therapeutic considerations. The patient received atropine and was paced initially for profound bradycardia. These therapies may have poor response in the hyperkalemic bradycardic patient. In fact, chronically paced patients have been known to lose capture in acute hyperkalemic states [2]. In this case, medical management was ineffective and the patient responded to a singular dialysis treatment with restoration of a stable rate and rhythm.

Acknowledgments

We would like to acknowledge the generous contributions of Drs Kenneth Smith and Shadi Mourad who provided ECGs.

References

1 Acker CG, Johnson JP, Palevsky PM, *et al.* Hyperkalemia in hospitalized patients: causes, adequacy of treatment, and results of an attempt to improve physician compliance with published therapy guidelines. *Arch Intern Med* 1998;**158**(8):917–24.

2 Alfonzo AV, Isles C, Geddes C, *et al.* Potassium disorders – clinical spectrum and emergency management. *Resuscitation* 2006; **70**(1):10–25.

3 Van Mieghem C, Sabbe M, Knockaert D. The clinical value of the ECG in noncardiac conditions. *Chest* 2004;**125**(4):1561–76.

4 Diercks DB, Shumaik GM, Harrigan RA, *et al.* Electrocardiographic manifestations: electrolyte abnormalities. *J Emerg Med* 2004;**27**(2):153–60.

5 Dittrich KL, Walls RM. Hyperkalemia: ECG manifestations and clinical considerations. *J Emerg Med* 1986;**4**(6):449–55.

6 Helfant RH. Hypokalemia and arrhythmias. *Am J Med* 1986; **80**(4A):13–22.

7 Mattu A, Brady WJ, Robinson DA. Electrocardiographic manifestations of hyperkalemia. *Am J Emerg Med* 2000;**18**(6):721–9.

8 Commerford PJ, Lloyd EA. Arrhythmias in patients with drug toxicity, electrolyte, and endocrine disturbances. *Med Clin North Am* 1984;**68**(5):1051–78.

9 Cohen HC, Gozo EG, Jr., Pick A. The nature and type of arrhythmias in acute experimental hyperkalemia in the intact dog. *Am Heart J* 1971;**82**(6):777–85.

10 Scarabeo V, Baccillieri MS, Di Marco A, *et al.* Sine-wave pattern on the electrocardiogram and hyperkalaemia. *J Cardiovasc Med (Hagerstown)* 2007;**8**(9):729–31.

11 Webster A, Brady W, Morris F. Recognising signs of danger: ECG changes resulting from an abnormal serum potassium concentration. *Emerg Med J* 2002;**19**(1):74–7.

12 Martinez-Vea A, Bardaji A, Garcia C, *et al.* Severe hyperkalemia with minimal electrocardiographic manifestations: a report of seven cases. *J Electrocardiol* 1999;**32**(1):45–9.

13 Szerlip HM, Weiss J, Singer I. Profound hyperkalemia without electrocardiographic manifestations. *Am J Kidney Dis* 1986;**7**(6): 461–5.

14 Ahmed J, Weisberg LS. Hyperkalemia in dialysis patients. *Semin Dial* 2001;**14**(5):348–56.

15 Aslam S, Friedman EA, Ifudu O. Electrocardiography is unreliable in detecting potentially lethal hyperkalaemia in haemodialysis patients. *Nephrol Dial Transplant* 2002;**17**(9):1639–42.

16 Esposito C, Bellotti N, Fasoli G, *et al.* Hyperkalemia-induced ECG abnormalities in patients with reduced renal function. *Clin Nephrol* 2004;**62**(6):465–8.

17 Hall JB, Schmidt GA, Wood LDH. *Principles of Critical Care.* 3rd ed. New York: McGraw-Hill, 2005; xxvii, 1778 pp.

18 Bellazzini MA, Meyer T. Pseudo-myocardial infarction in diabetic ketoacidosis with hyperkalemia. *J Emerg Med* 2007. [Epub ahead of print] last accessed August 30 2008.

19 Campistol JM, *et al.* Electrographic alterations induced by hyperkalaemia simulating acute myocardial infarction. *Nephrol Dial Transplant* 1989;**4**(3):233–5.

20 Levine HD, Wanzer SH, Merrill JP. Dialyzable currents of injury in potassium intoxication resembling acute myocardial infarction or pericarditis. *Circulation* 1956;**13**(1):29–36.

21 Wrenn KD, Slovis CM, Slovis BS. The ability of physicians to predict hyperkalemia from the ECG. *Ann Emerg Med* 1991;**20**(11): 1229–32.

Chapter 42 | What is the role and impact of the ECG in the patient with electrolyte abnormalities other than hyperkalemia?

Benjamin Holland[1], Franklin McGuire[2]
[1]University of Virginia, Charlottesville, VA, USA
[2]University of South Carolina, Columbia, SC, USA

Case presentations

Case 1: A 61-year-old male with well-controlled hypertension presents to the emergency department (ED) with 3 days of nausea, vomiting, and diarrhea. He also reports several more days of abdominal discomfort and little to eat or drink. He reports one episode of fainting at home, which prompted his visit to the ED. His other complaints include severe muscle weakness and dizziness. Upon examination, the patient is in mild distress and hypotensive. His blood pressure is 90/60 mmHg and he is tachycardic with a heart rate of 105 beats per minute (bpm). Other physical findings include dry mucous membranes and a tender abdomen without rebound. His electrocardiogram (ECG) shows non-specific T wave inversions followed by prominent U waves (Figure 42.1). An initial chemistry panel reveals serum potassium of 2.2 mmol/dL.

Case 2: A 41-year-old with end-stage renal disease, who is dialysis-dependent, is hospitalized following elective parathyroidectomy. He has recently been diagnosed with hyperparathyroidism related to his renal disease. He undergoes surgery that involves total parathyroidectomy with reimplantation of parathyroid tissue in the left sternocleidomastoid muscle. Postoperatively, he is noted to have an expanding neck swelling at the implantation site. Surgical re-exploration leads to drainage of a hematoma requiring reintubation. He is admitted to the intensive care unit (ICU) still on the ventilator for respiratory care and management. His remaining history is notable for peripheral vascular disease. He is successfully extubated the morning of his second ICU day. He initially complains of fatigue, muscle cramps in his legs, and numbness in his fingers and around his mouth. His vitals are all normal with an oxygen saturation of 98% on room air. A concerning new finding of prolonged QT interval on rhythm monitoring prompts a 12-lead ECG. Comparison with his admission ECG of 24 h earlier, confirms a widened QT interval (Figure 42.2 a and b). His initial calcium level of 7.8 mg/dL has dropped to 5.9 mg/dL with an ionized calcium nadir of 2.6 mg/dL. He is repleted with IV and oral calcium supplementation and given a diagnosis of hungry bone syndrome.

Case 3: A 66-year-old female with a history of end-stage renal disease on dialysis and coronary artery disease is admitted to the ICU with a non-ST elevation myocardial infarction and exacerbation of her heart failure. She had undergone coronary catheterization 1 day earlier, which revealed the grafts from her previous three-vessel bypass were all patent with additional diffuse disease that required no intervention. On hospital day #3, while receiving continuous veno-venous hemodialysis, an error is made in the calcium concentration added and 10 g of calcium chloride is infused over a 90-min period. The initial presenting symptom that led to identification of this error was profound tachycardia and hypertension. The maximum level of ionized calcium measured is 10.5 mg/dL. A significant change is noted in her ECG (Figure 42.3a) with identification of a new intraventricular delay. A rhythm strip captures a run of monomorphic ventricular tachycardia (Figure 42.3b) that initiated a cardiopulmonary resuscitation. Her morning and discharge ECGs are shown, with narrowing and eventual normalization of the QRS interval (Figure 42.3c).

Critical Decisions in Emergency and Acute Care Electrocardiography,
1st edition. Edited by W.J. Brady and J.D. Truwit. © 2009 Blackwell Publishing, ISBN: 9781405159067.

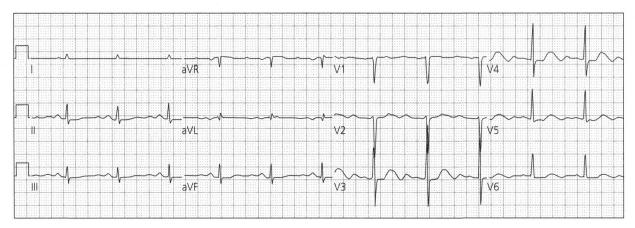

Figure 42.1 Sinus rhythm with flattening of T waves and prominent U waves in lead V2–V6.

(a)

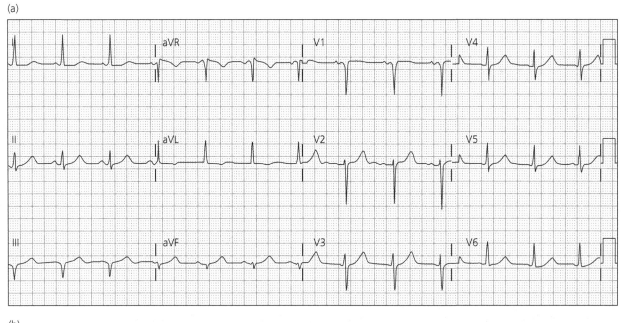

(b)

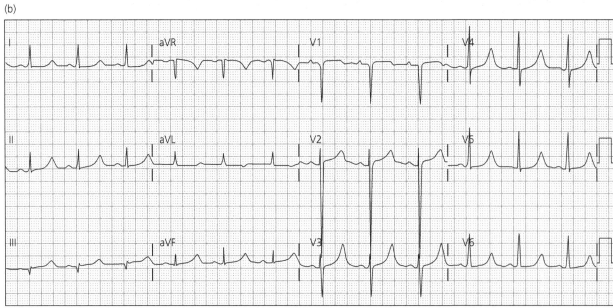

Figure 42.2 (a) Sinus rhythm preoperative with QTc of 440 ms. (b) ECG with new prolonged QT interval 18 h after parathyroidectomy with QTc 516 ms.

(a)

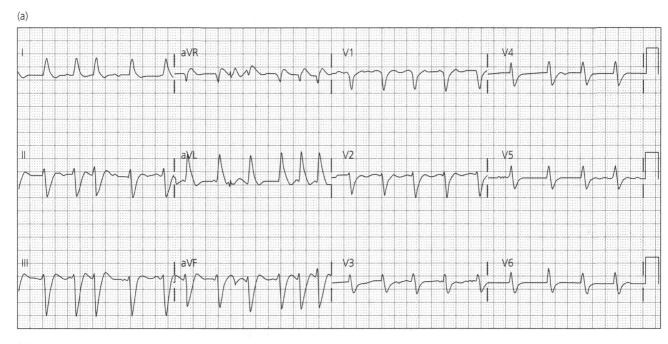

(b)

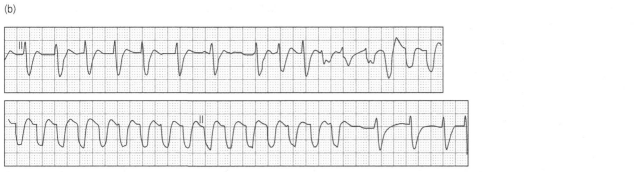

(c)

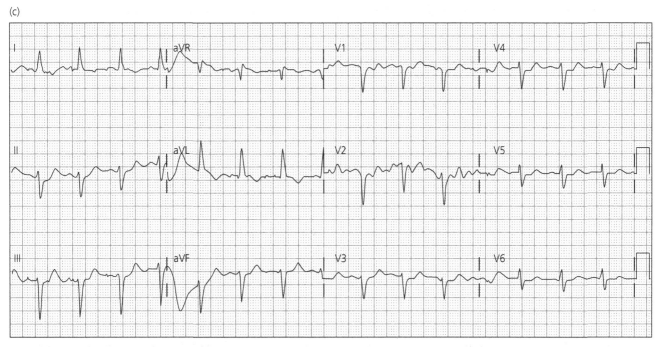

Figure 42.3 (a) Initial ECG during episode of tachycardia and hypertension with atrial fibrillation with a ventricular rate of 115 bpm and widened QRS (154 ms), QTc normal at 430 ms. (b) rhythm strip 15 min later showing episode of ventricular tachycardia. (c) After 5 h of corrected Continuous Veno-Venous Hemofiltration (CVVH) calcium regulation, rhythm is normal sinus with a QRS duration now 113 ms and QTc 472 ms.

The role and impact of the ECG in the patients with non-hyperkalemic electrolyte abnormalities

The three cases above represent cases who can be admitted to an ICU for close monitoring, identification and correction of electrolyte disturbances. The ECG findings in each are abnormal. What is the impact of these findings and what role do they play in the management of these cases?

Hypokalemia

Hypokalemia is commonly encountered in routine laboratory evaluation and can lead to life-threatening conditions. The differential is broad and can be viewed in a few general categories just as in hyperkalemia. Poor potassium intake is often not the sole reason for hypokalemia and will likely occur over a period of time where the individual is unable to normally eat or drink. More commonly, hypokalemia associated with poor intake will coincide with other pathologic potassium metabolism involving excretion or transcellular shifts. Excretion of potassium is normally via renal and gastrointestinal (GI) losses [1]. Renal losses are most commonly augmented by the increased delivery of sodium to the collecting duct. Mineralocorticoid use/excess and thiazide diuretic use are well known to enhance sodium concentrations in the distal nephron [2]. Also, osmotic diuresis will lead to low serum potassium by this same mechanism. Diarrhea will cause potassium excretion from the GI track itself, but vomiting produces a secondary hypokalemia. Vomiting gastric fluid produces a loss of protons and volume. The resultant volume contraction and metabolic alkalosis enhances the transcellular shift of potassium passively into cells in exchange for protons. This volume depletion also works to increase mineralocorticoid concentration and proton presentation to the kidney, resulting in further potassium losses. Laboratory diagnosis of hypokalemia is common in routine and critical presentations. The physical findings of muscle weakness, flaccid paralysis, and ileus are non-specific.

The ECG manifestations of hypokalemia may be a sign of an unstable myocardium in the critically ill patient with a host of other electrolyte derangements. The effect of hypokalemia on the cell membrane is to increase the negativity of the resting membrane potential, and increase the duration of the action potential and refractory period, which are potentially arrhythmogenic [3]. Classical ECG manifestations are non-specific but well documented. U waves, usually seen in the precordial leads, are positive deflections immediately after T waves. The magnitude of the U wave can be associated with the severity of the hypokalemia. The T wave itself can be seen to flatten as well (Figure 42.1). To differen-

tiate between peaked T waves and giant U waves the following rules can be used to aid the diagnosis. The peaked T waves in hyperkalemia tend to have a narrow base, and are tall with a prominent peak, the QT interval is normal or decreased. U waves tend to be broad-based and there may be an apparent prolongation of the QT interval, which is really a QU interval [3]. These ECG findings are typically absent in mild to moderate hypokalemia and seen only when serum potassium falls below 2.7 mmol/L. However, ventricular extrasystoles are not uncommon in patients with potassium of 2.5–3.0 mmol/L [4].

In addition, patients who present with hyperglycemic states commonly experience electrolyte abnormalities such as hypokalemia and hypophosphatemia. Despite normal to slightly elevated serum potassium concentrations, these patients have a net potassium deficit that is more clearly recognized after fluid and insulin administration. Electrocardiogram manifestations of hypokalemia in these cases are the same as above and include broad, flat T waves, ST depression, QT interval prolongation, and ventricular arrhythmias (Figure 42.4) [4].

Hypokalemia has been associated with an increased risk of developing a life-threatening arrhythmia. Oral potassium replacement is usually effective for correcting mild hypokalemia [5]. However, severely low serum potassium should be aggressively replaced with intravenous therapy, especially within the context of critical illness.

Calcium

Calcium is an essential mineral divalent cation in the body and is relatively abundant. The average adult body contains approximately 1 kg of calcium, and nearly all of this is stored in bone as hydroxyapatite. Calcium is absorbed through the small intestine and eventually is excreted in the urine. Extracellular and intracellular calcium are tightly regulated through parathyroid hormone, calcitriol, and calcitonin. The amount of total serum calcium varies with the level of serum albumin and the biologically active form of calcium is ionized, which is not protein-bound [6]. Calcium is important in a myriad of regulatory mechanisms, skeletal muscle contraction, and control of enzymatic reactions, and is a key ion in myocyte electrical activity and myocardial contraction [7].

Hypercalcemia: Hypercalcemia is commonly encountered in the context of hyperparathyroidism and malignancy; however, calcium may also be elevated on routine laboratory evaluation. Non-specific physical findings may present at mildly elevated calcium levels (more than 12 mg/dL) such as: fatigue, depression, confusion, anorexia, nausea, vomiting, constipation, pancreatitis, or urinary frequency. An elevation of serum calcium of more than 14 mg/dL is commonly associated with the acute signs and symptoms of hyper-

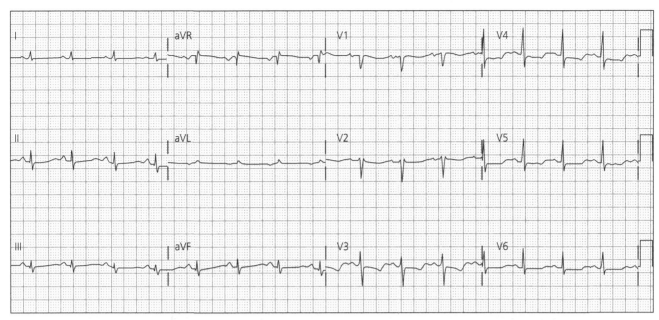

Figure 42.4 ECG shown of patient with diabetic ketoacidosis, initial serum potassium 4.3 mmol/dL, but there is ECG evidence of hypokalemia including QTc duration of 520 ms; flattened T waves in lateral precordial leads and suggestion of U waves best seen in leads V3 and V4. Significant potassium replacement was required to maintain normokalemia as management ensued.

calcemia, and should be considered a medical emergency [7]. Therapy for hypercalcemia should primarily focus on treating the underlying cause, though direct calcium-lowering therapy is often started at levels of 14 mg/dL even in the asymptomatic patient.

Electrocardiogram manifestations are related to altered membrane potentials affecting action potential conduction. Phase 2 of the action potential is shortened. Therefore, in contrast to hypocalcemia, corrected QT (QTc) interval shortening is considered the hallmark of hypercalcemia. Prolongation of the PR interval will sometimes occur with subsequent varying degrees of atrioventricular nodal blockade as seen. Conduction abnormalities manifest electrically usually only by a widened QRS as seen in Case 3 (Figure 42.3a and 3b). Repolarization abnormalities are sometimes encountered with flattened, notched, or inverted T waves [8]. Osborn J waves have been reported in the normothermic patient with extremely high calcium levels [9]. Fortunately, large concentrations of calcium are not often associated with malignant arrhythmias [7].

It is possible to see a long QT interval in the face of hypercalcemia. Potential confounders that contribute to this effect include concomitant anti-arrhythmic therapy (i.e. amiodarone, sotalol), hypokalemia, and hypomagnesemia [10]. If these conditions exist, caution should be taken in correcting calcium alone and causing ventricular arrhythmia. ST segment elevation has also been reported on several occasions in patients with profound hypercalcemia and subsequent normal coronary inspection. In these instances, this ECG finding resolves with electrolyte normalization [11,12].

Hypocalcemia: Hypocalcemia is commonly seen in critically ill patients, with a reported incidence of as many as 50% of this population [13]. Besides symptoms of lethargy, oral parasthesia, seizures, and tetany, laryngeal spasm and acute heart failure have been reported. Bedside examination should include assessment of Chvostec's sign and Trousseau's sign.

Some conditions associated with hypocalcemia include hypoparathyroidism, pseudo-hypoparathyroidism, hypomagnesemia, Vitamin D deficiency (nutritional deficiency, decreased intestinal absorption, hepatobiliary disease, pancreatic disease, renal failure), hyperphosphatemia, drugs, and critical illness. In case two, a less commonly encountered cause is manifest. Hungry bone syndrome occurs after thyroidectomy or parathyroidectomy. In patients with hyperparathyroidism, bone disease manifests due to chronic increases in bone resorption induced by preoperative elevations of parathyroid hormone. Postoperatively dramatic drops in serum calcium level result from an abrupt cessation of this process after surgical resection [14].

The ECG manifestation of hypocalcemia is most commonly QTc interval prolongation because of lengthening of the ST segment. This phenomenon is directly proportional to the magnitude of hypocalcemia. The exact opposite holds true for hypercalcemia [15]. Hypocalcemia prolongs phase 2 of the action potential with the impact modulated by the rate of change of serum calcium concentration and function of the myocyte calcium channels. A prolonged QTc is associated with early after-repolarizations and triggered dysrhythmias [3]. Torsade de pointes has been linked to hypocalcemia but is seen more frequently with hypokalemia or hypomagnesemia [16].

These ECG anomalies are frequently associated with hypocalcemia, yet fortunately life-threatening malignant arrhythmias are uncommon. The critically ill patient suffering from symptomatic hypocalcemia will require aggressive replacement with calcium salt. Also, this condition is frequently associated with other metabolic derangements that may exacerbate the manifestations of hypocalemia, such as acidosis and hypomagnesemia.

The prevalence of hypocalcemia in the ICU is dramatic [17]. Clear etiologies for the cause of this metabolic process are elucidated in less than half of these individuals. It remains controversial whether it should be uniformly treated in the asymptomatic ICU patient. It has been suggested that serum hypocalcemia may avoid significant intracellular hypercalcemia, and therefore occur as protective mechanism by attenuating tissue damage when it occurs. The evidence for avoiding replacement therapy in asymptomatic hypocalcemia of critical illness is best supported in the septic patients [18,19]. When treated in the ICU setting, hypocalcemia can occasionally precipitate additional issues. Arrhythmia has been noted in the patient on digitalis, and hypotension, pancreatitis and vasospasm have all been reported [20].

Other electrolytes

Hypernatremia has been shown to shorten the QRS duration, likely related to its effect on resting membrane potential, and increase slope of phase 0 of the action potential. Hypomagnesemia often occurs in conjunction with abnormalities in potassium and calcium. It is often seen in the context of hypokalemia and manifests identical ECG findings [21].

Case conclusions

Many critically ill patients experience metabolic derangements with multiple electrolyte disturbances. Understanding the effect of these ions on the action potential of the myocyte is helpful in predicting the effect on cardiac excitability and irritability. In addition, the ECG provides insight into the chance of arrhythmia.

In the first case, profound hypokalemia is found in a patient with severe dehydration. The ECG finding of prominent U waves is not accompanied by significant prolongation of the QTc or QRS. While this is reassuring, the absolute value of potassium depletion suggested by the low serum potassium value requires therapy and ECG monitoring.

In the second case, identification of an interval change following surgery prompted identification and monitoring of a precipitous decline in calcium. Given the patient's stability and the likelihood that parathyroid function would return within a week, the patient was discharged the following day with mild oral supplementation.

In the third case, profound iatrogenic hypercalcemia was manifest in the ECG with a widened QRS and apparent bundle branch block. While it is tantalizing to suspect that the hypercalcemia may have mediated the following ventricular arrhythmia via some direct effect, this has not been previously described. The monomorphic nature of the ventricular rhythm and subsequent marked elevation in serum troponin levels suggest that myocardial injury occurred related to a stress-induced acute coronary syndrome. It is worth reiterating that ECG findings of an electrolyte abnormality should be considered in the context of medications, underlying coronary history or risk, and other concomitant metabolic derangements (electrolyte, hypothermia, or endocrine) that can also impact the ECG.

Acknowledgments

We would like to acknowledge the generous contributions of Drs Victor Froelicher and Michael Lipinski, who provided ECG images.

References

1 Blumberg A, Weidmann P, Ferrari P. Effect of prolonged bicarbonate administration on plasma potassium in terminal renal failure. *Kidney Int* 1992;**41**(2):369–74.

2 Webster A, Brady W, Morris F. Recognising signs of danger: ECG changes resulting from an abnormal serum potassium concentration. *Emerg Med J* 2002;**19**(1):74–7.

3 Helfant RH. Hypokalemia and arrhythmias. *Am J Med* 1986; **80**(4A):13–22.

4 Slovis C, Jenkins R. ABC of clinical electrocardiography: Conditions not primarily affecting the heart. *BMJ* 2002;**324**(7349): 1320–3.

5 Van Mieghem C, Sabbe M, Knockaert D. The clinical value of the ECG in noncardiac conditions. *Chest* 2004;**125**(4):1561–76.

6 Ariyan CE, Sosa JA. Assessment and management of patients with abnormal calcium. *Crit Care Med* 2004;**32**(Suppl 4):S146–54.

7 Ziegler R. Hypercalcemic crisis. *J Am Soc Nephrol* 2001;**12** (Suppl 17):S3–9.

8 Ahmed R, Yano K, Mitsuoka T, *et al.* Changes in T wave morphology during hypercalcemia and its relation to the severity of hypercalcemia. *J Electrocardiol* 1989;**22**(2):125–32.

9 Wald DA. ECG manifestations of selected metabolic and endocrine disorders. *Emerg Med Clin North Am* 2006;**24**(1):145–57, vii.

10 Ortega-Carnicer J, Ceres F, Sanabria C. Long QT interval in severe hypercalcaemia. *Resuscitation* 2004;**61**(2):242–3.

11 Nishi SP, Barbagelata NA, Atar S, *et al.* Hypercalcemia-induced ST-segment elevation mimicking acute myocardial infarction. *J Electrocardiol* 2006;**39**(3):298–300.

12 Turhan S, Kilickap M, Kilinc S. ST segment elevation mimicking acute myocardial infarction in hypercalcaemia. *Heart* 2005; **91**(8):999.

13 Carlstedt F, Lind L. Hypocalcemic syndromes. *Crit Care Clin* 2001;**17**(1):139–53, vii–viii.

14 Brasier AR, Nussbaum SR. Hungry bone syndrome: clinical and biochemical predictors of its occurrence after parathyroid surgery. *Am J Med* 1988;**84**(4):654–60.

15 RuDusky BM. ECG abnormalities associated with hypocalcemia. *Chest* 2001;**119**(2):668–9.

16 Kasper DL, Harrison TR. *Harrison's Principles of Internal Medicine*. 16th ed. New York: McGraw-Hill, 2005; 2 v. (xxvii, 2607, [15, 128] pp.).

17 Zivin JR, Gooley T, Zager RA, *et al.* Hypocalcemia: a pervasive metabolic abnormality in the critically ill. *Am J Kidney Dis* 2001;**37**(4):689–98.

18 Hall JB, Schmidt GA, Wood LDH. *Principles of Critical Care*. 3rd ed. New York: McGraw-Hill, 2005; xxvii, 1778 pp.

19 Zaloga GP. Ionized hypocalcemia during sepsis. *Crit Care Med* 2000;**28**(1):266–8.

20 Jankowski S, Vincent JL. Calcium administration for cardiovascular support in critically ill patients: when is it indicated? *J Intensive Care Med* 1995;**10**(2):91–100.

21 Commerford PJ, Lloyd EA. Arrhythmias in patients with drug toxicity, electrolyte, and endocrine disturbances. *Med Clin North Am* 1984;**68**(5):1051–78.

Chapter 43 | What is the role of the ECG in the hypothermic patient?

Raed Wahab[1], Clay A. Cauthen[1], Daniel Grinnan[2]
[1]University of Virginia, Charlottesville, VA, USA
[2]Virginia Commonwealth University, Richmond, VA, USA

Case presentations

Case 1: A 72-year-old homeless male with an unknown past medical history is found altered outside a local food shelter during a winter month. The patient is intubated in the field due to lack of airway protection. In the emergency department (ED), the patient's physical exam is notable for an irregularly slow rhythm and core body temperature (CBT) was 28 °C. The patient is otherwise hemodynamically stable. During rewarming, the ECG recorded a slow rhythm with a rate of 40–45 beats per minute (bpm) and first-degree heart block with diminished P waves. Additionally, J waves are also observed on the 12-lead electrocardiogram (ECG) (Figure 43.1a). The patient is transferred to the intensive care unit (ICU) and actively warmed to the goal CBT of 32 °C that resulted in the restoration of sinus rhythm with a rate in the 80s and loss of the J wave deflection (Figure 43.1b).

Case 2: A 41-year-old male is brought into the ED after emergency medical services (EMS) was activated for respiratory distress. His initial ECG had findings consistent with a right bundle branch block and right axis deviation (Figure 43.2a). Lower extremity doppler examination shows left common femoral vein thrombus bolstering the pretest diagnosis of pulmonary embolism. After two witnessed arrests in the ED, a protocol aiming for intentional mild hypothermia is initiated. Anti-coagulation, volume resuscitation and mechanical ventilation along with hypothermia are continued in the ICU. Electrocardiograms obtained at a CBT of 32.5 °C show interval resolution of right axis and right bundle patterns and new J waves in anterolateral precordial and inferior leads (Figure 43.2b). The QT duration is increased from 370 to 428 ms. Intermittent wide complex arrhythmia is noted by bedside staff and a separate 12-lead ECG captures a run of this wide complex rhythm. The cooling protocol is abandoned, and, with passive warming, there is resolution of

J waves and return to a normal sinus rhythm with a normal QT interval duration (Figure 43.2c).

Case 3: A 49-year-old female is hospitalized for community-acquired pneumonia. She is admitted to the ICU after a cardiopulmonary arrest, with the predominant rhythm being pulseless electrical activity. She is quickly resuscitated to an organized sinus tachycardia, and, following the arrest, a mild hypothermia protocol is instituted. Her temperature erroneously overshoots to a CBT of 30.8 °C. Her troponin I returns elevated and her second of serial ECG evaluations shows J waves in inferior and anterolateral precordial leads and new ST segment elevations in V4–V6 (Figure 43.3). Anti-coagulation is initiated, and cardiac catheterization is contemplated. After the patient's temperature returns to 34.3 °C, ST segment elevation is less prominent with J waves still appreciated.

The role of the ECG in the hypothermic patient

These three patients have electrocardiographic evidence of hypothermia. For the intensivist, what is the role of identification and monitoring of these findings?

Hypothermia is defined as a CBT less than 35 °C (95 °F) and is classified as either accidental (also known as primary) or secondary to an underlying condition or intervention. Hypothermia is graded as mild (35–32 °C), moderate (32–28 °C) and severe (< 28 °C) [1]. Jolly and Ghezzi suggest that 3.5% of the elderly males hospitalized present with hypothermia [2]. Accidental hypothermia is associated with a high mortality and typically affects the extremes of ages during the winter months [3]. Additional risk factors include mental retardation, unattended children, cold-water exposure and being under the influence of a substance of abuse (most notably alcohol). Intentional hypothermia has become more commonplace as a therapeutic modality for in-house and out-of-hospital cardiac arrest, as the neurologic benefits have been rediscovered over the last decade [4]. Table 43.1 provides a more complete list of causes and contributors to accidental and secondary hypothermia.

Critical Decisions in Emergency and Acute Care Electrocardiography, 1st edition. Edited by W.J. Brady and J.D. Truwit. © 2009 Blackwell Publishing. ISBN: 9781405159067

(a)

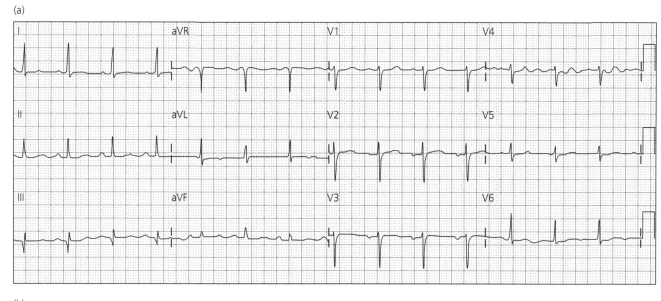

(b)

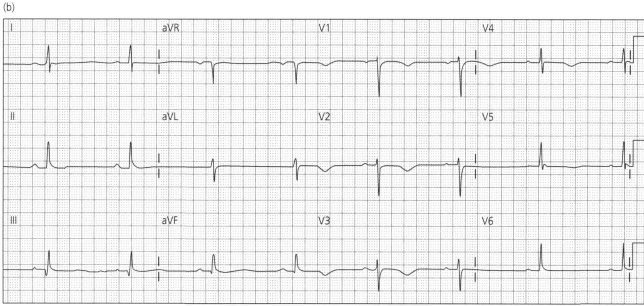

Figure 43.1 (a) ECG during active warming from a core body temperature of 28 °C. It shows sinus bradycardia at a rate of 45 bpm and first-degree heart block. (b) After rewarming, ECG shows normal sinus rhythm at 85 bpm with normal intervals.

Hypothermia has been shown to induce morphologic, interval, conduction, and rhythm abnormalities present on the ECG that are predictable by the grade of severity [5]. Electrocardiogram abnormalities in hypothermia were first observed at the end of the nineteenth century by Bayliss and Starling [6], and later were systematically described by Osborn in animal studies that correlated characteristic ECG abnormalities and core body temperature (CBT) cooling [7]. The classic ECG changes associated with hypothermia include atrial dysrhythmias and prolongations of the PR, QRS, and QT intervals, as well as the presence of J waves [8,9]. While

first formally described by Tomasjewski in 1938 [10], the J wave carries the famous moniker, the "Osborn wave," based on the latter's extensive studies during the 1950s.

In addition, hypothermia has been associated with more ominous and lethal electrocardiographic abnormalities such as atrioventricular blocks, ventricular tachycardia, ventricular fibrillation, and asystole. We will discuss the wave morphologies, interval changes, and rhythm disturbances characteristic to hypothermia with emphasis on their diagnostic accuracy, and prognostic values at different grades of hypothermia.

(a)

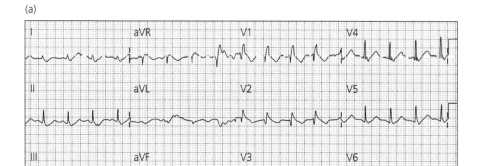

(b)

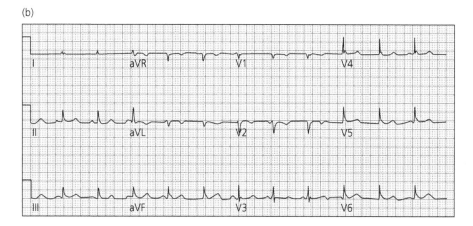

(c)

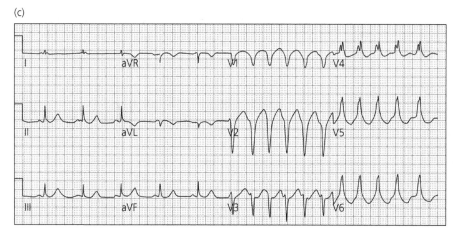

(d)

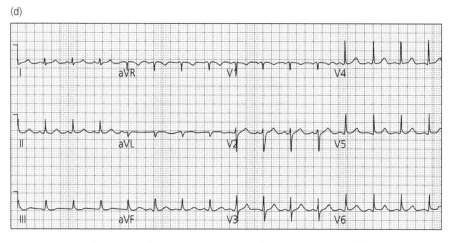

Figure 43.2 (a) Admission ECG with right bundle branch and sinus tachycardia. (b) After intentional hypothermia there is a reduction in rate and the initial presence of J waves in anterolateral precordial and inferior leads. (c) Prominent wide complex tachycardia is captured in the second half of this ECG tracing. J waves are still noted in inferior leads. (d) After passive rewarming, all rhythm and waveform abnormalities are resolved except for the subtle persistence of small J waves.

(a)

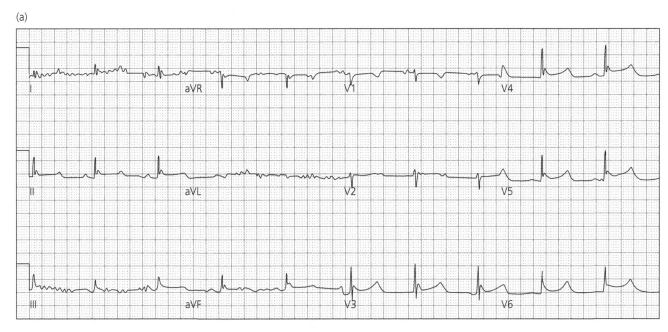

(b)

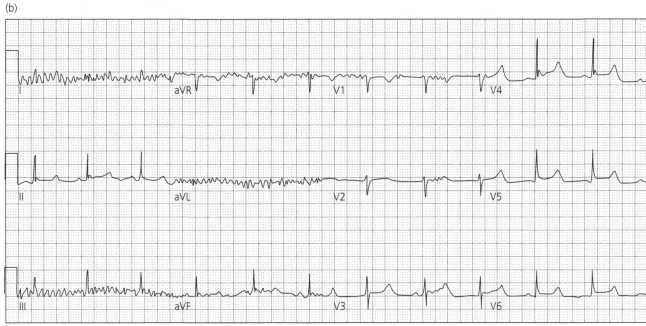

Figure 43.3 (a) During intentional hypothermia overshoot to a core body temperature (CBT) of 30.8 °C, ECG reveals prominent J waves in anterolateral precordial and inferior leads along with ST segment elevations in leads V4–V6. (b) When CBT is raised to above 34 °C, J waves have not entirely resolved and there is more prominent shiver artifact.

Electrocardiographic morphology of hypothermia

The earliest morphologic abnormality in patients with mild hypothermia is a tremor artifact due to the shiver response [11]. This is non-specific and becomes uncommon at CBT < 32 °C as the body's ability to generate a shiver response diminishes [7,9]. As CBT approaches moderate hypothermia, the appearance of the J waves (Osborn waves, camel hump sign, or J deflection) can be detected [12]. A J wave (Figures 43.1 and 43. 2) is characterized as an extra-deflection of the terminal junction of the QRS complex and the start of the ST segment. J waves are detected in up to 80% of patients presenting with moderate to severe hypothermia [8], and, in one study, were seen in 86% of presenting ECGs in patients with a CBT ≤ 30.5 °C [13].

J waves are more prominent in inferior and lateral precordial leads, and tend to appear more anteriorly as CBT continues to fall [14]. The onset of J waves was originally thought to

Table 43.1 Causes and contributors to hypothermia

Mechanism	Diseases
Heat loss	Environment
	Vasodilated state
	Sepsis
	Decompensated cirrhosis
	Drugs and alcohol
	Skin abnormalities
	Psoriasis
	Toxic shock syndrome
	Toxic epidermal necrolysis
	Iatrogenic
	Cold saline
	Massive bleeding resuscitation
	Neuromuscular blockade
	Postoperative
Decreased heat production	Endocrinopathy
	Hypothyroid
	Adrenal failure
	Hypopituitarism
	Metabolic disarray
	Malnutrition
	Starvation
	Hypoglycemia
	Advanced age and inactivity
Altered thermoregulation	Drugs
	Alcohol
	Barbiturates
	Tricylic anti-depressants
	Stroke
	Trauma
	Degenerative neurologic state
	Parkinson's disease
	Multiple sclerosis
	Anorexia nervosa
Miscellaneous	Sepsis
	Uremia
	Pancreatitis

Adapted from Chapter 110 of reference [1].

herald ventricular fibrillation and the prominence of the deflection to be of prognostic value [7], but subsequent studies have demonstrated that there is no correlation between the onset or prominence of the deflection with ventricular fibrillation or prognosis, respectively [15]. Furthermore, unlike early reports, J waves appear to have no relationship to pH, sodium, potassium, or chloride concentrations [16]. It is believed that J waves result from the prominent action potential notch of the epicardium that generates a voltage gradient as the intrathoracic temperature decreases [17].

J waves can be considered highly suggestive of hypothermia, but are not considered to be pathognomonic. J waves have also been described in a variety of other clinical settings, such as hypercalcemia, central nervous system

events, myocardial ischemia, post cardiac arrest, Brugada's disease, sepsis, and with certain drugs [9,18–20]. While J waves most often resolve with return to normothermia, they have been reported to persist as in Case 3 [13].

Other ECG morphologic abnormalities are more concerning for coronary infarct and ischemia, such as ST elevation, ST depression, and T wave inversion [21,22]. As these are case-reportable entities, they should still prompt immediate investigation for an acute coronary syndrome. It has also been suggested that T wave inversions associated with hypothermia can veil competing ECG evidence of cardiac irritability associated with hyperkalemia [22].

Interval prolongation has been well documented in animal and human studies. The cooling heart demonstrates a dramatic decrease in the ability to spread electrical potentials, or excitation, resulting in the prolongation of PR, QRS, and QTc intervals. These findings are noted in each of the three cases above. The interval prolongations appear to be a function of temperature [15]. The clinical significance is still unclear, and some authors suggest lethal arrythmias in hypothermic patients with prolonged QRS and QT intervals are secondary to concomitant metabolic processes [5]. However, QTc prolongation in hypothermia has been reported to precipitate torsade de pointes in the absence of secondary contributors [23].

Sinus rhythm predominates mild hypothermia [13], whereas atrial dysrhythmias are more common in moderate and severe hypothermia. With moderate hypothermia, sinus rhythm is slowed and atrial activity becomes increasingly disorganized [9]. Slowing of the sinus rate occurs in a non-linear, inverse relationship to temperature [24]. The resultant bradycardia is likely due to decreased depolarization of the atrial pacemaker cells, and is thought to be refractory to atropine stimulation [11]. As the atrial activity becomes increasingly disorganized, the risk for atrial dysrhythmias with slow ventricular responses increases. The risk of developing a supraventricular tachycardia (SVT) is more common with a CBT < 30 °C. Case series and prospective studies of accidental hypothermia observed that the most common SVT was atrial fibrillation, which was found to be absent in mild hypothermia, common in patients with moderate hypothermia, and occurred in 50% of patients with severe hypothermia [13,14]. As the majority of reported cases with hypothermia associated atrial dysrhythmias resolved with rewarming, it is felt that these rhythms are transient and benign, not associated with more lethal dysrhythmias, and do not warrant anti-arrhythmic treatment in the absence of hemodynamic destabilization [3,13,14].

In severe hypothermia, the risk of terminal arrythmias increases. When CBT < 25 °C, asystole is the predominant terminal arrhythmia [22]. Even though atrioventricular blocks, ventricular tachycardia (VT), and ventricular fibrillation (VF) are of concern in patients with hypothermia, the incidence and association with hypothermia has been less consistently described in the literature. As the mechanism and direct association of VF in patients with severe hypothermia has yet to be fully elucidated, it may still be the terminal complication in patients with severe hypothermia. However, compelling evidence supports that VT and VF associated with hypothermia are precipitated by secondary causes including metabolic disarray, alkalosis, acidosis, or hypocapnia [5].

The hypothermic patient is a challenge to the intensivist. The ECG provides diagnostic value by demonstrating temperature-specific morphologic abnormalities such as the tremor artifact in mild hypothermia and J waves in moderate and severe hypothermia, as well as providing temperature-specific rhythm and rate abnormalities such as sinus bradycardia in mild hypothermia and slow supraventricular rhythms in moderate hypothermia and SVT in severe hypothermia. The direct association with lethal ventricular rhythms is not clear but is associated with hypothermia and its precipitating conditions.

Case conclusions

In the first case, the patient with severe accidental hypothermia experienced sinus bradycardia with prolonged intervals without progression to a more serious arrhythmia or arrest. Prompt restoration of normothermia resulted in restoration of hemodynamic and electrocardiographic stability. Unfortunately, intentional mild hypothermia in Case 2 was associated with a wide complex arrhythmia. The patients underlying acute thromboembolic insult likely contributed significantly to myocardial irritability. Unfortunately, after 3 days of no neurologic progress and development of a severe aspiration pneumonia, the patient's care was transitioned to comfort only. In the last case, ECG suspicion of myocardial injury as a cause of the arrest was attenuated as troponin levels plateaued at a mild increased level and ECG abnormalities resolved after cooling was finished. Subsequent cardiology work-up after resolution of her critical illness included a normal nuclear stress test.

While the intensivist never diagnoses hypothermia from an ECG alone, it remains an important adjunct to critical care. Attention to pharmacologic therapies that may interact with consequent prolonged QT intervals should be noted to avoid torsade de pointes as a complication. Furthermore, significant bradyarrhythmias rarely respond to atropine administration and most stable arrhythmias respond to passive rewarming alone. Finally, hypothermic effects on the ECG may confound clinical discernment of hyperkalemia and acute coronary syndromes.

References

1 Hall JB, Schmidt GA, Wood LDH. *Principles of Critical Care.* 3rd ed. New York: McGraw-Hill, 2005; xxvii, 1778 pp.

2 Jolly BT, Ghezzi KT. Accidental hypothermia. *Emerg Med Clin North Am* 1992;**10**(2):311–27.

3 Rankin AC, Rae AP. Cardiac arrhythmias during rewarming of patients with accidental hypothermia. *Br Med J (Clin Res Ed)* 1984;**289**(6449):874–7.

4 Alzaga AG, Cerdan M, Varon J. Therapeutic hypothermia. *Resuscitation* 2006;**70**(3):369–80.

5 Aslam AF, *et al.* Hypothermia: evaluation, electrocardiographic manifestations, and management. *Am J Med* 2006;**119**(4):297–301.

6 Bayliss WM, Starling EH. On some points in the innervation of the mammalian heart. *J Physiol* 1892;**13**(5):407–418.

7 Osborn JJ. Experimental hypothermia; respiratory and blood pH changes in relation to cardiac function. *Am J Physiol* 1953;**175**(3):389–98.

8 Mustafa S, *et al.* Electrocardiographic features of hypothermia. *Cardiology* 2005;**103**(3):118–9.

9 Slovis C, Jenkins R. ABC of clinical electrocardiography: Conditions not primarily affecting the heart. *BMJ* 2002;**324**(7349):1320–3.

10 Tomasjewski W. Changements electrographique observes chez un homme mort de froid. *Arch Mal Coeur* 1938;**31**:525–8.

11 Mallet ML. Pathophysiology of accidental hypothermia. *QJM* 2002;**95**(12):775–85.

12 Gussak I, *et al.* ECG phenomenon called the J wave. History, pathophysiology, and clinical significance. *J Electrocardiol* 1995;**28**(1):49–58.

13 Vassallo SU, Delaney KA, Hoffman RS, *et al.* A prospective evaluation of the electrocardiographic manifestations of hypothermia. *Acad Emerg Med* 1999;**6**(11):1121–6.

14 Okada M. The cardiac rhythm in accidental hypothermia. *J Electrocardiol* 1984;**17**(2):123–8.

15 Gould L, Reddy CV. Effect of cold isotonic glucose infusion on A-V nodal conduction. *J Electrocardiol* 1976;**9**(1):23–8.

16 Schwab RH, Lewis DW, Killough JH, *et al.* Electrocardiographic changes occurring in rapidly induced deep hypothermia. *Am J Med Sci* 1964;**248**:290–303.

17 Yan GX, Antzelevitch C. Cellular basis for the electrocardiographic J wave. *Circulation* 1996;**93**(2):372–9.

18 Cardenas GA, Ventura HO, Francis JE. Osborn waves in sepsis. *South Med J* 2006;**99**(11):1302–3.

19 Jain U, Wallis DE, Shah K, *et al.* Electrocardiographic J waves after resuscitation from cardiac arrest. *Chest* 1990;**98**(5):1294–6.

20 Salerno D, Vahid B, Marik PE. Osborn wave in hypothermia from Vibrio vunificus sepsis unrelated to exposure. *Int J Cardiol* 2007;**114**(3):e124–5.

21 Glusman A, Hasan K, Roguin, N. Contraindication to thrombolytic therapy in accidental hypothermia simulating acute myocardial infarction. *Int J Cardiol* 1990;**28**(2):269–72.

22 Mattu A, Brady WJ, Perron AD. Electrocardiographic manifestations of hypothermia. *Am J Emerg Med* 2002;**20**(4):314–26.

23 Huang CH, Tsai MS, Hsu CY, *et al.* Images in cardiovascular medicine. Therapeutic hypothermia-related torsade de pointes. *Circulation* 2006;**114**(14):e521–2.

24 Kossmann CE. General cryotherapy: cardiovascular aspects. *Bull N Y Acad Med* 1940;**16**:317.

Chapter 44 | What are the non-ACS "deadly" ECG presentations?

Adam Helms, Clay A. Cauthen, Ajeet Vinayak
University of Virginia, Charlottesville, VA, USA

Case presentations

Case 1: A 44-year-old female presents to the emergency department (ED) with worsening dyspnea over the prior 4 days. On the day of admission, she described feeling lightheaded with standing and has had severe fatigue. She has had no chest discomfort or palpitations. In the ED, she becomes progressively more hypotensive, despite 3 L of intravenous fluids, and pressors are started. She is admitted to the intensive care unit (ICU). On exam, she is alert and oriented with a blood pressure of 85/50 on 10 mcg/kg/min of dopamine. Her heart is quiet but with no murmurs, rubs, or gallops, and her lungs are clear to auscultation. Her radial pulse is noted to decrease with inspiration, corresponding with a pulsus paradoxus of 15 mmHg. Her electrocardiogram (ECG) (Figure 44.1) shows diffuse low voltages and varying amplitudes of the QRS waveforms. An echocardiogram reveals a large pericardial fluid collection and features of tamponade.

Case 2: A 35-year-old man is monitored in the ICU following thrombolytic therapy for an acute hemodynamically unstable pulmonary embolism (PE). His medical condition stabilizes over a period of 6 h following thrombolysis, and he is weaned from vasoactive drugs. Suddenly, he loses consciousness. In the evaluation, an ECG is performed (Figure 44.2), which shows anterior ST segment elevations. These findings were transient. A computed tomography (CT) scan of the brain reveals a large subarachnoid hemorrhage.

Case 3: A 42-year-old female is brought to the ED. She has been experiencing worsened fatigue over the past 3 months. For 1 week, she has also complained of worsening shortness of breath. Her primary care physician was worried about the

possibility of PE, and a CT pulmonary angiogram was done the day prior to admission. Over the 24 h following the CT scan, which was negative for PE, she became increasingly short of breath and agitated. In the ED, she is found to be hypotensive with a blood pressure of 82/40 and febrile with a temperature of 39 °C. An ECG shows sinus tachycardia with a rate of 120. On exam, she is agitated and mildly confused; her lungs are notable for bilateral crackles halfway up her lung fields; cardiac auscultation reveals a 2/6 early peaking systolic murmur at the left upper sternal border; and her jugular venous pulse is elevated to 12 cm water. She is admitted to the ICU where she is fluid-resuscitated, but continues to exhibit hypotension. A dopamine infusion is started, and shortly thereafter her heart rate increases to 150 beats per minute (bpm) and the ECG is repeated (Figure 44.3). Laboratory evaluation reveals an undetectable thyroid-stimulating hormone.

Case 4: A 68-year-old male arrives at the ED with sharp substernal pain for the last 3 h. While he denies any known coronary disease, his risk factors include hypertension and a significant smoking history. On examination, his blood pressure is 95/63 in his right arm, and his heart rate is 125 bpm. His ECG reveals ST segment elevation in leads II, III, and aVF (Figure 44.4). A chest x-ray is unremarkable. However, based on the clinical presentation, a CT angiogram of the chest is obtained rather than proceeding to thrombolysis. A large ascending aortic aneurysm dissection is revealed.

Characteristic non-ACS deadly presentations

These four cases illustrate catastrophic diagnoses that lead to the requirement of critical care. Characteristic ECG findings are present in each case. What are the non-acute coronary syndrome (ACS) deadly ECG presentations?

While the most common use of the ECG in the acute care setting remains the identification of an ACS, several other acute disease states are associated with high immediate

Critical Decisions in Emergency and Acute Care Electrocardiography, 1st edition. Edited by W.J. Brady and J.D. Truwit. © 2009 Blackwell Publishing, ISBN: 9781405159067

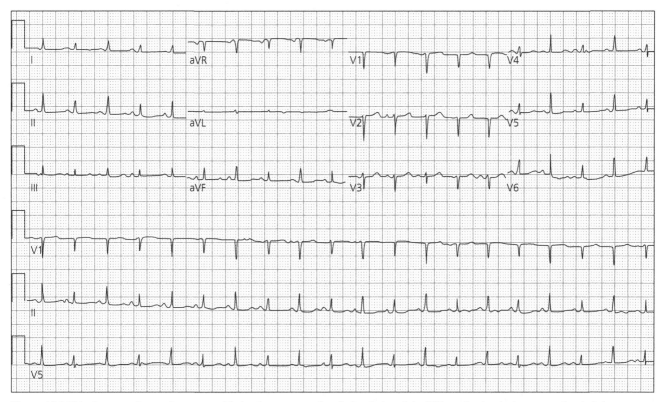

Figure 44.1 This electrocardiogram is most notable for the presence of cyclical variation of the QRS amplitude, also known as electrical alternans. This finding suggests cardiac tamponade.

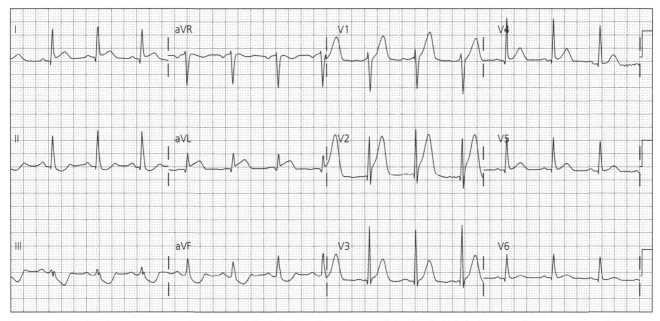

Figure 44.2 ST elevation occurred acutely after onset of sudden loss of mental status following fibrinolytic therapy. Tall T waves are noted. The patient's heart rate remained in the low 80s and blood pressure was significantly elevated.

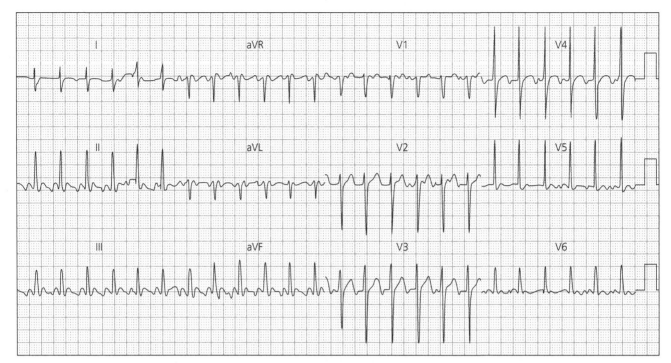

Figure 44.3 Atrial flutter is present with a characteristic ventricular rate of approximately 150, corresponding to an atrial rate of near 300 with a 2 : 1 atrial-to-ventricular conduction. While sometimes difficult to appreciate atrial flutter when 2 : 1 conduction is present, in this case, negative saw-tooth atrial waveforms are appreciated in the inferior leads.

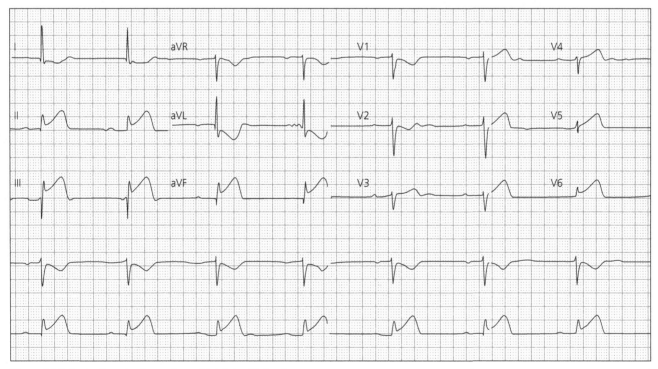

Figure 44.4 Aortic dissection in a patient with inferior ST elevations.

mortality. In this chapter, we characterize ECGs associated with several of these processes.

Cardiac tamponade and pericardial disease

Case 1, above, describes a patient presenting with cardiac tamponade. Patients with tamponade often present with subtle signs, making the diagnosis elusive in some cases. The most important symptom is dyspnea, though non-specific signs such as fatigue may also be present [1]. Some patients may have chest pain if an underlying pericarditis is present. The cardiac examination characteristically reveals distant heart sounds, and a pericardial rub may or may not be appreciated. A pulsus paradoxus should be present in most cases, and, thus, the pulsus should be measured in any patient with unexplained hypotension. The ECG, while not a sensitive test for tamponade, may provide important clues for the diagnosis. The most common sign present on the ECG in cardiac tamponade is sinus tachycardia, though tachycardia may not be present when the pericardial effusion is due to uremia or hypothyroidism [1]. The more specific signs on ECG are low QRS voltage, electrical alternans, and findings of underlying pericarditis.

Low QRS voltage and electrical alternans are only present when the pericardial effusion causing tamponade is moderate to large. Most etiologies of tamponade fall into this category. In the acute setting the volume may be moderate, defined as a volume of 300–600 ml [1]. The important exception is hemorrhagic pleural effusions, which develop rapidly and may cause tamponade despite a small effusion size. Low QRS voltage is defined as less than 5 mm of QRS amplitude in the limb leads or less than 10 mm in the precordial leads. The sensitivity of low QRS voltage is approximately 42% based on a recent metanalysis (see Table 44.1), making it a more sensitive finding than electrical alternans [2]. However, the specificity of low QRS voltage is lower as the differential diagnosis of low voltage is broad, including conditions

such as left ventricular dysfunction, increased chest wall size, emphysema, and hypothyroidism.

Electrical alternans, as seen in Figure 44.1, is defined as waveforms on the ECG that are alternately of smaller voltage and reversed polarity. The mechanism of electrical alternans is swinging of the heart within the pericardial sack. While any of the ECG waveforms may be affected, the involvement of both the QRS and P waveforms is most specific [3]. The most common finding is alternation of the voltage and polarity of the QRS complex alone. The specificity of this ECG finding for the presence of tamponade is high, but the sensitivity is limited to 16–21% (see Table 44.1) [2].

When pericardial inflammation is present, ECG findings of pericarditis may also be present. These findings include ST segment elevations, found in 30% of patients with tamponade, and PR segment depressions, found in 18% of patients [4,5]. When tamponade progresses, pulseless electrical activity may develop, in which electrical activity is observed on the ECG in the absence of blood pressure. At this point, death is imminent without emergent drainage.

Pericardial and myocardial disease: The most common pericardial disease is pericarditis, defined as inflammation of the pericardium in association with infections, connective tissue disorders, metabolic abnormalities, trauma, neoplasms, or iatrogenic causes [6]. Pericarditis may be associated with pericardial effusions and myocarditis, and can be categorized as acute or chronic. The hallmark symptom of pericarditis is the abrupt onset of pleuritic chest pain, which often radiates to the back and is often alleviated by sitting upright and leaning forward. Clinical signs include a pericardial friction rub that is best heard during exhalation and distant heart sounds if the pericarditis is also associated with a pericardial effusion [6].

Characteristic ECG manifestations of acute pericarditis are observed more commonly than physical exam findings. Diffuse ST segment elevations in both the limb and precordial leads signifies extensive ventricular involvement, distinguished from myocardial infarction (MI) by the involvement of more

Table 44.1 Sensitivity of the electrocardiogram in the diagnosis of cardiac tamponade

	Reddy et al., 1978 [43] (n = 19)	Guberman et al., 1981 [4] (n = 53)*	Singh et al., 1984 [44] (n = 16)	Levine et al., 1991 [5] (n = 50)	Cooper et al., 1995 [45] (n = 23)	Gibbs et al., 2000 [46] (n = 46)*	Pooled sensitivity (95% CI)
Low voltage	NA	40	50	56	22	39	42 (32–53)
Atrial arrhythmia	0	9	NA	4	NA	NA	6 (1–11)
Electrical alternans	NA	21	NA	16	NA	NA	NA
ST segment elevation	NA	30	18		NA	NA	NA
PR segment depression	NA	NA	NA	18	NA	NA	NA

*Not all patients had documentation of clinical findings.

CI, confidence interval.

Table developed from *JAMA*, 2007;**297**:1810–18. Copyright © 2007.

than one vascular domain, while PR segment depression (or elevation in aVR) reflects an atrial injury current [7]. Characteristic ECG patterns tend to change over time reflecting the evolution of the disease process.

The first phase of ECG changes with pericarditis is ST segment elevation that results from diffuse pericardial inflammation involving the contiguous subepicardial ventricular walls. This finding is seen in up to 90% of cases of proven pericarditis [8]. The most common ECG pattern is ST elevations in leads I, II, V5, and V6, and this pattern can be seen in up to 70% of patients. With more diffuse involvement, additional ST elevations include III, aVL, aVF, V3, and V4. The ST segment elevations observed in pericarditis are rarely greater than 5 mm, while acute infarctions *may* exceed this threshold. In addition to the pattern of ST elevation in different leads, the morphology of the ST elevation is also important. The ST elevation most frequently involves elevation of the J point (junction of where the QRS complex ends and ST segment begins) with a concave elevation of the ST segment. These changes are important to recognize when determining if ECG findings are more consistent with pericarditis or an acute infarction.

A few important exceptions to the above generalizations are notable. First, pericarditis occasionally involves only a small region (i.e. focal pericarditis), and the ECG patterns may localize to this region, resembling an infarction [7]. Second, the intrinsic axis of the heart may be tilted, in which case comparisons of amplitude of ST elevations in leads II and III may be inaccurate. Last, early in acute MI the J point frequently elevates associated with a concave elevation in the ST segment, appearing similar to pericarditis. The history (i.e. the time of pain onset) is helpful in these cases to distinguish whether the pattern is more likely to represent an acute infarction or pericarditis. In any case, if the correlation of clinical presentation and ECG are not clear, an echocardiogram or cardiac catheterization should be performed to solidify the diagnosis.

PR depression is common to pericarditis but is not specific as it is seen with both atrial infarction and early repolarization [7]. As in determining ST segment changes, PR depression is determined by comparison with the TP segment, which may be difficult to assess in the presence of tachycardia or pronounced ST segment elevation [9]. PR segment depressions may be seen in all leads but are most commonly identified in leads II, aVR, aVF, and V4–V6. Interestingly, PR segment elevation can be seen in aVR as well.

The next phase of ECG changes that occurs with evolution of pericarditis is T wave alteration [9]. Biphasic, notched, and inverted T waves are characteristic [9]. Importantly, the T wave inversions do not occur in the early phase of ST elevation, such that if concurrent TW inversion and ST elevation are observed, acute MI should be suspected. Supraventricular dysrhythmias have also been associated with pericarditis, but, in general, dysrhythmias are uncommon in pericarditis. Advanced atrioventricular (AV) or intraventricular conduction blocks, as well as ventricular arrhythmias, should alert the intensivist to the advancement of inflammation into the myocardium or to another disease process [9].

Myocarditis is defined as inflammation of the myocardium and is most commonly due to infection [10]. The clinical spectrum includes asymptomatic, self-limited disease, subacute heart failure, dysrhythmias (sometimes associated with sudden death), and acute fulminant heart failure [9]. Electrocardiogram abnormalities commonly manifest as diffusely inverted T waves without ST segment changes. However, as myocarditis and pericarditis can occur as a part of the same disease process, diffuse ST elevations may occur [7]. Pathologic Q waves have been described and may represent the development of fulminant disease [9].

Transient conduction abnormalities are also associated with myocarditis, as demonstrated by ECG abnormalities such as incomplete AV block and intraventricular conduction blocks. Conduction abnormalities are typically short-lived and rarely present as a complete AV block [9].

Acute neurologic conditions

Case 2 above demonstrates the marked ECG changes that may occur with an acute neurologic event, such as intracranial hemorrhage or ischemic stroke. One must be aware of this possibility to avoid confusion with acute MI, as the initial urgent management of these two conditions is clearly very different. However, the ECG interpretation is complicated by several factors. First, the patient presenting with an embolic stroke may have underlying cardiac disease and correspondingly have an abnormal ECG at baseline. In addition, patients at risk for stroke due to atherosclerosis or hypertension are likewise at risk of cardiac disease, and they may have ECG changes due to underlying cardiac disease rather than from the acute neurologic event. Last, an abnormal ECG in the presence of a neurologic event does not rule out that the patient may also be suffering from an acute MI – myocardial and cerebral infarction may be co-incident in some cases, and the MI may be otherwise clinically silent [11]. Thus, considerable caution should be exercised before ascribing ECG changes completely to the neurologic event. Yet, at the same time, caution should also be exercised prior to treating ECG changes as ischemic cardiac events with anticoagulants and anti-anginal medications, which may cause hemorrhagic conversion of an ischemic stroke, worsen existing hemorrhage, or decrease cerebral perfusion pressure.

The pathophysiology and importance of ECG changes in the presence of an acute neurologic event are still topics of debate. Sympathetic dysregulation has been thought to play a role in cardiac injury as (1) patients with ECG changes have higher catecholamine levels, (2) reversal of ECG changes occurs with propranolol administration, and (3) the severity of ECG changes correlates with the level of catecholamine secretion [12,13]. The effect of an increased sympathetic response is cardiac myocyte damage with resultant alteration of cardiac repolarization and arrhythmogenesis [14]. Coronary vasospasm may also be induced by this process, resulting in true ischemia. Several studies indicate that strokes involving the insular cortex, particularly the right insular cortex, are most likely to result in reflex cardiac injury with ECG changes [14–16]. As a sign of myocardial injury, 10–20% of patients with acute ischemic stroke have troponin elevations, which may correlate with epinephrine levels and ischemic ECG changes [17,18].

Electrocardiogram findings of intracranial hemorrhage or stroke include QT interval prolongation, T wave inversions, U waves, ST segment elevations or depressions, and dysrhythmias. When only new ECG changes are taken into account compared with a baseline ECG, QT interval prolongation is the most common finding (32%), followed by T wave inversion (15%), ST depression (13%), and U waves (13%) [19]. ST elevations are much less common. The classic finding of combined QT prolongation, T wave inversion, and a U wave (see Figure 44.5) is present only in a minority of patients (8%), but is very specific for acute stroke. The T wave inversions that occur with a neurologic event are classically deep and asymmetric. The presence of these ECG changes is more likely in those who have had a subarachnoid or intracerebral hemorrhage compared with those who have had an ischemic stroke, and also is more likely in those who present with moderate to severe hypertension [19]. Dysrhythmias may also occur and include bradyarrhythmias, atrial fibrillation, and ventricular tachycardia.

Thyrotoxicosis

Case 3 exhibits a case of thyroid storm complicated by atrial flutter and cardiovascular compromise. Thyroid storm is a severe form of thyrotoxicosis, and it is diagnosed based on clinical factors, including agitation, confusion, fever, congestive heart failure, new-onset atrial arrhythmia, sinus tachycardia, and gastrointestinal (GI) dysfunction [20]. While only 1–2% of patients admitted to the hospital with a diagnosis of thyrotoxicosis have true thyroid storm, rapid identification

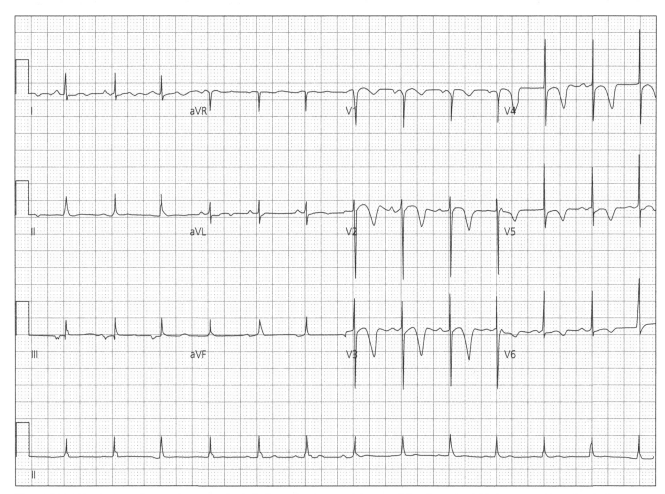

Figure 44.5 This electrocardiogram shows the classic findings of an intracranial event – QT prolongation with deep T wave inversions in the precordial leads. A subtle U wave is appreciated at the end of the T wave in the precordial leads.

is crucial, as thyroid storm carries a high mortality rate of 20–30% if left untreated [21]. A precipitant, such as acute illness, infection, or iodine load, is usually present. In Case 3, the patient had smoldering thyrotoxicosis for months that was acutely worsened when she received iodinated contrast for the CT pulmonary angiogram study.

Thyroid hormone has many effects on the cardiovascular system, including decreased systemic vascular resistance, increased heart rate, increased contractility, and increased cardiac output [22]. In otherwise healthy individuals, hyperthyroidism is typically well tolerated; however, some patients with severe, longstanding hyperthyroidism will develop congestive heart failure with a low cardiac output. Patients with pre-existing hypertensive or ischemic heart disease are more likely to have a clinical course complicated by congestive heart failure [22]. In addition, some patients with no underlying cardiac disease may develop congestive heart failure from thyrotoxicosis, as suggested by several case reports [23]. The pathophysiology of cardiomyopathy in these cases is unclear.

The ECG is an important clue to the presence of thyrotoxicosis and thyroid storm. The presence of sinus tachycardia alone should trigger a consideration of hyperthyroidism, as sinus tachycardia is frequently present in thyrotoxicosis [20]. Moreover, atrial tachydysrhythmias have a particularly strong correlation with thyrotoxicosis, most commonly atrial fibrillation, which has an incidence of 5–15% in these patients. Because thyroid storm is an uncommon problem, and because the symptoms (fever, dyspnea, GI complaints and confusion) are non-specific, the finding of an atrial tachydysrhythmia on initial evaluation should prompt immediate thyroid function testing as rapid diagnosis and management are imperative.

Other endocrinopathies

Other endocrinopathies may also have associated ECG changes, as discussed earlier in this section. However, the only other endocrinopathy clearly associated with ECG that can potentially be lethal is hypothyroidism. In its most severe form, hypothyroidism leads to myxedema coma, which is a true medical emergency. Myxedema coma is rare, can be difficult to diagnose, and is associated with a mortality of 60–70% if not aggressively treated [21]. Therefore, in addition to the clinical signs of hypotension, hypothermia, intestinal hypomotility, and slowed mentation, the ECG may provide valuable clues. The key changes on ECG are bradycardia, decreased voltage, and flat or inverted T waves; less common changes include bundle branch block, AV block and QT prolongation [24]. Bradycardia is the most common finding. Decreased QRS voltage is likely due to a combination of both the hypocontractile effects of thyroid hormone deficiency and the dampening effects of pericardial effusion [25,26]. Pericardial effusion is present in 30% of untreated

patients, but only rarely progresses to cardiac tamponade [27,28]. In cases of tamponade, a paradoxic tachycardia may actually be present [29].

Aortic aneurysm dissection

Dissection of the thoracic aorta may cause chest pain and hemodynamic instability. When not directly associated with trauma, the relatively low frequency of this catastrophic event, can make correct diagnosis elusive. In one retrospective surveillance study, less than 50% of aortic aneurysm dissection (AAD) cases were suspected after initial emergency room evaluation [30]. The presence of classic back pain along with chest discomfort improved clinical acumen. Confounding diagnosis further, risk factors for aortic dissection, such as advanced age, hypertension, and male sex, are also risk factors for the much more common diagnosis of acute coronary syndrome. In younger patients, groups at risk include pregnant women and those with inherited conditions, such as Marfan's syndrome, Ehlers-Danlos syndrome or Turner's syndrome.

Aortic aneurysm dissections are most commonly classified as Stanford type A or B. Type A dissections involve the ascending aorta and have been associated with far more frequent ECG abnormalities than type B dissections, which affect only the descending thoracic aorta. The most common ECG abnormalities were patterns associated with left ventricular hypertrophy (LVH) and only a minority of patients had normal ECGs. The incidence of ST elevation is roughly 5% and occurs when a type A dissection extends proximally along the aortic root to one of the coronary artery ostia, directly causing myocardial ischemia [31]. The vast majority of these ST elevations occur in an inferior distribution because the location of the right coronary artery ostia is most commonly located in the path of an extending aortic intimal tear. However, involvement of a coronary ostium does not result in ST elevation in all cases [32].

As both AAD and patterns of ST elevation infrequently occur together, the overall incidence of erroneously administered thrombolysis is fortunately low. A large European survey reported that this error occurs in 0.33% of cases of thrombolytic administration for presumed MI [33]. Thrombolytic administration in AAD risks worsening hemodynamics by propagating intimal tear or causing cardiac tamponade.

While the ECG is limited in its diagnostic accuracy for AAD, patterns of LVH suggesting hypertension and the absence of ST segment elevation in patients with remarkable chest pain may provide clinicians with adjunctive clues. Identification of asymmetric blood pressure on exam and the co-existence of back and chest pain add clinical support for AAD. Yet, it requires high suspicion and awareness of these infrequent inferior MI patterns to avoid what could be the potentially catastrophic administration of thrombolysis in patients with AAD.

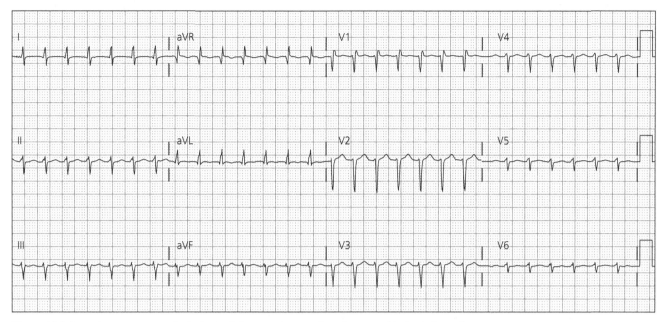

Figure 44.6 A regular, narrow complex tachycardia is present, suggestive of supraventricular tachycardia.

New-onset atrial tachydysrhythmias

New-onset atrial tachydysrhythmias (e.g. atrial fibrillation, atrial flutter, AV node re-entrant tachycardia, atrial tachycardia) may be the presenting feature of a potentially life-threatening non-cardiac illness in the ICU. In addition to treating the arrhythmia, the differential diagnosis of the precipitating event must be considered. Figure 44.6 shows a supraventricular tachycardia that was precipitated by a pulmonary embolism. The diagnosis was suspected after telemetry revealed a supraventricular tachycardia. Clinical suspicion led to definitive testing with CT pulmonary angiogram. Right axis deviation can be helpful in the diagnosis of PE but is often not present.

Probably the most common cause of a new atrial tachydysrhythmia in the ICU is sepsis. Evolving sepsis should be strongly considered when a patient suddenly develops tachycardia, and early goal-directed therapy should be aggressively pursued. Conditions other than sepsis that cause the systemic inflammatory response syndrome (SIRS) may also cause tachydysrhythmias, for example, pancreatitis. Other precipitants include thyrotoxicosis (as described previously), alcohol intoxication, hemorrhage, and congestive heart failure.

Pneumothorax in the ICU

While typically diagnosed radiographically or by clinical examination, pneumothorax can be a precipitous cause of clinical decline in the critically ill patient. Pneumothorax develops in 0.1–0.2% of internal jugular and 1.5–3.1% of subclavian central line placements, as well as in 1.3–6.7% of thoracenteses in mechanically ventilated patients [34–36].

Patients presenting with pneumothorax can display a variety of ECG patterns, ranging from decreased QRS amplitude to ST segment deviations that may be confused with myocardial ischemia or infarction. The ECG differs depending on the affected side. Left-sided pneumothoraces are more commonly associated with characteristic ECG changes, while right-sided pneumothoraces may have subtle ECG changes [37,38]. The classic ECG pattern of a left-sided pneumothorax consists of a decreased QRS amplitude, rightward shift of the frontal QRS axis, inverted precordial T waves, and decreased R wave progression [37,38]. All four findings occur in less than a third of cases, whereas two to three of the four ECG findings are present in most cases. This ECG pattern is frequently misdiagnosed as an anterior MI and, thus, can delay correct diagnosis.

Proposed mechanisms for the left-sided pneumothorax ECG pattern include cardiac rotation about the posteroanterior or longitudinal axis, and volume conduction abnormalities within the thoracic cavity generating an insulation of the heart. The majority of pneumothorax cases that present with ECG abnormalities demonstrate normalization of the ECG with resolution of the pneumothorax. In addition, laboratory and echocardiographic studies have indicated no signs of cardiac damage.

In addition to these classic ECG findings, isolated reports have demonstrated transient ST segment elevation and PR segment elevations in the inferior leads [39,40]. Similarly, one case report demonstrated reversible ST segment elevation in a patient with complete atelectasis of the left lung

(a)

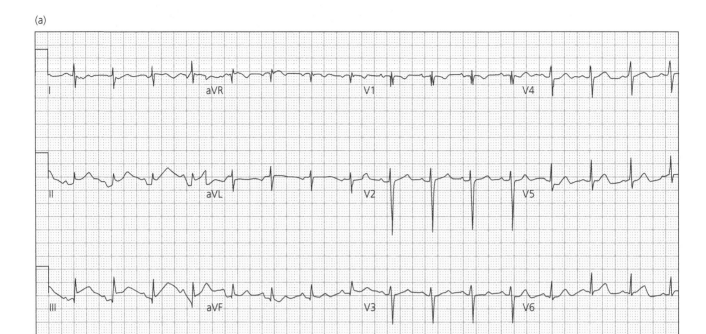

(b)

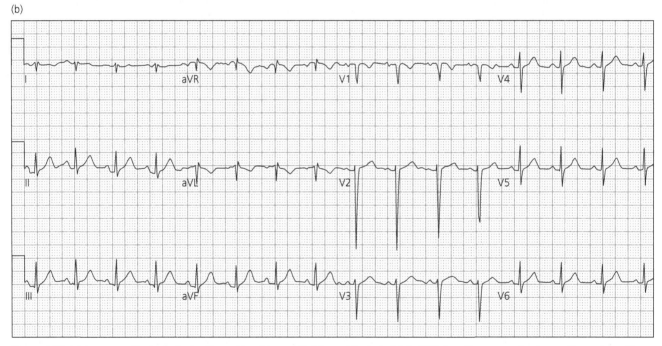

Figure 44.7 (a) A young patient who had radiographic evidence of left lung atelectasis. (b) An ECG from the same patient several hours later after reversal of atelectasis. There have been interval normalization prior findings correlating with radiographic resolution of atelectasis.

(Figure 44.7) [41]. While the ECG abnormalities associated with left-sided pneumothorax may be misinterpreted for an acute coronary event, nonetheless, the ECG may provide early diagnostic clues, in the correct clinical context, to the potentially life-threatening diagnosis of a pneumothorax.

Electrocardiogram findings occurring with right-sided pneumothoraces are more subtle and less specific. The most consistent finding is diminished QRS amplitude [38]. An isolated report describes the transient development of the $S_1Q_3T_3$ pattern that is more characteristically seen with PE [42]. As seen with a left-sided pneumothorax, the ECG may provide early diagnostic clues of right-sided pneumothorax in the correct clinical context. While the definitive diagnosis of pneumothorax rests on the clinical exam and chest radiography, awareness that pneumothorax may present with concerning ECG findings is important both to avoid confusion with other diagnoses and also to recognize potentially early clues that will lead to the correct diagnosis.

Case conclusions

While primary coronary events are the most frequent deadly acute presentation screened for routinely by ECG, other catastrophic events can lead to abnormal ECGs. Certain presentations are immediately discernible, as in Case 1, with characteristic findings of pericardial disease. Other presentations may mimic coronary syndromes and clinical clues such as a sudden change in mental status (Case 2) or a widened mediastinum on chest x-ray (Case 4) can assist in identifying alternative diagnoses. The presence of atrial tachycardia is frequent in the ICU and can herald a multitude of associated diagnoses. Given its accessibility and reliability, ECG may often be the first clue for one of these processes.

References

1 Spodick DH. Acute cardiac tamponade. *N Engl J Med* 2003; **349**:684–90.

2 Roy CL, Minor MA, Brookhart MA, Choudhry NK. Does this patient with a pericardial effusion have cardiac tamponade? *JAMA* 2007;**297**:1810–18.

3 Spodick D. Pericardial diseases. In: Braunwald E, Zipes DP, Libby P, editors. *Heart Disease: a Textbook of Cardiovascular Medicine.* 6th ed. Vol. 2. Philadelphia: W.B. Saunders, 2001: 1823–76.

4 Guberman BA, Fowler NO, Engel PJ, *et al.* Cardiac tamponade in medical patients. *Circulation* 1981;**64**:633–40.

5 Levine MJ, Lorell BH, Diver DJ, Come PC. Implications of echocardiographically assisted diagnosis of pericardial tamponade in contemporary medical patients: detection before hemodynamic embarrassment. *J Am Coll Cardiol* 1991;**17**:59–65.

6 Lange RA, Hillis LD. Clinical practice. Acute pericarditis. *N Engl J Med* 2004;**351**:2195–202.

7 Wang K, Asinger RW, Marriott HJ. ST-segment elevation in conditions other than acute myocardial infarction. *N Engl J Med* 2003;**349**:2128–35.

8 Surawicz B, Lasseter KC. Electrocardiogram in pericarditis. *Am J Cardiol* 1970;**26**:471–4.

9 Demangone D. ECG manifestations: noncoronary heart disease. *Emerg Med Clin North Am* 2006;**24**:113–31.

10 Feldman AM, McNamara D. Myocarditis. *N Engl J Med* 2000; **343**(19):1388–98.

11 Badui E, Estanol B, Garcia-Rubi D. Coincidence of cerebrovascular accident and silent myocardial infarction. *Angiology* 1982;**33**:702–9.

12 Cruickshank JM, Dwyer GN. Proceedings: Electrocardiographic changes in subarachnoid haemorrhage: role of catecholamines and effects of beta-blockade. *Br Heart J* 1974;**36**:395.

13 Feibel JH, Campbell RG, Joynt RJ. Myocardial damage and cardiac arrhythmias in cerebral infarction and subarachnoid hemorrhage: correlation with increased systemic catecholamine output. *Trans Am Neurol Assoc* 1976;**101**:242–4.

14 Oppenheimer SM. Neurogenic cardiac effects of cerebrovascular disease. *Curr Opin Neurol* 1994;**7**:20–4.

15 Christensen H, Boysen G, Christensen AF, Johannesen HH. Insular lesions, ECG abnormalities, and outcome in acute stroke. *J Neurol Neurosurg Psychiatry* 2005;**76**:269–71.

16 Abboud H, Berroir S, Labreuche J, *et al.* Insular involvement in brain infarction increases risk for cardiac arrhythmia and death. *Ann Neurol* 2006;**59**:691–9.

17 Jensen JK, Kristensen SR, Bak S, *et al.* Frequency and significance of troponin T elevation in acute ischemic stroke. *Am J Cardiol* 2007;**99**:108–12.

18 Barber M, Morton JJ, Macfarlane PW, *et al.* Elevated troponin levels are associated with sympathoadrenal activation in acute ischaemic stroke. *Cerebrovasc Dis* 2007;**23**:260–6.

19 Goldstein DS. The electrocardiogram in stroke: relationship to pathophysiological type and comparison with prior tracings. *Stroke* 1979;**10**:253–9.

20 Wartofsky L. *Thyrotoxic Storm.* Philadelphia, PA: Lippincott Williams & Wilkins, 2000.

21 Sarlis NJ, Gourgiotis L. Thyroid emergencies. *Rev Endocr Metab Disord* 2003;**4**:129–36.

22 Klein I, Ojamaa K. Thyroid hormone and the cardiovascular system. *N Engl J Med* 2001;**344**:501–9.

23 Ladenson PW. Recognition and management of cardiovascular disease related to thyroid dysfunction [see comment]. *Am J Med* 1990;**88**:638–41.

24 Slovis C, Jenkins R. ABC of clinical electrocardiography: Conditions not primarily affecting the heart. *BMJ* 2002;**324**:1320–3.

25 Fazio S, Biondi B, Lupoli G, *et al.* Evaluation, by noninvasive methods, of the effects of acute loss of thyroid hormones on the heart. *Angiology* 1992;**43**:287–93.

26 Tajiri J, Morita M, Higashi K, *et al.* The cause of low voltage QRS complex in primary hypothyroidism. Pericardial effusion or thyroid hormone deficiency? *Jpn Heart J* 1985;**26**:539–47.

27 Kerber RE, Sherman B. Echocardiographic evaluation of pericardial effusion in myxedema. Incidence and biochemical and clinical correlations. *Circulation* 1975;**52**:823–7.

28 Manolis AS, Varriale P, Ostrowski RM. Hypothyroid cardiac tamponade. *Arch Intern Med* 1987;**147**:1167–9.

29 Lee KO, Choo MH. Low voltage electrocardiogram with tachycardia in hypothyroidism – a warning sign of cardiac tamponade. *Ann Acad Med Singapore* 1993;**22**:945–7.

30 Sullivan PR, Wolfson AB, Leckey RD, Burke JL. Diagnosis of acute thoracic aortic dissection in the emergency department. *Am J Emerg Med* 2000;**18**:46–50.

31 Hagan PG, Nienaber CA, Isselbacher EM, *et al.* The International Registry of Acute Aortic Dissection (IRAD): new insights into an old disease. *JAMA* 2000;**283**:897–903.

32 Bossone E, Mehta RH, Trimarchi S, *et al.* Coronary artery involvement in patients with acute type A aortic dissection: Clinical characteristics and in-hospital outcomes. *J Am Col Cardiol* 2003;**41**(6, Suppl 1):235.

33 Group TEMIP. Prehospital thrombolytic therapy in patients with suspected acute myocardial infarction. *N Engl J Med* 1993;**329**: 383–9.

34 McGee DC, Gould MK. Preventing complications of central venous catheterization. [see comment]. *N Engl J Med* 2003;**348**: 1123–33.

35 Mayo PH, Goltz HR, Tafreshi M, Doelken P. Safety of ultrasound-guided thoracentesis in patients receiving mechanical ventilation. *Chest* 2004;**125**:1059–62.

36 Gervais DA, Petersein A, Lee MJ, *et al.* US-guided thoracentesis: requirement for postprocedure chest radiography in patients who receive mechanical ventilation versus patients who breathe spontaneously. *Radiology* 1997;**204**:503–6.

37 Walston A, Brewer DL, Kitchens CS, Krook JE. The electrocardiographic manifestations of spontaneous left pneumothorax. *Ann Intern Med* 1974;**80**:375–9.

38 Alikhan M, Biddison JH. Electrocardiographic changes with right-sided pneumothorax. *South Med J* 1998;**91**:677–80.

39 Slay RD, Slay LE, Luehrs JG. Transient ST elevation associated with tension pneumothorax. *J Am Col Emerg Phys* 1979;**8**:16–18.

40 Strizik B, Forman R. New ECG changes associated with a tension pneumothorax: a case report. *Chest* 1999;**115**:1742–4.

41 Sampson M, Rose CE, Jr. Reversible ST-segment elevation associated with atelectasis of the left lung. *South Med J* 2005;**98**: 950–2.

42 Goddard R, Scofield RH. Right pneumothorax with the S1Q3T3 electrocardiogram pattern usually associated with pulmonary embolus. *Am J Emerg Med* 1997;**15**(3):310–12.

43 Reddy PS, Curtiss EI, O'Toole JD, Shaver JA. Cardiac tamponade: hemodynamic observations in man. *Circulation* 1978;**58**:265–72.

44 Singh S, Wann LS, Schuchard GH, *et al.* Right ventricular and right atrial collapse in patients with cardiac tamponade – a combined echocardiographic and hemodynamic study. *Circulation* 1984;**70**:966–71.

45 Cooper JP, Oliver RM, Currie P, *et al.* How do the clinical findings in patients with pericardial effusions influence the success of aspiration? [see comment]. *Br Heart J.* 1995;**73**:351–4.

46 Gibbs CR, Watson RD, Singh SP, Lip GY. Management of pericardial effusion by drainage: a survey of 10 years' experience in a city centre general hospital serving a multiracial population. *Postgrad Med J* 2000;**76**:809–13.

Part 6 | **The Toxicologic ECG**

Chapter 45 | How useful is the ECG in the evaluation of the poisoned patient?

Nathan P. Charlton

University of Virginia School of Medicine, Charlottesville, VA, USA

Case presentations

Case 1: In resuscitation room 1, a 67-year-old male arrives at the emergency department (ED) by emergency medical services (EMS) with altered mental status. He was found at home unresponsive by concerned neighbors. When EMS arrived they found him poorly responsive to painful stimuli and with shallow respirations. On presentation, one large bore IV is established while the patient is being supported with bag-valve-mask ventilation and a cardiac monitor is attached. Initial vital signs show a heart rate of 47 beats per minute (bpm), a blood pressure of 68/42 mmHg and spontaneous respirations of 4. While intubation supplies are being prepared, the rhythm strip is noted to show a wide complex bradydysrhythmia (Figure 45.1). Friends arrive at the ED and explain they have found a suicide note from the patient. He was known to have a history of chronic hip pain and his wife had recently passed away.

Case 2: Next door, in resuscitation 2, triage nurses have rushed back a 23-year-old female who was brought to the ED by her boyfriend after he was unable to wake her this morning. The boyfriend had returned home at 8:00 am after playing pool all night. As the patient is put in the room, vital signs are assessed and she is found to have a blood pressure of 84/50, a heart rate of 124 and respirations of 12. She is poorly responsive to painful stimuli. A brief exam is performed to find miotic pupils, but no track marks or skin lesions, clear lungs and tachycardia. While naloxone is being titrated up to 2 mg, an electrocardiogram (ECG) is performed that reveals sinus tachycardia with a narrow QRS interval and a QTc interval of 540 ms.

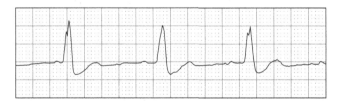

Figure 45.1 Bradycardia and QRS prolongation associated with propoxyphene overdose.

Utilizing the ECG as a diagnostic tool in the poisoned patient

The ECG is an essential diagnostic tool in the evaluation of the poisoned patient. Up to 70% of poisoned patients may exhibit some degree of ECG abnormality [1]. Cardiovascular drugs are the thirteenth most common exposure in all age groups and the sixth most common in adults [2]. These medications are the fifth leading cause of poisoning mortality in all age groups [2]. In addition, many medications of which the primary therapeutic use is not cardiovascular may alter cardiac physiology and contribute to morbidity and mortality that are not factored into these data. While these cardiotoxic medications may vary widely in their therapeutic action, their effects on cardiac physiology follow typical patterns that may be grouped together as a diagnostic tool. When evaluating the ECG, abnormal findings may include tachycardia, bradycardia, or PR, QRS, or QT interval prolongation. These changes reflect five primary cardiac toxicities that occur: sodium channel-blockade, potassium efflux-blockade, Na^+/K^+-ATPase pump-blockade, beta-blockade, and calcium channel-blockade. To a lesser extent, sympathomimetic and anti-cholinergic agents can also be included in these categories; however, these both lead to tachycardia which can be non-specific in an ill patient. When the constellation of symptoms along with the ECG findings are taken into consideration, the physician can then narrow the diagnosis and help guide further management.

Sodium channel-blockade

After examining the rate and rhythm, evaluation of the QRS complex is of primary importance. During myocardial

Critical Decisions in Emergency and Acute Care Electrocardiography, 1st edition. Edited by W.J. Brady and J.D. Truwit. © 2009 Blackwell Publishing, ISBN: 9781405159067

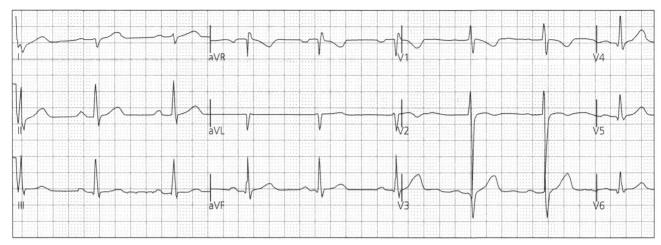

Figure 45.2 Typical pattern of cyclic anti-depressant toxicity with: S wave in aVL and III with terminal R wave in aVR.

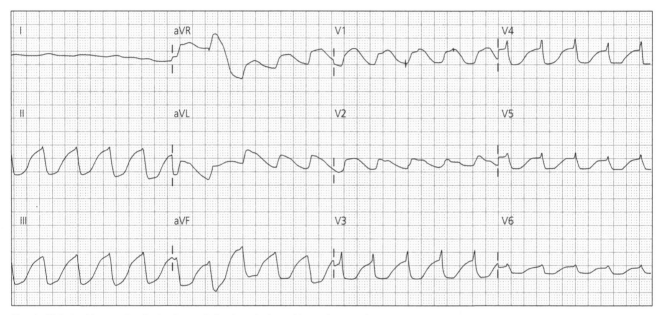

Figure 45.3 A wide complex rhythm is seen following a hydroxychloroquine overdose.

depolarization membrane sodium channels open, allowing sodium to flow down its concentration gradient into the cell. This is phase 0 of the action potential and the net voltage of ventricular depolarization is reflected as the QRS complex on the ECG. Sodium channels exist in three phases: resting, activated, and inactivated [3]. Sodium channel-blockers generally bind in the inactivated or activated phase, and slow recovery of these channels [3]. Consequently, a decreased amount of sodium per unit time enters into the cell. This delays the upslope of depolarization, prolonging the time for the ventricles to depolarize resulting in a widening of the QRS on the ECG. The degree of widening depends on the number of sodium channels poisoned. Medications that block these channels have been used in the treatment of arrhythmias and are listed as Type 1 in the Vaughan-Williams classification scheme. The prototypical sodium

channel-blocking agent is quinidine. Many chemicals act as sodium channel-blockers, and in overdose these effects are magnified. These agents are often referred to as having membrane-stabilizing or quinidine-like effects. The standard QRS duration is listed as less than 120 ms [4]; however, when evaluating a suspected poisoned patient > 100 ms of QRS duration is considered wide as the potential for dysrhythmia begins to increase above this duration. More specifically, sodium channel-blockers may result in prolongation of the terminal 40 ms of the QRS complex, which results in right axis deviation and may resemble a right bundle branch block (Figure 45.2) [5–7]. When evaluating a suspected poisoning, a QRS interval duration greater than 100 ms should clue the physician in to a potential sodium channel-blocker (Figure 45.3). A few classic examples of sodium channel-blockers include tricyclic anti-depressants

Table 45.1 Na⁺ channel-blocking drugs

Amantidine	Diltiazem
Carbamazepine	Diphenhydramine
Chloroquine	Hydroxychloroquine
Class IA anti-dysrhythmics	Loxapine
Disopyramide	Orphenadrine
Quinidine	Phenothiazines
Procainamide	Mesoidazine
Class IC anti-dysrhythmics	Thioridazine
Encainide	Propanolol
Flecainide	Propoxyphene
Propafenone	Quinine
Citalopram	Verapamil
Cocaine	
Cyclic anti-depressants	
Amitriptyline	
Amoxapine	
Desipramine	
Doxepin	
Imipramine	
Nortriptyline	
Maprotiline	

Table 45.2 K⁺ efflux channel-blocking drugs

Anti-histamines	Class III anti-dysrhythmics
Astemizole	Amiodarone
Diphenhydramine	Dofetilide
Loratidine	Ibutilide
Terfenadine	Sotalol
Anti-psychotics	Cyclic anti-depressants
Chlorpromazine	Amitriptyline
Droperidol	Amoxapine
Haloperidol	Desipramine
Mesoridazine	Doxepin
Pimozide	Imipramine
Quetiapine	Nortriptyline
Risperidone	Maprotiline
Thioridazine	Fluoroquinolones
Ziprasidone	Ciprofloxacin
Arsenic trioxide	Gatifloxacin
Bepridil	Levofloxacin
Chloroquine	Moxifloxacin
Cisapride	Sparfloxacin
Citalopram	Halofantrine
Class IA anti-dysrhythmics	Hydroxychloroquine
Disopyramide	Levomethadyl
Quinidine	Macrolides
Procainamide	Clarithromycin
Class IC anti-dysrhythmics	Erythromycin
Encainide	Pentamidine
Flecainide	Quinine
Moricizine	Tacrolimus
Propafenone	Venlafaxine

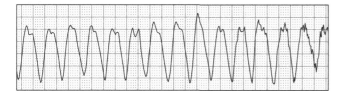

Figure 45.4 A rhythm strip demonstrating a diphenhydramine-induced wide complex tachydysrhythmia.

(TCAs), propoxyphene and diphenhydramine; others can be obtained from many published lists such as those listed in Table 45.1. Sodium channel-blockade predisposes to re-entrant arrhythmias, particularly ventricular tachycardia. Unfortunately, with sodium channel-blockade, the resultant ECG may look similar to a pre-existing conduction delay or bundle branch block, and in a tachycardic patient it may be difficult to differentiate between a ventricular tachycardia versus a supraventricular rhythm with aberrant conduction (Figure 45.4) [4]. Sodium channel-blockade not only leads to conduction abnormalities, but may also lead to inotropic depression and hypotension as delayed sodium entry into the cell may also delay the release of calcium from intracellular stores [8].

Potassium efflux blockade

QT interval prolongation is a common side effect of many medications noted in Table 45.2 [9]. QT interval prolonga-

tion results primarily from potassium efflux-blockade [1,10]. In the cardiac action potential, repolarization of myocytes is dependent on potassium. Potassium is a positively charged ion that is heavily concentrated inside the myocyte. Potassium channels initially open in response to depolarization (sodium channel opening) of the myocyte. This efflux of potassium, along with continued influx of calcium, is responsible for the plateau of the action potential. Potassium channels are open in phases 1 through 3 of the action potential [10], and the resulting flow of positive ions out of the cell helps to return the cell to its normal resting potential. Medications that block the efflux of potassium during repolarization increase the length of time the myocyte is in the repolarization phase and, therefore, result in prolonged QTc duration. Normal intervals have been described as greater than 440 ms in men and greater than 460 ms in women [10]. Intervals greater than 500 ms appear to predispose to dysrhythmias; however, this is variable as dysrhythmias have occurred at lengths less than 500 ms and patients have remained dysrhythmia-free at intervals longer than this [10]. The inability of potassium to leave the cell increases the amount of positive ions in the cell and, therefore, raises the membrane potential. This may result in early myocyte firing, termed "early after depolarization," which is the mechanism behind the initiation of torsade de pointes. There are two primary formulations for calculating the QT interval. The most common is Bazett's formula (QTc – QT/RR1/2), but this formula may be inaccurate in tachycardia and bradycardia. In these instances, Fridericia's formula may be more appropriate (QTc = QT/RR1/3) [11]. However, the QTc may vary from beat to beat and from lead to lead so the computer-calculated QTc may in fact be the most accurate calculation. Medications that typically cause QT prolongation are in the psychiatric, anti-arrhythmic, or anti-infective classes. An extensive list of potassium efflux-blockers can be found in Table 45.2. Finding QTc prolongation on the ECG should prompt evaluation for any of these medications.

Na⁺/K⁺-ATPase blockade

While cardiac glycoside toxicity may not be as common, digoxin is still prescribed on a regular basis and the potential for ECG abnormalities is substantial. Cardiac glycosides inhibit the Na⁺/K⁺-ATPase, which results in an increase in sodium inside the cell. This potentiates the Na⁺/Ca²⁺-transporter, which is a non-ATP-dependent transporter located on the cell membrane. Through this channel, intercellular sodium is exchanged for extracellular calcium. The end result is increased calcium inside the cell, which therapeutically serves to increase myocardial contractility. Therapeutic dosing may result in the scooped ST segments [1,12]. Cardiac glycosides also slow atrioventricular (AV) nodal conduction, which may result in bradycardia or AV block (Figure 45.5). Increased calcium inside the myocytes raises the resting membrane potential and lowers their firing threshold. As a result, the cells become more irritable and increase their automaticity [12,13]. Resulting dysrhythmias come from a combination of these two features: tachydysrhythmias with AV block. Classic dysrhythmias with digoxin toxicity are biventricular tachycardia and atrial tachycardia with AV block, although the most common dysrhythmia is frequent premature ventricular contractions (PVCs) [12]. While almost any dysrhythmia may occur with digoxin toxicity, supraventricular tachycardias with rapid ventricular response are usually not seen. Scooped T waves with PVCs or evidence of automaticity with a block are useful diagnostic tools for the physician in diagnosing digoxin toxicity.

Calcium channel- and beta-blockade

Both calcium channel-antagonists (CCAs) and beta-blockers (BBs) are prevalent as therapeutic medications and, therefore, the likelihood of toxic ingestion is high. In therapeutic use, as well as in overdose, they may have similar ECG findings. The typical finding in symptomatic patients for both classes is bradycardia with varying degrees of AV block (Figure 45.6) [1,14,15]. This is mediated by direct (CCA) and indirect (BB) blockade of the L-type (ligand-gated) calcium channel in the cell membrane [16]. In therapeutic dosing, first-degree AV block may be noted without the presence of bradycardia and manifests as a PR interval greater than 200 ms. Bradycardia and hypotension are the predominant findings with BBs and non-dihydropyridine classes of CCAs. Dihydropyridine CCAs can present with reflex tachycardia in response to peripheral vasodilation early in the course of poisoning or with mild poisoning; however, with high doses selectivity is lost and direct cardiodepressant effects are seen. Lipophilic beta-blockers and calcium channel-blockers may also prolong the QRS interval [1,14]. Propranolol in particular is a highly active sodium channel-blocker. Poisoning with this agent may cause the bradycardia and AV block associated with beta-blocker toxicity, as well as QRS interval prolongation typical of sodium channel-blockade [3,14]. Centrally acting alpha-2-agonists, such as clonidine and imidazolines, also produce bradycardia.

While calcium channel-blockers and beta-blockers often produce bradycardia in poisoning, many other drugs may produce tachycardia in poisoning. Sympathomimetics and anti-cholinergics are well-known causes of tachycardia. Sympathomimetics primarily produce tachycardia by activation of beta-receptors while anti-cholinergics block vagal tone. Peripheral alpha-blocking agents can produce tachycardia by a reflex mechanism as they cause hypotension. Conversely, peripheral alpha-agonists may cause reflex bradycardia secondary to induction of hypertension.

Case conclusions

In the first case, the patient presents with bradycardia, respiratory depression, altered mental status and a wide QRS after

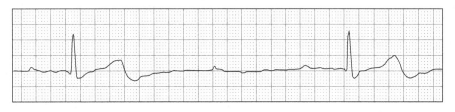

Figure 45.5 A rhythm strip demonstrating a third-degree heart block induced by digoxin toxicity.

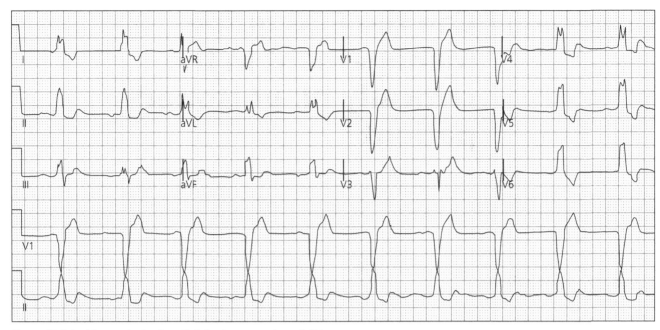

Figure 45.6 A wide complex bradycardia following an overdose of diltiazem.

a suicide attempt. In reviewing a list of sodium channel-blockers, anti-cholinergic agents can be ruled out as they will cause tachycardia. Calcium channel-blockers, propanolol, and propoxyphene could all cause a similar picture. As this patient had only a history of chronic back pain, propoxyphene is a likely choice. Secondary to the widened QRS, standard treatment with sodium bicarbonate was initiated with 150 mEq administered through IV push. After treatment, the QRS interval narrowed and blood pressure improved. The patient's mental status improved after titrating naloxone to effect.

The female patient did not respond to naloxone. Review of her medications revealed that she had been prescribed quetiapine, an atypical anti-psychotic that produces QT prolongation, CNS depression and peripheral alpha-adrenergic-blockade in overdose. The patient was given 2 g of IV magnesium to help protect against dysrhythmia. She did not respond to initial fluid bolus so an infusion of phenylephrine was begun to combat quetiapine's vasodilatory effects. The patient was admitted to the ICU and recovered without sequelae the subsequent day.

References

1 Holstege CP, Eldridge DL, Rowden AK. ECG manifestations: the poisoned patient. *Emerg Med Clin North Am* 2006;**24**(1):159–77.
2 Lai MW, Klein-Schwartz W, Rodgers GC, *et al.* 2005 Annual Report of the American Association of Poison Control Centers' national poisoning and exposure database. *Clin Toxicol (Phila)* 2006;**44**(6–7):803–932.
3 Kolecki PF, Curry SC. Poisoning by sodium channel blocking agents. *Crit Care Clin* 1997;**13**(4):829–48.
4 Brady WJ, Skiles J. Wide QRS complex tachycardia: ECG differential diagnosis. *Am J Emerg Med* 1999;**17**(4):376–81.
5 Harrigan RA, Brady WJ. ECG abnormalities in tricyclic antidepressant ingestion. *Am J Emerg Med* 1999;**17**(4):387–93.
6 Liebelt EL, Francis PD, Woolf AD. ECG lead aVR versus QRS interval in predicting seizures and arrhythmias in acute tricyclic antidepressant toxicity. *Ann Emerg Med* 1995;**26**(2):195–201.
7 Fernandez-Quero L, Riesgo MJ, Agusti S, *et al.* Left anterior hemiblock, complete right bundle branch block and sinus tachycardia in maprotiline poisoning. *Intensive Care Med* 1985;**11**(4):220–2.
8 Seger DL. A critical reconsideration of the clinical effects and treatment recommendations for sodium channel blocking drug cardiotoxicity. *Toxicol Rev* 2006;**25**(4):283–96.
9 De Ponti F, Poluzzi E, Montanaro N, *et al.* QTc and psychotropic drugs. *Lancet* 2000;**356**(9223):75–6.
10 Kao LW, Furbee RB. Drug-induced q-T prolongation. *Med Clin North Am* 2005;**89**(6):1125–44, x.
11 Yap YG, Camm AJ. Drug induced QT prolongation and torsades de pointes. *Heart* 2003;**89**(11):1363–72.
12 Ma G, Brady WJ, Pollack M, *et al.* Electrocardiographic manifestations: digitalis toxicity. *J Emerg Med* 2001;**20**(2):145–52.
13 Kerns W. Management of beta-adrenergic blocker and calcium channel antagonist toxicity. *Emerg Med Clin North Am* 2007;**25**(2):309–31; abstract viii.
14 Katz AM. Selectivity and toxicity of antiarrhythmic drugs: molecular interactions with ion channels. *Am J Med* 1998;**104**(2):179–95.
15 Love JN, Enlow B, Howell JM, *et al.* Electrocardiographic changes associated with beta-blocker toxicity. *Ann Emerg Med* 2002;**40**(6):603–10.

Chapter 46 | Can the ECG guide management in the critically ill, poisoned patient?

Nathan P. Charlton
University of Virginia School of Medicine, Charlottesville, VA, USA

Case presentations

Case 1: A 72-year-old male with a history of depression and previous suicide attempts presents to the emergency department (ED) via emergency medical services with acute alteration of mental status. He vocalizes incomprehensible sounds upon stimulation, but rapidly drifts back to sleep. His gag is intact with clear but shallow breaths sounds. His presenting pulse is 150 beats per minute (bpm), respirations 12 per minute, and blood pressure 81/34 mmHg. The remainder of the exam is significant for mydriasis, dry skin, lack of bowel sounds, and, on placement of the bladder catheter, a return of 1.5 L of urine. The initial electrocardiogram (ECG) shows a sinus tachycardia at a rate of 153 with a QRS interval of 182 ms and a QTc interval of 473 ms (Figure 46.1).

Case 2: A 57-year-old male with history of hypertension only arrives at the ED by emergency medical services with altered mental status. A suicide note was found at the scene. Initial vital signs reveal a heart rate of 40 bpm, a blood pressure of 68/42 mmHg and spontaneous respirations of 12 breaths per minute. His initial blood sugar at bedside is 357 mg/dL. His ECG is seen in Figure 46.2.

Utilizing the ECG to guide management in the critically ill, poisoned patient

The critically ill, poisoned patient can present a unique medical management problem. The histories of poisoned patients are typically unreliable, especially in the setting of an intentional overdose. Subsequently, clinicians must utilize

physical examination and diagnostic testing to help narrow the potential etiologies. Management may differ from other critically ill patients. At times, conventional advanced life support (ALS) therapy may be ineffective or may even lead to harm in the poisoned patient. Current literature reveals that cardiovascular drugs are responsible for 8.7% of all reported poisoning fatalities [1]. In addition, poisoning fatalities due to non-cardiovascular drugs are commonly secondary to dysrhythmias.

During the initial assessment of the poisoned patient, the clinician must ensure that the patient's airway is patent and with adequate ventilation. If necessary, endotracheal tube intubation should be performed. Physicians are often falsely reassured when a patient's oxygen saturations are adequate on high-flow oxygen. If the patient has inadequate ventilation, the patient may be at risk for subsequent CO_2 narcosis, declining mental status, development of a respiratory acidosis, and subsequent dysrhythmias. The patient who has a poor gag reflex or is not handling secretions adequately is at risk for aspiration and prolonged hospitalization. Intubation should be performed in such patients. As patients with cardiac toxicity have the potential to rapidly decline, extra care should be taken to insure a secure airway. Because laryngoscopy has been reported to induce a vagal response, administration of atropine should be considered in the bradycardic poisoned patient prior to intubation.

Patients who have taken an overdose of a potential cardiovascular toxin must be placed on continuous cardiac monitoring with pulse oximetry. All patients should receive a large bore peripheral intravenous line and all symptomatic patients should have a second line placed, either peripheral or central. If the patient is a potential candidate for an intravenous pacemaker, central line placement is preferentially placed in the right internal jugular or the left subclavian. The initial treatment of hypotension consists of intravenous fluids. Close monitoring of the patient's pulmonary exam needs to be performed to assure that pulmonary edema does not develop as fluids are infused. Placement of a urinary catheter should be considered early in the care of symptomatic

Critical Decisions in Emergency and Acute Care Electrocardiography,
1st edition. Edited by W.J. Brady and J.D. Truwit. © 2009 Blackwell Publishing, ISBN: 9781405159067

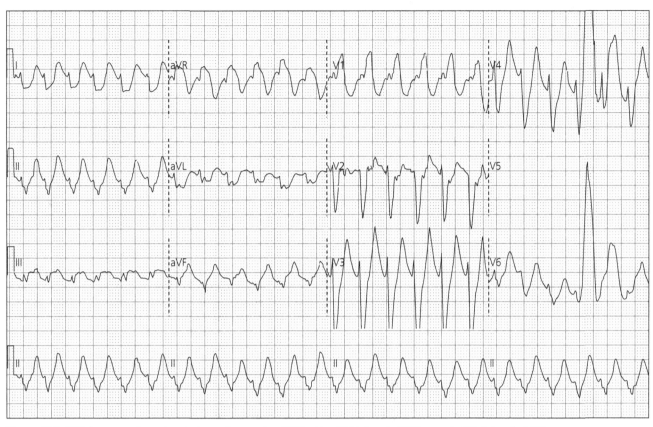

Figure 46.1 ECG demonstrating a sinus tachycardia at a rate of 153 with a QRS interval of 182 ms and a QTc interval of 473 ms.

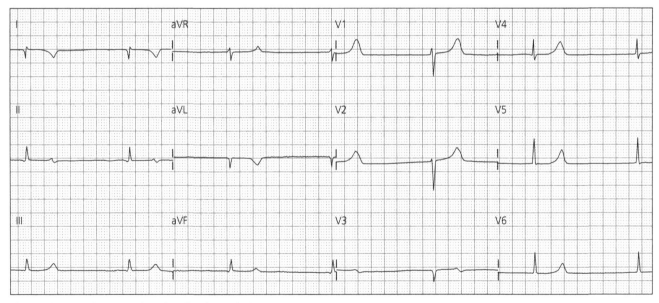

Figure 46.2 ECG demonstrating a junctional rate of 40.

patients to monitor urinary output as an indicator of adequate renal perfusion.

In order to understand the cardiac complications of various agents, physicians must have a clear understanding of basic myocardial cell function. The myocardial cell membrane in its resting state is impermeable to Na^+. The Na^+/K^+-ATPase

actively pumps three Na^+ out of cardiac cells while pumping in two K^+, in order to maintain a negative electric potential in the myocyte of approximately -90 mV (phase 4). Depolarization of the cardiac cell membrane is due to the rapid opening of Na^+ channels and the subsequent massive Na^+ influx (phase 0). This Na^+ influx causes the rapid upstroke of the cardiac action potential as it is conducted through the ventricles and is directly responsible for the QRS interval of the ECG. The peak of the action potential is marked by the closure of Na⁺ channels and the activation of K⁺ efflux channels (phase 1). Calcium influx then occurs, allowing for a plateau in the action potential (phase 2) and continued myocardial contraction. The cardiac cycle ends with closure of the Ca^{2+} channels and activation of K⁺ efflux channels causing the potential to again approach −90 mV (phase 3). It is this K⁺ efflux from the myocardial cell that is directly responsible for the QT interval of the ECG.

Severely poisoned patients often have ECG abnormalities [2]. Wide complex tachycardias are a common dysrhythmia encountered in the overdose setting. These rhythms may initially be difficult to differentiate. When the cardiac sodium channel is inhibited, less sodium per unit time enters the cardiac myocyte and is reflected as QRS widening on the ECG [3,4]. In addition, when sodium entry into the cell is delayed, less calcium is released from intracellular stores [4]. This decreased calcium results in a subsequent decrease in inotropy as the interaction of calcium with troponin mediates muscle contraction. Hypotension may then occur. Many sodium channel-blockers also have separate mechanisms that promote tachycardia, including sympathomimetic and anti-cholinergic properties [3,5,6]. The resultant supraventricular tachycardia with a prolongation of the QRS complex with associated hypotension may present a clinical picture identical to a ventricular tachydysrhythmia [7]. This pattern of tachycardia with QRS widening in the setting of a poisoning should prompt the treating physician to administer intravenous sodium bicarbonate.

There have been multiple studies on the effects of sodium bicarbonate. As sodium bicarbonate may act to overcome sodium channel-blockade, it then shortens the action potential of the myocardial cell and increases calcium influx into the cell. This improves dromotropy and inotropy and, therefore, may be used as therapy for both tachydysrhythmias and hypotension in patients with a widened QRS [3,4,6,8]. Administering sodium bicarbonate to the poisoned hypotensive patient may increase cardiac output and directly improve hypotension. In the unstable patient, ALS principles still apply as to cardioversion and defibrillation; however, sodium bicarbonate should be given concomitantly to treat the source of the problem and restore normal sodium channel function. A typical practice is to administer sodium bicarbonate in IV boluses, usually in 1–2 mEq/kg increments, and monitor the ECG, with the primary endpoint being QRS interval narrowing and/or resolution of hypotension. Depending on physician preference, a sodium bicarbonate infusion may be started after the initial bolus [3]. Three ampoules of sodium bicarbonate in 1 L of 5% dextrose in water (D5W) will provide about 150 mEq of sodium per liter. This infusion may then be run at two times the maintenance rate and should have the inclusion of 40 mEq KCl to prevent the development of hypokalemia. An alternative practice is to forego the sodium bicarbonate infusion and perform serial ECGs,

administering sodium bicarbonate as needed for QRS intervals greater than 100 ms and/or hypotension.

There is currently a preponderance of patients receiving medications that have the ability to block myocardial potassium efflux channels and consequently prolong the QTc interval. Patients presenting with prolonged QT intervals are at risk of dysrhythmia, predominantly torsade de pointes (TdP). Generally, QTc prolongation is secondary to potassium efflux channel-blockade, resulting in prolongation of myocardial repolarization [9]. Normal QTc intervals are less than 440 ms for men and less than 460 ms in women [9]. As QTc intervals rise to greater than 500 ms, the risk of TdP appears to rise [3,9,10].

QT interval prolongation predisposes to TdP. Susceptibility to TdP is not only a function of the length of the QTc interval, but is also likely secondary to increased QT interval dispersion, which reflects interbeat variability [11]. To help stabilize the myocyte, 1–2 g of IV magnesium sulfate is recommended for any QTc interval exceeding 500 ms after a suspected poisoning or overdose in adults [9]. This usually does not shorten the interval, but prevents the onset of dysrhythmias. While TdP often spontaneously resolves, it may also degenerate to ventricular fibrillation. Consequently, for any episode of TdP, patients should be given an IV bolus of 1–2 g magnesium sulfate, which can be repeated for refractory dysrhythmias. A second option for treatment is overdrive pacing using chemical or electrical means. This treatment is typically reserved for refractory bouts of TdP. Isoproterenol, a beta-receptor agonist, is the classic drug of choice for overdrive pacing. For either method, treatment consists of increasing the heart rate to 90–140 bpm, which acts to decrease the risk of TdP by narrowing and homogenizing the QT interval [12].

In patients presenting with ECG changes and hyperkalemia, cardiac glycosides should be considered in the differential diagnosis. In a patient with acute or chronic poisoning by digoxin, one of the primary clinical manifestations may be cardiac dysrhythmias. Digoxin causes both myocardial cell irritability and blockade of the atrioventricular (AV) node. The resulting dysrhythmias can be almost any type, the only exclusion is that supraventricular tachycardias with rapid ventricular conduction are usually not seen [13,14]. The two well-established guidelines for initiating treatment with digoxin-specific Fab fragments depend on dysrhythmias and hyperkalemia [14]. In the setting of acute digoxin toxicity, a measured potassium greater than 5 mEq/L and/or dysrhythmias that threaten or result in hemodynamic compromise should prompt treatment with digoxin Fab fragments [14]. In chronic digoxin poisoning, cardiac toxicity as evidenced on ECG or other cardiovascular symptomatology should prompt treatment with digoxin Fab fragments [14]. The number of vials needed for the treatment of digoxin poisoning can be estimated by the formula: digoxin level (ng/mL) × weight of patient (kg)/100 [14]. As one 40 mg vial binds about 0.6 mg of digoxin, the amount of Fab fragments given can be calculated from the dose taken in an acute poisoning. In severely poisoned patients who have taken unquantified overdose, treatment with 5–10 vials can be given initially while the digoxin level is pending. Care must be taken to monitor exacerbation of congestive heart failure and underlying atrial fibrillation after treatment with digoxin Fab fragments [15]. In patients with renal failure, the clearance of digoxin-bound Fab fragments will be prolonged, and, consequently, dissociation and rebound toxicity may occur [14,16]. Potassium replacement may be beneficial in chronic poisoning with hypokalemia; however, caution is needed as many of these patients will also have renal insufficiency.

Patients presenting with a new bradydysrhythmia may be manifesting either calcium channel-antagonist (CCA) toxicity or beta-blocker (BB) toxicity. Calcium channel-antagonists and BBs have similar mechanisms of toxicity on the heart. Both CCAs (directly) and BBs (indirectly) inhibit calcium entry into the myocyte. Classically, toxicity can be recognized on the ECG by bradydysrhythmia and AV block with associated hypotension. Junctional or ventricular escape rhythms may occur. The treatment for these two types of poisonings is similar. Atropine may be given initially, but its efficacy is expected to be limited. For mild symptoms, intravenous calcium may be used to help overcome the blockade of the calcium channel. Intravenous calcium gluconate or chloride may be given to raise the ionized calcium to two to three times its normal limit. Glucagon appears to be particularly useful in the management of beta-blocker toxicity. Glucagon possesses its own receptor site on the myocardial cell separate from the beta receptor. Independently increasing intracellular cAMP may help to increase inotropy.

Five milligrams of glucagon is the standard intravenous starting dose for adult patients. A common side effect to glucagon administration is vomiting, so the clinician must assure airway protection prior to administration. Adrenergic receptor-agonists also may be of use to overcome competitive blockade. Direct acting agents (norepinephrine/epinephrine) are usually preferred. Hyperinsulinemia-euglycemia therapy is a recent development in the treatment of both CCA and BB toxicity. The mechanism of action is based on evolving knowledge of cellular physiology. In times of stress, cardiac cells switch their preferred energy substrate from free fatty acid to carbohydrates [17–19]. It has been found that CCAs block insulin release from pancreatic beta islet cells and inhibit the action of insulin on tissue, thereby resulting in a state of insulin deficiency. Hyperinsulinemia-euglycemia therapy supplies the insulin necessary to deliver substrate to the cell. Initial studies used up to 2.5 units/kg of regular insulin per hour; however, it has been found that a reasonable dose is 0.5–1.0 U/kg regular insulin bolus followed by an infusion of 0.5 U/kg/h and titrated up to effect [18,20].

Case conclusions

In Case 1, anti-cholinergic signs and symptoms coupled with the ECG changes prompted consideration for cyclic anti-depressant overdose. The patient received 150 mEq of sodium bicarbonate bolus IV. A repeat ECG is seen in Figure 46.3. He

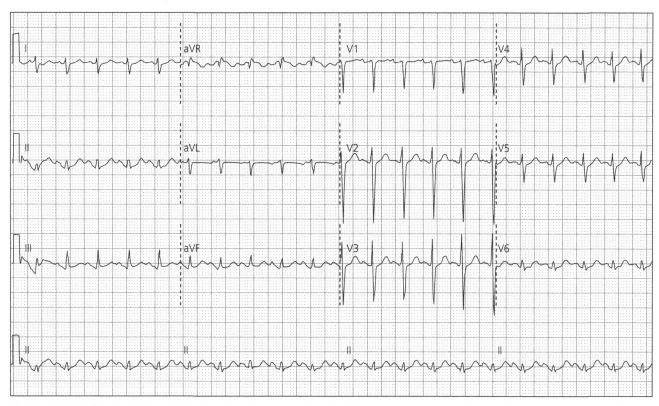

Figure 46.3 ECG demonstrating a sinus tachycardia with a narrowing of the QRS complex, compared with Figure 46.1, following administration of sodium bicarbonate.

was intermittently given 50 mEq of IV sodium bicarbonate while in the intensive care unit over the ensuing 24 h. The patient's condition gradually improved over the following day and he was discharged 48 h later. The patient admitted to an intentional overdose of doxepin, which he had been taking for depression.

In Case 2, based upon the ECG and other clinical factors suggestive of calcium-antagonist exposure, a presumptive diagnosis of CCA toxicity was made. The patient was intubated, placed on mechanical ventilation, and central and arterial lines were inserted. Intravenous fluids were administered, 2 g of calcium chloride was infused through the central line, and insulin was titrated to maintained euglycemia. The patient's blood pressure responded well to therapy. An empty bottle of diltiazem was found by police at the scene. Two days following the overdose, the patient was discharged to a psychiatric facility.

References

1 William AW, Toby LL, George CR, *et al.* 2004 Annual report of the American Association of Poison Control Centers Toxic Exposure Surveillance System. *Am J Emerg Med* 2005;**23**(5):589–666.

2 Homer A, Brady W, Holstege C. *The Association of Toxins and ECG Abnormality in Poisoned Patients.* Paper presented at Mediterranean Emergency Medicine Congress, Nice, France, 2005.

3 Holstege CP, Eldridge DL, Rowden AK. ECG manifestations: the poisoned patient. *Emerg Med Clin North Am* 2006;**24**(1):159–77.

4 Kolecki PF, Curry SC. Poisoning by sodium channel blocking agents. *Crit Care Clin* 1997;**13**(4):829–48.

5 Harrigan RA, Brady WJ. ECG abnormalities in tricyclic antidepressant ingestion. *Am J Emerg Med* 1999;**17**(4):387–93.

6 Sharma AN, Hexdall AH, Chang EK, *et al.* Diphenhydramine-induced wide complex dysrhythmia responds to treatment with sodium bicarbonate. *Am J Emerg Med* 2003;**21**(3):212–15.

7 Brady WJ, Skiles J. Wide QRS complex tachycardia: ECG differential diagnosis. *Am J Emerg Med* 1999;**17**(4):376–81.

8 Wasserman F, Brodsky L, Dick MM, *et al.* Successful treatment of quinidine and procaine amide intoxication; report of three cases. *N Engl J Med* 1958;**259**(17):797–802.

9 Kao LW, Furbee RB. Drug-induced q-T prolongation. *Med Clin North Am* 2005;**89**(6):1125–44.

10 Yap YG, Camm AJ. Drug induced QT prolongation and torsades de pointes. *Heart* 2003;**89**(11):1363–72.

11 Gowda RM, Khan IA, Wilbur SL, *et al.* Torsade de pointes: the clinical considerations. *Inter J Cardiol* 2004;**96**(1):1–6.

12 Keren A, Tzivoni D, Gavish D, *et al.* Etiology, warning signs and therapy of torsade de pointes. A study of 10 patients. *Circulation* 1981;**64**(6):1167–74.

13 Ma G, Brady WJ, Pollack M, *et al.* Electrocardiographic manifestations: digitalis toxicity. *J Emerg Med* 2001;**20**(2):145–52.

14 Kirk MA, Judge B, eds. *Digitalis Poisoning.* 5th ed. Baltimore: Lippincott Williams & Wilkins, 2003.

15 Smith TW. Review of clinical experience with digoxin immune Fab (ovine). *Am J Emerg Med* 1991;**9**(2, Suppl 1):1–6.

16 Mehta RN, Mehta NJ, Gulati A. Late rebound digoxin toxicity after digoxin-specific antibody fab fragments therapy in anuric patient. *J Emerg Med* 2002;**22**(2):203–6.

17 Yuan TH, Kerns WP, Tomaszewski CA, *et al.* Insulin-Glucose as Adjunctive Therapy for Severe Calcium Channel Antagonist Poisoning. *Clin Toxicol* 1999;**37**(4):463–74.

18 Kerns W. Management of beta-adrenergic blocker and calcium channel antagonist toxicity. *Emerg Med Clin North Am* 2007;**25**(2):309–31

19 Kline JAMD, Leonova EMS, Raymond RMP. Beneficial myocardial metabolic effects of insulin during verapamil toxicity in the anesthetized canine. *Crit Care Med* 1995;**23**(7):1251–63.

20 Daubert P. *A Bitter Sweet Surrender in Calcium Channel Antagonist Poisoning: the End of Calcium, the New Era or Insulin.* Paper presented at North America Congress of Clinical Toxicology, New Orleans, Louisiana, 2007.

Chapter 47

Do characteristics of the QRS complex in the poisoned patient correlate with outcome?

Stephen D. Lee, Nathan P. Charlton, Christopher P. Holstege
University of Virginia School of Medicine, Charlottesville, VA, USA

Case presentations

Case 1: A 32-year-old female with history of depression presents to the emergency department (ED) 1 h after an overdose of amitriptyline. Upon arrival, she is agitated, screaming that she does not want help and that the staff should just "let me die." Her initial vitals reveal a blood pressure of 100/60 mmHg, a pulse of 105 beats per minute (bpm), and respirations of 26 breaths per minute. Her initial electrocardiogram (ECG) is noted in Figure 47.1. Over the ensuing hour, her mentation steadily declines and she becomes progressively somnolent. Two hours post-ingestion her blood pressure drops to 75/30 and her pulse increases to 130 bpm, despite infusion of intravenous fluids. A second ECG is noted in Figure 47.2. The patient sustains a brief seizure 2.5 h after post-ingestion requiring intubation, and, following her intubation, the ECG in Figure 47.3 is noted.

Case 2: A 47-year-old transvestite with a history of chronic drug abuse presents following an acute overdose of imipramine. The patient's initial vital signs are significant for a blood pressure of 140/85 mmHg, a pulse of 140 bpm, and respirations of 16 breaths per minute. He is fully anti-cholinergic with mumbling speech, agitation, mydriasis, anhydrosis, lack of bowel sounds and cutaneous flushing. His initial ECG is noted in Figure 47.4. Twenty minutes later, the rhythm depicted in Figure 47.5 is observed. A total of 200 mEq of sodium bicarbonate are infused and the patient converts to a sinus tachycardia with a rate of 130 bpm. He is subsequently placed on a sodium bicarbonate continuous infusion (3 amps of sodium bicarbonate [50 mEq per amp of sodium] in 1 L of 5% dextrose in water [D5W] with 40 mEq of KCl infused at a rate of 200 cc/h to maintain an arterial pH of 7.50–7.55) and he develops no further dysrhythmias. He is discharged to a

psychiatric facility 3 days later, after resolution of all signs and symptoms.

The QRS complex in the poisoned patient

Overdoses of tricyclic anti-depressants (TCAs) are among the most extensively studied toxic overdoses with regards to the significance of ECG findings. Literature on the value of the ECG in predicting outcomes in TCA toxicity has been thoroughly examined in the past decade [1–3]; however, the utility of the QRS interval duration specifically in predicting patient outcomes such as seizures or dysrhythmias still remains a point of contention. While literature on the subject is somewhat confounding, the literature appears to support the finding that as TCA toxicity increases, the QRS duration lengthens, making the ECG a useful tool in management of the TCA poisoned patient.

One of the earliest and most cited publications is the 1985 prospective study by Boehnert and Lovejoy of 49 acute TCA overdoses, which found that no seizures or arrhythmias occurred in those with a maximal QRS < 100 ms (n = 13). However, TCA overdoses with a QRS > 100 ms (n = 36) had a 34% and 14% incidence of seizures and ventricular arrhythmias, respectively [4]. Furthermore, while seizures were seen with QRS durations > 100 ms, ventricular arrhythmias were only observed with QRS intervals > 160 ms (50% incidence) [4], suggesting that the QRS duration could potentially be used to predict the risk of seizures and arrhythmias in acute TCA overdose. Another prospective cohort study of 36 acute TCA overdose patients suggested similar potential, as patients with seizures and/or arrhythmias had significantly (P < 0.01) greater initial and maximal QRS intervals (approximately 150 ms, range 60–260, n = 16) than those without those complications (approximately 100 ms, range 80–150, n = 20) [5].

An extensive meta-analysis looked at three specific outcomes of TCA overdose (seizures, arrhythmias, death) and

Critical Decisions in Emergency and Acute Care Electrocardiography,
1st edition. Edited by W.J. Brady and J.D. Truwit. © 2009 Blackwell
Publishing, ISBN: 9781405159067

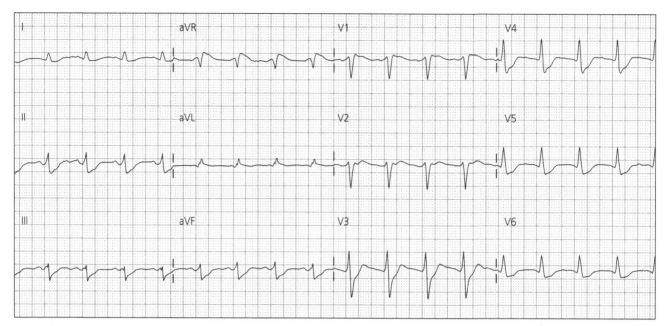

Figure 47.1 Initial ECG reveals QRS prolongation of 120 ms and tachycardia.

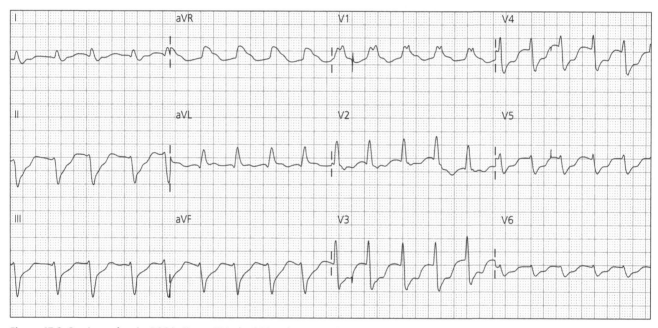

Figure 47.2 One hour after the ECG in Figure 47.1, the QRS prolongs to 140 ms.

calculated pooled sensitivities and specificities to examine the value of a QRS duration ≥ 100 ms in predicting those outcomes. Results are shown in Table 47.1 [3]. While the above analysis supports a positive correlation between a QRS duration ≥ 100 ms and the complications of seizure, ventricular arrhythmias and death, the authors concluded that the QRS duration was a relatively poor individual predictor of outcome, but was better suited for categorizing low-risk patients, given higher sensitivities and lower specificities [3].

Alternately, several investigators have questioned the utility of established QRS interval cutoffs for predicting arrhythmias in TCA overdose. One 1987 retrospective review of 102 patients found no significant difference in the occurrence of ventricular arrhythmias (VAs) or seizures between controls and those with QRS intervals ≥ 100 ms. In this study, 5% (3/57) of control subjects versus 6% (3/45) of those with a QRS ≥ 100 ms had VAs, while 7% (4/57) versus 11% (5/45) experienced seizures [6]. More recently, Buckley and colleagues reported a similar lack of support for

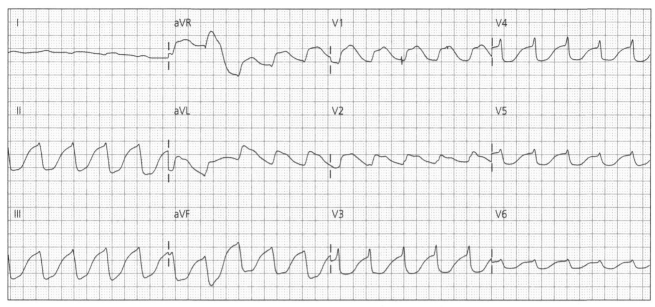

Figure 47.3 Following a seizure, and subsequent acidosis, cardiac sodium channel-blocking activity has worsened resulting in a sinusoidal wave form with marked QRS prolongation and slowing of the heart rate – ominous signs.

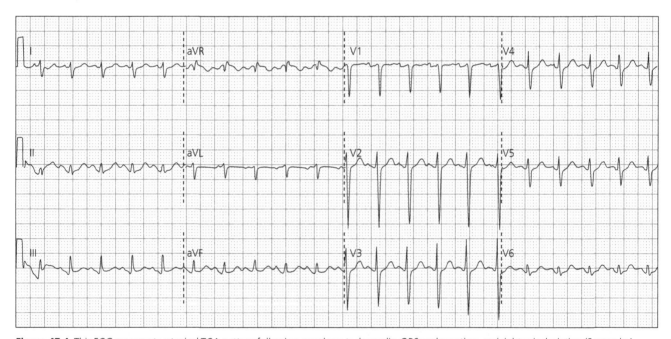

Figure 47.4 This ECG represents a typical TCA pattern following overdose: tachycardia, QRS prolongation, and right axis deviation (S wave in I, S wave in aVL, and R in terminal aVR).

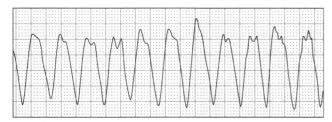

Figure 47.5 Wide complex tachydysrhythmia following TCA overdose representing ventricular tachycardia.

pre-established QRS interval cutoffs, finding 76% of controls (n = 117) and 82% of psychotropic drug overdoses with serious arrhythmias (n = 39) had a QRS ≥ 100 ms. Also, a QRS ≥ 160 ms only occurred in 2% of controls and in 13% of those with arrhythmias [7]. This suggests that a QRS of 160 ms is not an absolute predictor of dysrhythmias as inferred in the Boehnert and Lovejoy study, although there was a correlation between the incidence of arrhythmia and prolonged QRS [7].

Table 47.1 Pooled statistical data for QRS ≥ 100 ms, adapted from meta-analysis by Bailey *et al.* [3]

Criteria	# of studies included	# of subjects included	Pooled sensitivity (95% CI)	Pooled specificity (95% CI)
QRS to predict death	5	599	0.81 (0.54–0.94)	0.62 (0.55–0.68)
QRS to predict seizures	11	1334	0.69 (0.57–0.78)	0.69 (0.58–0.78)
QRS to predict ventricular arrhythmia	7	587	0.79 (0.58–0.91)	0.46 (0.35–0.59)

An early retrospective study by Hulton and Heath observed an increased incidence of respiratory depression, coma, and convulsions in TCA overdoses with a QRS > 100 ms [8], and a more recent prospective cohort series of 79 patients with TCA overdoses showed a prolonged mean QRS interval (147 ms, SD = 57) in those with seizure or arrhythmia (17/79 cases) compared with controls (96 ms, SD = 28) [9]. However, Liebelt and colleagues found that the QRS ≥ 100 ms produced a sensitivity of 82% and specificity of 58% for seizures or arrhythmias, with a PPV of only 35%, and thus concluded that QRS interval was not a significant independent predictor of those outcomes. This study did show a negative predictive value (NPV) of 92% for seizures or arrhythmias with a QRS > 100 ms, similar to those values in a study by Buckley and colleagues, who calculated NPVs of approximately 94.7%, 94.4%, and 93.7% for QRS intervals > 100, > 120, and > 160 ms, respectively – values initially proposed as predictors of outcome in the oft-referenced Boehnert and Lovejoy study [4]. While those statistics cannot be used to rule out seizure/arrhythmia risk, they suggest a potential role in lowering one's clinical suspicion of such outcomes in cases of TCA toxicity with a QRS < 100 ms.

There has also been some discussion on the reliability of measured QRS intervals in the clinical setting. One study that considered observer variation in manually measured QRS intervals in TCA poisoning found that three blinded interpreters disagreed on whether the QRS interval was greater or less than 100 ms in approximately 20% of cases (45/231). Thus, this cautioned against over-reliance on specific QRS interval cutoffs in determining the need for seizure or arrhythmia monitoring [7]. Additionally, the authors suggested that results from previous studies associating measured QRS interval lengths with risk of complications should also be interpreted with caution, as many did not blind ECG interpreters to outcome nor consider inter-rater variation.

Ultimately, many of these studies involve statistical analysis on a relatively small number of cases. While the meta-analysis by Bailey and colleagues provides a useful gestalt by which to infer risk of certain outcomes using the QRS duration, the existing literature unfortunately cannot be used to provide an absolute answer in the clinical setting. At best, the QRS interval duration can be used to stratify high risk versus low risk of outcomes such as seizure, arrhythmia, and or death, to be used in conjunction with other clinical findings to guide management of TCA overdoses.

Literature does exist regarding outcome compared with QRS duration for a few other medications outside of TCAs, with much of the remaining studies focusing on beta-blockers. Beta-blocker toxicity commonly manifests as bradycardia and/or hypotension, resulting mainly from the antagonist effect at beta-adrenergic receptor sites. However, some beta-blockers such as acebutolol, betaxolol, oxprenolol, and propranolol also have "membrane-stabilizing" activity via sodium channel-blockade [10]. Therefore, in cases of suspected beta-blocker overdose, there remains a possibility for cardiac conduction delays and subsequent QRS prolongation, suggesting the utility of determining a correlation between QRS length and outcomes in cases of beta-blocker toxicity.

A retrospective review of 52,156 beta-blocker-related exposures with 164 fatalities found that propranolol was responsible for the greatest number of exposures (44%) and a relatively high percentage of fatalities (71%) in beta-blocker toxicity [11]. Similarly, a prospective cohort study of 280 beta-blocker exposures noted that in the 16 cases with cardiovascular morbidities not complicated by a cardioactive co-ingestant, 94% (15/16) involved beta-blockers with membrane-stabilizing activity, with the most significant fraction (8/16) of these cases due to propranolol overdose [11]. Though based on a relatively small number of morbid cases, both studies suggest propranolol, and its sodium channel-blocking activity, may be associated with a greater risk of negative outcomes in isolated beta-blocker overdose.

One study by Reith and colleagues involving 55 admissions for beta-blocker poisoning found that propranolol (ingested in 28/55 cases) was the only beta-blocker in the study associated with seizure or death [12]. Furthermore, there was a significant association between a widened QRS interval and risk of seizures, with the sensitivity and specificity of a QRS > 100 ms for predicting seizure calculated at 62% and 90%, respectively [12]. However, given the relatively high specificity and lower sensitivity noted in the aforementioned study, researchers proposed that while a QRS > 100 ms indicates a higher risk of seizure, a QRS < 100 ms cannot be used to rule out such risk in the clinical setting [12].

Case conclusions

In Case 1, a total of 8 amps of sodium bicarbonate are infused IV over the ensuing hour at which time her ECG in Figure 47.6

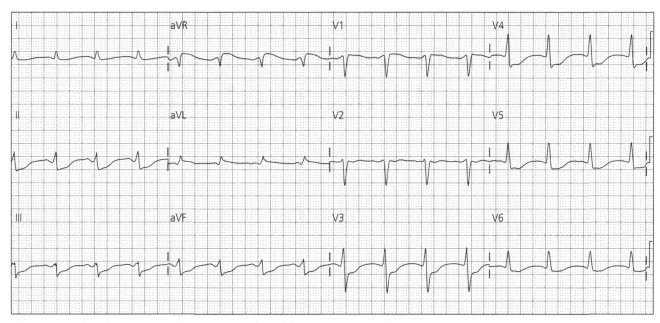

Figure 47.6 Sodium bicarbonate results in narrowing of QRS from previous ECG noted in Figure 47.3.

was noted. She was placed on a sodium bicarbonate continuous infusion consisting of 3 amps of sodium bicarbonate (50 mEq per amp of sodium) in 1 L of D5W with 40 mEq of KCl given at a rate of 200 cc/h to maintain an arterial pH of 7.50–7.55. The patient stabilized hemodynamically and was extubated 48 h later without complication. She was subsequently admitted to the psychiatric service.

In Case 2, a total of 4 amps of sodium bicarbonate were infused and the patient converted to a sinus tachycardia with rate of 130 bpm. He was subsequently placed on a sodium bicarbonate continuous infusion (3 amps of sodium bicarbonate [50 mEq per amp of sodium] in 1 L of D5W with 40 mEq of KCl infused at a rate of 200 cc/h to maintain an arterial pH of 7.50–7.55) and he develops no further dysrhythmias. He is discharged to a psychiatric facility after resolution of all signs and symptoms.

References

1 Woolf AD, Erdman AR, Nelson LS, *et al.* Tricyclic antidepressant poisoning: an evidence-based consensus guideline for out-of-hospital management. *Clin Toxicol (Phila)* 2007;**45**(3):203–33.

2 Harrigan RA, Brady WJ. ECG abnormalities in tricyclic antidepressant ingestion. *Am J Emerg Med* 1999;**17**(4):387–93.

3 Bailey B, Buckley NA, Amre DK. A meta-analysis of prognostic indicators to predict seizures, arrhythmias or death after tricyclic antidepressant overdose. *J Toxicol Clin Toxicol* 2004;**42**(6):877–88.

4 Boehnert MT, Lovejoy FH, Jr. Value of the QRS duration versus the serum drug level in predicting seizures and ventricular arrhythmias after an acute overdose of tricyclic antidepressants. *N Engl J Med* 1985;**313**(8):474–9.

5 Liebelt EL, Francis PD, Woolf AD. ECG lead aVR versus QRS interval in predicting seizures and arrhythmias in acute tricyclic antidepressant toxicity. *Ann Emerg Med* 1995;**26**(2):195–201.

6 Foulke GE, Albertson TE. QRS interval in tricyclic antidepressant overdosage: inaccuracy as a toxicity indicator in emergency settings. *Ann Emerg Med* 1987;**16**(2):160–3.

7 Buckley NA, O'Connell DL, Whyte IM, Dawson AH. Interrater agreement in the measurement of QRS interval in tricyclic antidepressant overdose: implications for monitoring and research. *Ann Emerg Med* 1996;**28**(5):515–19.

8 Hulten BA, Adams R, Askenasi R, *et al.* Predicting severity of tricyclic antidepressant overdose. *J Toxicol Clin Toxicol* 1992;**30**(2):161–70.

9 Liebelt EL, Ulrich A, Francis PD, Woolf A. Serial electrocardiogram changes in acute tricyclic antidepressant overdoses. *Crit Care Med* 1997;**25**(10):1721–6.

10 Shepherd G. Treatment of poisoning caused by beta-adrenergic and calcium-channel blockers. *Am J Health Syst Pharm* 2006;**63**(19):1828–35.

11 Love JN, Howell JM, Litovitz TL, Klein-Schwartz W. Acute beta blocker overdose: factors associated with the development of cardiovascular morbidity. *J Toxicol Clin Toxicol* 2000;**38**(3):275–81.

12 Reith DM, Dawson AH, Epid D, *et al.* Relative toxicity of beta blockers in overdose. *J Toxicol Clin Toxicol* 1996;**34**(3):273–8.

Chapter 48 | What is the treatment for wide complex dysrhythmias in the poisoned patient?

David T. Lawrence

University of Virginia School of Medicine, Charlottesville, VA, USA

Case presentations

Case 1: A 49-year-old female presents to the emergency department (ED) following an overdose of amitriptyline. She is obtunded and requires intubation for airway protection. She has a heart rate of 110 and a blood pressure of 64/36, which does not improve after an intravenous fluid bolus. The electrocardiogram (ECG) is noted in Figure 48.1.

Case 2: A 34-year-old male arrives at the ED after an overdose of sotolol and ethanol. He is lethargic, with a heart rate of 38 and a blood pressure of 81/42. His ECG reveals a QTc interval of 660 ms (Figure 48.2). After administration of intravenous fluids and 5 mg of glucagon, the patient's blood pressure increases to 105/61. The patient begins to have frequent episodes of polymorphic ventricular tachycardia (PVT) as noted in Figure 48.3. Despite the infusion of 6 g of magnesium sulfate, the patient continues to have frequent runs of PVT.

Treatment for wide complex dysrhythmias in the poisoned patient

There are two main drug-induced etiologies for wide complex dysrhythmias in the poisoned patient. First, blockage of the cardiac sodium channels results in prolongation of phase 0 of depolarization and subsequent widening of the QRS. This also decreases inotropy by reducing the amount of calcium entering the myocytes [1] and contributes to hypotension. The majority of cardiac sodium channel-blockers are also sympathomimetic or anti-cholinergic, resulting in tachycardia. The electrocardiographic pattern (tachycardia with QRS prolongation) with associated hypotension is difficult to distinguish from a ventricular arrhythmia (Figure 48.4).

Critical Decisions in Emergency and Acute Care Electrocardiography,
1st edition. Edited by W.J. Brady and J.D. Truwit. © 2009 Blackwell Publishing, ISBN: 9781405159067.

Second, blockage of cardiac potassium efflux-channels results in the prolongation of phase 3 of depolarization and subsequent prolongation of the QT interval. This can lead to PVT (torsade de pointes).

Sodium channel-blockade

Serum alkalinization and/or the administration of sodium are the accepted treatments for cardiotoxicity secondary to a sodium channel-blocking agent. There are numerous animal studies and human case reports of intravenous sodium bicarbonate being used successfully after poisoning with sodium channel-blocking agents [2–7]. There are several proposed mechanisms for the efficacy of sodium bicarbonate. First, the sodium load overcomes the sodium channel-blockade. Second, serum alkalinization prevents binding of the toxin to the sodium channel [8]. Evidence supporting both mechanisms comes from animal and *in vitro* experiments.

Sodium loading: There are a number of case reports describing the utilization of hypertonic saline (3% NaCl) in the management of cardiac sodium channel-blocker toxicity. For example, there is a report of hypertonic saline improving hypotension and decreasing QRS duration in a patient poisoned with nortriptyline. The decision to utilize hypertonic saline was made because the patient had already developed significant alkalemia due to hyperventilation and sodium bicarbonate administration [9]. There have been multiple animal experiments demonstrating successful reversal of sodium channel-blockade with hypertonic saline, but with varying results when compared with other therapies. Hypertonic sodium chloride was found to be more effective than sodium bicarbonate or respiratory alkalosis in improving hypotension and reducing QRS duration in a swine model of nortriptyline poisoning [10]. However, a study utilizing a rat model of desipramine poisoning showed equal efficacy between hypertonic saline and sodium bicarbonate [11].

Alkalinization: Studies attempting to treat cardiotoxicity with alkalinization alone have had mixed results. In a study using a canine model of amitriptyline toxicity, alkalinization

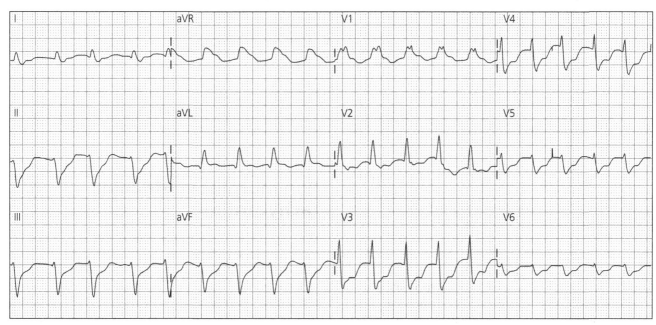

Figure 48.1 ECG demonstrating sinus tachycardia with marked prolongation of the QRS complex (160 ms).

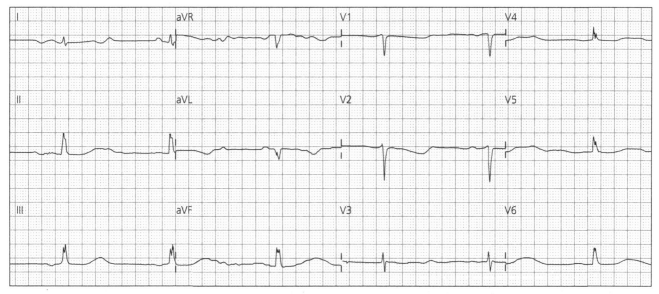

Figure 48.2 ECG demonstrating sinus bradycardia with marked QT prolongation (660 ms).

with a sodium-free buffer was effective in reversing QRS widening [12]. Studies comparing the benefit of hypertonic sodium chloride, sodium bicarbonate, and hyperventilation have found hyperventilation not to be effective [10,11], although respiratory acidosis did exacerbate toxicity [11].

Sodium bicarbonate: A study using canine models poisoned with amitriptyline showed that sodium bicarbonate infusion could convert ventricular tachycardia to sinus rhythm [13]. Another canine model revealed sodium bicar-

bonate to be superior to placebo in treating ECG changes due to cocaine poisoning [14]. A canine model of amitriptyline poisoning found sodium bicarbonate more effective in preventing ventricular arrhythmias than hypertonic saline [15]. Another canine model showed that sodium bicarbonate was superior to sodium chloride in reducing ECG changes due to cocaine, suggesting that alkalinization provides added benefit [16]. Multiple other animal models of tricyclic antidepressant poisoning have shown superiority of sodium bicarbonate over hypertonic saline or hyperventilation.

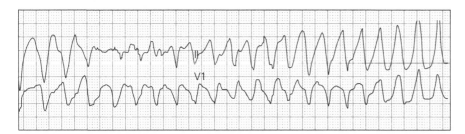

Figure 48.3 Rhythm strip of Case 2 demonstrating PVT.

A review of the above evidence leads to the recommendation that intravenous sodium bicarbonate should be the treatment of choice for cardiac toxicity secondary to cardiac sodium channel-blocker poisoning. Sodium bicarbonate administration should be considered for either: a QRS interval over 100 ms, hypotension refractory to intravenous fluids in the presence of a sodium channel-blocking drug, or dysrhythmias [17]. It is reasonable to add hypertonic saline if a patient is still demonstrating cardiac dysfunction despite adequate alkalinization. Hyperventilation may add benefit by increasing alkalinization in a patient who is hypernatremic and not a candidate for further sodium loading. Care must be taken to achieve a pH of between 7.45 and 7.55, inducing excessive alkalemia can be detrimental [18]. This can be due to cerebral vasoconstriction [19] impaired tissue oxygen delivery, hypokalemia, and reduction of ionized calcium [20].

Anti-dysrhythmics: The class 1b anti-dysrhythmics phenytoin and lidocaine have been used to treat arrhythmias caused by sodium channel-blocking agents [21,22]. This is likely because combining two agents with different binding kinetics will reduce the effect of the agent with slower-binding kinetics by competing for a binding site on the sodium channel or allosteric modulation [23]. One study showed less dramatic and more transient arrhythmia reversal with lidocaine compared with sodium bicarbonate [15]. An animal model showed an increase in toxicity when phenytoin was used to prevent toxicity secondary to amitriptyline [24]. Lidocaine increased seizures and death in a rat model of cocaine poisoning [25]. Amiodarone has been tested in two animal models of tricyclic anti-depressant poisoning without showing significant benefit [26,27]. Due to the unproven efficacy and potential dangers of using anti-dysrhythmics to treat arrhythmias secondary to sodium channel-blockade, and the proven benefit of sodium bicarbonate, the use of anti-dysrhythmics cannot be recommended.

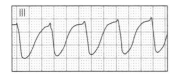

Figure 48.4 A rhythm strip of a wide complex dysrhythmia following a hydroxychloroquine overdose due to marked QRS prolongation.

Polymorphic ventricular tachycardia

Most reported episodes of drug-induced PVT are self-limited. However, these episodes can become sustained and have the potential to deteriorate into hemodynamically unstable ventricular tachycardia or ventricular fibrillation [28]. If this occurs, defibrillation is necessary to restore a perfusing rhythm. Defibrillation can convert PVT to a sinus rhythm, but recurrence of PVT is likely. Recognizing the cause and discontinuing any QT prolonging medicines is an important action in preventing PVT. Potassium should be maintained in the high normal range, as hypokalemia will reduce the rapid component of the delayed rectifying current [29]. Two treatments can be utilized to treat drug-induced PVT: magnesium and overdrive pacing.

Magnesium: Magnesium has been used successfully to treat drug-associated PVT [28,30,31] and should be considered the primary treatment. Magnesium administration is beneficial even in patients with normal serum magnesium [28]. Administration of magnesium does not shorten the QT interval [31]. The mechanism behind magnesium's efficacy is either its ability to act as a calcium channel-blocker preventing afterdepolarization, or by facilitating potassium influx into cells through its action as a co-factor in Na^+/K^+-ATPase activity [32].

Pacing: Overdrive pacing can be effective in treating drug-induced PVT that is resistant to other treatments [33]. This modality is effective due to several proposed mechanisms, including decreasing the QT dispersion [34]. Typically, the goal is to achieve a heart rate of 90–110 bpm. In situations where pacing is unavailable or contraindicated, isoproterenol can be administered with a goal of achieving a heart rate of over 90 bpm [28].

Case conclusions

In Case 1, 3 amps of sodium bicarbonate (150 mEq) were administered to the patient and the blood pressure improved to 89/42 mmHg and the QRS interval narrowed (Figure 48.5). The patient remained unresponsive on the ventilator. Sodium

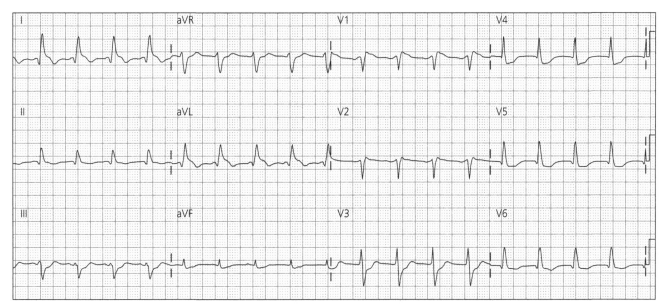

Figure 48.5 Subsequent ECG from Case 1 demonstrating sinus tachycardia with narrowing of the QRS complex (~140 ms) after 100 mEq of sodium bicarbonate.

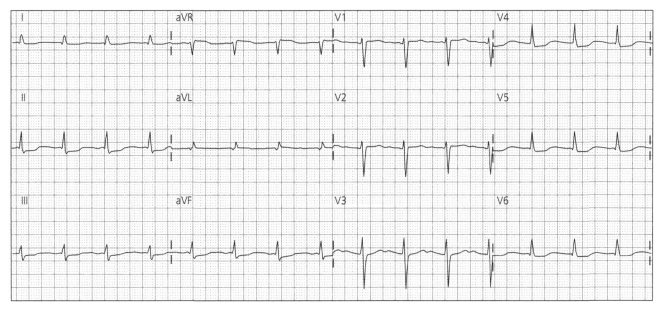

Figure 48.6 Final ECG from Case 1 demonstrating narrowed QRS complex (100 ms) after a total of 250 mEq of sodium bicarbonate.

Figure 48.7 Rhythm strip of Case 2 following administration of isoproterenol, bringing the patient's heart rate to 75. The patient ceased having runs of PVT.

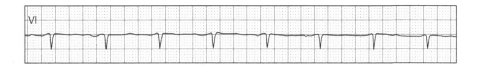

bicarbonate boluses were administered to maintain a pH of 7.5. The patient's blood pressure stabilized at 136/72 and the QRS continued to narrow (Figure 48.6). On the hospital day #3, the patient was alert, co-operative, and had normal vital signs.

The patient in Case 2 continued to have frequent episodes of PVT despite treatment with magnesium sulfate. The deci-

sion to initiate overdrive pacing was made. Due to previous cardiac surgery, the patient was not a candidate for transvenous pacing. Therefore, isoproterenol was administered and titrated to a heart rate of 75 (Figure 48.7). The patient had no further episodes of ventricular arrhythmia. The patient's QT interval and heart rate normalized and he was discharged from the medical service on hospital day #3.

Reference

1 Kolecki P, Curry S. Poisoning by sodium channel blocking agents. *Crit Care Clin* 1997;**13**(4):829–48.

2 Kerns W, Garvey L, Owens J. Cocaine-induced wide complex dysrhythmia. J Emerg Med 1997;**15**(3):321–9.

3 Ortega-Carnicer J, Bertos-Polo J, Gutirrez-Tirado C. Aborted sudden death, transient Brugada pattern, and wide QRS dysrrhythmias after massive cocaine ingestion. *J Electrocardiol* 2001; **34**(4):345–9.

4 Stork CM, Redd JT, Fine K, *et al.* Propoxyphene-induced wide QRS complex dysrhythmia responsive to sodium bicarbonate: a case report. *Clin Toxicol* 1995;**33**(2):179–83.

5 Donovan KD, Gerace RV, Gerace R, *et al.* Acebutolol-induced ventricular tachycardia reversed with sodium bicarbonate. *Clin Toxicol* 1999;**37**(4):481–4.

6 Sharma AN, Hexdall AH, Chang EK, *et al.* Diphenhydramine-induced wide complex dysrhythmia responds to treatment with sodium bicarbonate. *Amer J Emerg Med* 2003;**21**(3):212–15.

7 Goldman MJ, Mowry JB, Kirk MA. Sodium bicarbonate to correct widened QRS in a case of flecainide overdose. *J Emerg Med* 1997;**15**(2):183–6.

8 Seger DL. A critical reconsideration of the clinical effects and treatment recommendations for sodium channel blocking drug cardiotoxicity. *Toxicol Reviews* 2006;**25**(4):283–96.

9 McKinney PE, Rasmussen R. Reversal of severe tricyclic antidepressant-induced cardiotoxicity with intravenous hypertonic saline solution. *Annals Emerg Med* 2003;**42**(1):20–4.

10 McCabe JL, Cobaugh DJ, Menegazzi JJ, *et al.* Experimental tricyclic antidepressant toxicity: a randomized, controlled comparison of hypertonic saline solution, sodium bicarbonate, and hyperventilation. *Annals Emerg Med* 1998;**32**(3):329–33.

11 Pentel P, Benowitz N. Efficacy and mechanism of action of sodium bicarbonate in the treatment of desipramine toxicity in rats. *J Pharmacol Exp Ther* 1984;**230**(1):12–19.

12 Stone CK, Kraemer CM, Carroll R, *et al.* Does a sodium-free buffer affect QRS width in experimental amitriptyline overdose? *Annals Emerg Med* 1995;**26**(1):58–64.

13 Sasyniuk BI, Jhamandas V, Valois M. Experimental amitriptyline intoxication: Treatment of cardiac toxicity with sodium bicarbonate. *Annals Emerg Med* 1986;**15**(9):1052–9.

14 Wilson LD, Shelat C. Electrophysiologic and hemodynamic effects of sodium bicarbonate in a canine model of severe cocaine intoxication. *Clin Toxicol* 2003;**41**(6):777–88.

15 Nattel S, Mittleman M. Treatment of ventricular tachyarrhythmias resulting from amitriptyline toxicity in dogs. *J Pharmacol Exp Ther* 1984;**231**(2):430–5.

16 Parker RB, Perry GY, Horan LG, *et al.* Comparative effects of sodium bicarbonate and sodium chloride on reversing cocaine-induced changes in the electrocardiogram. *J Cardiovasc Pharmacol* 1999;**34**(6):864–9.

17 Holstege CP, Dobmeier S. Cardiovascular challenges in toxicology. *Emerg Med Clin North Am* 2005;**23**(4):1195–217.

18 Bradberry SM, Thanacoody HKR, Watt BE, *et al.* Management of the cardiovascular complications of tricyclic antidepressant poisoning: role of sodium bicarbonate. *Toxicol Reviews* 2005; **24**(3):195–204.

19 Apkon M, Boron WF. Extracellular and intracellular alkalinization and the constriction of rat cerebral arterioles. *J Physiol* 1995; **484**:743–53.

20 Wrenn K, Smith BA, Slovis CM. Profound alkalemia during treatment of tricyclic antidepressant overdose: A potential Hazard of combined hyperventilation and intravenous bicarbonate. *Am J Emerg Med* 1992;**10**(6):553–5.

21 Bauman JL, Gallastegui J, Tanenbaum SR, *et al.* Flecainide-induced sustained ventricular tachycardia successfully treated with lidocaine. *Chest* 1987;**92**(3):573–5.

22 Hagerman GA, Hanashiro PK. Reversal of tricyclic-antidepressant-induced cardiac conduction abnormalities by phenytoin. *Annals Emerg Med* 1981;**10**(2):82–6.

23 Barber MJ, Starmer CF, Grant AO. Blockade of cardiac sodium channels by amitriptyline and diphenylhydantoin. Evidence for two use-dependent binding sites. *Circ Res* 1991;**69**(3):677–96.

24 Callaham M, Schumaker H, Pentel P. Phenytoin prophylaxis of cardiotoxicity in experimental amitriptyline poisoning. *J Pharmacol Exp Ther* 1988;**245**(1):216–20.

25 Derlet RW, Albertson TE. Lidocaine potentiation of cocaine toxicity. *Annals Emerg Med* 1991;**20**(2):135–8.

26 Barrueto F, Chuang A, Cotter BW, *et al.* Amiodarone fails to improve survival in amitriptyline-poisoned mice. *Clin Toxicol* 2005;**43**(3):147–9.

27 Barruteo F, Murr I, Meltzer A, *et al.* Effects of amiodarone in a swine model of nortriptyline toxicity. *J Med Toxicol* 2006;**2**(4): 147–51.

28 Gupta A, Lawrence AT, Krishnan K, *et al.* Current concepts in the mechanisms and management of drug-induced QT prolongation and torsade de pointes. *Am Heart J* 2007;**153**(6):891–9.

29 Kannankeril PJ, Roden DM. Drug-induced long QT and torsade de pointes: recent advances. *Curr Opin Cardiol* 2007;**22**(1): 39–43.

30 Gowda RM, Khan IA, Wilbur SL, *et al.* Torsade de pointes: the clinical considerations. *Int J Cardiol* 2004;**96**(1):1–6.

31 Kao LW, Furbee RB. Drug-induced Q-T prolongation. *Med Clin* 2005;**89**(6):1125–44.

32 Tzivoni D, Banai S, Schuger C, *et al.* Treatment of torsade de pointes with magnesium sulfate. *Circulation* 1988;**77**(2):392–7.

33 Paris DG, Parente TF, Bruschetta HR, *et al.* Torsades de pointes induced by erythromycin and terfenadine. *Am J Emerg Med* 1994;**12**(5):636–8.

34 Thomsen MB, Volders PA, Beekman JM, *et al.* Beat-to-beat variability of repolarization determines proarrhythmic outcome in dogs susceptible to drug-induced torsades de pointes. *J Am Coll Cardiol* 2006;**48**(6):1268–76.

Part 7 | **Electrocardiographic Differential Diagnosis**

Chapter 49 | What is the ECG differential diagnosis of ST segment elevation?

Richard A. Harrigan[1], Theodore C. Chan[2]
[1]Temple University, Philadelphia, PA, USA
[2]University of California, San Diego, CA, USA

Case presentations

Case 1: A 74-year-old diabetic woman presents to the emergency department (ED) after a near-syncopal event at home. This occurred without prodrome, and there was no history of chest pain, dyspnea, nausea, or dizziness. She has no history of volume loss, melena, or other blood loss. On evaluation, her vital signs are: temperature 98 °F, heart rate 78 beats per minute (bpm), respiration 24 breaths per minute, and blood pressure 100/68 mmHg; there are no significant changes on orthostatic measurement. Her oxygen saturation is 98%. There is no diaphoresis or conjunctival pallor. The heart examination is normal, the lungs demonstrate fine rales at the bases, and the abdominal examination is normal. Her electrocardiogram (ECG) on presentation to the ED is shown in Figure 49.1.

Case 2: A 56-year-old female with chronic kidney disease, on hemodialysis, presents to the ED with dyspnea, nausea, and fatigue. She has missed her last two hemodialysis appointments. The patient has no history of chest pain, vomiting, or diaphoresis. On physical examination, her temperature is normal, her heart rate is 70 bpm, her respiratory rate is 28 breaths per minute, and her blood pressure is 196/112 mmHg in both arms. Her neck shows jugular venous distention, her heart has a II/VI systolic murmur without a rub, and her lungs have bilateral rales. The abdomen is non-tender, and the legs show symmetric pedal edema without erythema or cords. The sensorium is clear, and there is no neurologic focality. The patient's initial ECG is seen in Figure 49.2.

ST segment elevation

Elevation of the ST segment on the 12-lead ECG is potentially one of the most ominous findings in electrocardiography.

Critical Decisions in Emergency and Acute Care Electrocardiography, 1st edition. Edited by W.J. Brady and J.D. Truwit. © 2009 Blackwell Publishing, ISBN: 9781405159067.

Causes range from life-threatening entities such as acute ST segment elevation myocardial infarction (STEMI) to non-pathologic normal variants, such as benign early repolarization (BER). Indeed, it has been argued that as most men have some degree of ST segment elevation (STE) on their normal, symptom-free resting ECG, some degree of STE is a normal finding, rather than a normal variant, in this population [1]. Two large studies have found that over 90% of healthy men have some degree of STE on their ECG, more commonly in their younger adult years, and more commonly in the mid-to-right precordial leads (V1–V4). By age 76, only 30% of men still have this STE. Women less frequently exhibit this normal finding – with about 20% displaying STE of 1 mm or more – a figure that does not vary with age [1–3]. Due to the ubiquity of STE, the emergency physician (EP) must learn to distinguish the many different causes of STE for two reasons: to recognize and appropriately treat pathology when it occurs, and to not treat STE that is either normal, or normally found as part of a non-STEMI, STE syndrome.

ECG differential diagnosis of ST segment elevation

The ST segment represents that part of the cardiac cycle that occurs after the ventricle has been depolarized (the QRS complex), but before the ventricle is repolarized (the T wave). It runs from the J point, which marks the junction of the QRS complex and the ST segment, to the beginning of the T wave. The ST segment should be examined for deviation from the baseline, although there is some dispute over what portion of the waveform should be used as the baseline for purposes of comparison. Classically, the *TP segment* is used (that portion of the tracing that approximates an isoelectric course, from the end of the T wave of the preceding cardiac cycle to the beginning of the P wave of the next cardiac cycle). Others have argued that the *end of the PR segment* should be used as the baseline for measurement of STE; more precisely, it should be measured from the upper edge of the PR segment to the upper edge of the J point (which marks the beginning of the ST segment). The PR segment may be

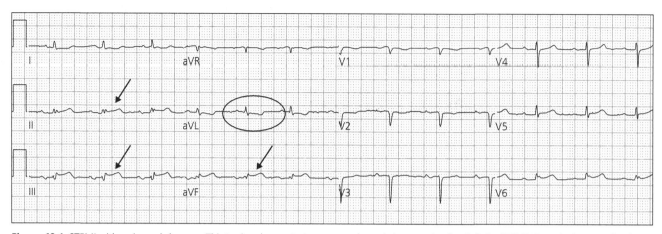

Figure 49.1 STEMI with reciprocal changes. This tracing demonstrates a somewhat subtle example of an inferior STEMI. Note the low-amplitude STE in the inferior leads (*bold arrows*), greatest in lead III. The ST depression in lead aVL is a reciprocal change (*circle*), and is a key to the cause of the STE.

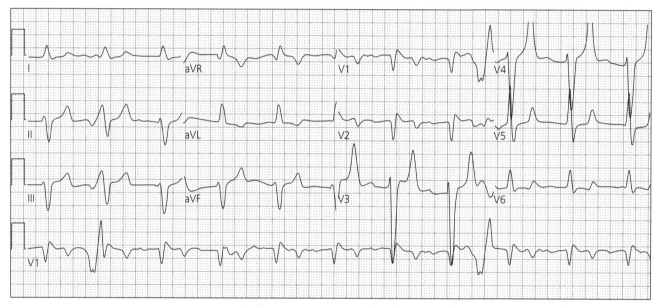

Figure 49.2 Hyperkalemia. Note the downsloping STE in leads V1 and V2, and the more horizontal-to-concave STE in leads V3 and V4 – where the classic peaked T waves of hyperkalemia are best seen in this tracing. The PR, QRS, and QT intervals are all prolonged. The ECG normalized after treatment with calcium salts, nebulized beta adrenergic agonists, and insulin/glucose.

slightly depressed below the isoelectric line (and thus below the TP segment) due to the atrial repolarization wave that follows atrial depolarization (manifested by the P wave) [4,5].

Amplitude, contour, and distribution of STE: Like ST segment depression, STE is measured in millimeters (mm). In addition to quantifying the *amplitude* of STE in mm, the *contour of the STE* must also be analyzed. ST elevation contour can be termed "concave," meaning upwardly scooped with the open aspect directed upward (able to "hold water"), or "convex," meaning upwardly domed with the open aspect directed downward (unable to "hold water"). Lastly, the ST segment may be "obliquely straight," meaning the course

from the end of the QRS complex to the apex of the P wave is an ascending horizontal line (Figure 49.3). Finally, the *distribution* of the morphologic changes in STE syndromes is paramount to determining the cause of that STE. ST elevation that occurs in a regional distribution – e.g. inferiorly, in leads II, III, and aVF – is suggestive of STEMI. Similarly, the distribution of STE in other STE syndromes discussed below bears an important clue as to the etiology of that STE.

Although amplitude, contour, and distribution are all important characteristics of STE, there is significant overlap between STE syndromes with respect to these characteristics. That is to say, the EP must consider these characteristics as generalities and not absolutes. Furthermore, the ST segment must also be examined in the context in which it occurs; this

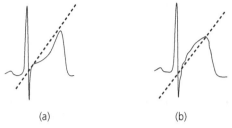

(a)   (b)

Figure 49.3 Morphology of ST segment elevation. Note the differing contours of the ST segments in the figure. The waveform in (a) demonstrates concave STE, highlighted by its coved, scooped pitch below the imaginary diagonal. The waveform in (b) features convex STE, with its domed ascent above the imaginary diagonal.

includes the *clinical context* (how the patient appears; the history of the present illness), and the *morphologic context* of the ECG. ST elevation in the morphologic context of a widened QRS complex (duration > 0.12 s) in the clinical context of an asymptomatic person should invoke consideration of bundle branch block (see below), given it occurs in the proper distribution. Conversely, seemingly trivial 1 mm STE in the inferior leads (II, III, and aVF) in a patient with a compelling story for an acute myocardial infarction who is diaphoretic on examination deserves consideration for an evolving STEMI.

Differential considerations in ST segment elevation

The causes of STE on the ECG are myriad; differentiation can be confusing. Furthermore, two or more coincident processes may occur on one tracing (e.g. a STEMI in a patient with a prior BER pattern). Table 49.1 displays the differential diagnosis for STE, with a somewhat arbitrary division of syndromes into those encountered more commonly versus those seen more rarely. This discussion will focus on those entities listed in the "more common" list, in addition to Brugada syndrome and ventricular aneurysm. The remainder of the syndromes found in the "less common" list are usually made apparent by the clinical context.

Acute myocardial infarction: ST elevation in the context of an acute myocardial infarction (AMI) may signify a STEMI. The hallmarks of a STEMI begin with regional distribution of ST segment changes (Table 49.2). Although the first evidence of STEMI on the ECG is the hyperacute T wave, this is closely followed in time by STE, and the two may coincide on the tracing. Classically, the STE of AMI is convex, with this morphology being more specific for AMI. However, the *contour* may be concave (especially early on) or obliquely straight. In one series, 43% of angiographically proven STEMIs involving the left anterior descending coronary artery had a concave contour, whereas 32% had an obliquely straight contour, and the remaining 24% had the classic convex

Table 49.1 Differential diagnosis of ST segment elevation

Relatively common and/or commonly manifests STE	Relatively uncommon and/or uncommonly manifests STE
Acute myocardial infarction	Brugada syndrome
Benign early repolarization	Ventricular aneurysm
Acute pericarditis	Central nervous system injury
Left ventricular hypertrophy	Pulmonary embolism
Bundle branch block	Myocarditis
Ventricular paced rhythm	Cardiomyopathy
Hyperkalemia	Post-cardioversion
Hypothermia	Cardiac contusion

The division by frequency in this table is somewhat arbitrary; it should be remembered that any syndrome, or ECG finding, may be encountered by the EP at any time.

The syndromes in the "common" list are either common (e.g. BER, LVH, acute MI) or, when encountered, they commonly manifest STE (e.g. pericarditis). The syndromes in the "uncommon" list may be uncommonly seen (e.g. Brugada syndrome, ventricular aneurysm) – yet they nevertheless will manifest STE – or they may be common syndromes themselves (e.g. central nervous system injury, pulmonary embolism), which uncommonly manifest STE on the ECG.

Table 49.2 Regional distribution of ST segment elevation myocardial infarction

Region	STE leads
Anterior	V3, V4
Septal	V1, V2
Anteroseptal	V1, V2, V3, V4
Lateral	V5, V6, I, aVL
Anterolateral	V1–V6, I, aVL
Inferior	II, III, aVF
Posterior	V8, V9 (with ST depression in V1, V2)
Right ventricular	V4R; V3R–V6R; sometimes V1

shape [6]. At times, the STE of AMI will *distort the terminal portion of the QRS complex*, actually elevating before the R wave returns to baseline (Figure 49.4). This serves as a further clue that the STE is due to a STEMI [6]. The presence of *reciprocal changes* also increases the specificity for STE due to STEMI. Reciprocal changes are manifested as ST depression in a region that approximates the vector (at or nearly) 180 degrees opposite to the major vector of injury. For example, if lead aVL demonstrates ST depression while leads II, III, and aVF are demonstrating STE, this is suggestive of an inferior AMI. The vector of lead aVL (−30 degrees) is 150 degrees away from the major vector of most right coronary artery-mediated STEMIs, as the principal vector of injury in these cases is along the vector of lead III (+120 degrees) (Figure 49.1). Another harbinger of STE due to STEMI is a *change in the ECG tracing over time*. Coronary ischemia is a dynamic phenomenon, so one would expect the STE of AMI to change over time along with the clinical picture; serial ECGs or ST

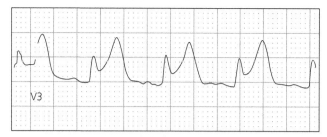

Figure 49.4 STEMI with distortion of the terminal portion of the QRS complex. In this lead V3 tracing, the downward leg of the R wave never reaches the baseline before the STE begins.

segment trend monitoring are useful in demonstrating this phenomenon. Finally, the *presence or emergence of Q waves* in the company of new STE increases the likelihood of STEMI as the cause for the STE, although ventricular aneurysm must also be considered in such circumstances (see below); as always, an old tracing for comparison is helpful in these situations.

Benign early repolarization: This is a fairly common, non-pathologic finding on the ECG, seen in approximately 1% of the population – mostly in individuals less than 50 years of age, rarely seen in those greater than 70 years of age [7,8]. In one series, it was found in 13% of ED patients presenting with STE, approximating that of STEMI at 15% [9]. Clearly, differentiation of STEMI from BER is important. In a study where EPs examined only the initial ECG from patients with chest pain, tracings showing BER were misinterpreted as AMI in 28% of cases, whereas ECGs demonstrating AMI were misdiagnosed as BER in 10% of cases [10].

Characteristics of STE due to BER (Figure 49.5) include the following: diffuse STE, usually seen more in the precordial (especially lead V4) than limb leads; J point elevation; notching or irregularity of the J point; concave contour of the elevated ST segments; prominent precordial T waves of large amplitude; and stability over time (and certainly during the clinical evaluation) [11]. Reciprocal ST depression can be seen in lead aVR, but not lead aVL, when the limb leads are involved with BER [1].

Pericarditis: This pathologic cause of STE can be difficult to distinguish from both BER and STEMI. Like BER, *many leads are involved* in pericarditis (it being a diffuse disease) as opposed to the usual regional pattern of STE seen in STEMI (Figure 49.6). ST segments are usually of the concave contour, and the J point is maintained. Using lead V6 as a discriminator, the *ratio of the amplitude of ST segment onset/T wave amplitude* has been found to be greater than 25% (or > 1 : 4) in acute pericarditis, and less than 25% in BER – where T waves are characteristically taller [12]. In diffuse pericarditis, the ST segment axis is closest to +45 degrees in the frontal plane, thus yielding *greater STE in lead II than in lead III*. This finding would be less common with inferior STEMI, which is most commonly due to occlusion of the right coronary artery – the vector axis of which is closer to that of lead III, thus resulting in a greater degree of STE in that lead compared with lead II. In the less common inferior AMIs due to proximal left circumflex disease, the ST segment vector is closer to that of lead aVF, yielding STE of equivalent height in leads II and III, with reciprocal ST depression in leads aVR and aVL. BER (with inferior lead involvement) and diffuse pericarditis should not manifest reciprocal ST depression in lead aVL on the ECG – although it may be seen in lead aVR [1]. PR segment depression (or PR segment elevation in lead aVR) is also seen with pericarditis, and, although present in some cases of BER and atrial infarction, it is also suggestive of pericarditis as the cause of STE on the ECG. Lastly, STE is rarely > 5 mm in pericarditis – but it may be so in AMI [1].

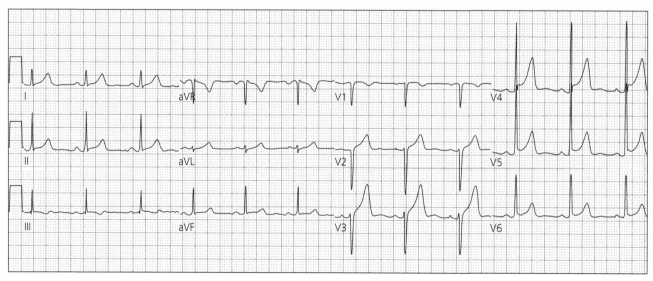

Figure 49.5 Benign early repolarization. Note the diffuse nature of the STE, although it is greater in the precordial leads, especially lead V4 where notching of the J point is seen. The T waves are characteristically large.

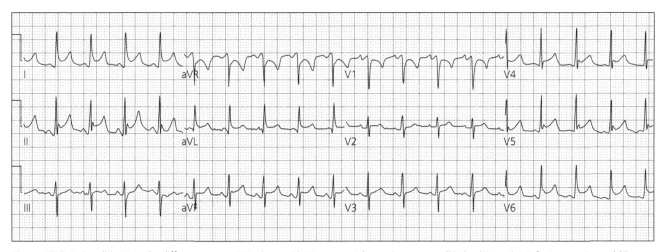

Figure 49.6 Pericarditis. Note the diffuse, concave STE, along with PR segment depression, seen well in lead II. Lead aVR features reciprocal ST depression and PR segment elevation.

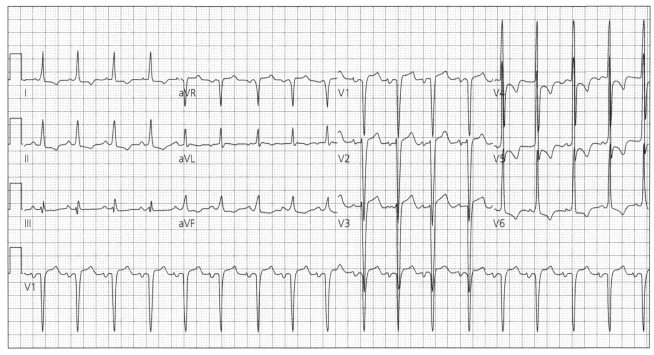

Figure 49.7 Left ventricular hypertrophy. In the right precordial leads (V1–V3), there is concave ST segment elevation; there are prominent upright T waves, and there are large QS (lead V1) and rS (leads V2, V3) waves. The left precordial leads (V5, V6, and in this tracing, V4) demonstrate large R waves with depressed ST segments and asymmetrically inverted T waves. The ST segment findings in V1–V3 seem to mirror those of V4–V6.

Left ventricular hypertrophy: Hypertrophy of the left ventricular wall, frequently resulting from longstanding hypertension, can present with STE (and ST depression) on the ECG. Approximately 30% of ED patients with chest pain were found to have left ventricular hypertrophy (LVH) on their ECG – this was the most frequently encountered cause of STE in this group [13,14]. This high frequency of LVH on the ECG has been reported in the prehospital population as well [15]. In LVH, the STE is seen in the right precordial leads (V1–V3), is concave in contour, and is associated with large amplitude QS or rS waves (due to the accentuated left-sided forces) as well as tall T waves. The STE is usually 2–4 mm, or at most 5 mm, in height [16]. The mirror image of this should appear in the left precordial leads (V6, sometimes V5) and the left-sided limb leads (I, aVL): ST depression with asymmetric T wave inversion (Figure 49.7). ST elevation due to left LVH, like that of BER and pericarditis, should be stable over the time of the clinical encounter; the ST changes seen

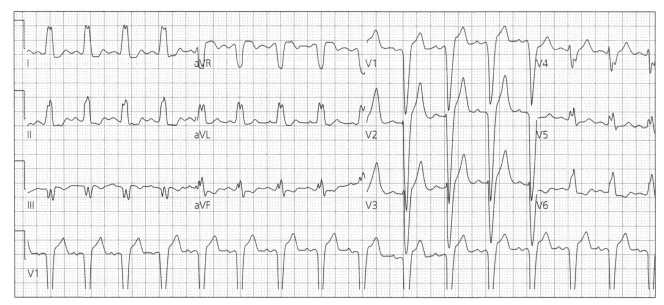

Figure 49.8 Left bundle branch block. The large QS and rS waveforms in leads V1–V3 are accompanied by discordantly elevated ST segments and large T waves in the same leads. Note the classic notched, monophasic R wave and discordant/depressed ST segment T wave complex in the left-sided leads as well (V5, V6, I, and aVL).

with STEMI are dynamic. Other clues to LVH on the ECG include QRS complex widening, left atrial enlargement, and left axis deviation; although none of these entities is necessary to diagnose LVH on the ECG, their presence implies significant left-sided chamber enlargement and wall thickness.

Bundle branch block: Similar to LVH, bundle branch block (BBB) patterns may present with ST segment changes on the ECG; left BBB (LBBB) features STE that is non-pathologic and part of the expected morphology due to the ventricular conduction delay. Characteristics of this LBBB pattern include a widened QRS complex (by definition > 0.12 s); large rS or QS complexes in the right precordial leads (V1–V2 or V3) with STE and large T waves; absence of septal Q waves (especially lead V6); and notched, monophasic R waves with discordant ST segment depression and T wave inversion in the left precordial and limb leads (V5, V6, I, and aVL). This STE in the right precordial leads resembles the changes seen in acute anteroseptal MI; key to distinguishing the two is recognition of the classic BBB pattern on the tracing (Figure 49.8). Criteria have been proposed to detect acute STEMI in the presence of LBBB (Table 49.3) [17]; these demonstrate good

Table 49.3 Sgarbossa criteria: acute MI with left bundle branch block [17]

ST segment elevation ≥ 1 mm *concordant* with the QRS complex
ST segment depression ≥ 1 mm in leads V1, V2, or V3
This will be *concordant* with the QRS complex as well
ST segment elevation ≥ 5 mm *discordant* with the QRS complex

specificity but inadequate sensitivity for acute STEMI. Basically, concordant (i.e. the ST segment is on the same side of the isoelectric line as the major portion of the QRS complex) STE or concordant ST depression in the affected leads with LBBB is suggestive of acute STEMI, and overly discordant (> 5 mm) STE in the affected leads (V1–V3) is suggestive (but not as robustly as the concordant changes) of acute STEMI.

Ventricular paced rhythm: Like BBB, the ventricular paced rhythm (VPR) will present a wide QRS complex (as the impulse originates in the ventricle) and discordant STE as part of the normal baseline tracing. Pacemaker spikes, which make recognition of this rhythm easy, are not always evident on the ECG tracing. Like LBBB, a right ventricular paced rhythm will demonstrate large QS complexes across the right precordial leads, which may persist all the way through lead V6. And, like LBBB and LVH with repolarization abnormality, there is some degree of non-pathologic STE in the right precordial leads (which also may persist through lead V6) – and indeed, in any lead that shows a negative QS paced complex (Figure 49.9). Not surprisingly, as this entity bares resemblance to LBBB, there are parallel ECG criteria for detection of acute STEMI in the presence of VPR [18]. These criteria are the same as those with LBBB and acute MI (Table 49.3) [17]; however, Sgarbossa and colleagues found (in a rather small sample group of 17 patients with VPR and acute MI compared with a like number of patients with stable coronary artery disease and VPR) that the finding of discordant STE > 5 mm was the best of the three criteria for the prediction of acute STEMI with VPR on the ECG – unlike LBBB where that criterion has been the least predictive. Serial

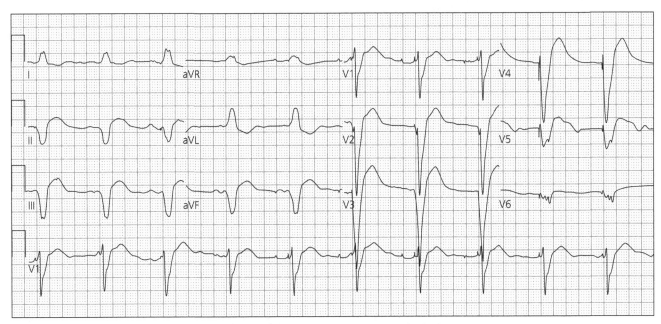

Figure 49.9 Ventricular paced rhythm. The pacemaker spikes, seen best in lead V1 on this tracing, are more subtle in other leads. Note the STE that is discordant to the major QRS complex vector in the precordial leads (V1–V6 here) and the inferior limb leads (II, III, and aVF). This dual-chamber pacemaker is an AV sequential pacemaker (note atrial and ventricular spikes).

ECGs looking for dynamic changes are recommended to enhance the sensitivity of the ECG for acute STEMI when any one of these confounding patterns (LVH, LBBB, VPR) is present.

Hyperkalemia: Elevation of serum potassium can result in myriad changes on the ECG, including STE. As the earliest electrocardiographic change of hyperkalemia is peaking of the T waves, that finding is uniformly present when there is also STE. The peaked T waves of hyperkalemia are usually narrow and pointed (Figure 49.2), whereas the hyperacute T waves of acute MI are usually broad-based and bulky (Figure 49.4). The elevated ST segment in hyperkalemia can take on multiple morphologies, some of which are evident in Figure 49.2. The STE may mimic acute STEMI and has been termed a "pseudo-infarction pattern" [19]. ST elevation in hyperkalemia may follow a downsloping contour, often seen in the septal leads (V1 and V2) [19,20]. Widening of the intervals (PR, QRS, and QT) provides a further clue that the STE is due to hyperkalemia; at times conduction disturbances, usually bradydysrhythmic, may occur as well.

Hypothermia: Osborn, or J, waves are positively directed notches that occur at the terminal portion of the R wave on the ECG of some hypothermic patients – simulating STE. Osborn waves usually appear at core temperatures below 90 °F, are generally larger with lower temperatures, and usually disappear sometime (although at times not immediately) after the core temperature normalizes. They are best seen in leads V2–V4, which include those leads, not coincidentally,

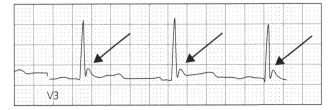

Figure 49.10 Hypothermia. The notched wave (*arrow*) immediately following the downward leg of the R wave is the Osborn wave, or J wave, of hypothermia. A large Osborn wave such as this gives the appearance of STE.

that normally feature the largest R waves (Figure 49.10) [21]. Other features of hypothermia on the ECG include bradydysrhythmia (sinus bradycardia; atrial fibrillation with a slow ventricular response) and QT prolongation.

Brugada syndrome: This syndrome features key electrocardiographic findings in individuals with structurally normal hearts who are at risk for dysrhythmia-mediated sudden death [22,23]. The tracing will demonstrate a complete or incomplete right BBB (RBBB) morphology (or will mimic RBBB) principally in leads V1 and V2, with either downsloping, or saddleback, STE terminating in an inverted T wave (Figure 49.11). The classic deep, wide S waves seen in the left-sided leads with RBBB are absent, however. The ECG findings can be transient, and have been found to be unmasked by sodium channel-antagonists [1,24]. These findings, especially in the clinical context of syncope or averted sudden death, should prompt the EP to consider Brugada syndrome.

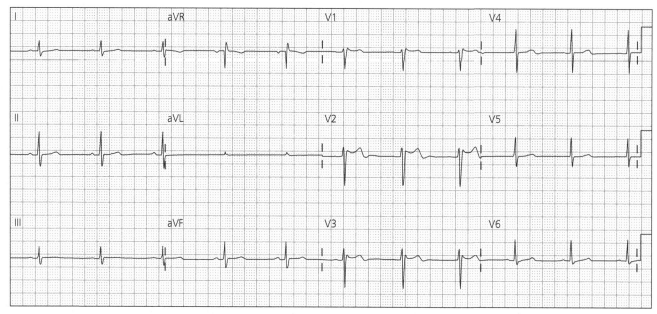

Figure 49.11 Brugada syndrome. Note the saddleback deformity STE in leads V1 and V2, with a pattern similar to an incomplete RBBB (rSr′ complex), yet no deep, wide S waves in the left-sided leads (V6, I, and aVL).

Ventricular aneurysm: A final entity, rather uncommon but worthy of mention in a discussion of STE – due to its similarity to STEMI – is left ventricular aneurysm (LVA). Usually, LVA occurs in the anterior wall of the left ventricle due to occlusion and infarction in the territory of the left anterior descending coronary artery. Although best detected by echocardiography, LVA can be suspected based upon certain ECG findings including: persistent STE (classically ≥ 1 mm for more than 4 weeks), usually in the anterior precordial leads and of variable morphology (concave or convex), with pathologic Q waves (as seen at times with STEMI) but without reciprocal changes (and therefore unlike some STEMIs). Like so many other STEMI-mimics, these changes do not change over the course of the clinical evaluation [25]. In a study that looked at physician interpretation of STE on the ECG (outside the actual clinical context), the entity most commonly misdiagnosed as STEMI was LVA (by 72% of participants) [26], highlighting the similarity between LVA and acute STEMI. T wave changes are variable with LVA, but recently Smith and associates looked at the ratio of amplitudes of the T wave relative to the QRS complex in LVA. If any lead demonstrated a T wave/QRS complex amplitude greater than 0.36, it was likely to be a STEMI; conversely, if all leads had that ratio fall below 0.36, the diagnosis of LVA was likely [27].

Case conclusions

The patient in Case 1 had right-sided ECG leads performed, which demonstrated STE in lead V4R as well. She was treated with aspirin, heparin, and beta-adrenergic blockers, and taken emergently to the cardiac catheterization laboratory, where her right coronary artery contained a 99% stenosis that was successfully opened, with subsequent placement of an intracoronary stent. The patient was ultimately discharged to home. The patient in Case 2 had a potassium level of 8.0 mEq/L, secondary to her chronic renal failure, in the context of a 1-week hiatus from hemodialysis. In the ED, she was treated with intravenous calcium chloride, insulin and glucose, and nebulized beta-adrenergic agonists, with improvement of her ECG. She then was admitted to the hospital for urgent hemodialysis; serial cardiac enzymes were negative for myocardial infarction. She was discharged to home in good condition.

References

1 Wang K, Asinger RW, Marriott HJL. ST-segment elevation in conditions other than acute myocardial infarction. *N Engl J Med* 2003;**349**:2128–35.

2 Hiss RG, Lamb LE, Allen MF. Electrocardiographic findings in 67,375 asymptomatic subjects. *Am J Cardiol* 1960;**6**:200–31.

3 Surawicz B, Parikh SR. Prevalence of male and female patterns of early ventricular repolarization in the normal ECG of males and females from childhood to old age. *J Am Coll Cardiol* 2002;**40**: 1870–6.

4 Tranchesi J, Adelardi V, de Oliverira JM. Atrial repolarization: Its importance in clinical electrocardiography. *Circulation* 1960;**22**: 635–44.

5 Smith SW, Whitwam W. Acute Coronary Syndromes. *Emerg Med Clin North Am* 2006;**24**:53–89.

6 Smith SW. Upwardly concave ST segment morphology is common in acute left anterior descending coronary occlusion. *J Emerg Med* 2006;**31**:105–9.

7 Brady WJ, Perron AD, Ullman EA, *et al.* Electrocardiographic ST

segment elevation: a comparison of AMI and non-AMI syndromes. *Am J Emerg Med* 2002;**20**:609–12.

8 Mehta MC, Jain AC. Early repolarization on scalar electrocardiogram. *Am J Med Sci* 1995;**309**:305–11.

9 Brady WJ, Perron AD, Martin ML, *et al.* Cause of ST segment abnormality in ED chest pain patients. *Am J Emerg Med* 2001; **19**:25–28.

10 Turnipseed SD, Bair AE, Kirk D, *et al.* Electrocardiogram differentiation of benign early repolarization versus acute myocardial infarction by emergency physicians and cardiologists. *Acad Emerg Med* 2006;**13**:961–6.

11 Brady WJ, Chan TC. Electrocardiographic manifestations: benign early repolarization. *J Emerg Med* 1999;**17**:473–8.

12 Ginzton LE, Laks MM. The differential diagnosis of acute pericarditis from the normal variant: new electrocardiographic criteria. *Circulation* 1982;**65**:1004–9.

13 Brady WJ, Syverud SA, Beagle C, *et al.* Electrocardiographic ST segment elevation: The diagnosis of AMI by morphologic analysis of the ST segment. *Acad Emerg Med* 2001;**8**:961–7.

14 Brady WJ, Perron AD, Syverud SA, *et al.* Reciprocal ST segment depression: Impact on the electrocardiographic diagnosis of ST segment elevation acute myocardial infarction. *Am J Emerg Med* 2002;**20**:35–8.

15 Otto LA, Aufderheide TP. Evaluation of ST segment elevation criteria for the prehospital electrocardiographic diagnosis of acute myocardial infarction. *Ann Emerg Med* 1994;**23**:17–24.

16 Brady WJ, Pollack ML. Acute myocardial infarction: Confounding patterns. In: Chan TC, Brady WJ, Harrigan RA, *et al.* editors. *ECG in Emergency Medicine and Acute Care.* Philadelphia: Elsevier Mosby, 2005: 181–7.

17 Sgarbossa EB, Pinski SL, Barbagelata A, *et al.* Electrocardiographic diagnosis of evolving acute myocardial infarction in the presence of left bundle branch block. *N Engl J Med* 1996;**334**:481–7.

18 Sgarbossa EB, Pinski SL, Gates KB, *et al.* Early electrocardiographic diagnosis of acute myocardial infarction in the presence of ventricular paced rhythm. *Am J Cardiol* 1996;**77**:423–4.

19 Wang K. "Pseudoinfarction" pattern due to hyperkalemia. *N Engl J Med* 2004;**351**:593.

20 Abrahamian FM. ACS mimics: non-AMI causes of ST-segment elevation. In: Mattu A, Tabas JA, Barish RA editors. *Electrocardiography in Emergency Medicine.* Dallas: American College of Emergency Physicians, 2007:119–32.

21 Vassallo SU, Delaney KA, Hoffman RS, *et al.* A prospective evaluation of the electrocardiographic manifestations of hypothermia. *Acad Emerg Med* 1999;**6**:1121–6.

22 Brugada P, Brugada J. Right bundle branch block, persistent ST segment elevation and sudden cardiac death: a distinct clinical and electrocardiographic syndrome: a multicenter report. *J Am Coll Cardiol* 1992;**20**:1391–6.

23 Wilde AA, Antzelevitch C, Borggrefe M, *et al.* Proposed diagnostic criteria for the Brugada syndrome: consensus report. *Circulation* 2002;**106**:2514–9.

24 Brugada P, Brugada J, Antselevitch C, *et al.* Sodium channel blockers identify risk for sudden death in patients with ST-segment elevation and right bundle branch block but structurally normal hearts. *Circulation* 2000;**101**:510–5.

25 Harper RJ. Ventricular aneurysm. In: Chan TC, Brady WJ, Harrigan RA, *et al. ECG in Emergency Medicine and Acute Care.* Philadelphia: Elsevier Mosby, 2005:213–5.

26 Brady WJ, Perron A, Chan T. Electrocardiographic ST-segment elevation: Correct identification of acute myocardial infarction (AMI) and non-AMI syndromes by emergency physicians. *Acad Emerg Med* 2001;**8**:349–60.

27 Smith SW, Nolan M. Ratio of T wave amplitude to QRS amplitude best distinguishes acute anterior MI from anterior ventricular aneurysm [abstract]. *Acad Emerg Med* 2003;**10**:516–7.

Chapter 50 | What is the ECG differential diagnosis of ST segment depression?

Richard A. Harrigan[1], Theodore C. Chan[2]
[1]Temple University, Philadelphia, PA, USA
[2]University of California, San Diego, CA, USA

Case presentations

Case 1: A 56-year-old female presents to the emergency department (ED) with complaints of intermittent "sharp" left-sided chest pain for the past week. There is no dyspnea, diaphoresis, dizziness, or nausea. There are no clear exacerbating or alleviating symptoms. She has a history of hypertension and congestive heart failure, but no known coronary artery disease. Current medications include enalapril, furosemide, digoxin, aspirin, and amlodipine. Her vital signs and physical examination are within normal limits. Her electrocardiogram (ECG) on presentation to the ED is shown in Figure 50.1.

Case 2: A 67-year-old male presents to the ED with severe substernal chest "pressure" for several hours. The pressure waxes and wanes, and is worse with exertion. There is no radiation. Associated symptoms include dyspnea and diaphoresis. The patient has a history of hypertension, smoking, and hypercholesterolemia. On physical examination, his temperature is normal, his heart rate is 100 beats per minute (bpm), his respiratory rate is 24, and his blood pressure is 100/58 mmHg. He is mildly diaphoretic. His lungs are significant for bibasilar rales. The heart sounds are normal, and there is no abdominal tenderness. The extremities feature equal pulses bilaterally, and there is no lower extremity edema. The initial ECG is seen in Figure 50.2.

Case 3: A 29-year-old male presents to the ED with complaints of severe global weakness since he awakened that morning. The previous night, he had snorted an unspecified quantity of an unknown drug that he believed to be heroin. He noticed that instead of a sedated, euphoric effect, he became anxious and agitated – a feeling that persisted for hours. In the morning, he noticed diffuse muscle weakness, with difficulty walking. He finally summoned the assistance

of emergency medical services when he could no longer work the television remote control. There is no syncope, vomiting, or diarrhea. He has been previously healthy. On physical examination, his vital signs are normal. His examination is normal with the exception of 2–3/5 muscle strength diffusely without disturbance of his reflexes. Figure 50.3 shows his ECG on presentation.

ECG differential diagnosis of ST segment depression

Depression of the ST segment is a potentially portentous finding on the ECG. Due to its association with myocardial ischemia, it has taken the position behind ST segment elevation (STE) in the list of significant morphologic changes on the ECG that are associated with acute coronary syndrome (ACS). Although ST segment depression can signify both myocardial ischemia and myocardial infarction (MI), depending upon the context, it is associated with a number of other clinical entities – some serious, and others benign (see Table 50.1). As with STE, the emergency physician (EP) should have a ready differential diagnosis for ST depression, so as to institute testing and intervention when appropriate, and also to withhold unnecessary diagnostics and treatment when the ST depression is recognized as a non-pathologic finding.

The ST segment

Normally isoelectric, the ST segment reflects that portion of the cardiac cycle which follows ventricular depolarization (the QRS complex) and precedes ventricular repolarization (the T wave). The J point, which marks the junction of the QRS complex and the ST segment, marks the initial portion of the ST segment, which ends at the beginning of the T wave. The ST segment should be scrutinized for deviation from this isoelectric baseline, although there is some disagreement over what part of the cardiac waveform should be used as the baseline for purposes of comparison. Classically,

Critical Decisions in Emergency and Acute Care Electrocardiography,
1st edition. Edited by W.J. Brady and J.D. Truwit. © 2009 Blackwell Publishing, ISBN: 9781405159067

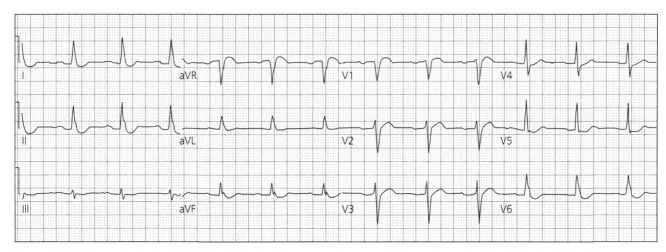

Figure 50.1 ST depression due to digitalis effect. Note the diffuse, scooped, concave ST depression, most evident in leads with large R waves – inferiorly (leads II and aVF; lead III as a right-sided lead, is typically spared) and laterally (I, aVL, V5, and V6). This is a typical example of digitalis effect, which is a pharmacologic ECG finding, rather than a toxicologic one.

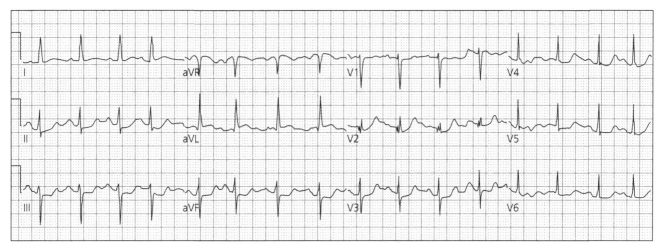

Figure 50.2 ST depression due to left main coronary artery disease. The most striking thing about this ECG is the diffuse ST depression – inferiorly (leads II, III, and aVF), and anteroseptally with lateral involvement (leads V1–V6). The STE in leads aVR and aVL is the clue to the culprit vessel; this patient had critical left main coronary artery stenosis.

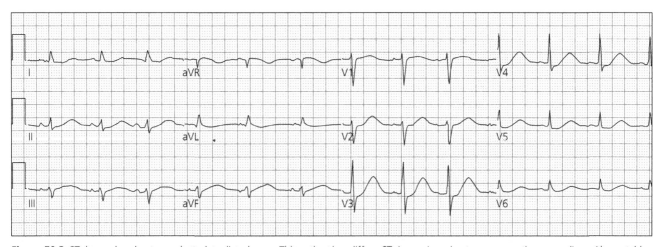

Figure 50.3 ST depression due to an electrolyte disturbance. This patient has diffuse ST depression – best seen across the precordium. Also notable are QT prolongation and prominent T waves – the latter may represent TU fusion. The potassium was 1.6 mEq/L.

Table 50.1 Differential diagnosis of ST segment depression

Acute coronary syndrome
  Non-ST segment elevation MI (NSTEMI)
  Posterior MI
  Reciprocal changes with STEMI*
  Left main coronary artery disease*
Bundle branch block
  Right
  Left*
Ventricular hypertrophy
  Right (leads V1, V2 with "strain" pattern)
  Left (leads V5, V6, perhaps 1, aVL with "strain" pattern)*
Ventricular paced rhythm*
Digitalis effect (may or may not have ST segment elevation in leads aVR, V1)
Rate-related ST segment depression
Electrolyte abnormalities
Post-electrical cardioversion
Myocarditis (may or may not have ST segment elevation, T wave changes)
Pulmonary embolism (may or may not have ST segment elevation, T wave changes)
Central nervous system event (may or may not have ST segment elevation, T wave changes)

*Expect ST segment elevation to occur elsewhere on the ECG as well.

the *TP segment* is used (that portion of the tracing which approximates an isoelectric course, from the end of the T wave of the preceding cardiac cycle to the beginning of the P wave of the next cardiac cycle). Others have argued that the *end of the PR segment* should be used as the baseline for measurement of STE; more precisely, it should be measured from the upper edge of the PR segment to the upper edge of the J point (which marks the beginning of the ST segment). The PR segment may be slightly depressed below the isoelectric line (and thus below the TP segment) due to the atrial repolarization wave that follows atrial depolarization (manifested by the P wave) [1,2].

Amplitude, contour, and distribution of ST depression: Like STE, ST depression is measured in millimeters (mm). Generally speaking, ST depression of at least 1 mm in *amplitude* is considered significant, when measured at the J point – but any degree of ST depression that is different from the baseline ECG should be regarded as potentially significant, recognizing the dynamic phenomenon of cardiac ischemia [3]. In addition to measuring the amplitude of ST depression in millimeters, the *contour* of the ST depression must also be analyzed. ST depression contour is generally considered in terms of direction, and classified as either downsloping, horizontal, or upsloping. Downsloping or horizontal ST depression, especially when associated with at least 1 mm of J point depression, is more suggestive of cardiac ischemia, whereas upsloping ST depression is not

suggestive of cardiac ischemia [3]. Finally, the *distribution* of the morphologic changes in ST depression syndromes is important in determining the cause of that ST depression. This will be discussed below in the various sections describing causes of ST depression.

Although amplitude, contour, and distribution are all important characteristics of ST depression, the EP must consider these characteristics in the general sense – not in the absolute. In the *clinical context* of ACS, ST depression should be considered an ominous finding, and thus treated aggressively. Furthermore, the *morphologic context* of the ST depression is helpful when trying to interpret these changes; for example, in the morphologic context of a broad QRS complex (duration > 0.12 s) in a clinically asymptomatic person, bundle branch block (BBB) or ventricular paced rhythm (VPR) should be considered (see below) – given diagnostic ECG criteria are met for those entities. Conversely, seemingly trivial, < 1 mm ST depression in the patient who appears to be having an acute MI should lead to treatment of that patient with appropriate ACS therapy, as well as serial ECGs or ST segment trend monitoring.

Differential diagnosis of ST segment depression

There are many causes of ST depression on the ECG; differentiation of these entities can be difficult. Furthermore, two or more processes may coincide temporally on one tracing, each causing ST depression, complicating the interpretation of that ECG (e.g. acute coronary ischemia in a patient with underlying left ventricular hypertrophy [LVH] with repolarization abnormality). Table 50.1 displays the differential diagnosis for ST depression.

Acute coronary syndrome: ST depression should first invoke consideration of acute myocardial ischemia – either in the presence or absence of serum marker evidence of acute MI. Primary ST depression – meaning that which occurs without evidence of STE or posterior MI on the tracing (see below) – is consistent with unstable angina or a non-ST segment elevation MI (NSTEMI). A recent study using the database of the National Registry of Myocardial Infarction (NRMI) found that patients with isolated ST depression (deemed consistent with an ischemic pattern) on the initial ECG had an inpatient mortality rate of 16% – approximating that of those patients with STE or left BBB (LBBB). Furthermore, the ST depression subgroup had an in-hospital cardiac complication rate of 33% – again virtually the same as that found in the STE-or-LBBB cohort [4]. Patients with acute MI and no deviation of the ST segment have been reported to be at lower risk [5]. Thus, ST depression should be treated aggressively in the setting of ACS.

Posterior MI is another key consideration in the clinical context of a patient with ACS symptoms and ST depression

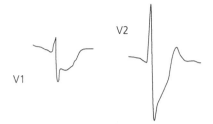

Figure 50.4 ST depression in posterior myocardial infarction. In posterior MI, there is ST depression in leads V1 and V2 (and perhaps in lead V3) that is typically horizontal in orientation, as it is here. Also note the abnormally large R wave in lead V2.

on the ECG. Due to the fact that the posterior wall of the heart is fed by either the right coronary or left circumflex arteries, true posterior MIs seldom happen in isolation, and are usually seen concurrently with inferior or lateral STEMIs [6,7]. Posterior MI deserves mention in a discussion of ST depression, however, because that is the principal manifestation of that entity on the 12-lead ECG. Cardinal features include: horizontal ST depression in leads V1, V2, and V3 with associated upright T waves; greater than expected R waves; and an R/S ratio of > 1 in lead V2 (Figure 50.4) [6]. If posterior leads (V8, V9) are applied, STE will be seen in acute posterior MI, as these leads image the posterior surface of the heart; the ST depression that is seen in leads V1–V3 is really a reciprocal change of the STE occurring in V8 and V9, just as the growth of an R wave in V1 and V2 is the anterior manifestation of a posterior Q wave.

A third situation in which ST depression occurs with ACS is in the *reciprocal changes* that sometimes accompany STEMI. True reciprocal changes are the electrocardiographic mirroring, on one surface of the myocardium, of the transmural injury occurring on the opposite side of the heart

(Figure 50.5). Reciprocal ST depression does not reflect true ischemia in that territory, and is not accompanied by regional wall motion abnormalities in the same territory on echocardiogram. Its presence identifies a subset of patients with more extensive disease, and increases the specificity of the STE for acute coronary ischemia [3]. About 80% of inferior STEMIs demonstrate reciprocal ST depression in lead aVL, and sometimes lead I, whereas approximately 30% of anterior STEMIs show reciprocal ST depression in the inferior leads II, III, and aVF [3]. Reciprocal changes are not 100% specific for STEMI (e.g. they can occur in lead aVR in pericarditis). When considering ECGs without confounding patterns (LVH, VPR, BBB) in chest pain patients, ST depression had a sensitivity of 69% and a specificity of 93% for acute MI [8].

Last, the significant presence of diffuse ST depression in patients with acute MI due to *left main disease* is worthy of mention (Figure 50.2). Patients with diffuse ST depression in the usual culprit leads – inferior (II, III, and aVF), anterior (V3, V4), perhaps septal (V1, V2) and lateral precordial (V5, V6) might lead the EP to conclude that the ECG reflects an NSTEMI, and that the patient is not a candidate for percutaneous coronary intervention (PCI). Lead aVR should not be ignored in these cases. ST elevation in aVR, or in aVL and aVR (or in aVR > V1), is highly suggestive of, though not diagnostic for, acute left main occlusion – although such tracings may be dominated by diffuse ST depression which may draw the eye away from lead aVR (Figure 50.2) [10–12]. Thus, it is important to consider lead aVR – indeed, all the leads – when reviewing the 12-lead ECG for evidence of STEMI.

Bundle branch block: Both left and right BBB feature some degree of ST depression in the non-ischemic state. The

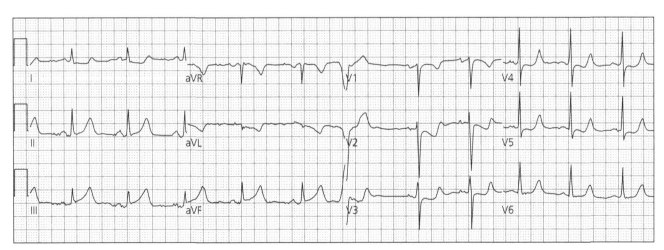

Figure 50.5 Reciprocal ST depression. This tracing shows an acute inferior MI, with STE in leads II, III, and aVF. Note also the *reciprocal ST depression* – best seen in lead aVL, but also present in lead I in this tracing. The borderline STE in lead V1, along with the ST depression in lead V2 – in the setting of an acute inferior STEMI with STE greater in lead III than in lead II – all point to right ventricular involvement as well. The cardiac catheterization showed a proximal 99% right coronary artery stenosis.

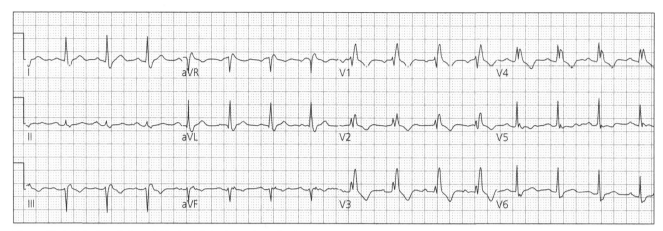

Figure 50.6 Right bundle branch block with ST depression. The characteristic rSR' morphology of RBBB is seen here – although its persistence beyond leads V1 and V2 into leads V3, and even V4, is unusual, and may be due to precordial electrode misplacement issues. Those leads with the rSR' pattern have ST depression that blends immediately into an inverted T wave. This is part of the RBBB pattern. Note also the slurred, wide S wave in left-sided leads V6 and I – also typical of RBBB.

hallmark of both left and right BBB is a widened (> 0.12 s) QRS complex; however, there are other key morphologic features that must be committed to memory. In LBBB, the ECG also features prominent rS or QS waves followed by STE and large T waves in the right precordial leads, as well as monophasic, often notched, R waves with discordant ST depression and T wave inversions in the left-sided leads (some combination of leads V5, V6, I, and aVL). It is important to remember that this ST depression in the left-sided leads, blending sharply into an inverted T wave, is not reflective of coronary ischemia. Rather, it is due to the altered repolarization vectors that follow the altered ventricular depolarization, attributable to the delayed depolarization seen in BBB (in LBBB – loss of the initial left-to-right septal forces, followed by the delayed, but normal, right-to-left depolarization of the ventricle) [12]. ST depression should *not* be seen in the right-sided precordial leads (V1–V3) in LBBB; if it exceeds 1 mm, it is suggestive (but not diagnostic) of an acute MI in the presence of LBBB [13]. In RBBB, the characteristic rSR' broad QRS complex pattern (or broad qR pattern, or broad, monophasic R wave pattern) seen in the right precordial leads is followed by a discordant and depressed ST segment blending quickly into an inverted T wave. Again, this discordant ST depression is not ischemic ST depression, but is due to altered ventricular repolarization vectors (Figure 50.6) [12]. The deep, wide S wave that appears in the left-sided leads as part of the pattern of right BBB bears a resemblance to ST depression, but is, in actuality, simply a slurring of the S wave due to the delayed depolarization of the right side of the heart (Figure 50.6) [12].

Ventricular hypertrophy: Both right and left ventricular hypertrophy may feature ST depression as part of the repolarization abnormality, or strain pattern, that can represent this process on the ECG. The classic repolarization abnormality, when seen, occurs in the left-sided leads (V5, V6, perhaps I

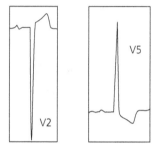

Figure 50.7 Left ventricular hypertrophy with repolarization abnormality. Single QRS complexes from leads V2 and V5 are shown here. Lead V5, a left-sided lead, shows the classic changes of repolarization abnormality seen in some cases of LVH. The ST segment is depressed, beginning with a slightly depressed J point. The ST depression is downsloping. The T wave is inverted, with a slow descending limb followed by a rapidly ascending limb. Lead V2, a right-sided precordial lead, shows the mirror opposite: STE with a concave contour, followed by a somewhat tall but asymmetric upright T wave.

and aVL) in LVH (Figure 50.7), and the right-sided leads (V1–V2) in RVH. It includes downsloping ST depression, usually without J point depression, in the leads that feature prominent R waves (reflecting the large ventricular mass overlying those electrodes). The T wave is inverted asymmetrically, with a gradual descent followed by a sharper ascent to the baseline, which it may overshoot, leading to slight terminal positivity of the inverted T wave. T wave inversion tends to be greater in lead V6 than in lead V4 [3]. This can be quite difficult, especially with LVH, to differentiate from coronary ischemia. Clues to LVH being the cause of ST depression may emerge from examination of old tracings, and finding the changes to be stable over time despite a changing clinical picture in the ED.

Ventricular paced rhythm: In that right VPR bears a resemblance to LBBB on the ECG, it is not surprising that

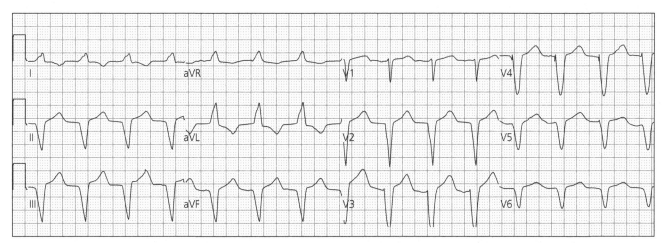

Figure 50.8 Right ventricular paced rhythm. There is a predominance of STE on this tracing, which features 100% paced beats from a ventricular pacemaker operating from the right ventricular base. The leads with upright QRS complexes – leads I and aVL here – feature ST depression appropriately. The relationship here between predominantly negatively oriented complexes and principally positively oriented complexes (they mirror one another) is parallel to that seen with LVH/repolarization (see Figure 50.7). Also, note the pacemaker spikes are hard to see (they are most evident in lead V4).

some ST depression, as well as STE, can be seen on "normal" tracings when the pacemaker is functioning. ST depression can be seen in those leads where the major vector of the paced QRS complex is upright. In many right ventricular paced ECGs that feature a left QRS axis deviation, this may be restricted to leads I and aVL, and perhaps lead V6 (Figure 50.8). As with LBBB, ST depression > 1 mm in leads V1–V3 is unexpected, and is suggestive of acute MI [14]. As with any of the ECG patterns that potentially confound the diagnosis of STEMI (e.g. LVH, LBBB), serial ECGs over time, and comparison of the current tracing with those from the past, is advisable when the patient with an underlying VPR presents with symptoms consistent with ACS.

Digitalis effect: The presence of the drug digoxin – even in therapeutic levels (the so-called digoxin effect or digitalis effect) – can cause several characteristic changes on the ECG, including ST depression. These are not a manifestation of digitalis toxicity, but may persist if the drug reaches toxic levels in the bloodstream. Findings include: "scooped" ST segment depression, a short QT interval, and T wave flattening or inversion, as well as PR segment prolongation and possibly U waves. The ST depression tends to be most evident in those leads with the tallest R waves [16]. The ST segment, in its depression, may be almost indistinguishable from the T wave. It is characteristically smooth, and may show the reciprocal effect (smooth, domed, STE) in leads aVR and V1 (Figure 50.1).

Pre-excitation: Electrocardiograms that show evidence of pre-excitation, such as in Wolff-Parkinson-White (WPW) syndrome, may also show some degree of ST depression. The classic findings of WPW include a short PR interval (< 0.12 s),

and a slurred upstroke of the QRS complex – the delta wave – with an associated slight widening of the QRS complex (0.11–0.12 s); the delta waves may mimic Q waves in the inferior or lateral leads, and may appear as large R waves in the right precordial leads. Repolarization changes of the ST segment/T wave complex may also be evident. These changes may include a depressed ST segment and an inverted T wave, although the location of these changes is dependent upon the location of the bypass tract. These changes are similar to those discordant changes seen in LVH with repolarization abnormality and in BBB (Figure 50.9).

Rate-related ST segment depression: ST segments are often depressed during episodes of supraventricular tachycardia (Figure 50.10). This ST depression does not necessarily reflect myocardial ischemia – a finding that has also been verified in the stress-testing arena as well as in cases of *de novo* supraventricular dysrhythmia [16,17,18]. J point depression and upsloping ST depression are seen often in these scenarios, and usually represent non-ischemic ST depression. Clinical correlation is warranted.

Electrolyte abnormalities: Hypokalemia (Figure 50.3) may cause ST depression, QT prolongation, T wave changes, and the appearance of U waves on the ECG. Fusion of the T and U waves may occur. Disturbances of calcium and hyperkalemia should not depress the ST segment. Coincident QT prolongation with the ST depression should invoke consideration of hypokalemia, especially in the presence of U waves [18]. Digitalis effect can cause ST depression and U waves as well, but the QT interval is shortened in the presence of digitalis, whereas it would be prolonged in hypokalemia.

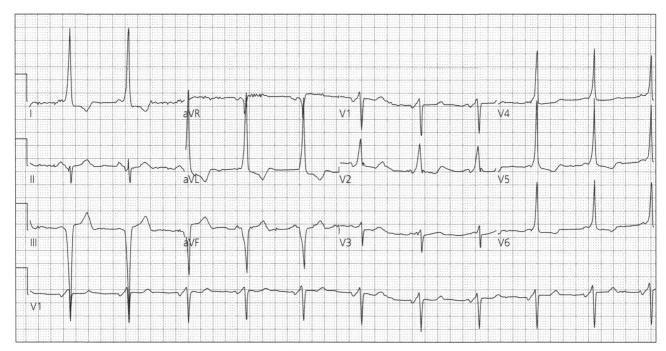

Figure 50.9 Wolff-Parkinson-White syndrome. Non-ischemic ST depression is seen in leads I, aVL, V5, and V6. This patient has an accessory bypass tract. Note the short PR intervals and widened QRS complexes due to the initial slurred upstrokes forming delta waves. Note also the pseudo-infarct pattern inferiorly – these apparent Q waves are in actuality delta waves.

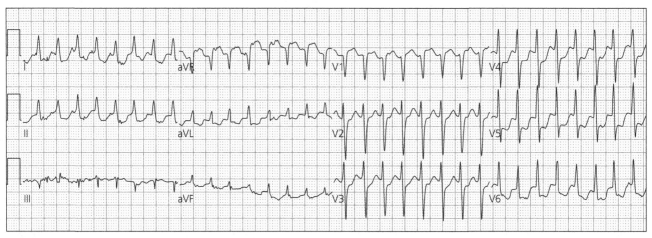

Figure 50.10 Rate-related ST segment depression. The ST depression is diffuse and upsloping in this ECG from an 8-year-old girl who presented with a supraventricular tachycardia. Although ischemia must always be considered, this was not the case here.

Case conclusions

In Case 1, the patient's ECGs were static over time, and her cardiac serum markers remained normal through serial sampling. Her digoxin level was 0.7 mcg/mL. She had a pharmacologic stress test that revealed no cardiac ischemia, and the patient was discharged to home after she had had no further chest pain. In Case 2, the patient was treated with aspirin, followed by intravenous heparin, nitroglycerin, and beta-adrenergic blockers in the ED, and taken promptly to

the cardiac catheterization suite, where multivessel coronary disease, including critical left main stenosis, was found. Emergency coronary bypass surgery was performed successfully. Lastly, in Case 3, the patient was found to have a serum potassium level of 1.6 mEq/L. His serum magnesium and calcium levels were normal. The patient's symptoms improved with intravenous and oral potassium replacement. Initial toxicologic screens, including a theophylline level as well as those of common drugs of abuse, were negative, and the patient left the hospital against medical advice before further testing could be performed.

References

1 Tranchesi J, Adelardi V, de Oliverira JM. Atrial repolarization: Its importance in clinical electrocardiography. *Circulation* 1960;**22**: 635–44.

2 Smith SW, Whitwam W. Acute Coronary Syndromes. *Emerg Med Clin North Am* 2006;**24**:53–89.

3 Pollehn T, Brady WJ, Perron AD, Morris F. The electrocardiographic differential diagnosis of ST segment depression. *Emerg Med J* 2002;**19**:129–35.

4 Pitta S, Grzybowski M, Welch RD, *et al.* ST-segment depression on the initial electrocardiogram in acute myocardial infarction – prognostic significance and its effect on short-term mortality: A report from the National Registry of Myocardial Infarction (NRMI-2, 3, 4). *Am J Cardiol* 2005;**95**:843–8.

5 Welch RD, Zalenski RJ, Frederick PD, *et al.* Prognostic value of a normal or nonspecific initial electrocardiogram in acute myocardial infarction. *JAMA* 2001;**286**:1977–84.

6 Zalenski RJ, Cooke D, Rydman R, *et al.* Assessing the diagnostic value of an ECG containing leads V4R, V8, and V9: the 15-lead ECG. *Ann Emerg Med* 1993;**22**:786–93.

7 Brady WJ. Acute posterior myocardial infarction: electrocardiographic manifestations. *Am J Emerg Med* 1998;**16**:409–13.

8 Brady WJ, Perron AD, Syverud SA, *et al.* Reciprocal ST segment depression: Impact on the electrocardiographic diagnosis of ST segment elevation acute myocardial infarction. *Am J Emerg Med* 2002;**20**:35–8.

9 Yamaji H, Iwasaki K, Kusachi S, *et al.* Prediction of acute left main coronary artery obstruction by 12-lead electrocardiography. ST segment elevation in lead aVR with less ST segment elevation in lead V1. *J Am Coll Cardiol* 2001;**38**:1348–54.

10 Kosuge M, Kimura K, Ishikawa T, *et al.* Predictors of left main or three-vessel disease in patients with have acute coronary syndromes with non-ST segment elevation. *Am J Cardiol* 2005; **95**:1366–9.

11 Rostoff P, Piwowarska W, Gackowski A, *et al.* Electrocardiographic prediction of acute left main coronary artery occlusion (letter). *Am J Emerg Med* 2007;**25**:852–5.

12 Harrigan RA. Intraventricular conduction abnormalities. In: Mattu A, Tabas JA, Barish RA editors. *Electrocardiography in Emergency Medicine*. Dallas: American College of Emergency Physicians, 2007:13–9.

13 Sgarbossa EB, Pinski SL, Barbagelata A, *et al.* Electrocardiographic diagnosis of evolving acute myocardial infarction in the presence of left bundle branch block. *N Engl J Med* 1996;**334**: 481–7.

14 Sgarbossa EB, Pinski SL, Gates KB, *et al.* Early electrocardiographic diagnosis of acute myocardial infarction in the presence of ventricular paced rhythm. *Am J Cardiol* 1996;**77**:423–4.

15 Holstege CP, Kirk MA. Digitalis. In: Chan TC, Brady WJ, Harrigan RA, *et al.* editors. *ECG in Emergency Medicine and Acute Care*. Philadelphia: Elsevier Mosby, 2005:255–60.

16 Kastor JA. *Arrhythmias*. 2nd edn. Philadelphia: WB Saunders, 2000:198–268.

17 Kontos MC. The electrocardiogram and stress testing. In: Chan TC, Brady WJ, Harrigan RA, *et al.* editors. *ECG in Emergency Medicine and Acute Care*. Philadelphia: Elsevier Mosby, 2005: 351–9.

18 Shumaik GM. Electrolyte abnormalities. In: Chan TC, Brady WJ, Harrigan RA, *et al.* editors. *ECG in Emergency Medicine and Acute Care*. Philadelphia: Elsevier Mosby, 2005:282–7.

Chapter 51 | What is the ECG differential diagnosis of the abnormal T wave?

Theodore C. Chan[1], Richard A. Harrigan[2]

[1]University of California, San Diego, CA, USA
[2]Temple University, Philadelphia, PA, USA

Case presentations

Case 1: A 63-year-old man presents to the emergency department (ED) complaining of substernal chest pain of 2 h duration, associated with shortness of breath, fatigue and lightheadedness. He has a history of hypertension, but no prior cardiac disease. His vital signs on arrival are pulse rate of 90 beats per minute (bpm), blood pressure of 146/88 mmHg, and respiratory rate of 16 breaths per minute. On examination, he appears in moderate distress, his skin is diaphoretic, and his extremities are cool to touch. His chest is clear on auscultation and cardiac examination reveals a regular rate with no rubs, murmurs or gallops. His electrocardiogram (ECG) reveals a sinus rhythm with a number of morphologic abnormalities (Figure 51.1).

Case 2: A 64-year-old man with history of diabetes mellitus and end-stage renal disease on hemodialysis presents to the ED complaining of weakness after missing his dialysis 2 days ago. His vital signs are notable for a pulse rate of 36 bpm, blood pressure 82/54 mmHg, respiratory rate of 24 breaths per minute, and temperature of 96.7°F. On examination, his chest is notable for bibasilar crackles, but good air movement, and cardiac auscultation reveals a regular bradycardic rhythm with no murmurs or rubs. The ECG demonstrates a marked bradycardia at a rate of 29 bpm, widened QRS complexes, and prominent T waves over the precordial leads (Figure 51.2).

Case 3: A 72-year-old man with a history of coronary artery disease and hypertension presents to the ED with 4 hours of substernal chest pain. He suffered a myocardial infarction 5 years ago and underwent stenting of his left anterior descending coronary artery without complication at that time. His vital signs are notable for a regular pulse rate of 112 bpm, blood pressure 142/88 mmHg, and respiratory rate of 12

breaths per minute. An ECG obtained while the patient is having chest pain (Figure 51.3) reveals a wide QRS complex tachycardia with a left bundle branch block (LBBB) pattern at a rate of 117 bpm and abnormal T wave morphology.

Differential diagnosis of the abnormal T wave

The T wave deflection on ECG represents electrical repolarization of the ventricles during the cardiac cycle. Under normal circumstances, repolarization of cardiac tissue follows the same path or direction as depolarization. As a result, the T wave deflection has a similar orientation to the QRS complex in a given lead. The T wave axis is directed toward the apex of the heart. In leads I, II, and V3 through V6, the T wave is normally upright or a positive deflection; in lead aVR the T wave is normally inverted or a negative deflection. For the other leads (III, aVL, aVF, V1, V2) the T wave is variable and may be upright, inverted or biphasic [1].

Both cardiac disease and non-cardiac conditions can cause abnormalities in the T wave on the ECG. These abnormalities can appear in a variety of different morphologies. T waves can increase in amplitude and appear more prominent. Inversion of the T waves can occur in leads where this morphology is not expected normally. Abnormal T waves can also appear as biphasic or flattened deflections following the QRS complex.

Cardiac conditions

Acute coronary syndrome: Acute coronary syndrome (ACS), including myocardial ischemia and infarction, can cause a variety of different T wave abnormalities over time. In the setting of ST elevation myocardial infarction (STEMI), prominent T waves with a marked increase in amplitude, also known as "hyperacute" T waves, may be present as early as 30 min after onset. These T waves are asymmetric with a broad base and occur just before and at the start of ST elevation (indicated by an elevated J point) (Figure 51.1). These

Critical Decisions in Emergency and Acute Care Electrocardiography, 1st edition. Edited by W.J. Brady and J.D. Truwit. © 2009 Blackwell Publishing, ISBN: 9781405159067

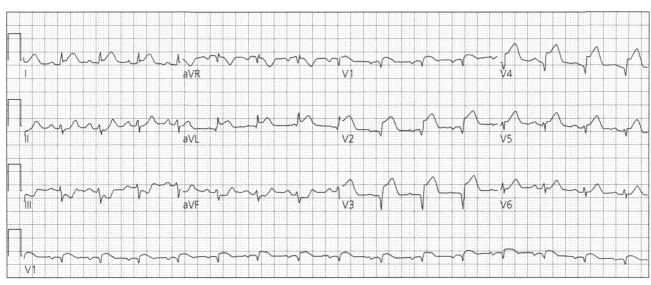

Figure 51.1 Twelve-lead ECG from Case 1. The ECG demonstrates marked ST segment and T wave abnormalities consistent with an acute myocardial infarction. In particular, there are ST segment elevations with prominent asymmetric T waves in the mid-precordial leads.

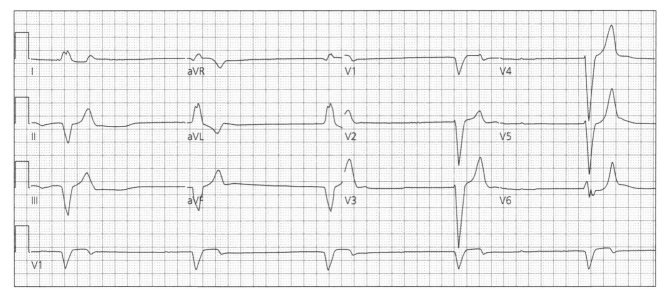

Figure 51.2 The 12-lead ECG from the patient of Case 2 demonstrates a marked bradycardia and wide QRS complex. This rhythm is consistent with a sinoventricular rhythm as a result of severe hyperkalemia. The T waves are symmetrically peaked in leads V3 thru V6.

hyperacute T waves are transient and resolve or transition to other T wave ACS morphologies over a short period of time. In the setting of non-acute myocardial infarction (AMI) ACS or non-STEMI (NSTEMI) AMI, the T waves may flatten or diminish in amplitude early in the presentation [1].

Abnormal T wave inversions are a common electrocardiographic finding in ACS including STEMI, NSTEMI, and myocardial ischemia (Figure 51.4). Typically, these inversions occur in a regional pattern reflective of the ischemic or infarcting myocardium. Classically, the T waves produced by ischemia or infarction are narrow and symmetric, but can vary in morphology. In STEMI, T waves invert as the ST elevations resolve. Persistent shallow T wave inversions,

particularly in the presence of deep QS waves, may indicate a completed infarction from prolonged coronary artery occlusion. Alternatively, inverted T waves may revert back to baseline indicating transient ischemia.

T wave inversions also may occur during reperfusion, whether spontaneous or as a result of treatment. The typical evolution as reperfusion occurs is an initial inversion of the terminal portion of the T wave. This terminal inversion may occur in combination with ST segment elevation giving the appearance of biphasic T waves. This change is followed by a deeper T wave inversion (> 3 mV) that, when combined with resolution of the ST segment elevation, appears as a symmetric, deeply inverted T wave.

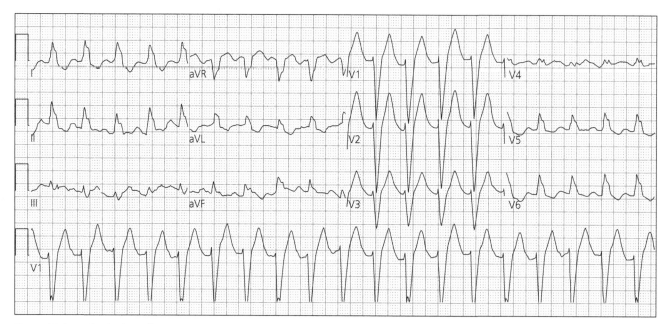

Figure 51.3 Twelve-lead ECG from Case 3. The ECG demonstrates abnormal T wave inversions in the lateral leads including I, aVL, and V6. In addition, prominent T waves are noted in the right precordial leads (V1–V3). In the setting of the wide QRS complex morphology consistent with LBBB, these T wave findings are appropriately discordant due to changes in repolarization following the abnormal depolarization.

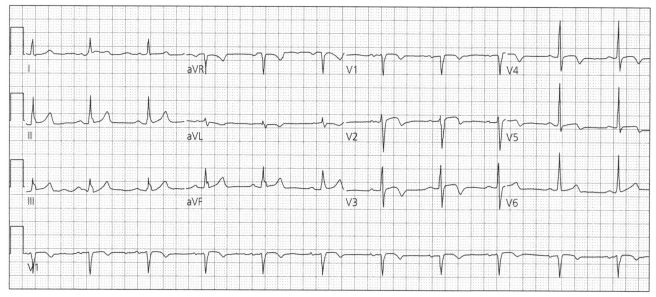

Figure 51.4 Twelve-lead ECG of patient with acute myocardial ischemia. Note the T wave inversions in the anterior precordium particularly leads V3 and V4. The ST elevation in V2 combined with the T wave inversion gives the appearance a biphasic T wave.

In leads where the T wave is normally inverted (e.g. leads V1 and sometimes V2), these changes in T wave morphology may appear opposite; that is, ACS may result in abnormal upright T waves in these leads. In addition, in the presence of abnormal T wave inversions from ACS, acute reocclusion of the coronary artery may actually result in reversal of these inversions and a "pseudo-normalization" of the T waves [2].

Wellens' syndrome: Wellens' syndrome represents a subgroup of ACS patients who have a critical stenosis of a coronary artery (classically the left anterior descending artery), evidence of non-infarction ACS, and abnormal T wave findings on ECG. Typically, these patients demonstrate markedly abnormal T wave inversions in the precordial leads, particularly V2–V4, usually during the pain-free state. These T wave inversions can appear as deep, symmetric inversions or biphasic T wave abnormalities (Figure 51.4). In Wellens' syndrome, these precordial T wave inversions are also associated with QT interval prolongation > 0.42 s [2].

Bundle branch block: Because ventricular activation takes place abnormally with bundle branch block (BBB), repolarization of the ventricles likewise occurs abnormally. As a result, morphologic changes in the T waves are expected and, in fact, establish a "new normal" on the ECG for patients with BBB [3]. Classically in BBB, the T wave axis is directed in the opposite direction to the major, terminal portion of the QRS complex with respect to the isoelectric baseline, in those leads showing the characteristic changes of the BBB. That is, in leads with a prominent upright or positive QRS complex, the T wave will be inverted or negative (often associated with ST segment depression). In leads with a negative QRS complex (e.g. QS or rS wave), the T wave will be upright (often associated with ST segment elevation). This relationship is known as QRS complex/T wave axis discordance or "rule of appropriate discordance" [4].

For example, in left BBB (LBBB), leads with mainly negative QS or rS waves (i.e. precordial leads V1–V3) will have discordant upright T waves (with ST segment elevation). In leads with large, upright QRS or R wave complexes (i.e. the lateral leads I, aVL, V6, and possibly V5), the T waves will be discordant and inverted (with ST segment depressions) (Figure 51.3) [4]. In right BBB (RBBB), a parallel pattern is found. In leads with predominant upright QRS complexes (e.g. anterior precordial leads V1 and V2), the T waves will be inverted. Classically, the T wave morphologies (prominent or inverted) associated with BBB are asymmetric; there is a longer initial deviation away from the isoelectric baseline (downstroke for inversion, upstroke for the prominent T wave), followed by a more rapid terminal return to the isoelectric baseline.

These discordant ST segment/T wave abnormalities can mimic ischemic and infarction patterns electrocardiograph-ically. In the case of LBBB, the ST segment/T wave discordance pattern can obscure acute ischemia. Prediction rules have been developed relating to the degree of ST segment elevation/depression in terms of determining whether these abnormalities represent true acute ischemia and infarction or the expected repolarization abnormalities with BBB, particularly LBBB (see AMI chapters) [5].

Ventricular pacing: Pacemakers that pace the heart through the ventricular chambers (usually the right ventricle) result in an ECG pattern similar to that of LBBB. Following the pacer spike on the ECG, ventricular depolarization produces wide, predominantly negative QS or rS waves with poor R wave progression across the precordium. QS complexes may also be seen in the inferior leads II, III, and aVF. Large positive R waves may be present in leads I and aVL. Similar to BBB, the rule of appropriate discordance applies to the ST segment/T wave complex in ventricular pacing. In leads with predominantly negative QRS complexes, ST elevation and upright T waves will be seen; in leads with predominantly positive QRS complexes, ST depression and asymmetric T wave inversions will be seen (Figure 51.5) [6].

Ventricular hypertrophy: Similar to BBB and ventricular pacing, repolarization is abnormal in patients with ventricular hypertrophy because depolarization is altered by the hypertrophied myocardium. In fact, ST segment and T wave changes are seen in approximately 70% of left ventricular hypertrophy (LVH) cases [3]. Similar to the rule of appropriate discordance in BBB, prominent T waves along with ST segment elevations are seen in leads with large QS or rS complexes (e.g. leads V1–V3). Asymmetric T wave inversions

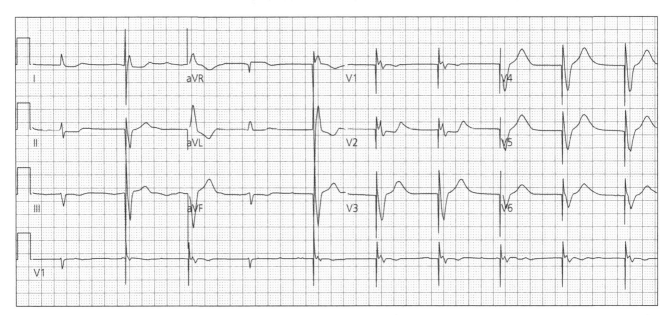

Figure 51.5 Twelve-lead ECG from patient with ventricular pacing. Note the discordant T waves – prominent and upright in precordial leads with rS or QS complexes; inverted in lateral leads with predominantly positive or upright QRS complexes (aVL). This discordance is only seen following paced ventricular beats (denoted by the pacing spike).

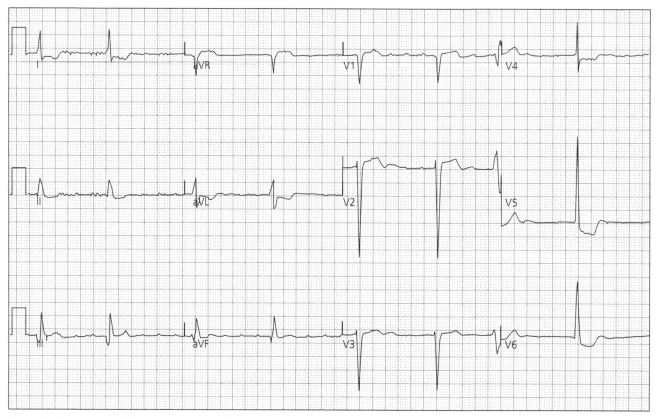

Figure 51.6 Twelve-lead ECG of patient with LVH by voltage criteria. Also, note the appropriately discordant T waves. T wave inversions in leads with prominent positive and upright QRS complexes laterally (leads I, aVL, V5, V6); upright T waves with in leads with prominent negative QRS complexes of increased amplitude in the anterior leads (leads V1, V2, V3).

and ST depressions are seen in leads with large amplitude QRS complexes and R waves (e.g. lateral leads V4–V6, possibly I, aVL). These inversions are usually most prominent in lead V6. The morphology of the T wave inversion is typically asymmetric with a gradual downward sloping, followed by a rapid return to baseline (Figure 51.6). The terminal T wave may actually "overshoot" the baseline and is termed "terminal positivity" [3]. However, the T wave may assume other morphologies including minimal inversion or flattening.

Pre-excitation: When an accessory pathway (AP) exists in addition to the atrioventricular (AV) node, impulses can potentially propagate down the AP and activate or "pre-excite" the ventricle prior to the normal impulse via the AV node. Wolff-Parkinson-White (WPW) syndrome is one type of pre-excitation syndrome caused by the presence of an AP. Because of the abnormal depolarization from pre-excitation, repolarization is altered and can result in T wave changes on the ECG. Typically, there can be ST segment and T wave abnormalities, such as discordant T waves (Figure 51.7). These findings, in addition to PR shortening and slurring of the initial portion of the QRS complex (delta wave) on the ECG are indicative of pre-excitation.

Benign early repolarization: Benign early repolarization (BER) is a normal electrocardiographic variant more commonly seen in younger and middle-aged men [7]. The exact mechanism of the electrocardiographic abnormalities seen in BER is unclear. The T waves in BER are of large amplitude, usually symmetric, although slight asymmetry may be present, and concordant with the QRS axis in a given lead. These findings are most prominent in the precordial leads, where the T wave may even appear "peaked." Other electrocardiographic findings include J point elevation and concave ST segment elevation. These ECG findings are marked by temporal stability over years and can be observed over prolonged periods of time in an individual. They are usually best seen in the precordial leads, but may also appear in other leads (e.g. inferior leads).

Acute myopericarditis: Up to 90% of patients with acute myopericarditis, an inflammation of the pericardial sac and superficial myocardium, can have evidence of electrocardiographic abnormalities. These abnormalities occur as a progression, which includes diffuse PR segment depression, ST elevation and normalization, T wave flattening followed by inversion, and normalization of the ECG to baseline. The

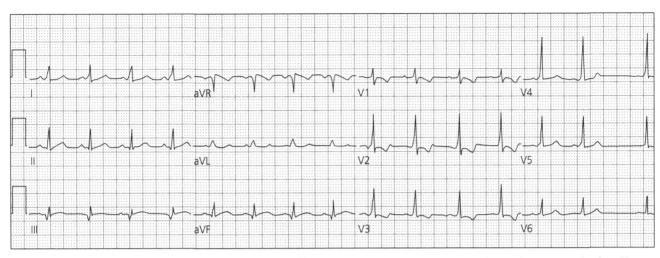

Figure 51.7 Twelve-lead ECG of patient with WPW syndrome. The patient is in sinus rhythm with evidence of pre-excitation. Note the short PR interval and slurring of the QRS complex with the delta wave (most prominent in lead I). Abnormal repolarization is evident by the T wave inversions seen in leads V2 and V3.

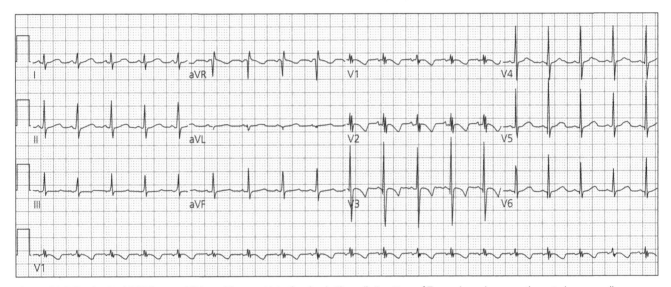

Figure 51.8 Twelve-lead ECG from a child aged 8 years. Note the classic "juvenile" pattern of T wave inversions over the anterior precordium, including leads V1 and V3. This is a normal finding up to adolescence.

T wave abnormalities are typically seen in stage 3, 3 or more weeks after the onset of disease. ST elevation resolves before the onset of the discordant T wave inversions. These inversions resolve over several weeks, but persistent or very gradual resolution of the abnormal deflection is indicative of post-infarct pericardial inflammation [8].

Persistent juvenile T wave pattern: Numerous electrocardiographic alterations occur in children over time as a result of underlying changes in normal cardiac physiology with age. These changes include the switch from right ventricular dominance to left ventricular dominance over the first year of life. The T waves in the pediatric ECG are quite variable. In the first few days of life, the T wave may be upright or inverted. After the first week, T wave inversions are commonly seen, particularly in leads V1 through V3, and last until approximately 8 years of age. This ECG finding is referred to as the juvenile T wave pattern, which usually normalizes during early adolescence, but may persist during the teenage years (Figure 51.8).

Toxic/metabolic conditions

Digitalis effect: Cardiac glycosides are associated with a number of electrocardiographic changes at therapeutic levels. In particular, the T wave can be altered with digitalis at therapeutic levels well below the toxic range. These changes include T wave flattening, inversion, and biphasic morphologies. The classic digitalis effect finding is an inverted or biphasic T wave with preceding ST segment "sagging" depression. The ST/T wave complex displays a "scooped" or "hockey stick" appearance, most pronounced in the leads with tall R waves. The QT interval is characteristically short with digitalis effect.

Hyperkalemia: Potassium is a predominantly intracellular cation that plays an important role in depolarization and repolarization of cardiac cells. Hyperkalemia can have significant electrophysiologic effects on the heart and result in changes on the ECG. Early evidence for elevated serum potassium levels includes changes in the T waves. Classically, hyperkalemia can result in tall, symmetric T waves, particularly across the precordium on the ECG. These changes have been described as "peaked" T waves or "tenting" of the T waves (Figure 51.2). These changes are the result of alterations in the normal transmembrane gradient resulting in acceleration of the terminal repolarization [9]. Other electrocardiographic findings at moderate levels of hyperkalemia include PR segment lengthening and decreased amplitude, and even loss of the P wave. With severe hyperkalemia, widening of the QRS complex may occur, which can degenerate into a "sine wave" pattern and malignant ventricular dysrhythmia.

Non-cardiac conditions

Pulmonary embolism: Pulmonary embolism (PE) can produce a number of ECG abnormalities. Findings reported in the literature include rhythm changes (e.g. sinus tachycardia, RBBB), QRS axis changes, and ST segment and T wave abnormalities. On occasion, T wave inversions may be present in the anterior precordial leads (e.g. V1–V4). These inversions are typically symmetric in appearance. Deeper T wave inversions with wider anatomic distribution across the leads may be seen related to the severity of the PE and may be an indication of right ventricular strain [10]. Similarly, right ventricular strain may be seen in other pulmonary diseases, such as pulmonary hypertension, and manifest electrocardiographically with T wave inversions across the anterior precordial leads.

Central nervous system events: Electrocardiographic abnormalities can be seen in variety of central nervous system (CNS) events, including subarachnoid hemorrhage, cerebrovascular accident (CVA), and intracranial hemorrhage. The pathophysiology behind these alterations remains unclear, but may be related to changes in sympathetic and vagal tone, hypothalamic damage, and possible myocardial injury leading to aberrant repolarization. T wave changes associated with a CNS event include increased T wave amplitude, as well as T wave inversions. These changes have been termed the "CVA T wave pattern." The inversions are often

deep with variable duration width, and are generally symmetric. However, there can be a bulge on the ascending limb, which can give an asymmetric appearance to the T wave inversions.

Gastrointestinal diseases: Electrocardiographic abnormalities have been reported in patients presenting with complaints of abdominal pain and other gastrointestinal diseases including cholecystitis, pancreatitis, peptic ulcer disease, inflammatory bowel disease, liver disease, and even renal colic. The mechanism of these abnormalities is likely multifactorial. Various gastrointestinal disorders are known to present with T wave inversions electrocardiographically and may appear as a pseudo-ischemic ECG pattern. In particular, inflammatory conditions such as cholecystitis and pancreatitis have been associated with transient deep T wave inversions.

Case conclusions

In all these cases, the critical issue electrocardiographically is the underlying cause of the abnormal T wave indicative of abnormal ventricular repolarization. In Case 1, the findings of ST elevation with prominent "hyperacute" asymmetric T waves in the precordial leads, along with reciprocal changes in the inferior leads were indicative of acute myocardial ischemia. The patient underwent cardiac catheterization that revealed a 100% occlusion of his left anterior descending coronary artery, which was successfully treated with stenting.

In Case 2, the ECG demonstrated a sinoventricular rhythm with abnormally peaked T waves caused by hyperkalemia ($K^+ = 8.2$ mEq/L) as a result of the patient missing hemodialysis. He was treated with intravenous calcium gluconate, sodium bicarbonate, and insulin/glucose in the ED. His rhythm improved and QRS complexes narrowed. He was admitted to the intensive care unit and underwent hemodialysis, after which time he markedly improved and was discharged from the hospital 4 days later in good condition.

In Case 3, the ECG demonstrated a classic LBBB pattern with repolarization abnormalities. Given the patient's history of ACS, a prior ECG was obtained from 1 year previously, which also demonstrated the same LBBB with repolarization abnormalities. The T wave changes were felt to be appropriately discordant from the primary QRS complex axis that would be expected normally with BBB.

References

1 Brady W. T Wave. In: Chan TC, Brady WJ, Harrigan RA, *et al.* editors. *ECG in Emergency Medicine and Acute Care* Chan TC, Brady WJ, Harrigan RA, Ornato JP, Rosen P. Philadelphia: Elsevier/ Mosby, 2005:66–69.

2 Smith SW, Whitwam W. Acute coronary syndromes. *Emerg Med Clinics North Am* 2006;**24**:53–89.

3 Brady WJ. ST segment and T wave abnormalities not caused by acute coronary syndromes. *Emerg Med Clinics North Am* 2006;**24**: 91–111.

4 Brady WJ, Pollack ML. Acute Myocardial Infarction: Confounding Patterns. In: Chan TC, Brady WJ, Harrigan RA, *et al.* editors. *Emergency Medicine and Acute Care*. Philadelphia: Elsevier/Mosby, 2005:181–87.

5 Sgarbossa FB, Pinski SL, Barbagelata A, *et al.* Electrocardiographic diagnosis of evolving acute myocardial infarction in the presence of left bundle branch block. *N Engl J Med* 1996;**334**:481–5.

6 Cardall TY, Chan TC, Brady WJ, *et al.* Permanent cardiac pacemakers: Issues relevant to the emergency physician, Part I. *J Emerg Med* 1999;**17**(3): 479–89.

7 Brady WJ, Chan TC. Electrocardiographic manifestations: benign early repolarization. *J Emerg Med* 1999;**17**:473–8.

8 Chan TC, Brady WJ, Pollack M. Electrocardiographic manifestations: acute myopericarditis. *J Emerg Med* 1999;**17**:865–72.

9 Diercks DB, Shumaik GM, Harrigan RA, *et al.* Electrocardiographic manifestations: electrolyte abnormalities. *J Emerg Med* 2004;**27**:153–60.

10 Chan TC, Vilke GM, Pollack M, Brady WJ. Electrocardiographic manifestations: pulmonary embolism. *J Emerg Med* 2001;**21**:263–70.

Chapter 52 | What is the ECG differential diagnosis of narrow complex tachycardia?

Theodore C. Chan[1], *Richard A. Harrigan*[2]
[1]University of California, San Diego, CA, USA
[2]Temple University, Philadelphia, PA, USA

Case presentations

Case 1: A 47-year-old woman presents to the emergency department (ED) complaining of palpitations, lightheadedness, chest pain with pounding in the neck and chest, shortness of breath, and anxiety of 6 h duration. She has no prior history of cardiac or pulmonary disease. Vital signs are notable for a pulse rate that the triage nurse reports is "too fast to count," blood pressure 112/68 mmHg, and respiratory rate 16 breaths per minute. Chest examination is notable for clear breath sounds bilaterally and cardiac auscultation reveals a regular tachycardia with no rubs, gallops or murmurs. The initial electrocardiogram (ECG) demonstrates a regular tachycardia with narrow QRS complexes at a rate of 195 beats per minute (BPM) (Figure 52.1).

Case 2: A 30-year-old woman presents to the ED complaining of progressive fatigue, palpitations, and anxiety over the past 2 weeks. She notes weight loss and "feeling hot off and on" over the same time period. Her past medical history is unremarkable. Her vital signs are pulse rate 132 bpm, blood pressure 128/72 mmHg, and respiratory rate 12 breaths per minute. Her examination is notable for a mildly anxious appearing woman with slight tremors of her extremities, diaphoretic skin, clear lungs on auscultation, and a regular tachycardia with a systolic flow murmur on cardiac evaluation. Her ECG reveals a sinus tachycardia at a regular rate of 131 bpm (Figure 52.2).

Case 3: A 38-year-old man is brought to the ED for medical clearance prior to booking at the local jail. The patient was placed under arrest for suspicion of illicit drug trafficking. At the time of his apprehension, the patient was in a bizarre and agitated state, resulting in physical confrontation with the police. On arrival to the ED, vital signs at triage are remarkable for a pulse rate of 160 bpm, blood pressure 148/92 mmHg, and respiratory rate of 24 breaths per minute. On examination, the patient has minor soft tissue traumatic injuries over his extremities. His cardiac examination is notable for a regular tachycardia with no rubs, murmurs or gallops. Because of his tachycardia, an ECG is obtained (Figure 52.3).

Differential diagnosis of the narrow QRS complex tachycardia

Tachycardias are defined as heart rates above the normal rate expected for age. There are three main mechanisms that can result in tachycardia: enhanced automaticity, re-entry circuit, and triggered activity. Enhanced automaticity occurs when the rate of depolarization for certain myocytes increases and overcomes the normal sinus rhythm rate. Re-entry occurs when two pathways exist that allow anterograde and retrograde impulse conduction, creating a circuit loop and recurrent reactivation. Triggered activity occurs when depolarization takes place during the repolarization period of the myocytes. The keys to determining the etiology of a tachycardic rhythm are the width of the underlying QRS complex (narrow or wide) and the regularity of the rate (regular or irregular).

QRS complex width

The QRS complex on the 12-lead ECG represents depolarization and activation of the ventricles. Normal depolarization of the ventricles occurs when impulses are conducted from the atria through the atrioventricular (AV) node to the bundle of His, and down both the right and left bundle branches, the latter of which divides into anterior and posterior fascicles. The Q wave is the initial negative deflection, followed by the R wave as the first positive deflection, and concluding with the S wave, the negative deflection following the R wave (if another positive deflection occurs after the S wave, it is known as the R' wave). Actual morphology depends on the

Critical Decisions in Emergency and Acute Care Electrocardiography,
1st edition. Edited by W.J. Brady and J.D. Truwit. © 2009 Blackwell Publishing, ISBN: 9781405159067

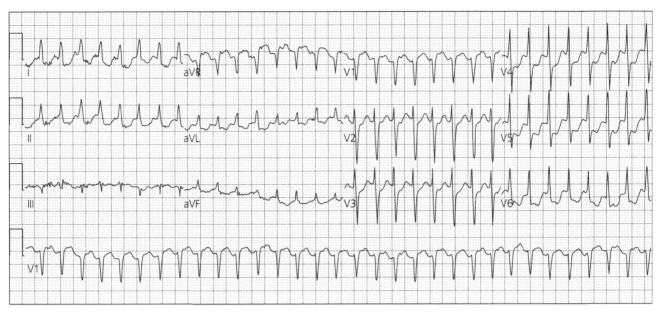

Figure 52.1 Twelve-lead ECG from Case 1. The patient has a regular NCT at a rate of 195 bpm. There is no clear preceding atrial activity, consistent with the diagnosis of supraventricular tachycardia. Diffuse, upsloping ST segment depression is likely "rate-related," and is not predictive of coronary ischemia.

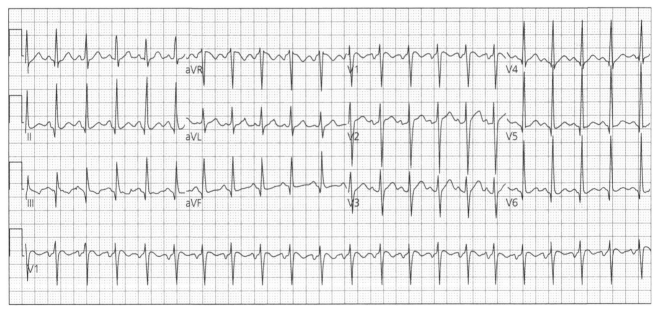

Figure 52.2 Twelve-lead ECG from Case 2. The ECG demonstrates a regular NCT at a rate of 131 bpm. There is a uniform P wave preceding each QRS complex consistent with the diagnosis of sinus tachycardia, most likely as a result of the patient's hyperthyroidism.

underlying vector of depolarization of the ventricles, any existing ventricular pathology or other metabolic abnormalities that affect electrical activity of the myocytes, and the actual electrocardiographic lead examined [1,2]. The normal duration of ventricular depolarization in adults is 0.06–0.11 s [2]. Accordingly, the normal width of the QRS complex is 0.06–0.11 s. Because morphology can vary between electrocardiographic leads, the width or duration should be measured in the lead in which the QRS complex is widest – usually one of the precordial leads, typically V2 or V3. A normal, or so-

called narrow, QRS complex width implies that ventricular activation is occurring down the normal conduction pathways.

Regular narrow complex tachycardia

Narrow complex tachycardias (NCTs) are differentiated by the regularity of the rhythm. Regular tachycardias with narrow QRS complexes are most commonly the result of

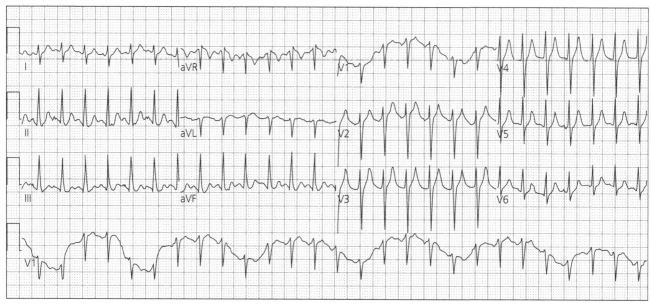

Figure 52.3 Twelve-lead ECG from Case 3. The ECG demonstrates a rapid, regular NCT at a rate of 165 bpm. There is P wave activity preceding the QRS complex. These findings were felt to be consistent with a marked sinus tachycardia from sympathomimetic drug use.

tachycardias generated from atrial or AV nodal tissue, with impulse transmission down the normal conduction pathways of the ventricles (producing narrow QRS complexes). Clinicians frequently use the term supraventricular tachycardia (SVT) or paroxysmal SVT (PSVT) when referring to a subset of NCTs with sudden onset and termination. These rhythms are commonly seen in patients presenting to the ED [3]. However, SVTs technically refer to a much more broad category of atrial tachycardias and atrioventricular (AV) tachycardias.

Atrial tachycardias

Atrial tachycardias are tachycardias that arise in atrial tissue above the AV node, usually as a result of abnormal automaticity or triggered activity. These tachycardias are also known as AV node-independent; that is, they may be present in the setting of AV block and do not terminate with AV blockade.

Sinus tachycardia: This can arise from any physiologic stress including volume depletion, fever, anxiety, exertion, or sympathomimetic drugs. The rate of onset is usually progressive rather than sudden, and the ECG demonstrates clear uniform P wave activity preceding each narrow QRS complex at the tachycardic rate. There are usually no morphologic changes on ECG with the faster rate when compared with the normal sinus rhythm (Figure 52.2).

Inappropriate sinus tachycardia: This resembles sinus tachycardia, but occurs without, or as an exaggerated response

to, a physiologic stimulus. Typically, inappropriate sinus tachycardia can be seen in young healthy women with no structural heart disease as an elevated resting heart rate or marked increase with minimal exertion.

Sinus node re-entrant tachycardia: This is the result of a re-entry circuit within the sinus node that results in a NCT at a rate of 100–150 bpm. The ECG is indistinguishable from sinus tachycardia as P wave and QRS complex morphology are normal due to the normal conduction of impulses down the atria and ventricles.

Atrial tachycardia: Regular NCTs produced by atrial tachycardias (ATs) are generally the result of a single ectopic atrial pacemaker generating rapid atrial impulses. These rapid impulses can be the result of increased automaticity at the ectopic focus, a re-entry circuit loop at the ectopic site, or triggered atrial activity from some other stimulus such as digoxin toxicity. While the atrial rate ranges between 100 and 250 bpm, the corresponding ventricular rate may be slower depending on whether impulses are blocked at the AV node. A regular NCT results from rapid, regular atrial impulses that are conducted to the ventricles at a 1 : 1 ratio or, more commonly if AV block is present, at some conduction ratio (e.g. 2 : 1 conduction) producing a tachycardic ventricular response (Figure 52.4).

Electrocardiographically, ATs from a single ectopic focus produce abnormal, but uniform, non-sinus P waves. The location of the focus can be determined by the morphology of the abnormal P wave. A positive ectopic P wave in lead V1 suggests a left atrial focus; a positive ectopic P wave in lead aVL suggests a right atrial focus. In the setting of rapid rates, it

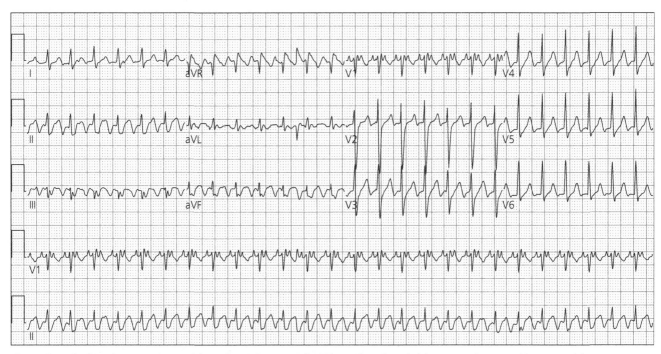

Figure 52.4 The ECG demonstrates a rapid, regular NCT at a rate of 162 bpm. There is underlying narrow P wave activity at an atrial rate near 300 bpm (best seen in the lead V1 rhythm strip) in a 2 : 1 conduction ratio with QRS activity. This finding is consistent with atrial flutter, with a constant 2 : 1 conduction resulting in a regular ventricular rate. The lack of upright atrial activity in lead II (note the "saw-tooth" pattern) – makes atrial flutter most likely, as does the ventricular rate approximating 150 bpm.

can be difficult to detect atrial activity because of overlying ventricular depolarization and repolarization on the ECG. The speed rate of the ECG can be modified (usually increasing from 25 mm/s to 50 mm/s) to artificially "slow" the cardiac cycle electrocardiographically and reveal underlying atrial activity.

Atrial flutter: This is a specific type of AT produced by a large re-entry circuit in the atrial tissue. As a result of this macro-re-entry circuit loop, atrial activity appears as a "saw-tooth" pattern at an atrial rate of 250–350 bpm with no isoelectric baseline. A regular NCT results when there is a consistent AV conduction ratio, most commonly 2 : 1, but possibly 4 : 1, 3 : 1 or 1 : 1 (Figure 52.4).

Atrioventricular tachycardias

Atrioventricular tachycardias are tachycardias that involve the AV node, usually as a result of increased nodal automaticity or a re-entry circuit loop. These tachycardias are also known as AV node-dependent; that is, they are not present in the setting of AV block and can be terminated with AV blockade.

Junctional tachycardias: Junctional tachycardias, such as non-paroxysmal junctional tachycardia and junctional ectopic tachycardia, occur as a result of increased automaticity or triggered activity at the AV node and junction. The electro-cardiographic result is a NCT, typically with no discernable preceding P waves.

Atrioventricular nodal re-entrant tachycardia: This is produced by the presence of a re-entry circuit loop with two pathways within the AV node [4]. The tachycardia is precipitated when a premature atrial impulse is conducted antegrade down one pathway in the AV node to activate the ventricles, and retrograde up the other pathway in the node to reactivate the atria. The impulse is then propagated down the antegrade pathway to reactivate the ventricles, thus creating the re-entry circuit. This circuit results in a rapid, recurrent nearly simultaneous activation of the vent-ricles and atria.

Electrocardiographically, atrioventricular nodal re-entrant tachycardia (AVNRT) appears as a regular tachycardia at heart rates of 120–250 bpm. The QRS complex is narrow, as AVNRT does not involve any changes in the ventricular conduction system (so long as there is no underlying aberrant conduction). Because of the near simultaneous depolarization of atria and ventricles, the P wave is often "buried" within the QRS complex and not detectable on ECG. Occasionally, atrial activity can cause a slight distortion of the QRS complex, known as the pseudo-S wave in inferior leads or pseudo-R′ wave in lead V1. Occasionally, a P wave can be detected just before or after the QRS complex depending on the rate and speed of the re-entry circuit. Because the atria

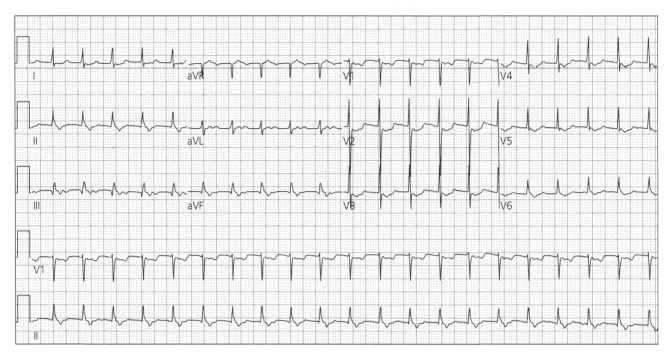

Figure 52.5 Twelve-lead ECG from a patient with AVNRT. There are inverted P waves at the terminal portion of the QRS complexes most prominent in the inferior leads, consistent with retrograde atrial activity.

are activated from the AV node, the atrial activity on the ECG when present will appear as an abnormal retrograde P wave (inverted in the inferior leads) (Figure 52.5) [5].

Atrioventricular re-entry tachycardia – orthodromic conduction: Atrioventricular re-entry tachycardias (AVRTs) occur when a macro-re-entry circuit loop exists because of the presence of an accessory pathway (AP) that bypasses the AV node [4]. As a result of this circuit, impulses are conducted from the atria down (antegrade) either the AV node or AP to activate the ventricles, then conducted back up (retrograde) the alternative pathway (AP or AV node) to reactivate the atria, forming the recurrent circuit loop. In orthodromic conduction, antegrade conduction to the ventricles occurs down the AV node and retrograde conduction back to the atria occurs up through the AP. As a result, the ventricles are depolarized down the normal His-Purkinje conduction pathway from the AV node. The re-entry circuit loop and retrograde AP impulse causes recurrent activation of the atria. This impulse is then conducted down the AV node again, completing the macro-re-entry circuit loop and resulting in a rapid regular NCT.

Electrocardiographically, the QRS complex is narrow (provided there is no underlying aberrant ventricular conduction) in orthodromic AVRT. Atrial activity is delayed as activation occurs from retrograde impulse conduction up the AP. As a result, P waves may be detected following the normal QRS complex. The P wave may appear normal or abnormal (inverted or flat) depending on the location of the AP in relation to the atria. Evidence of an AP may be detected

on the baseline ECG when the re-entry circuit is not active in AVRT. These findings can include evidence of pre-excitation with the presence of a delta wave, widened QRS complex, shortened PR interval and abnormal repolarization T wave.

Narrow complex ventricular tachycardia

Rarely, ventricular tachycardia (VT) can produce a regular NCT with QRS complexes of normal width. This occurs when the ectopic focus ventricular activation is located at or near the AV node and His-Purkinje conduction pathway. Fascicular tachycardia is a rare form of VT associated with digoxin toxicity that produces a regular NCT because it originates near the AV node along the fascicles.

Irregular Narrow Complex Tachycardias

Irregular tachycardias with narrow QRS complexes can result from irregular rhythms produced by abnormal or irregular supraventricular automaticity, or from variable block of supraventricular tachycardias, usually at the level of the AV node.

Atrial fibrillation: This is the most common cause of an irregularly irregular heart rate. Atrial fibrillation occurs when there is no organized activation of the atria, resulting in

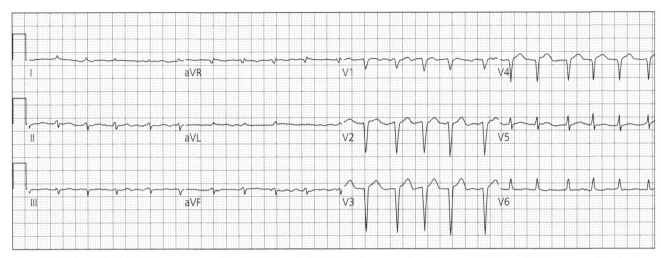

Figure 52.6 The 12-lead ECG demonstrates an irregularly, irregular NCT. There is no organized P wave activity. These findings are consistent with the diagnosis of atrial fibrillation with rapid ventricular response.

chaotic depolarization of atrial tissue. Electrocardiographically, the atrial activity appears as fibrillatory waves of varying amplitude and duration rather than distinct P waves. As a result, the baseline is not isoelectric, but oscillates with the fibrillatory waves. Fine atrial fibrillation (AF) occurs when the fibrillatory waves are of low amplitude (< 0.5 mV); coarse AF occurs when the fibrillatory waves are of larger amplitude (> 0.5 mV).

While the atrial fibrillatory rate is typically irregular at 400 bpm, impulses are blocked at the AV node, resulting in a slower, irregular ventricular response rate. In untreated patients with AF, the typical ventricular response rate is 110–130 bpm [6]. With no underlying aberrant conduction, the resulting electrocardiographic rhythm is an irregular NCT (Figure 52.6).

Occasionally, even without underlying chronic aberrant ventricular conduction, there can be a wide QRS complex beat as a result of Ashman's phenomenon. In this case, a prolonged RR interval results in a prolonged ventricular refractory period. If the next atrial impulse is conducted through the AV node during this time at a relatively short RR interval, the ventricular activation is abnormal due to ventricular refractoriness, and results in a wide, aberrant QRS complex (usually right bundle branch block [RBBB] pattern). Ashmann's phenomenon is best remembered by this "long-short" RR cycle.

Multifocal atrial tachycardia: Also known as chaotic atrial rhythm, this occurs from increased atrial automaticity when there is no dominant atrial pacemaker. As a result, multiple ectopic atrial foci are active producing an irregular rhythm. Multifocal atrial tachycardia is commonly associated with chronic pulmonary disease, atrial enlargement, hypoxia, and congestive heart failure [7].

Electrocardiographically, multifocal atrial tachycardia (MAT) manifests as an irregular NCT (provided there is no aberrant

conduction) with at least three morphologically different P wave morphologies in a given lead. The variable P wave morphology is often best detected in the leads II, III and V1. In addition, there is irregularity in the PP, PR, and RR intervals. Unlike AF, the baseline is isoelectric between P waves and the QRST complex (Figure 52.7).

Tachycardias with premature beats: Regular NCTs can appear irregular if premature beats occur. These beats can occur with premature atrial contractions (PACs), premature junctional contractions (PJCs) and premature ventricular contractions (PVCs). The first two (PAC and PJC) will result in narrow QRS complexes provided there is no underlying aberrant conduction. Premature ventricular contractions produce wide QRS complexes as a result of the ectopic ventricular activation. These premature beats can occur regularly, producing a regularly irregular rate; or they can occur irregularly, producing an irregularly irregular rate.

Atrial tachycardias with variable block: In the setting of any atrial tachycardia, rapid atrial impulses can overwhelm the AV node resulting in variable block and conduction to the ventricles. As a result, this variable block can produce an irregular NCT (provided there is no underlying aberrant ventricular conduction). Atrial flutter (usually at a regular rate of about 300 bpm) commonly results in altered AV conduction with variable block – such as 2 : 1 and 3 : 1 AV ratios. Electrocardiographically, the resulting rhythm is an irregular NCT (with no aberrant conduction present) (Figure 52.8).

Atrial tachycardia with block may occur with digitalis toxicity. Electrocardiographic manifestations of cardiac glycoside toxicity result from an exaggeration of its therapeutic actions: enhanced automaticity and increased AV blockade. Paroxysmal atrial tachycardia with variable AV block can

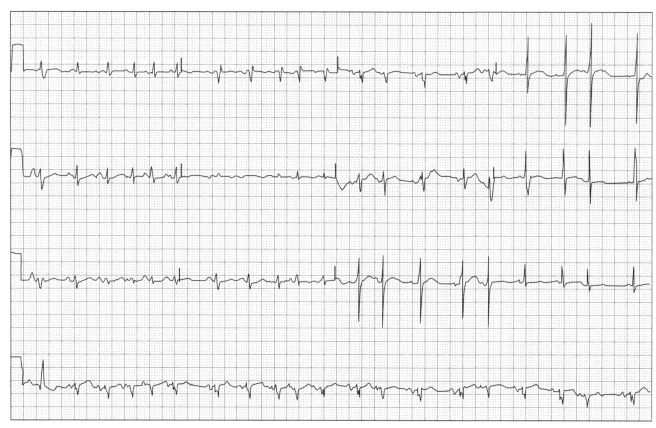

Figure 52.7 This 12-lead ECG demonstrates an irregular NCT as a result of MAT in a patient with chronic obstructive pulmonary disease. There are varying P wave morphologies occurring at irregular intervals resulting in the irregular rate.

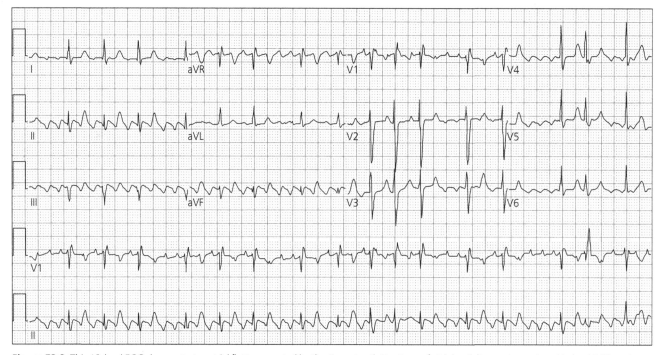

Figure 52.8 This 12-lead ECG demonstrates atrial flutter as noted by the "saw-tooth" pattern of atrial activity most prominent in lead II. There is variable conduction resulting in an irregular NCT as there is no aberrant ventricular conduction.

produce an irregular NCT and strongly suggests the diagnosis of digitalis toxicity [8].

Case conclusions

In the cases detailed in this chapter, the critical issue electrocardiographically is the underlying cause and management of the narrow complex tachycardia. In Case 1, the patient's ECG demonstrated a narrow complex regular tachycardia at a rate of 195 bpm. Because of the lack of clear P wave activity, he was diagnosed with a supraventricular tachycardia, mostly likely AVNRT. He was treated with adenosine and converted to sinus rhythm at a rate of 82 bpm. In Case 2, the ECG demonstrated a regular sinus tachycardia at a rate of 131 bpm. Clear P waves precede each of the narrow QRS complexes. The etiology of the patient's sinus tachycardia was revealed when laboratory testing determined the patient had a non-detectable serum thyroid-stimulating hormone level. The patient was subsequently diagnosed with hyperthyroidism, treatment was initiated with thyroid blocking and beta-adrenergic-antagonist agents and the patient was referred to endocrinology for follow-up. In Case 3, the ECG demonstrated a regular narrow complex tachycardia at a rate of 165 bpm. Given the patient's presentation, a toxicologic screen was obtained which confirmed the presence of methamphetamine. The patient's tachycardia was felt to be due to sympathomimetic toxicity. He was treated with benzodiazepine medications, admitted for observation to the hospital, and subsequently did well.

References

1 Mirvis DM, Goldberger AL. Electrocardiography. In: Braunwald E, Zipes DP, Libby P, editors. *Heart Disease: a Textbook of Cardiovascular Medicine*, 6th ed. Philadelphia: WB Saunders; 2001: 82–125.

2 Surawicz B, Knilans TK. *Chou's Electrocardiography in Clinical Practice: Adult and Pediatric*, 5th ed. Philadelphia: W.B. Saunders, 2001.

3 Murman DH, McDonald AJ, Pelletier AJ, Camargo CA. US emergency department visits for supraventricular tachycardia, 1993–2003. *Acad Emerg Med* 2007;**14**:578–81.

4 Delacretaz E. Supraventricular tachycardia. *N Engl J Med* 2006; **354**:1039–51.

5 Kazzi AA, Wong H. Other supraventricular tachydysrhythmias. In: Chan TC, Brady WJ, Harrigan RA, *et al.*, editors. *ECG in Emergency Medicine and Acute Care*. Philadelphia: Elsevier/Mosby, 2005:104–11.

6 Wrenn K. Wandering atrial pacemaker and multifocal atrial tachycardia. In: Chan TC, Brady WJ, Harrigan RA, *et al.*, editors. *ECG in Emergency Medicine and Acute Care*. Philadelphia: Elsevier/Mosby, 2005:101–3.

7 Kastor JA. Multifocal atrial tachycardia. *N Engl J Med* 1990;**322**: 1713–17.

8 Ma G, Brady WJ, Pollack M, Chan TC. Electrocardiographic manifestations: digitalis toxicity. *J Emerg Med* 2001;**20**:145–52.

Chapter 53 | What is the ECG differential diagnosis of wide complex tachycardia?

Theodore C. Chan[1], Richard A. Harrigan[2]
[1]University of California, San Diego, CA, USA
[2]Temple University, Philadelphia, PA, USA

Case presentations

Case 1: A 61-year-old male with a history of diabetes mellitus, coronary artery disease, and chronic kidney disease now dependent on hemodialysis presents to the emergency department (ED) with complaints of palpitations, chest pain, nausea, and dyspnea. Physical examination on presentation reveals a heart rate of 147 beats per minute (bpm), respiratory rate of 20 breaths per minute, and blood pressure of 128/88 mmHg. Lung fields are remarkable for bilateral rales, and the heart examination is tachycardic but without murmurs, gallops, or rubs. A 12-lead electrocardiogram (ECG) is obtained on ED presentation (Figure 53.1).

Case 2: A 20-year-old woman is brought to the ED by paramedics from an outside clinic complaining of palpitations and lightheadedness after a night of drinking alcohol. She denies chest pain, shortness of breath, or other complaints. She has no prior cardiac or other medical history. She denies any drug ingestions. On examination, her vital signs are blood pressure 112/72 mmHg, respiratory rate 20 breaths per minute, and pulse rate too fast to count per triage nurse. On examination, she is a young woman in mild distress, chest is clear on auscultation, and cardiac examination reveals a very rapid tachycardia that appears irregular. An ECG from the outside clinic is brought to you by the paramedics (Figure 53.2).

Case 3: A 72-year-old man with a history of coronary artery disease and hypertension presents to the ED with 4 h of substernal chest pain. He suffered a myocardial infarction 5 years ago and underwent stenting of his left anterior descending coronary artery without complication at that time. His vital signs are notable for a regular pulse rate at 112 bpm, blood pressure 142/88 mmHg, and respiratory rate of 12 breaths per minute. An ECG obtained while the patient is having

Critical Decisions in Emergency and Acute Care Electrocardiography,
1st edition. Edited by W.J. Brady and J.D. Truwit. © 2009 Blackwell Publishing, ISBN: 9781405159067

chest pain (Figure 53.3) reveals a wide QRS complex tachycardia with a left bundle branch block (LBBB) pattern at a rate of 117 bpm.

Differential diagnosis of the wide QRS complex tachycardia

Wide complex tachycardias (WCTs) refer to abnormally rapid cardiac rhythms with abnormally wide QRS complexes on the ECG. Tachycardias are themselves defined as heart rates above the normal rate expected for age. There are three main mechanisms that can result in tachycardia: enhanced automaticity, re-entry circuit, and triggered activity. Enhanced automaticity occurs when the rate of depolarization for certain myocytes increases and overcomes the normal sinus rhythm rate. Re-entry occurs when two pathways exist that allow anterograde and retrograde impulse conduction, creating a circuit loop and recurrent reactivation. Triggered activity occurs when depolarization takes place during the repolarization period of the myocytes. The keys to determining the etiology of a tachycardic rhythm are the width of the underlying QRS complex (narrow or wide) and the regularity of the rate (regular or irregular).

QRS complex width

The QRS complex on the 12-lead ECG represents depolarization and activation of the ventricles. Normal depolarization of the ventricles occurs when impulses are conducted from the atria through the atrioventricular (AV) node to the bundle of His, and down both the right and left bundle branches, the latter of which divides into anterior and posterior fascicles. The Q wave is the initial negative deflection, followed by the R wave as the first positive deflection, and concluding with the S wave, the negative deflection following the R wave (if another positive deflection occurs after the S wave, it is known as the R' wave). Not all electrocardiographic leads demonstrate each wave of the complex or the typical morphology. Actual morphology depends on the underlying

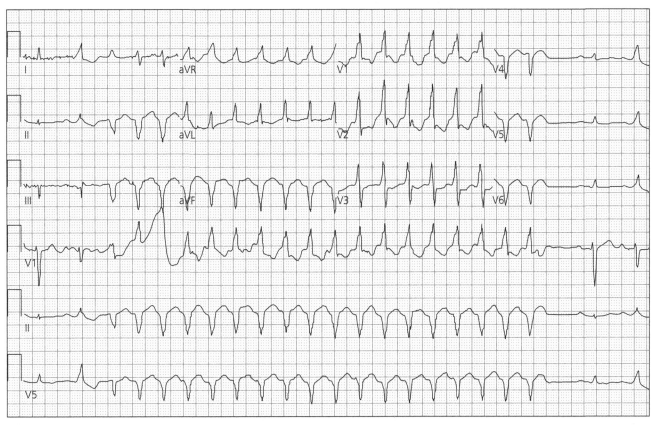

Figure 53.1 The ECG shows a predominant WCT, although a few native supraventricular beats are also evident. Note the frontal plane QRS axis deviation, while the wide complex rhythm is evident; the QRS axis is in the extreme (right superior) quadrant (i.e. the QRS vector is predominantly negative in leads II and aVF). The patient normally has a leftward QRS axis of approximately (−)25 degrees. The third ventricular complex may represent a fusion beat (see lead II rhythm strip).

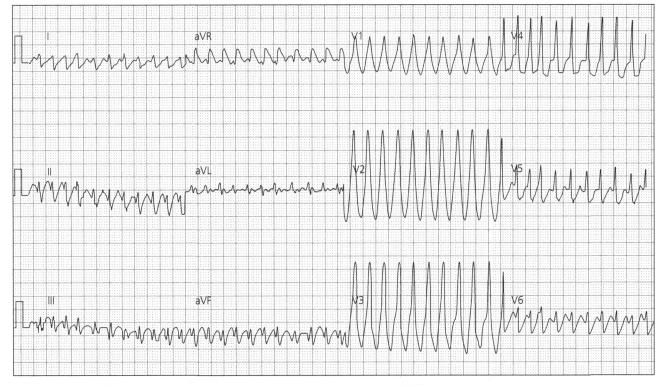

Figure 53.2 Twelve-lead ECG from Case 2. The ECG demonstrates a very rapid, irregular WCT.

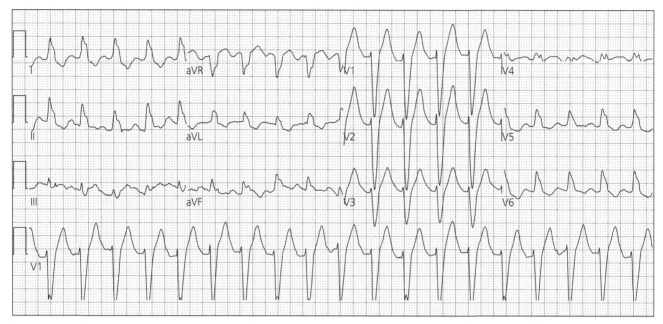

Figure 53.3 Twelve-lead ECG from Case 3. This ECG demonstrates a sinus tachycardia (note presence of regular P waves preceding each QRS complex, seen well in leads II, V5, and V6) with a LBBB resulting in a wide QRS complex.

vector of depolarization of the ventricles, any existing ventricular pathology or other metabolic abnormalities that affect electrical activity of the myocytes, and the actual electrocardiographic lead examined [1,2]. The normal duration of ventricular depolarization in adults is 0.06–0.11 s [2]. Accordingly, the normal width of the QRS complex is 0.06–0.11 s. Because morphology can vary between electrocardiographic leads, the width or duration should be measured in the lead in which the QRS complex is widest – usually one of the precordial leads, typically V2 or V3.

An abnormally wide QRS complex occurs when the duration of the ventricular activation exceeds 0.12 s. This prolongation can occur when the conduction of electrical impulses down the ventricular bundle branches and fascicles is delayed, disrupted, or bypassed. Thus, any rhythm that originates from an ectopic ventricular source outside the normal conduction pathways can result in a wide QRS complex – this includes naturally occurring ectopic beats as well as impulses originating from a ventricular pacemaker. In addition, supraventricular rhythms in which there is aberrant ventricular conduction (such as with bundle branch block) can result in a wide QRS complex. Conditions that can prolong or delay ventricular depolarization by disrupting the normal electrical impulse transmission and activation from myocyte-to-myocyte, such as occurs with severe toxicologic or metabolic abnormalities, can also result in an abnormally wide QRS complex.

Regular WCTs

Tachycardias are differentiated by the regularity of the rhythm. Wide complex tachycardias with a regular rhythm

indicate that while the depolarization of the ventricles is abnormal, the actual rhythm of depolarization is regular. This regularity can occur as a result of recurrent activation from a ventricular focus firing rapidly and regularly, a regular supraventricular tachycardic rhythm with aberrant ventricular conduction, or a re-entry circuit loop with abnormal ventricular depolarization.

Monomorphic ventricular tachycardia: Ventricular tachycardia (VT) is a common cause of WCT [3,4]. In VT, the ventricles are activated at an abnormally fast rate by a focus within the ventricular tissue outside the normal conduction system. This abnormal ventricular rhythm can occur as a result of ischemic heart disease (from active ischemic myocardium or chronic scar tissue), cardiomyopathy, proarrhythmic medications, or severe metabolic and electrolyte abnormalities. Ventricular tachycardia is defined as three or more consecutive ventricular beats at an abnormally fast rate. Ventricular tachycardia with regular wide QRS complexes that appear uniform in morphology over time on the ECG is known as monomorphic VT (Figure 53.1).

Clinically, it can be difficult to distinguish VT from supraventricular tachycardia (SVT) with aberrant ventricular conduction. Both can present with a wide QRS complex tachycardia rhythm on ECG. Common misconceptions are that VT cannot occur in an awake or hemodynamically stable patient. However, both VT and SVT with aberrancy can have minimal hemodynamic effects or present with marked cardiovascular instability.

Despite this difficulty, the 12-lead ECG can provide important clues as to the etiology of a WCT. Numerous criteria, which vary in reliability and applicability, have been developed to differentiate VT [3,4,5,6].

Atrioventricular dissociation: Dissociation of atrial activity (including sinus node impulses) from ectopic ventricular activity in WCTs is essentially diagnostic of VT. However, AV dissociation can be difficult to detect on the ECG particularly in the presence of a rapid VT. If P waves can be detected, it is important to demonstrate a true lack of relationship between atrial and ventricular activity; as ectopic ventricular impulses can give rise to intermittent retrograde P waves (V-A conduction).

Capture and fusion beats: Like AV dissociation, capture and fusion beats are rarely seen on the ECG, but when present are virtually diagnostic of VT. Capture beats occur when there is a narrow or normal appearing QRS complex beat in the midst of a run of WCT. This beat is the result of a supraventricular impulse that is successfully conducted down the normal conduction pathways of the ventricles; indicating that the WCT is otherwise of ventricular origin. Similarly, fusion beats occur when there is partial capture of the ventricles; that is, the successfully transmitted supraventricular impulse combines with an ectopic ventricular beat to activate the ventricles. The result is a fused or intermediate QRS complex that appears morphologically different from that of the WCT run or normal narrow QRS complex (Figures 53.1 and 53.4).

QRS complex morphology: The morphology of the QRS complex in VT depends on the location of the ventricular ectopic foci. The further the activation site from the His bundle and normal conduction pathways, the more abnormal appearing the QRS complex morphology. In general, the QRS complex in VT is often classified by its morphology in lead V1.

A positive QRS complex (V1-positive) implies a left-sided ectopic focus and resulting right bundle branch block (RBBB)-type QRS complex (because right ventricular depolarization occurs later from the left-sided focus). A monophasic or biphasic QRS complex in this case suggests VT. For triphasic complexes, rSR′ patterns are more likely supraventricular rhythms with RBBB aberrant ventricular conduction; whereas RSr′ ("reversed rabbit ears") are more likely VT. In the case of triphasic complexes, an R/S ratio < 1 or QS complex in lead V6 suggests the diagnosis of VT [6].

Ventricular tachycardia with a negative QRS complex in V1 (V1-negative) implies a right-sided focus and resulting LBBB-type QRS complex (because left ventricular depolarization occurs later from the right-sided focus). The presence of an R wave > 0.03 s in leads V1 or V2 suggests VT. Unlike LBBB aberrancy, the downstroke of the S wave can be slurred, notched, or prolonged in VT (> 0.06 s from the start of the QRS complex to nadir of the S wave). The presence of a Q wave, or S wave or QS amplitude > 15 mV deep in lead V6 suggests VT. QRS complexes with an indeterminant axis in lead V1 (neither positive nor negative) are more likely to be VT. In addition, the absence of RS complexes in any of the precordial leads has been suggested as virtually diagnostic of VT [4].

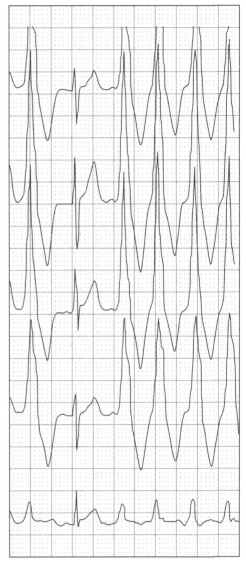

Figure 53.4 Capture beat. The second beat appears quite different from the surrounding wide QRS complexes. This narrow QRS complex appears normal and consistent with a capture beat, suggesting that the wide QRS complex runs are VT.

QRS complex width: It has been suggested that the wider the QRS complex (longer duration), the more likely the diagnosis of VT. In V1-positive patterns (RBBB morphology), a QRS complex width greater than 0.14 s suggests VT. In V1-negative patterns (LBBB morphology), a QRS complex width greater than 0.16 s suggests VT. However, there is significant overlap in QRS complex duration between VT and SVT with aberrancy [5]. For example, ectopic origins near the septum and bundle of His can result in VT with a more narrow QRS complex width.

QRS complex axis: The more abnormal location of the ventricular ectopic foci in VT, the more abnormal the QRS complex axis. As a result, an extreme QRS complex axis from

−90 degrees to +180 degrees (extreme superior) is highly suggestive of VT (Figure 53.1). Otherwise, the QRS complex axis cannot discriminate between VT and SVT with aberrancy.

Concordance: Concordance indicates a uniform axis for the QRS complex across the precordial leads from V1 through V6. Negative concordance implies the presence of negative QRS complexes across leads V1 through V6, whereas positive concordance is evidenced by predominantly positive QRS complexes across the precordium. Concordance is highly suggestive of VT, but can be seen in non-SVT rhythms such as pre-excitation or atrioventricular re-entry tachycardia.

Accelerated idioventricular rhythm: An accelerated idioventricular rhythm (AIVR) is a type of idioventricular rhythm that is rapid rather than being slow. Accelerated idioventricular rhythm can result in a regular tachycardia with wide QRS complexes similar in morphology to those seen in slow idioventricular rhythms.

Ventricular flutter: This is an extreme form of VT that produces a regular sine-wave pattern on the ECG. The impulse rate can exceed 200 bpm and, electrocardiographically, there are no clearly distinct QRS complexes, ST segments, or T waves.

Regular tachycardia with pre-excitation: Pre-excitation occurs when the ventricles are fully or partially activated earlier than would occur down the normal conduction pathways. Pre-excitation primarily occurs with the presence of an accessory pathway (AP), whereby an impulse can be transmitted from the atria to the ventricles outside the normal AV node pathway (such as in Wolff-Parkinson-White syndrome) (Figure 53.5). On the ECG, this pre-excitation

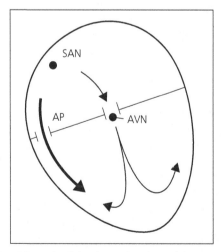

Figure 53.5 Schematic of the electrophysiology of the accessory pathway (AP) in Wolff-Parkinson-White syndrome. Depolarization is transmitted from the sinoatrial node (SAN) to the ventricles via both the AP and AV node (AVN) resulting in pre-excitation of the ventricle.

appears as an initial slurring (delta wave) and widening of the QRS complex. In addition, the PR interval is shortened to less than 0.12 s, and repolarization abnormalities such as T wave inversions may be seen. Wide complex tachycardias can occur in this setting with any supraventricular tachycardias transmitted down the normal conduction pathways in combination with the early pre-excitation of the ventricles (and resulting widening of the QRS complexes).

In addition, APs can lead to more serious WCTs by two mechanisms: rapid atrial rates are transmitted to the ventricles exclusively by the AP, or re-entry circuit loops formed by the AV node and AP that allow recurrent reactivation of the ventricles (atrioventricular re-entry tachycardia – see below). With the former, rapid atrial tachycardias can be directly transmitted to the ventricles primarily through the AP. Because these impulses bypass the normal delay and rate modulation of the AV node, the ventricles are activated not only abnormally (resulting in the wide QRS complexes), but also at the rapid rates of the atrial tachycardia (near 1 : 1 conduction). In the setting of atrial flutter, rapid transmission of impulses down the AP to the ventricles has the potential to result in WCT rates as high as 300 bpm.

Atrioventricular re-entry tachycardia – antidromic conduction: Atrioventricular re-entry tachycardias (AVRTs) occur when a circuit loop exists due to the presence of an AP that bypasses the AV node. As a result of this circuit, impulses are conducted from the atria down (antegrade) either the AV node or AP to activate the ventricles, then conducted back up (retrograde) the alternative pathway (AP or AV node) to re-activate the atria, forming the recurrent circuit loop [7]. In antidromic conduction, antegrade conduction to the ventricles occurs down the AP, and retrograde conduction back to the atria occurs up through the AV node. As a result, the ventricles are depolarized in an abnormal fashion from the AP resulting in a wide QRS complex. The re-entry circuit loop causes recurrent activation of the atria and ventricles resulting in a rapid tachycardia.

Regular SVT with aberrancy or bundle branch block: Supraventricular and atrial tachycardias can result in WCTs if ventricular depolarization is delayed or occurs abnormally outside the normal conduction system (Figure 53.3). The regularity of the WCT tachycardia depends on the regularity of the underlying SVT. Thus, regular SVTs such as sinus tachycardia, atrial tachycardia, junctional tachycardia, AV nodal tachycardia and atrial flutter, can produce a regular WCT in the setting of aberrant ventricular activation. The most common causes of this aberrancy or abnormal ventricular depolarization are LBBB and RBBB, as well as non-specific intraventricular conduction delay, which result in a widening of the QRS complex width.

Tachycardia with pacemakers: Pacemakers with ventricular pacing can cause WCTs in multiple ways. Because

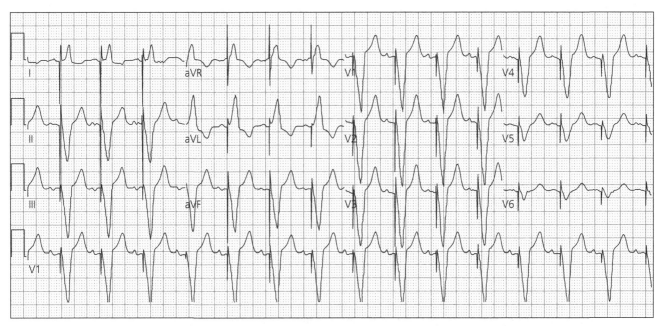

Figure 53.6 This regular, wide QRS complex tachycardia is the result of underlying physiologically appropriate tachycardia in a patient with ventricular pacing. Note the pacing spikes prior to each wide QRS complex that demonstrate a pseudo-LBBB pattern typical of ventricular pacing.

ventricular depolarization comes from the ectopic ventricular site where the pacemaker lead is placed, activation is abnormal and produces a wide QRS complex, most commonly in a LBBB pattern. Accordingly, any tachycardia with ventricular pacing will produce a WCT (Figure 53.6). These tachycardias include any appropriately paced tachycardia, sensor-induced tachycardia (whereby the pacemaker oversenses stimuli and triggers ventricular pacing), and runaway pacemaker (primary component pacemaker failure that results in inappropriate rapid ventricular pacing discharges).

Pacemaker-mediated tachycardia, also known as endless-loop tachycardia, is a re-entry dysrhythmia that can occur in dual-chamber pacemakers with atrial sensing and ventricular pacing. In pacemaker-mediated tachycardia, the pacemaker itself acts as part of the re-entry circuit. The normal ventricular paced beat produces retrograde atrial depolarization (retrograde P wave) that is sensed by the pacemaker as a native atrial stimulus, triggering recurrent ventricular pacing and, thus, forming the re-entry circuit loop [8].

Myocardial ischemia: Acute myocardial ischemia can cause both tachycardia and morphologic changes that produce a wide QRS complex in addition to the more classic ECG findings associated with ischemia and infarction patterns. These changes are the result of ischemic changes and disruption of the normal impulse conduction in the ventricular myocytes. As a result, WCT can be seen electrocardiographically in patients with acute severe myocardial ischemia (Figure 53.7). Similarly, WCT rhythms can be seen immediately following electrical cardioversion as a result of transient changes to the ventricular myocytes.

Hyperkalemia: Potassium is a predominantly intracellular cation that plays an important role in the action potential of myocytes. Severe changes in potassium levels can result in changes in the loss of the transmembrane gradient that can alter impulse propagation down the normal conduction pathways as well as impair electrical transmission from myocyte to myocyte. Hyperkalemia can result in marked widening of the QRS complex and the appearance of a WCT rhythm. Other findings include tall, symmetric T waves, particularly across the precordium, PR segment lengthening, and decreased amplitude and even loss of the P wave on the 12-lead ECG. At severe hyperkalemia, the QRS complex widens and merges with the T wave to produce a "sine-wave" pattern. Interestingly, in extreme circumstances, hypokalemia can also cause WCT rhythms and a sine-wave-type pattern (Figure 53.8).

Toxicologic and pharmacologic causes: Drugs that block sodium (Na^+) channels cause a delay in phase 0 of the cardiac action potential cycle, prolonging ventricular depolarization and widening the QRS complex. Medications that can produce a WCT include anti-dysrhythmics (e.g. procainamide) and non-cardiac medications (e.g. phenothiazines and tricyclic anti-depressants [TCAs]). Sympathomimetic drugs, such as cocaine, cause an increase in heart rate. Cocaine is unique among sympathomimetics because of its ability to block sodium channels. As a result, cocaine toxicity can result in widening of the QRS complex and WCT rhythms (Figure 53.9).

Tricyclic anti-depressants in particular can result in WCT rhythms. Tricyclic anti-depressants pose a unique threat

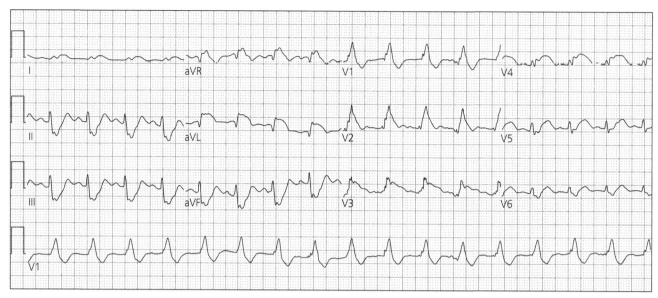

Figure 53.7 Twelve-lead patient with acute anterolateral myocardial infarction subsequently found to have acute occlusion of his left main coronary artery. The acute ischemia resulted not only in marked ST segment changes, but also a wide QRS complex tachycardia.

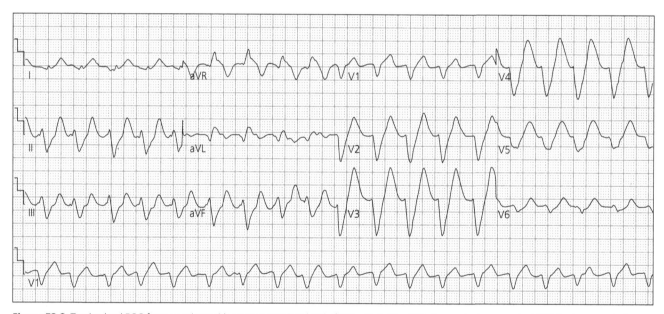

Figure 53.8 Twelve-lead ECG from a patient with serum potassium level of 8.2 mEq/L. The ECG demonstrates a regular WCT that appears to be approaching a sine-wave pattern seen in life-threatening hyperkalemia.

to cardiac function by their anti-cholinergic effect, alpha-adrenergic-blocking properties, inhibition of presynaptic neurotransmitter reuptake, and fast sodium channel-blockade. In addition to QRS widening (from the Na+ channel-block), tachycardia is often present (from the anti-cholinergic effect, catecholamine reuptake inhibition and vasodilation induced by alpha-adrenergic-blockade). A unique finding with QRS complex widening from TCA poisoning is the presence of rightward deviation of the terminal 0.04 s of the frontal plane QRS complex axis. On the 12-lead ECG, this can be detected as a terminal negative deflection S wave in lead I and terminal positive deflection R wave in lead aVR [9].

WCTs with an irregular rate

Wide complex tachycardias with an irregular rate indicate that the abnormal depolarization of the ventricles occurs irregularly. This irregularity can occur as a result of variability in the ventricular impulse foci causing the abnormal

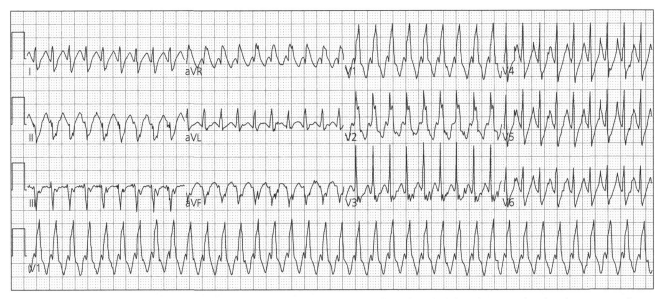

Figure 53.9 Twelve-lead ECG from patient after cocaine overdose resulting in a rapid, regular WCT. Like other sympathomimetic agents, cocaine can cause a regular tachycardia. Cocaine is unique amongst these agents because its sodium channel-blocking properties can result in QRS complex widening.

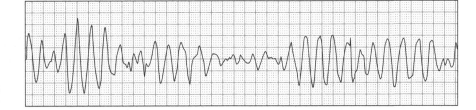

Figure 53.10 Rhythm strip from patient with torsade de pointes. This type of irregular WCT is characterized by the oscillatory nature of the polymorphic wide QRS complexes.

ventricular activation, or an irregular SVT that is conducted to the ventricles in an aberrant manner or via an AP.

Polymorphic ventricular tachycardia: This is a form of VT that originates from multiple different ventricular foci. As a result of this multifocal ventricular ectopy, the QRS complexes are not only abnormally wide, but also vary in morphology including amplitude, axis, and duration. Polymorphic ventricular tachycardia is often associated with ischemic heart disease.

Torsade de pointes: This is a form of polymorphic ventricular tachycardia (PVT) with QRS complex morphology varying beat-to-beat in both amplitude and polarity [10]. Classically, the QRS complex runs appear to "twist" around an isoelectric line (Figure 53.10). These cycles appear as runs of 5 to 20 complexes at a rate of 200–250 bpm. Torsade de pointes is initiated by a premature ventricular beat that falls on the preceding T wave (often there can be a series of premature ventricular beats beforehand, followed by a pause and then the supraventricular beat with the preceding T wave). In fact, underlying prolongation of the QT interval (congenital or acquired) predisposes toward the development of torsade de pointes.

Ventricular fibrillation: This occurs when there is no synchronous or coordinated activation of the ventricles. Electrocardiographically, ventricular fibrillation (VF) appears as an irregular and chaotic rhythm with fibrillatory waves and no discernable QRS complexes. So-called fine VF appears when the amplitude of the fibrillatory waves is so low that the rhythm mimics that of asystole or an isolelectric "flatline" electrocardiographically.

Irregular tachycardia with pre-excitation: As noted above, pre-excitation occurs when the ventricles are fully or partially activated earlier than would occur down the normal conduction pathways, resulting in an initial slurring (delta wave) and widening of the QRS complex. Accordingly, pre-excitation with an underlying irregular tachycardia can result in an irregular WCT. These irregular tachycardias include tachycardias with premature atrial, junctional or ventricular contractions, atrial fibrillation, and atrial flutter or other atrial tachycardias (such as paroxysmal atrial tachycardia) with variable block.

In addition, APs can lead to more serious irregular WCTs when rapid irregular atrial rates are transmitted to the ventricles exclusively by the AP. Because these impulses bypass the normal delay and rate modulation of the AV node, the ventricles are activated not only abnormally (resulting in the wide QRS complexes), but also at the rapid rates of the irregular atrial tachycardia (near 1 : 1 conduction). In the setting of atrial fibrillation, conduction through the AP can result in rapid, irregular ventricular activation at potentially extreme rates up to 300 bpm (Figure 53.2).

Irregular SVT with aberrancy or bundle branch block: Irregular supraventricular and atrial tachycardias can result in irregular WCTs if ventricular depolarization is delayed or occurs abnormally outside the normal conduction system. The regularity of the WCT tachycardia depends on the regularity of the underlying SVT. Thus, irregular SVTs such as atrial fibrillation or tachycardias with premature beats, can produce irregular WCTs in the setting of aberrant ventricular activation. The most common causes of this aberrancy or abnormal ventricular depolarization are left and right bundle branch block, as well as non-specific intraventricular conduction delay which results in a widening of the QRS complex width. In addition, supraventricular and atrial tachycardias with variable AV block can result in irregular rhythms. Again, when these rhythms with variable block are combined with abnormal aberrant ventricular activation or bundle branch block, an irregular WCT will be seen electrocardiographically.

Case conclusions

In all these cases, the critical issue electrocardiographically is the cause and management of the WCT. In Case 1, the WCT was diagnosed as VT. The patient's WCT responded to intravenous lidocaine, which was supplemented with oxygen and nitroglycerin. His serum markers were negative for acute myocardial infarction. The patient ultimately received an automatic implantable cardioverter-defibrillator for treatment of his ventricular tachycardia. In Case 2, the ECG demonstrated an irregular rapid WCT. In the ED, the patient underwent electrical cardioversion, which was successful in returning her to sinus rhythm. A follow-up ECG revealed evidence of pre-excitation including a slurred QRS complex delta wave, shortened PR segment, and repolarization abnormalities. She underwent electrophysiologic study, which demonstrated a left posterior AP that was ablated without complications. In Case 3, the ECG demonstrated a regular WCT with a classic LBBB pattern. Given the patient's prior history of acute coronary syndrome, a prior ECG was obtained from 1 year previously which also demonstrated a LBBB. Accordingly, the WCT was felt to be due to a SVT with aberrant ventricular BBB conduction.

References

1 Mirvis DM, Goldberger AL. Electrocardiography. In: Braunwald E, Zipes DP, Libby P, editors. *Heart Disease: A Textbook of Cardiovascular Medicine*, 6th ed. Philadelphia: WB Saunders; 2001:82–125.

2 Surawicz B, Knilans TK. *Chou's Electrocardiography in Clinical Practice: Adult and Pediatric*, 5th ed. Philadelphia: W.B. Saunders, 2001.

3 Gupta AK, Thakur RK. Wide QRS complex tachycardias. *Med Clin North Am* 2001;**85**:245.

4 Akhtar M. Clinical spectrum of ventricular tachycardia. *Circulation* 1990;**82**:1561.

5 Brugada P, Brugada J, Mont L, *et al.* A new approach to the differential diagnosis of a regular tachycardia with a wide QRS complex. *Circulation* 1991;**83**:1649–59.

6 Brady WJ, Skiles J. Wide QRS complex tachycardia: ECG differential diagnosis. *Am J Emerg Med* 1999;**17**:376–81.

7 Delacretaz E. Supraventricular tachycardia. *N Engl J Med* 2006; **354**:1039–51.

8 Cardall TY, Chan TC, Brady WJ, *et al.* Permanent cardiac pacemakers: issues relevant to the emergency physician, Part I. *J Emerg Med* 1999;**17**(3):479–89.

9 Harrigan RA, Brady WJ. ECG abnormalities in tricyclic antidepressant ingestion. *Am J Emerg Med* 1999;**17**:387–93.

10 Jensen S, Stahmer SA. Ventricular tachycardia and ventricular fibrillation. In: Chan TC, Brady WJ, Harrigan RA, *et al.*, editors. *ECG in Emergency Medicine and Acute Care*. Philadelphia: Elsevier/Mosby, 2005: 118–28.

Chapter 54 | What is the ECG differential diagnosis of bradycardia?

Richard A. Harrigan[1], Theodore C. Chan[2]
[1]Temple University, Philadelphia, PA, USA
[2]University of California, San Diego, CA, USA

Case presentations

Case 1: A 74-year-old woman is sent to the emergency department (ED) from her primary care office with complaints of postural lightheadedness for several days. There is no history of syncope, chest pain, shortness of breath, nausea, or diaphoresis. Her past medical history is remarkable for a history of hypertension treated with metoprolol. On physical examination, her temperature and respiratory rate are normal. Her heart rate is 40 bpm, and her blood pressure in the supine position is 96/60 mmHg. The remainder of her examination is normal. Her ECG is seen in Figure 54.1.

Case 2: A 69-year-old female presents to the ED with several hours of intermittent substernal chest tightness accompanied by shortness of breath and nausea. She felt dizzy. There is no syncope or blood loss. Her past history is significant for diabetes mellitus and high cholesterol. On physical examination, her vital signs are remarkable only for a mildly brady-cardic heart rate of 50 bpm. Her lungs are clear, her heart is without murmurs, gallops, or rubs, and her abdominal examination is normal. Her stool is negative for occult blood. Her initial ECG is seen in Figure 54.2.

Case 3: An 82-year-old woman presents to the ED following electrical countershock for ventricular fibrillation in the field. She had suffered a witnessed arrest with loss of pulse. The first ECG after presentation is shown in Figure 54.3a (with the baseline ECG shown in Figure 54.3b). The patient is intubated with full ventilatory support at the time of this tracing. She has a faint femoral pulse of 60 bpm. Her blood pressure is 86/60 mmHg. Physical examination is remarkable for diffuse crackles on lung examination, a soft abdomen, and no response to painful stimuli.

Critical Decisions in Emergency and Acute Care Electrocardiography, 1st edition. Edited by W.J. Brady and J.D. Truwit. © 2009 Blackwell Publishing, ISBN: 9781405159067

The ECG differential diagnosis of bradydysrhythmias

Bradycardia is usually defined as a heart rate of < 60 bpm (although some use a threshold of 50 bpm) [1]; yet to rigidly define this entity is to miss the key point that all bradycardias are not created equal. Heart rate is a continuous variable; it stands to reason that a heart rate of 61 is not much different than a heart rate of 59, yet only the latter would be brady-cardic if a stiff definition were employed. Most clinically significant bradycardias are below 45 bpm [2], but it is best to regard bradycardia in the context of the clinical situation. Some individuals will be asymptomatic with heart rates as low as 35–40 bpm due to adequate compensatory increases in stroke volume, whereas others will be symptomatic with heart rates in the vicinity of 60 bpm [3]. Symptoms may include syncope or near syncope, lightheadedness, weakness, chest pain with or without radiation, dyspnea, and nausea. Bradydysrhythmias are abnormal rhythms in the bradycardic range. They may result from cardiac ischemia, endocrinologic effects (e.g. hypothyroidism), pharmacologic effects (e.g. beta-adrenergic- or calcium channel-blockers), physiologic responses (e.g. vasovagal responses, hypothermia), infiltrative disease of the cardiac conduction system (e.g. sarcoidosis, amyloidosis), and chronic conduction system disease (e.g. Lev's and Lenegre's disease). Bradydysrhythmias may be subdivided into regular versus irregular varieties, and will be discussed as such below.

Regular bradydysrhythmias

If the QRS complexes appear on the ECG at a slow rate, but with equivalent RR intervals, the bradydysrhythmia is said to be regular. The most common of these is sinus bradycardia (Figure 54.1). Sinus bradycardias originate from the sinus node, which is located in the right atrium. For the rhythm to be sinus bradycardia, there must be a normal appearing P wave before each QRS, with a normal PR interval (range 0.12–0.20 s). Normal P waves are usually upright in leads I and II (at least), due to the major vector of atrial depolarization and subsequent normal P wave axis, which is usually

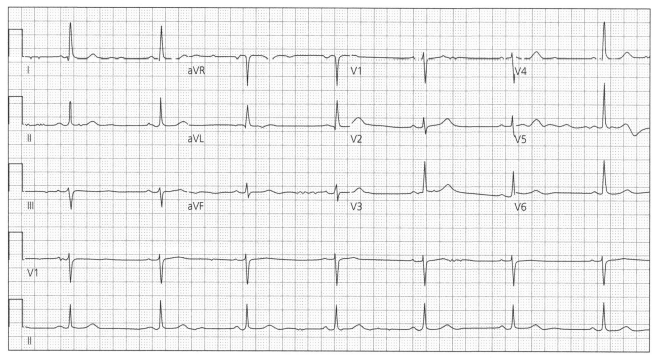

Figure 54.1 Sinus bradycardia. Note the consistent relationship of uniform P waves before every QRS in this regular rhythm. The PR intervals are logically constant as well, and < 0.20 s in this case (i.e. there is no first-degree AV block). The heart rate is 44 bpm.

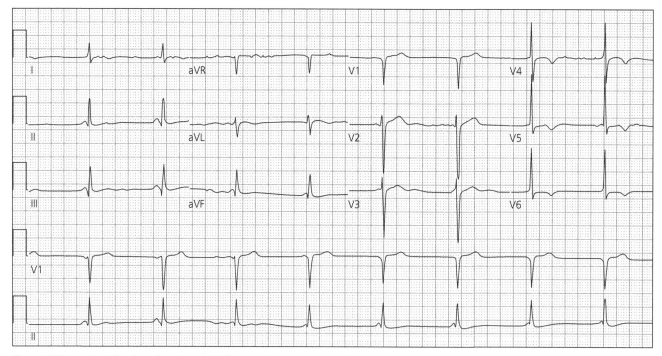

Figure 54.2 Junctional bradycardia. The atrial deflections that precede each of the QRS complexes are too close to the QRS to conduct (i.e. the PR interval is much less than 0.12 s). Note that these deflections are evident in some leads (e.g. lead II) but not others (e.g. V6). The T wave inversions in leads V4–V6 were new and suggestive of coronary ischemia. The heart rate is 52 bpm.

approximately +45 to +60 degrees; the vector axes of leads I and II in the hexaxial plane are 0 and +60 degrees, respectively. At +30 degrees lies the negative pole of the vector axis of lead aVR, so logically most P waves are negative in this lead (Figure 54.1). Sinus bradycardia can have a narrow or

wide QRS complex, depending on whether or not ventricular conduction is aberrant (wide complex).

A junctional rhythm (Figures 54.2 and 54.4) is usually, by definition, bradycardic, with most junctional rhythms ranging between 40 and 60 bpm. A junctional rhythm results

(a)

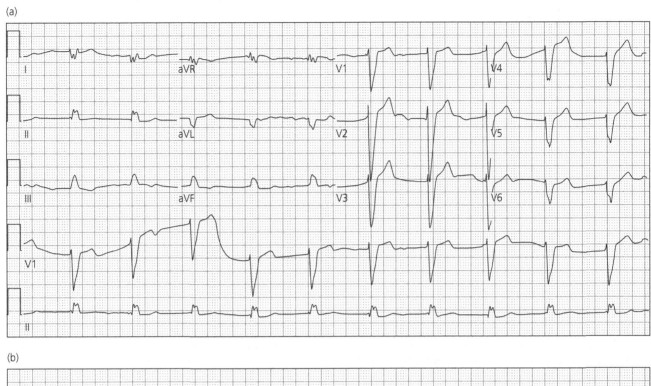

(b)

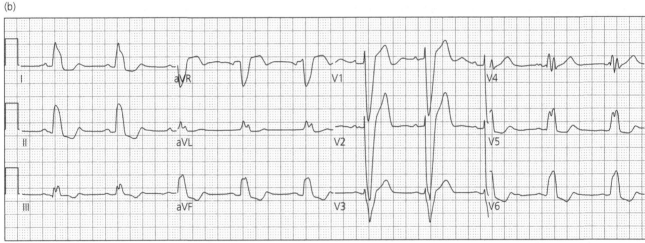

Figure 54.3 Idioventricular rhythm. (a) Note the wide QRS complex rhythm without P waves, at a rate of 60 bpm. The precordial QRS morphologies resemble those of a left bundle branch block, or a ventricular paced rhythm – but are emanating from a native ventricular source. (b) The patient's native rhythm, which is normal sinus with a left bundle branch block. Compare the precordial progression in (a) to that of (b) – the latter being classic for left bundle branch block. Note also the difference between the two tracings insofar as frontal plane QRS axis.

when a subsidiary pacemaker – the atrioventricular (AV) node – takes over the job of cardiac pacemaker boss, usually due to an absence of sinus node activity. As such, it is an escape rhythm when slower than the intrinsic sinus rate. It follows that junctional rhythms feature RR intervals longer than the native PP interval. The ventricle is depolarized by the AV node in junctional (or nodal) rhythms. True sinus P waves will be absent, but atrial waves may appear – before, during, or after the QRS complex – by retrograde conduction (Figures 54.2 and 54.4). These atrial waves reflect atrial depolarization – but this depolarization stems from a nodal impulse propagating "backwards" from the AV node to the atria. The timing of this depolarization reaching the atria

determines when the atrial wave appears on the ECG with respect to the QRS complex (which reflects the ventricular depolarization response to the nodal pacemaker). Atrial waves appearing before the QRS complex should be at an interval of less than 0.11 s [4]. Atrial waves appearing before or after the QRS complex may indeed appear to adjoin the QRS complex (Figure 54.2). These atrial waves, or P′ waves, may be inverted in certain leads – as may any atrial *ectopic* beat – depending on the site of atrial depolarization and its vector relationship to that particular lead. Junctional rhythms feature narrow QRS complexes, unless there is an underlying aberrant ventricular conduction. Healthy people, especially with high vagal tone, may experience periods of a junctional

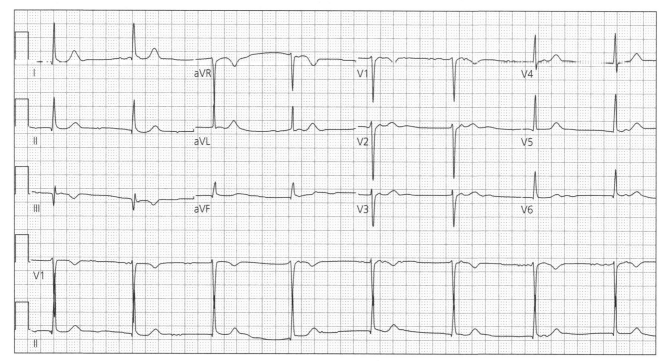

Figure 54.4 Junctional bradycardia. Here the atrial deflections, or P′ waves, are seen immediately after the QRS complex – before the T wave. Leads V2 and V3 demonstrate this well. The heart rate is 49 bpm.

rhythm; symptomatology and clinical milieu are very important in deciphering the degree of pathology in these rhythms.

Beware the sinoventricular rhythm seen with extreme hyperkalemia. This rhythm is usually regular with an apparent wide complex nodal rhythm, although QRS width will vary and the rhythm may appear nodal. In cases of sinoventricular rhythm, the P waves are absent despite the firing of the sinus node; the excess potassium poisons cell-to-cell transmission of the impulse and the P wave disappears. Usually, the potassium is high enough at this juncture to cause the electrocardiographic hallmark of hyperkalemia – peaked, tall T waves [5].

Idioventricular rhythms (Figure 54.3a) are, by definition, bradydysrhythmias with wide QRS complexes, and are usually regular. In these bradydysrhythmias, the role of cardiac pacemaker has passed from the sinoatrial (SA) node, to the AV node, and is now assumed by the ventricle in the form of the His bundle system. As such, the resultant ventricular rate is characteristically slower – usually in the range of 30–40 bpm; if it is faster, it may be termed an accelerated idioventricular rhythm. These rhythms do not occur in healthy people.

Complete heart block (or third-degree AV block) is the most advanced form of AV block (Table 54.1), yet is mentioned early in this discussion because it is in the differential diagnosis of a regular bradycardia. Due to the high degree of interference in AV conduction, the resultant ventricular rate is quite slow, so this rhythm is best considered in a discussion of bradydysrhythmias. When the block is uniform and not

evolving with the clinical situation, complete heart block is usually regular, but at times it has periods of irregularity (Figure 54.5). In complete heart block, the atria and ventricles are dissociated – they are functioning as independent pacemakers, at different rates (the atrial rate is generally faster) (Figure 54.5). As such, the PR interval varies, but the PP interval is constant as is the RR interval (and the PP interval is shorter than the RR interval). The QRS complex may be narrow (nodal escape) or wide (ventricular escape) depending on the level of the block.

Second-degree AV block is frequently irregular, due to the nature of the variable periodicity of the dropped QRS complex (see section on irregular bradydysrhythmias below). However, if it is 2 : 1 second-degree AV block variety (a ratio of two atrial beats for each QRS complex, or more simply stated, P-QRS-T followed by P, followed by P-QRS-T, followed by P, etc.), it may be regular (Figure 54.6). In that every other P wave is not followed by a QRS complex in this dysrhythmia, it is impossible to discern if pure 2 : 1 AV block is Mobitz I or Mobitz II, due to the fact that the PR interval does not have an opportunity to show constancy (Mobitz II) or progressive lengthening (Mobitz I) (Table 54.1).

Irregular bradydysrhythmias

If the QRS complexes appear on the ECG at a slow rate, but with variability in the RR intervals, the bradydysrhythmia is said to be irregular. Sinus arrhythmia is a benign irregular

Table 54.1 Atrioventricular (AV) block

First-degree
In the absence of other pathology, usually a non-bradycardic, regular rhythm
PR interval > 0.20 s
PP and RR intervals usually regular and constant

Second-degree, Mobitz Type I (Wenckebach)
Usually an irregular rhythm, and frequently bradycardic
PR interval gradually lengthening until at last a P wave appears without a corresponding QRS
  complex; the QRS complex is "dropped."
PR interval changes over time (lengthening)
RR interval shortens over time, until the dropped QRS complex (then there is a bigger RR gap); the
  appearance of "grouped beating" is present.
Usually narrow complex
May or may not be bradycardic depending upon the sinus rate and the degree of AV block

Second-degree, Mobitz Type II
Usually an irregular bradycardia rhythm
PR interval is constant, and may be normal or prolonged
RR interval is constant until a QRS complex is "dropped" – then there is a gap
The QRS complex is more frequently wide than narrow

Second-degree AV block, 2 : 1 conduction
Usually a bradycardic, regular rhythm (if the 2 : 1 conduction ratio is maintained)
PR interval is the same in every other beat, because the alternating beats are loan P waves without
  a QRS complex (P-QRS-T, followed by P, followed by P-QRS-T, followed by P, etc.)
The 2 : 1 conduction (two atrial beats for every one ventricular beat) prevents determination of
  whether the PR interval is lengthening, and thus prevents discrimination between Mobitz I and
  Mobitz II conduction

High-grade AV block
Usually an irregular, bradycardic rhythm
Not specifically second- or third-degree AV block
Clinically relevant in that it implies severe conduction system pathology
AV conduction ratio is at least 3 : 1 (three or more P waves for every QRS complex)
Multiple lone P waves without QRS complexes

Third-degree AV block
Usually a regular, bradycardic rhythm
Type of AV dissociation; but there are other types (e.g. accelerated junctional rhythm, ventricular
  tachycardia)
P waves are not linked to the QRS complexes (they are dissociated) – thus the PR interval varies,
  while the PP interval, and the RR interval, remain fixed (in its purest form) but not equal to each
  other
The PP interval is shorter than the RR interval (meaning the atrial rate is faster than the ventricular
  rate)

dysrhythmia that is often within the bradycardia range. Although the morphology of the P wave does not change in this dysrhythmia, the PP interval does – in an accordion-like fashion (lengthening/shortening/lengthening, etc.). In that the PR interval is fixed in sinus arrhythmia, the RR interval varies correspondingly. In healthy individuals (usually with high vagal tone rendering its effect on the SA node), this reflects the phasic variation of the respiratory cycle, with slowing of the rate (increasing PP intervals) during the inspiratory phase, and quickening of the rate (decreasing PP intervals) during the expiratory phase (Figure 54.7). In older individuals, sinus arrhythmia may be independent of the respiratory cycle, and be more indicative of pathology [4].

Sinus pause or sinus arrest generally does not follow a periodicity, and thus may present as an irregular bradydysrhythmia. The hallmark is an underlying sinus rhythm with periods of asystole. Sinus arrest is a longer version of sinus pause; the distinction being relative.

Second-degree AV block usually presents as an irregular dysrhythmia, but may or may not be bradycardic in rate. It will be discussed here for the sake of completeness, since third-degree AV block is so frequently bradycardic and is discussed above. Mobitz I second-degree AV block features a progressive lengthening of the PR interval, culminating in a P wave that occurs in isolation without a corresponding QRS complex. This so-called dropped QRS gives the rhythm its irregularity (Figure 54.8). The RR intervals progressively

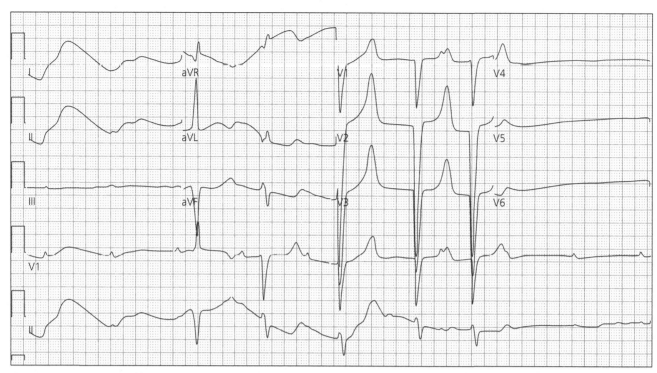

Figure 54.5 Complete heart block with evidence of high-grade AV block. The PP interval is shorter than the interval between the wide complex beats in the middle of the tracing, constituting the RR interval in this case of a patient with an unstable third-degree AV block. The P waves (best seen in the lead V1 rhythm strip) are dissociated from the QRS complexes, and the PR interval is, thus, variable. Note periods of ventricular asystole at the beginning and end of the tracing, where there are multiple P waves without QRS complexes. This is high-grade AV block.

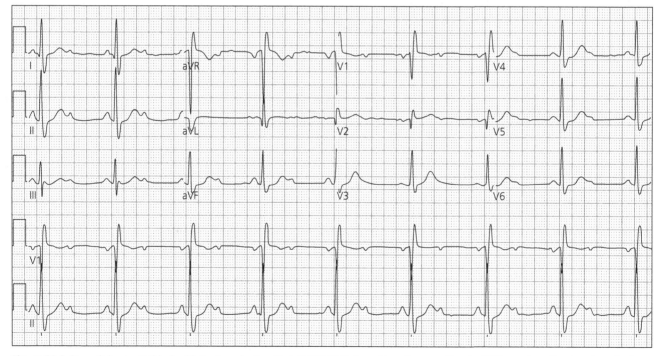

Figure 54.6 Second-degree AV block with 2 : 1 conduction. Each P-QRS-T is followed by a P wave without a QRS complex – thus meeting criteria for AV block (P waves with "dropped" QRS complexes). As every other QRS complex is absent, this is 2 : 1 conduction. In such cases, it is impossible to determine if the PR interval is lengthening (as in Mobitz I) or constant (as in Mobitz II). The ventricular rate is bradycardic at 50 bpm.

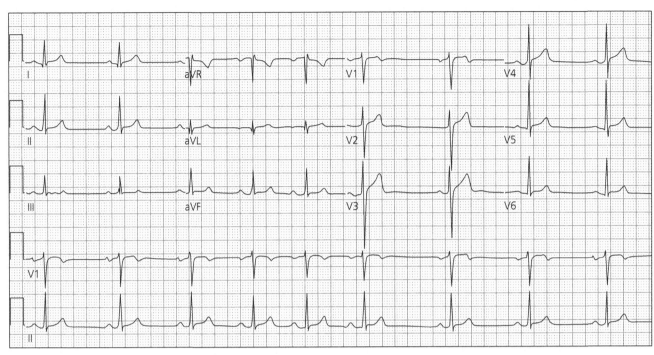

Figure 54.7 Sinus arrhythmia. This 27-year-old male was asymptomatic from a cardiac standpoint. Note the phasic variation in RR intervals without a change in the PR intervals. The heart rate is 54 bpm.

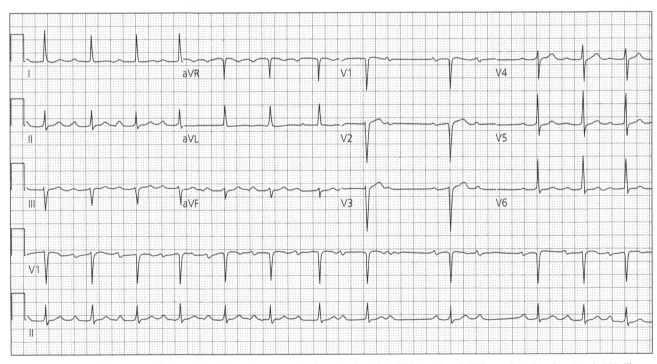

Figure 54.8 Second-degree AV block, Mobitz I. Note the progressive lengthening of the PR interval until QRS complex #9 is absent, as is #11. The ninth and eleventh P waves are still present, however. This tracing shows evidence of a baseline first-degree AV block (PR interval > 0.20 s) before progressing to the Wenckebach rhythm.

shorten prior to this dropped QRS (Table 54.1). The QRS complexes are generally narrow in this form of AV block, unless an underlying condition of aberrant ventricular conduction exists. Mobitz II second-degree AV block features the same hallmark as Mobitz I – an absent QRS complex – but differs from Mobitz I in that the PR interval is fixed (be it prolonged or not) prior to the loss of a QRS complex (Table 54.1) (Figure 54.9). The QRS complex may be of normal width, or prolonged. Mobitz II carries a graver prognosis than docs Mobitz I second-degree AV block.

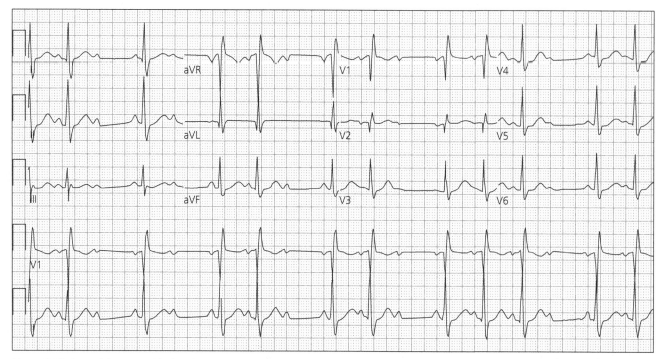

Figure 54.9 Second-degree AV block, Mobitz II. There is no progressive lengthening of the PR interval before the "dropped" QRS complexes in this tracing.

Case conclusions

In Case 1, the patient was not given any pharmacotherapy in the ED, as she was stable clinically. She was admitted for telemetric monitoring and a rule-out acute coronary syndrome protocol was instituted. It was discovered upon review of her medications that she had two bottles of metoprolol, and that she was taking pills from both. After an initial period of holding all metoprolol, she was restarted on her usual regimen and did well.

In Case 2, the patient was admitted and her cardiac enzymes were positive, thus suggestive of cardiac ischemia. She was admitted. Her junctional rhythm resolved. She refused cardiac catheterization, and was managed medically.

In Case 3, the patient's clinical status deteriorated over time in the ED. She had multiple periods of hypotension that were eventually not responsive to vasopressor therapy. Her Glasgow Coma Scale score was 3. After a discussion with her family, the decision was made to withdraw care, and the patient expired in the ED.

References

1 Kastor JA. *Arrhythmias.* 2nd ed. WB Saunders: Philadelphia, 2000.
2 Brown KR. Bradycardias and heart blocks. In: Mattu A, Tabas JA, Barish RA editors. *Electrocardiography in Emergency Medicine.* American College of Emergency Physicians: Dallas TX, 2007:27–44.
3 Ware CJ, Ufberg JW. Bradycardia and escape rhythms. In: Chan TC, Brady WJ, Harrigan RA, *et al.*, editors *ECG in Emergency Medicine and Acute Care.* Elsevier Mosby: Philadelphia, 2006:77–82.
4 Harrigan RA. Dysrhythmias at normal rates. In: Chan TC, Brady WJ, Harrigan RA, *et al.*, editors. *ECG in Emergency Medicine and Acute Care.* Elsevier Mosby: Philadelphia, 2006:31–5.
5 Shumaik GM. Electrolyte abnormalities. In: Chan TC, Brady WJ, Harrigan RA, *et al.*, editors. *ECG in Emergency Medicine and Acute Care.* Elsevier Mosby: Philadelphia, 2006:282–7.

Chapter 55 | What is the ECG differential diagnosis of the abnormally wide or large QRS complex?

Theodore C. Chan[1], *Richard A. Harrigan*[2]
[1]University of California, San Diego, CA, USA
[2]Temple University, Philadelphia, PA, USA

Case presentations

Case 1: A 36-year-old man in police custody is brought to the emergency department (ED) by paramedics for seizures. The police report pursuing the man for possession and trafficking of illicit drugs. At the time of apprehension, the patient reportedly swallowed a number of small bags containing a white substance. On arrival, the patient is experiencing intermittent seizures with no lucid interval. His examination is notable for vital signs of pulse 100 beats per minute (bpm), blood pressure 96/56 mmHg, respiratory rate of 36 breaths per minute and temperature of 101.4 °F. He is confused with lungs clear bilaterally on auscultation, and a tachycardic regular rate with occasional irregular beats and no murmurs or rubs on cardiac examination. The electrocardiogram (ECG) (Figure 55.1) demonstrates a marked abnormal wide QRS complex (0.18 s).

Case 2: A 58-year-old woman presents to the ED complaining of pleuritic chest pain. She has no prior history of coronary artery disease, but states "my doctor told me my ECG was abnormal in the past." She denies shortness of breath, arm, neck or back pain, or weakness. Her examination is notable for vital signs of pulse 107 bpm, blood pressure 138/82 mmHg, respiratory rate of 18 breaths per minute and temperature of 98.8°F. Her lungs are clear on examination, and cardiac auscultation reveals a tachycardic regular rate with no murmurs or gallops. The ECG (Figure 55.2) demonstrates a widened QRS complex (0.16 s) and a pattern consistent with left bundle branch block (LBBB).

Case 3: A 64-year-old man with history of diabetes mellitus and end-stage renal disease on hemodialysis presents to the ED complaining of weakness after missing his dialysis 2 days previously. His vital signs are notable for a pulse rate

of 36 bpm, blood pressure 82/54 mmHg, respiratory rate of 24 breaths per minute, and temperature of 96.7 °F. On examination, his chest is notable for bibasilar crackles, but good air movement, and cardiac auscultation reveals a regular bradycardic rate with no murmurs or rubs. The ECG (Figure 55.3) demonstrates a remarkable bradycardia at a rate of 29 bpm and widened QRS complexes (0.18 s).

Differential diagnosis of the abnormally large or wide QRS complex

Normal QRS complex: The QRS complex on the 12-lead ECG represents depolarization and activation of the ventricles. The Q wave is the initial negative deflection, followed by the R wave as the first positive deflection, and concluding with the S wave, the negative deflection following the R wave (if another positive deflection occurs after the S wave, it is known as the R' wave). If the QRS complex features only a negative deflection, it is termed a QS complex. Not all electrocardiographic leads demonstrate each wave of the complex or the typical morphology. The actual morphology of the QRS complex depends on the underlying vector of depolarization of the ventricles, any existing ventricular pathology or other metabolic abnormalities that affect electrical activity of the ventricular myocytes, and the actual electrocardiographic lead examined.

Normal depolarization of the ventricles occurs when impulses are conducted from the atria through the atrioventricular (AV) node to the bundle of His, and down both the right and left bundle branches, the latter of which divides into anterior and posterior fascicles. While depolarization is nearly simultaneous down both the right and left bundle branches, ventricular activation does occur as a two-phase event. The initial vector is in a left-to-right and slightly anterior direction as activation of the ventricular septum occurs. Second, the vector changes to a predominantly right-to-left and slightly inferior direction as depolarization of the right and much larger left ventricular free wall occurs. On the normal

Critical Decisions in Emergency and Acute Care Electrocardiography, 1st edition. Edited by W.J. Brady and J.D. Truwit. © 2009 Blackwell Publishing, ISBN: 9781405159067

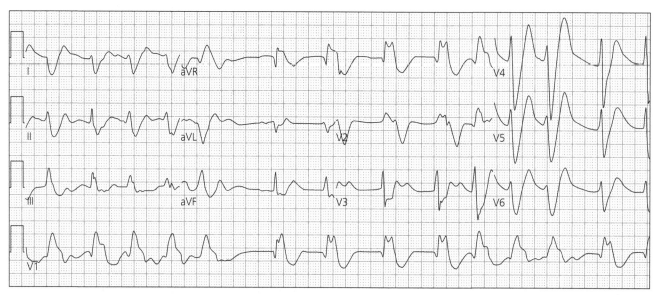

Figure 55.1 The 12-lead ECG from the patient of Case 1 demonstrates a wide QRS complex as a result of cocaine toxicity.

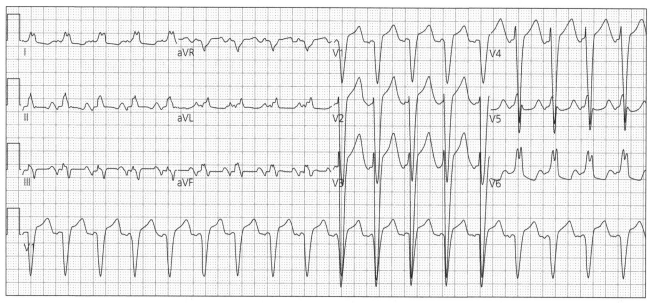

Figure 55.2 The 12-lead ECG from the patient of Case 2 demonstrates a wide QRS complex as a result of LBBB. Note the qS and rS waves in the right precordial leads, which simulate acute anteroseptal injury, and the appropriately discordant ST segment/T wave complexes.

12-lead ECG, the septal phase vector produces an initial small, low amplitude positive deflection (R wave) in the rightward and anterior leads (aVR, V1) and small negative deflection (Q wave) in the leftward leads (I, aVL, V5, V6). After this small deflection, the vector axis changes to produce a much larger amplitude negative deflection in the right-sided leads, resulting in an rS wave; as well as a large positive deflection in the left-sided leads, producing the qR or qRs pattern on the normal 12-lead ECG [1,2].

The normal duration of ventricular depolarization and width of the QRS complex in adults is 0.06–0.11 s [2]. Again,

because morphology can vary between electrocardiographic leads, the width or duration should be measured in the lead in which the QRS complex is widest – usually one of the precordial leads, typically V2 or V3. The intrinsicoid deflection is the interval on the electrocardiographic tracing representing the time till full depolarization of the ventricular free wall. The interval is measured from the beginning of the QRS complex to the peak of the R wave in positive leads, or nadir of the S wave in negative leads. In right precordial leads, the upper limit of normal for the intrinsicoid deflection is 0.035 s, while in the left precordial leads it is 0.045 s.

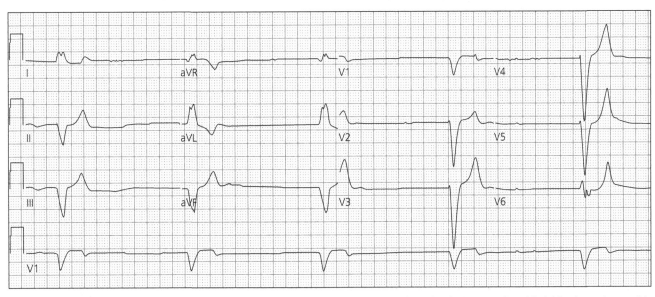

Figure 55.3 The 12-lead ECG from the patient of Case 3 demonstrates a marked bradycardia and wide QRS complex. This rhythm is consistent with a sinoventricular rhythm as a result of severe hyperkalemia. Note the peaked T waves as well.

Abnormally large QRS complex

QRS complex amplitude is determined by the vector of ventricular depolarization and, accordingly, varies by electrocardiographic lead. The amplitude of the normal Q wave is less than one-quarter of that of the corresponding R wave in the same lead, and generally less than 0.4 mV (with the exception of lead III where the Q wave may be larger). The normal R wave amplitude also varies based on electrocardiographic lead and is generally largest in the leads overlying the left ventricle. The R wave amplitude increases progressively across the precordium and is largest in lead V4. In contrast, the normal S wave amplitude decreases progressively across the precordium and is found at its maximum in leads aVR and V2.

The abnormally large QRS complex occurs when the amplitude of the QRS complex is markedly increased in a given electrocardiographic lead. The differential diagnosis of the abnormally large QRS complex includes a variety of pathologic and non-pathologic conditions. This differential can be further broken down by the width or duration of the QRS complex. The differential for large and wide QRS complexes will be addressed later in this chapter. The differential diagnosis for abnormally large amplitude, but normal duration or narrow QRS complexes includes ventricular hypertrophy, normal variants particularly in athletes and benign early repolarization, and other non-cardiac conditions such as hyperthyroidism. However, the most common cause of the large QRS complex that will be seen by the emergency physician (EP) is left or right ventricular hypertrophy.

Left ventricular hypertrophy: The increased left ventricular mass in left ventricular hypertrophy (LVH) results in a marked increase in amplitude on the QRS complex. In fact, the abnormally large QRS complex is the most characteristic finding for LVH on the 12-lead ECG. In addition, with LVH there is a change in the position of the heart such that the lateral free wall lies more directly below the anterior chest producing additional changes in the QRS complex. As a result of these changes, the dominant vector of depolarization is directed leftward and more posteriorly.

On the 12-lead ECG, this change in vector and ventricular mass results in an increase in the amplitude of the dominant R wave in the leads directed toward the left (I, aVL, V5 and V6). In fact, in these leads the QRS complex may appear as a large Rs wave or monophasic R wave. There is a large negative deflection or increase in the S wave in those leads on the right side (V1 and V2). In the precordial leads, there can be poor R wave progression and loss of the R wave in the septal leads, resulting in a QS pattern in leads V1 and V2.

Threshold voltage and QRS complex amplitude criteria have been developed for LVH on the 12-lead ECG (Table 55.1). These criteria are often specific but not sensitive for the diagnosis of LVH [3]. These criteria are defined by the amplitude of the R wave in a left-sided lead (such as R wave amplitude in lead aVL > 11 mV) or a combination of the amplitude of the R wave in a left-sided lead and the S wave in a septal lead (such as R wave amplitude in leads V5 or V6 plus S wave amplitude in leads V1 or V2 > 35 mV) to establish the diagnosis of LVH (Figure 55.4).

In addition, because of the increased cardiac muscle mass, activation may be slightly prolonged and produce widening or notching of the QRS complex. The intrinsicoid deflection may be greater than 0.05 s, particularly in leads V5 and V6, reflecting the longer duration to fully depolarize the myocardium in the setting of ventricular hypertrophy [1,2].

Table 55.1 Electrocardiographic criteria for LVH

S wave in V1 + (R wave in V5 or V6) > 35 mV [Sokolow–Lyon Index]

S wave in V3 + R wave in aVL > 28 mV (men) or > 20 mV (women) [Cornell Voltage Criteria]

R wave in I + S wave in III > 25 mV

R wave in aVL > 11 mV

Romhilt and Estes Point Score System

    1. Amplitude (3 points if any of the following):

        a. R wave or S wave in any limb lead ≥ 20 mV

        b. S wave in leads V1 or V2 ≥ 30 mV

        c. R wave in leads V5 or V6 ≥ 30 mV

    2. ST segment/T wave – typical repolarization abnormality without digitalis (3 points), with digitalis (1 point)

    3. Left atrial abnormality (3 points)

    4. Left axis deviation ≥ 30 degrees (2 points)

    5. QRS complex duration ≥ 0.09 s (1 point)

    6. Intrinsicoid deflection in V5 or V6 ≥ 0.05 s (1 point)

Total points = 4 points: LVH probable

Total points ≥ 5 points: LVH present

Beyond the QRS complex, there are additional ECG findings indicative of LVH. With increased muscle mass, marked changes in repolarization as well as depolarization can occur, resulting in abnormal findings in the ST segment and T waves. In the left-sided lateral leads with prominent R waves (I, aVL, V5, and V6), there can be ST segment depression and T wave inversion. In right-sided septal leads with prominent S waves (V1 and V2), there can be ST segment elevation and tall upright T waves. These findings are commonly referred to as a "strain pattern," but are more correctly termed "repolarization abnormality" associated with LVH (Figure 55.4).

The repolarization abnormality associated with LVH – ST segment depression or elevation, with T wave inversion or prominence, respectively – can be misdiagnosed as acute cardiac ischemia [4,5]. However, the ST segment elevation associated with LVH repolarization abnormality seen in those leads with prominent S or qS waves (V1 or V2) has an initial upsloping that is more typically concave rather than the flat or convex pattern classically seen in AMI. The ST segment depression in the lateral leads with prominent R waves is associated with J point depression and bowed or convex upward ST segment morphology in LVH. The T wave inversions seen in these same leads (most prominently in lead V6, often greater than 3 mm) are asymmetric with a slow or longer initial downslope, followed by a rapid upstroke, as opposed to the more symmetric T wave inversions of ischemia. In addition, there can be an "overshoot" of the terminal T wave (terminal positivity) that can produce the appearance of near biphasic T waves.

Other findings that can be associated with LVH include left axis deviation and left atrial abnormality. On the ECG, these findings can be detected with a negative QRS complex axis

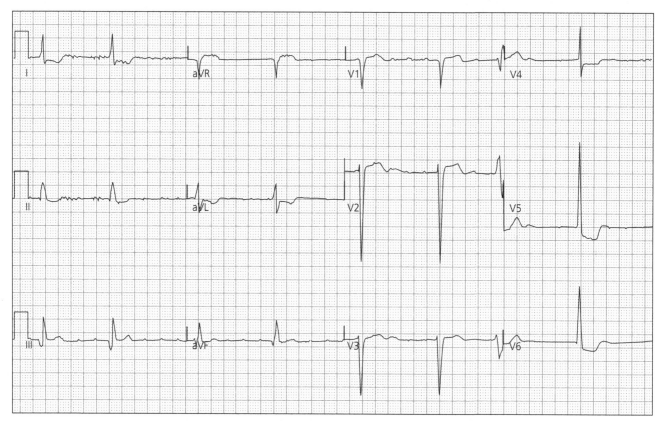

Figure 55.4 This 12-lead ECG shows an abnormally large S wave in V2 and R wave in V5 consistent with voltage criteria for LVH. Note the discordant ST segment and T wave repolarization abnormalities that are expected with LVH.

Table 55.2 Electrocardiographic criteria for RVH

R/S ratio in leads V5 or V6 < 1
R/S ratio in lead V1 > 1 (with R wave > 0.7 mV)
S wave in leads V5 or V6 > 0.7 mV
R wave in leads V5 or V6 < 0.4 mV with S wave in lead V1 < 0.2 mV
Right axis deviation > +110 degrees
P pulmonale
S wave in I, II, III pattern

more than −30 degrees and P wave in lead V1 with terminal negativity greater than 1 mm and 0.04 s in duration, respectively. A bifid or notched P wave in lead II is suggestive of left atrial abnormality as well.

Right ventricular hypertrophy: Because the left ventricle is normally larger than the right, findings of right ventricular hypertrophy (RVH) on the ECG are often not apparent until the right ventricle is two or three times its normal size. At that point, the mass of the RVH overcomes the electrical vector of the left ventricle electrocardiographically. The electrical forces of the hypertrophied right ventricle are directed anteriorly and rightward. As a result, RVH results in a positive vector in this direction, producing an increase in amplitude of the R waves in the rightward, septal leads (V1 and V2). In contrast, there are deep S waves in the leftward and lateral precordial leads (V5 and V6).

Similar to LVH, criteria have been developed for detecting RVH on the ECG that have excellent specificity, but low sensitivity (Table 55.2). These criteria include an R/S ratio greater than 1 in lead V1 and an R/S ratio less than 1 in leads V5 or V6, indicative of a change in the predominant electrical vector away from the normal left lateral direction to the anterior right and septal direction with RVH (Figure 55.5).

Other electrocardiographic findings include the rSr' or qR patterns in lead V1 in mild RVH, as well as the less specific $S_1S_2S_3$ pattern (predominant negative S waves or R/S ratio less than one in leads I, II, and III). Similar to LVH, repolariza-

tion abnormalities can also be seen in RVH. These findings include J point depression, ST segment depression with bowed convex upward morphology, and asymmetric T wave inversions in the right precordial leads (V1 and V2) and inferior limb leads. Right axis deviation with a QRS complex axis greater than +110 degrees and evidence of right atrial abnormality (prominent peaked P wave in lead II) can also be present on the ECG in the setting of RVH.

Abnormally wide QRS complex

An abnormally wide QRS complex occurs when the duration of the ventricular activation exceeds the normal 0.12 s. This prolongation can occur when the conduction of electrical impulses down the ventricular bundle branches and fascicles is delayed, disrupted, or bypassed. Thus, any rhythm in which there is aberrant ventricular conduction (such as with bundle branch block) can result in a wide QRS complex. In addition, conditions that can prolong or delay ventricular depolarization by disrupting the normal electrical impulse transmission and activation from myocyte to myocyte, such as occurs with severe hyperkalemia, can also result in an abnormally wide QRS complex.

Ventricular ectopy: Ectopic activation of the ventricles outside the normal conduction pathway results in wide, and at times bizarre, QRS complexes. Because activation from an ectopic focus within the ventricles occurs with little or no involvement of the normal electrical pathways, the resulting QRS complex can be extremely wide (> 0.14 s). Ectopic ventricular activation occurring between beats of normal depolarization is seen on the ECG as wide, abnormal QRS complexes, or premature ventricular contractions (PVCs), interspersed between normal QRS complexes. Increasing frequency of ectopic ventricular beats can result in couplets, triplets, bigeminy (alternating ectopic and normal beats of ventricular depolarization) and runs of idioventricular

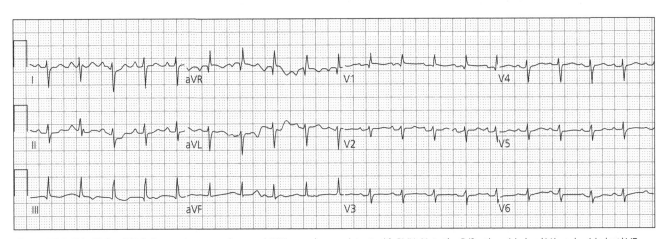

Figure 55.5 This 12-lead ECG demonstrates an abnormal QRS complex consistent with RVH. Note the R/S ratio > 1 in lead V1 and < 1 in lead V5. The ECG also demonstrates a right axis deviation.

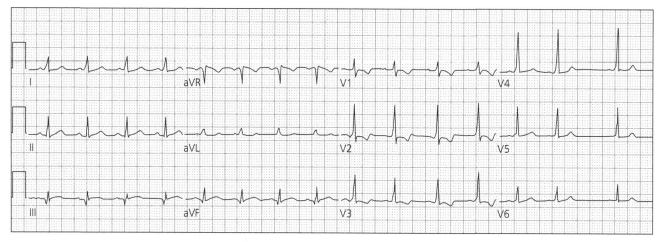

Figure 55.6 This 12-lead ECG shows a slurred upstroke on the QRS complex, shortened PR interval and slightly widened QRS complex. In addition, there are ST segment and T wave abnormalities (particularly in leads V1–V3) all consistent with the existence of an accessory pathway and pre-excitation. This patient has Wolff-Parkinson-White syndrome.

rhythms or even ventricular tachycardia. In addition, in the setting of complete AV block, ventricular escape beats will also produce similar wide, bizarre QRS complexes at a slow rate, usually less than 60 bpm.

Pre-excitation: When an accessory pathway (AP) exists in addition to the AV node, impulses can potentially propagate down the AP and activate or "pre-excite" the ventricle prior to the normal impulse via the AV node. Wolff-Parkinson-White (WPW) syndrome is one type of pre-excitation syndrome caused by the presence of an AP known as the Bundle of Kent. Accessory pathways are associated with significant tachydysrhythmias as a result of the rapid propagation of atrial tachycardias through the AP node (effectively bypassing the normal delay of the AV node), or by the creation of a re-entry loop between the atria and ventricles involving the AV node and AP circuits.

In many cases, however, the existence of an AP and WPW syndrome is detected by evidence of pre-excitation during sinus rhythm on the 12-lead ECG. In these cases, the QRS complex appears wide with an initial slurring of the complex known as the delta wave [6]. The delta wave occurs as a result of the ventricular pre-excitation caused by impulse conduction down the AP just ahead of the impulse transmitted through the AV node, which activates the remainder of the ventricles. Another electrocardiographic finding indicative of pre-excitation includes shortening of the PR interval to < 0.12 s as a result of the early activation and pre-excitation. In addition, there can be ST segment and T wave abnormalities, such as discordant T waves, because of the changes in repolarization following the abnormal depolarization that occurs with pre-excitation (Figure 55.6).

Bundle branch block: Intraventricular conduction abnormalities are common and can occur at any level of the

Table 55.3 Electrocardiographic findings in LBBB

QRS complex ≥ 0.12 s
QS or rS complex in right precordial leads (V1–V3)
No Q wave in lateral leads (I, V5, and V6)
Large prominent R wave in lateral leads (I, V5, and V6)

bundle branches or fascicles. In general, however, only blocks at the level of the left or right bundle branches result in an overall delay in ventricular activation and abnormal widening of the QRS complex. In these cases, the ventricles are not depolarized simultaneously, but rather sequentially. Thus, the QRS interval is prolonged.

In the setting of left bundle branch block (LBBB), depolarization of the left ventricle is delayed resulting in widening (in the case of complete LBBB) of the QRS complex to > 0.12 s. In addition, the intrinsicoid deflection in lead V6 is at least 0.08 s in duration. Typical abnormalities of the QRS complex in LBBB include a mostly negative deflection QS or rS complex in the right precordial leads (V1 and V2) and a large positive deflection or monophasic R wave in the left sided leads (I and V6) (Figures 55.2, 55.7 and Table 55.3). In fact, the presence of a Q wave in leads I or V6 makes the diagnosis of LBBB doubtful. Left axis deviation also may be present on the ECG.

Because of the abnormal depolarization, changes also occur in repolarization and abnormalities in the ST segment and T wave are expected with bundle branch blocks. In general, the appropriate abnormalities seen in the ST segment/ T wave complex are dictated by the major terminal portion of the QRS complex in a given lead. The rule of appropriate discordance dictates that ST segment depressions and T wave inversions are seen in leads with predominantly positive QRS complexes; ST segment elevations and prominent upright T waves are seen in leads with predominantly negative QRS

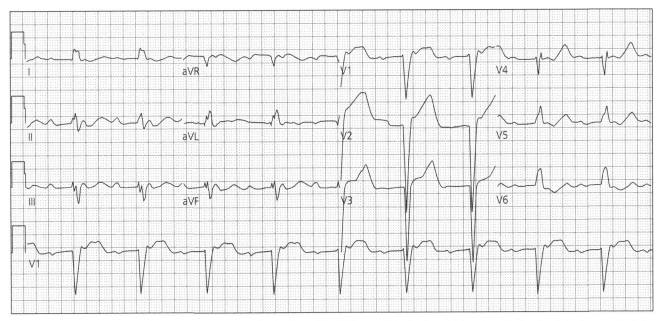

Figure 55.7 This 12-lead ECG shows another example of LBBB. The wide QRS interval is indicative of delayed ventricular depolarization, particularly in the lateral leads I, aVL, and V6 with monophasic R, rR' or Rr' waves. The ST segment and T waves are appropriately discordant in those leads with primarily negative QS complexes (precordial leads).

complexes [5]. Thus, in LBBB, ST segment depression and T wave inversion may be seen in the left lateral leads I and V6, whereas ST segment elevation (with upward concavity of the initial portion) and prominent upright T wave may be seen in the right precordial leads V1 and V2.

In complete right bundle branch block (RBBB), depolarization of the right side of the heart is delayed. The QRS complex is again wide (> 0.12 s) with an intrinsicoid deflection delayed to at least 0.08 s. In the right-sided precordial leads, particularly lead V1, the predominant deflection is positive, producing a large R wave. The R wave can be notched and form the classic rSR' pattern, but a monophasic, notched, or qR morphology also may be present (Figure 55.8). In the lateral leads I and V6, a wide, but shallow S or rS wave may be seen on the ECG (Table 55.4). As with LBBB, appropriate discordance of the ST segment and T wave may be associated with these changes. In particular, discordant ST segment depression and inverted and asymmetric T wave with a slow downslope and rapid return may be seen in the right precordial leads V1 through V3.

Ventricular paced beats: Pacemakers that pace the heart through the ventricular chambers (usually the right ventricle) result in a wide QRS complex similar to that of

Table 55.4 Electrocardiographic criteria for RBBB

QRS complex ≥ 0.12 s
Prominent R wave, qR wave or notched R wave (rSR') in lead V1
Wide S wave in lateral leads (I and V6)

LBBB. Following the pacer spike on the ECG, ventricular depolarization produces wide, predominantly negative QS or rS waves with poor R wave progression across the precordium. QS complexes may also be seen in the inferior leads II, III, and aVF. Large positive R waves may be present in leads I and aVL. Left axis deviation usually occurs as well, particularly if the pacing lead is placed near the apex of the heart. Similar to BBB, the rule of appropriate discordance applies for the ST segment/T wave complex in ventricular pacing. In leads with predominantly negative QRS complexes, ST segment elevation and upright T waves will be seen; in leads with predominantly positive QRS complexes, ST segment depression and asymmetric T wave inversions will be seen (Figure 55.9) [7].

Hyperkalemia: Potassium is a predominantly intracellular cation that plays an important role in depolarization and repolarization in the action potential of myocytes. Both hypokalemia and hyperkalemia can have significant electrophysiologic effects on the heart and result in changes on the ECG. QRS complex widening can be seen in the setting of severe hyperkalemia (> 8.0 mEq/L). Severe hyperkalemia results in the loss of the transmembrane gradient that can slow impulse propagation down the normal conduction pathways as well as impair electrical transmission from myocyte to myocyte. QRS complex widening with the appearance of intraventricular conduction delays may mimic BBB; loss of the P wave and emergence of a sinoventricular rhythm due to impaired sinoatrial automaticity, and AV nodal conduction can result (Figure 55.3). At extremely high potassium levels, the QRS complex widens and merges with the T wave

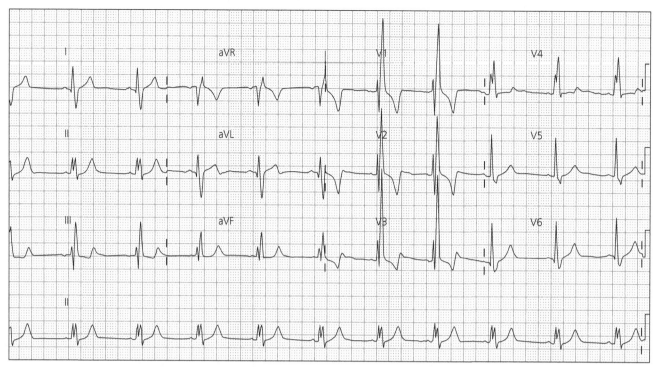

Figure 55.8 This 12-lead ECG demonstrates RBBB. Note the prominent rSR' wave in the right-sided precordial leads (particularly lead V1). In addition, note the wide S wave in lead V6. There is also evidence of ST segment and T wave repolarization abnormalities that are appropriately discordant.

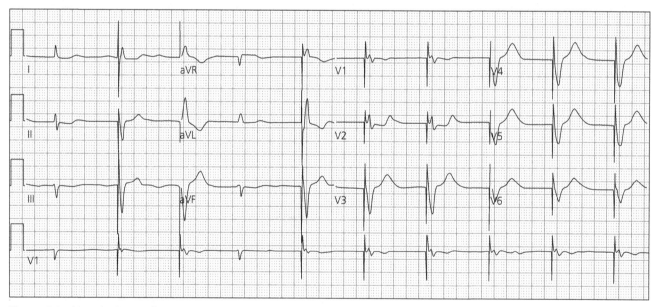

Figure 55.9 This 12-lead ECG is from a patient with a ventricular pacemaker. Note the pacer spikes followed by an abnormal, wide QRS complex with a morphology similar to that of LBBB.

to produce a "sine-wave" pattern, which can rapidly deteriorate into ventricular fibrillation and asystole.

Early evidence for hyperkalemia can be seen on the ECG prior to the QRS widening at higher potassium levels. These findings include tall, symmetric T waves particularly across the precordium, PR segment lengthening, and decreased amplitude and even loss of the P wave on the 12-lead ECG.

Toxicologic and pharmacologic causes: Many medications and drugs act on the ion channels of the cell membrane and can potentially affect the cardiac action potential, resulting in changes on the ECG. In particular, agents that block sodium (Na^+) channels cause a delay in phase 0 of the action potential cycle, prolonging ventricular depolarization and resulting in a widening of the QRS complex.

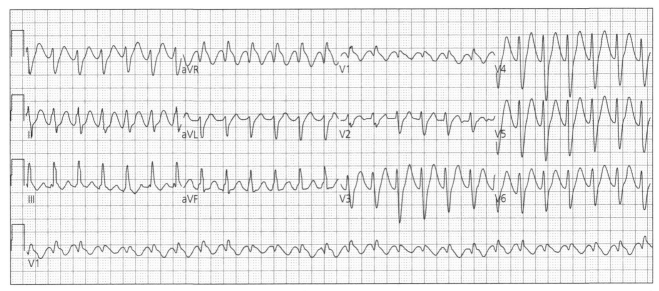

Figure 55.10 This 12-lead ECG is from a patient following a tricyclic anti-depressant overdose. Note the wide QRS complexes and tachycardiac rhythm. Of particular note is the R wave deflection in the terminal portion of the QRS complex in lead aVR, which is highly suggestive of TCA cardiotoxicity.

Medications that can result in QRS widening by this mechanism include a multitude of cardiac agents. These medications include type IA anti-dysrhythmics (e.g. disopyramide, procainamide, quinidine) and type IC anti-dysrhythmics (e.g. flecainide, propafenone). Certain beta-adrenergic-blocking agents also possess Na$^+$ blocking properties and include propranolol and acebutalol. Non-cardiac medications that can cause QRS complex widening by a similar mechanism include anti-psychotics (primarily piperidine phenothiazines), anti-malarial agents (quinine and chloroquine), propoxyphene, carbamazepine, diphenhydramine, and cyclobenzaprine. Many of these agents cause other electrocardiographic changes including a variety of potential dysrhythmias (e.g. bradycardia with beta-adrenergic-blocking agents) and QT interval prolongation (e.g. IA, IC, phenothiazines, diphenhydramine) that can be seen along with QRS complex widening.

Tricyclic anti-depressant (TCA) overdoses can cause a variety of electrocardiographic abnormalities in addition to QRS complex widening. Tricyclic anti-depressants pose a unique threat to cardiac function by their anti-cholinergic effect, alpha-adrenergic-blocking properties, inhibition of presynaptic neurotransmitter reuptake, and fast sodium channel-blockade. In addition to QRS widening (from the Na$^+$ channel-blockade), sinus tachycardia may be present (principally from the anti-cholinergic effect, but also from catecholamine reuptake inhibition and vasodilation induced by alpha-adrenergic blockade) and QT interval prolongation (at both toxic and therapeutic TCA levels). A unique finding with QRS complex widening from TCA poisoning is the presence of rightward deviation of the terminal 0.04 s of the frontal plane QRS complex axis. On the 12-lead ECG,

this can be detected as a terminal negative deflection S wave in lead I and terminal positive deflection R wave in lead aVR (Figure 55.10). This finding, along with QRS widening, has been reported to be predictive of risk for TCA-induced seizures and ventricular dysrhythmias [8,9].

Cocaine is unique among sympathomimetic drugs because of its ability to block sodium channels similar to class IA anti-dysrhythmic agents. As a result, use of cocaine (and cocaethylene) can result in widening of the QRS complex (Figure 55.1). Similar to TCAs, this widening can be accompanied by a rightward deviation of the terminal portion of the QRS complex, as represented by a prominent terminal R wave in lead aVR and larger S wave in leads aVL or I. Other electrocardiographic manifestations of sympathomimetic poisoning with cocaine include tachycardia (perhaps wide complex), QT interval prolongation, and ST segment abnormalities that can mimic or represent true cardiac ischemia.

Case conclusions

In all these cases, the critical issue electrocardiographically is the cause and management of the abnormal QRS complex. In Case 1, the widened QRS complex was caused by acute cocaine intoxication. The patient was treated in the ED with sodium bicarbonate and benzodiazepines and his QRS complex narrowed significantly. He was subsequently admitted to the ICU. He was hospitalized for 1 week for other manifestations of cocaine toxicity, after which he was discharged at baseline condition. In Case 2, the critical issue is whether the LBBB was old or new in the setting of a patient with chest pain (see Brady chapter). Fortunately, an ECG was obtained from the year prior, which also demonstrated LBBB. The patient was subsequently admitted to the hospital overnight and ruled out for myocardial infarction at that time. In Case 3, the ECG demonstrated a sinoventricular rhythm caused by hyperkalemia (K^+ = 8.2 mEq/L) as a result of the patient missing hemodialysis. He was treated with calcium gluconate, sodium bicarbonate, and insulin in the ED. His rhythm improved and QRS complexes narrowed. He was admitted to the intensive care unit and underwent hemodialysis, after which time he markedly improved and was discharged from the hospital 4 days later in good condition.

References

1 Mirvis DM, Goldberger AL. Electrocardiography. In: Braunwald E, Zipes DP, Libby P, editors. *Heart Disease: a Textbook of Cardiovascular Medicine*, 6th ed. Philadelphia: WB Saunders; 2001:82–125.

2 Surawicz B, Knilans TK. *Chou's Electrocardiography in Clinical Practice: Adult and Pediatric*, 5th ed. Philadelphia: W.B. Saunders, 2001.

3 Gazoni PM, Evans TC. Ventricular Hypertrophy. In: Chan TC, Brady WJ, Harrigan RA, *et al.*, editors. *ECG in Emergency Medicine and Acute Care*. Philadelphia: Elsevier/Mosby, 2005:188–94.

4 Brady WJ, Pollack ML. Acute Myocardial Infarction: Confounding Patterns. In: Chan TC, Brady WJ, Harrigan RA, *et al.*, editors. *ECG in Emergency Medicine and Acute Care*. Philadelphia: Elsevier/Mosby, 2005:181–7.

5 Brady WJ, Chan TC, Pollack M. Electrocardiographic manifestations: patterns that confound the EKG diagnosis of acute myocardial infarction – left bundle branch block, ventricular paced rhythm, and left ventricular hypertrophy. *J Emerg Med* 2000; **18**(1):71–8.

6 Rosner MH, Brady WJ, Kefer MP, Martin ML. Electrocardiography in the patient with Wolff-Parkinson-White syndrome: Diagnostic and initial therapeutic issues. *Am J Emerg Med* 1999;**17**:705–9.

7 Cardall TY, Chan TC, Brady WJ, *et al.* Permanent cardiac pacemakers: Issues relevant to the emergency physician, Part I. *J Emerg Med* 1999;**17**(3):479–89.

8 Harrigan RA, Brady WJ. ECG abnormalities in tricyclic antidepressant ingestion. *Am J Emerg Med* 1999;**17**:387–93.

9 Liebelt EL, Francis PD, Woolf AD. ECG lead aVR versus QRS interval in predicting seizures and arrhythmias in acute tricyclic antidepressant toxicity. *Ann Emerg Med* 1995;**26**:195–201.

Chapter 56 | What is the ECG differential diagnosis of a prolonged QT interval?

Richard A. Harrigan[1], Theodore C. Chan[2]
[1]Temple University, Philadelphia, PA, USA
[2]University of California, San Diego, CA, USA

Case presentations

Case 1: A 24-year-old female presents to the emergency department (ED) with a complaint of incessant nausea and vomiting for 1 month. She is pregnant for the first time, with a gestational age of approximately 9 weeks by dates. She denies fever, diarrhea, abdominal pain, or vaginal bleeding. On physical examination, her vital signs are normal with the exception of a heart rate of 106 beats per minute (bpm). Her sclera are anicteric and her conjunctiva are without pallor. Heart and lung examinations are normal. The abdomen is soft and non-tender. Her initial electrocardiogram (ECG) is seen in Figure 56.1.

Case 2: A 62-year-old female presents to the ED with a complaint of several days of increasing numbness in her hands, feet, and face. The distribution is non-lateralizing. There is no weakness, difficulty in speech, or gait disturbance. Her past medical history is significant for a thyroidectomy, during which her parathyroid glands were also removed. She is non-compliant with the calcium carbonate (Tums®) her primary physician had recommended she take daily. Her vital signs and physical examination are within normal limits, with the exception of a positive Chvostek's sign. Her admission ECG is seen in Figure 56.2.

ECG differential diagnosis of the long QT interval

On the ECG, the QT interval includes everything from the beginning of the Q wave to the end of the T wave – thus, it includes the QRS complex, the ST segment, and the T wave. This corresponds to the depolarization of the ventricles (QRS complex) as well as its recovery phase, followed by the period of ventricular repolarization (T wave). The QT interval features intertracing as well as intratracing variability. Between ECG tracings, it varies with age, gender, and heart rate. The QT interval tends to be longer with advancing age, in female patients, and at lower heart rates. Within a given tracing, QT interval variability will occur across the 12 leads on the ECG. By convention, the longest of these intervals serves as the QT interval for that tracing. The phenomenon of intratracing QT interval variability is termed QT dispersion. This dispersion has been linked to dysrhythmias due to variability across the myocardium in ventricular refractoriness [1–3]. These dysrhythmias may or may not stem from myocardial ischemia, as ischemic myocardium has been found to take longer to repolarize (i.e. have a longer QT interval) than normal tissue [3–6]. Alternatively, QT dispersion can be calculated, using the difference between the shortest and longest QT intervals on a given tracing; this can be done manually or by an automated system. QT interval dispersion is mostly calculated and put to use as a research tool at this juncture.

The QT interval may be normal, shortened, or prolonged. Pathologic ramifications are related to QT prolongation, and will be the focus of this discussion. Generally speaking, and in cases of normal heart rates, the QT interval should be less than half the preceding RR interval, i.e. the distance subtended by the QT interval can be fit twice within the preceding RR interval. The QT interval is often corrected for rate, and is termed the QTc. The QTc is determined by Bazett's formula, which is as follows: the QTc is equal to the QT interval divided by the square root of the RR interval. The QTc is automatically calculated by most ECG machines in use today. It is commonly listed with the rate, rhythm, and axis data found in the upper left portion of the tracing.

Measurement of the QT interval can be challenging when obscured by the terminal portion of the T wave, at times making a correct estimation of the QT interval difficult. If the T wave is flattened, or encroaches upon the next P wave or a U wave (if the latter appears on the tracing), accurate determination of the QT interval can be problematic. These same problems encountered in the correct determination of the QT interval obviously confound the accurate determination of QT dispersion as well.

Critical Decisions in Emergency and Acute Care Electrocardiography,
1st edition. Edited by W.J. Brady and J.D. Truwit. © 2009 Blackwell Publishing, ISBN: 9781405159067

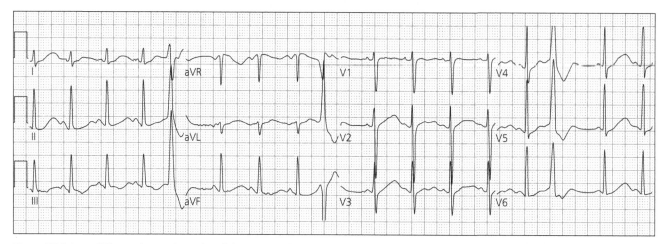

Figure 56.1 Long QT interval secondary to hypokalemia. Note the long QT interval, perhaps seen best in lead II, where the T wave terminus approaches the P wave. U waves can be seen following the T waves in lead V3, which is classically one of the best leads in which to see U waves. There appears to be some T-U fusion in lead V2. These are the electrocardiographic hallmarks of hypokalemia. Also note the ventricular ectopy.

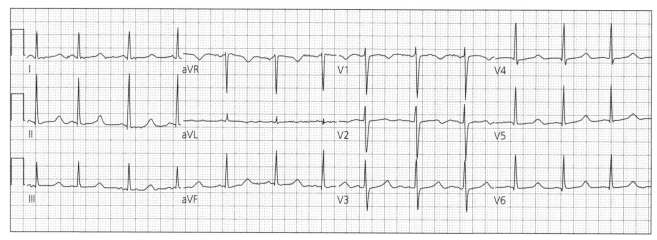

Figure 56.2 Long QT interval secondary to hypocalcemia. The QT interval is prolonged at 0.54 s, consistent with the diagnosis of severe hypocalcemia.

The QTc is generally considered to be prolonged if greater than 0.44 s in the male and 0.46 s in the female. The risk of potentially fatal dysrhythmias is related to the length of the QTc [7]. Mechanistically, the dysrhythmia results when an early afterdepolarization falls during a period of prolonged ventricular recovery (the long QT interval). Commonly referred to as the "R-on-T phenomenon," this may lead to a variety of ventricular dysrhythmias, including torsade de pointes (literally, "twisting of the points"). Commonly referred to as "torsade," this serious ventricular dysrhythmia is in actuality a multifocal ventricular tachycardia (see chapter on wide complex tachycardias). Clinical manifestations include sudden death, syncope, seizure-like activity, near-syncope, or dizziness [8].

Differential diagnosis of a long QT interval

The differential diagnosis of the long QT interval can be divided into cardiac or congenital forms and acquired, non-cardiac causes. A number of different genetic mutations have been discovered as causative for the former, whereas acquired forms are generally secondary to pharmacologic, endocrine, or metabolic disorders.

Congenital long QT syndromes: Interestingly, patients with these disorders may present with QT prolongation on their ECG – or the QT interval may be normal. Thus, a single normal ECG does not rule out this syndrome. Clinical history and family history heighten the index of suspicion. Catecholamine surges may precipitate the symptomatology, as with exertion or stress; epinephrine infusion has been used to unmask asymptomatic carriers [9]. The Romano Ward syndrome – long QT intervals, torsade de pointes, and normal hearing – is an autosomal dominant trait that was first described in the early 1960s. Jervell Lange-Nielsen syndrome – long QT intervals, torsade de pointes, and deafness – was first described in 1957, and is carried recessively. Generally, male patients with congenital long QT syndrome experience cardiac events more commonly until puberty,

Table 56.1 Pharmacologic classes linked to QT interval prolongation [12]

Cardiac agents
Anti-arrhythmics (Type Ia, Ic, and III)
Calcium channel-blockers (some) (e.g. bepridil, isradipine, nicardipine)
Anti-psychotic agents
Phenothiazines (some) (e.g. thioridazine, mesoridazine)
Butyrophenones (e.g. haloperidol, droperidol)
Anti-depressants (some) (e.g. tricyclics, fluoxetine, sertraline, venlafaxine)
Anti-infective agents
   Fluoroquinolones (some) (e.g. sparfloxacin, gatifloxacin, moxifloxacin)
   Macrolides (some) (e.g. erythromycin, clarithromycin)
Miscellaneous (pentamidine, amantadine, tetracyclines, foscarnet, quinine, chloroquine)
Neurologic agents
   Carbamazepine, fosphenytoin, sumatriptan, zolmitriptan, naratriptan
Organophosphates
Gastrointestinal agents (e.g. cisapride, ipecac, octreotide, dolasetron)
Other (e.g. cocaine, diphenhydramine, methadone, tacrolimus, tamoxifen, probucol, tizanidine, salmeterol)

whereas females will more likely present after age 14 years [10]. The annual rates of syncope and death have been reported to be 5% and 0.9%, respectively, in one series looking at congenital long QT syndrome over time [11].

Acquired long QT syndromes: A variety of pharmacologic, endocrine, and metabolic conditions may prolong the QT interval. Anyone with a long QT interval on their ECG should have their list of medications reviewed for possible offending agents. The list of drugs is vast (Table 56.1) and the strength of a causal relationship is variable; there are websites available (e.g. www.qtdrugs.org) to query regarding a the potential of a drug to prolong the QT interval.

Electrolyte disturbance must also be considered when a long QT interval is encountered on the ECG. Hypokalemia (Figure 56.1) may cause QT prolongation, as well as T wave flattening or inversion, ST segment depression, and U waves. There may be TU fusion, usually seen in more severe hypokalemia, and this further lengthens the QT (or QU) interval. Hypocalcemia is also known to cause QT interval prolongation. More precisely, low serum calcium levels cause ST segment prolongation, as calcium does not affect T wave duration because it influences phase 2, but not phase 3, of the action potential [13]. Hypomagnesemia is often linked to prolongation of the QT interval, and is associated with the development of torsade de pointes (see above). There is, however, no known direct electrocardiographic effect attributable to hypomagnesemia. Low magnesium is frequently associated with hypokalemia and hypocalcemia, and these electrolyte disorders do cause QT prolongation [14].

Hypothermia causes a variety of ECG abnormalities (bradydysrhythmias, Osborn waves), with QT prolongation

(specifically ST segment prolongation) being among them [13]. Hypothyroidism leads to diminution of the cardiac waveforms (P-QRS-T) as well as prolongation of the QT interval and bradydysrhythmias. Patients with hypoparathyroidism may have QT interval lengthening on their ECG, as this disorder is associated with low serum calcium levels (Figure 56.2). Vitamin B_1 (thiamine) deficiency is also associated with prolongation of the QT interval. Finally, the QT interval may be prolonged in certain central nervous system disorders, such as subarachnoid hemorrhage, intracerebral hemorrhage, and thromboembolic stroke. T wave changes, sometimes including profoundly deep, symmetric T wave inversions, may also be seen in patients with these disorders.

Case conclusions

The patient in Case 1 suffered from hyperemesis gravidarum. Her serum potassium was 2.0 mEq/L at the time of this tracing. The patient in Case 2 had symptomatic hypocalcemia secondary to iatrogenic hypoparathyroidism. The serum calcium in this patient was 5.0 mEq/L (her albumin was 4.1 mEq/L); her ionized calcium was 2.8 mEq/L (normal being 4.6–5.3 mEq/L). Both the patients in Cases 1 and 2 did well with replenishment of their potassium and calcium stores, respectively. The patient in Case 1 was discharged on anti-emetics, and the patient in Case 2 left the hospital on regular calcium supplementation.

References

1 Day CP, McComb JM, Campbell RWF. QT interval dispersion: An indicator of arrhythmia risk in patients with long QT intervals. *Br Heart J* 1990;**63**:342–4.
2 Franz MR, Zabel M. Electrophysiological basis of QT dispersion measurements. *Prog Cardiovasc Dis* 2000;**42**:311–24.
3 Perkiomaki JS, Koistinen J, Yli-Mayry S, *et al.* Dispersion of QT intervals in patients with and without susceptibility to ventricular tachydysrhythmias after previous myocardial infarction. *J Am Coll Cardiol* 1995;**26**:174–9.
4 Mirvis DM. Spatial variation of QT interval in normal persons and patients with acute myocardial infarction. *J Am Coll Cardiol* 1985;**5**:625–31.
5 Van de Loo A, Arendts W, Hohnloser SH. Variability of QT dispersion measurements in the surface electrocardiogram in patients with acute myocardial infarction and in normal subjects. *Am J Cardiol* 1994;**74**:1113–8.
6 Higham PD, Furniss SS, Campbell RW. QT dispersion and components of the QT interval in ischemia and infarction. *Br Heart J* 1995;**73**:32–6.
7 Moss AJ. Measurement of the QT interval and the risk associated with QT_c interval prolongation: a review. *Am J Cardiol* 1993;**72**:23B–25B.
8 Pines JM, Brady WJ. Long QT syndromes. In: Chan TC, Brady WJ, Harrigan RA, *et al.*, editors. *ECG in Emergency Medicine and Acute Care.* Philadelphia: Elsevier-Mosby, 2006; 235–8.
9 Shimuzu W, Noda T, Takaki H, *et al.* Epinephrine unmasks latent mutation carriers with LQT1 form of congenital long QT syndrome. *J Am Coll Cardiol* 2003;**41**:633–42.

10 Kastor JA. *Arrythmias*, 2nd edn. Philadelphia: W.B. Saunders, 2000:413–45.

11 Moss AJ, Schwartz PJ, Crampton RS, *et al.* The long QT syndrome: prospective longitudinal study of 328 families. *Circulation* 1999;**84**:1136–44.

12 Chan TC. Toxicology section: Introduction. In: Chan TC, Brady WJ, Harrigan RA, *et al.*, editors. *ECG in Emergency Medicine and Acute Care*. Philadelphia: Elsevier Mosby, 2006:253–4.

13 Abrahamian RM, Gupta M. Metabolic abnormalities: Effects of Electrolyte imbalances and thyroid disorders on the ECG. In: Mattu A, Tabas JA, Barish RA editors. *Electrocardiography in Emergency Medicine*. Dallas TX: American College of Emergency Physicians; 2007:193–202.

14 Surawicz B, Knilans TK. *Chou's Electrocardiography in Clinical Practice: Adult and Pediatric*, 5th edn. Philadelphia: WB Saunders, 2001.

Index

Page numbers in **bold** represent tables, those in *italics* represent figures.